The
Handbook

by Dagmar Ehling

with Steve Swart

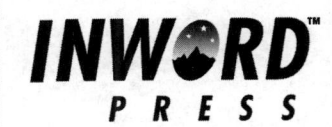

The Chinese Herbalist's Handbook

by Dagmar Ehling with Steve Swart

Published by:

InWord Press
2530 Camino Entrada
Santa Fe, NM 87505-4835 USA

Copyright © 1996 Dagmar Ehling

First Edition, 1994
Revised Edition, 1996
SAN 694-0269

10 9 8 7 6 5 4 3 2

Printed in the United States of America

Cataloging-in-Publication Data

Ehling, Dagmar
The Chinese Herbalist's Handbook

Includes index.

1. Herbs 2. Medicine, Chinese

ISBN 1-56690-312-2

Warning and Disclaimer

This book is intended as a professional reference volume only, not as a medical manual or a guide to self-treatment. We caution lay persons not to attempt diagnosis or to embark upon self-treatment of a serious illness without competent professional assistance.

The information presented here is not intended to substitute for any treatment that may have been prescribed by your physician. The information contained in this book is given in good faith, but the authors and publisher cannot be held responsible for any error or omission, nor can they be held in any way responsible for treatment given on the basis of information contained herein. If you are in doubt concerning any aspect of this book, consult a qualified, licensed practitioner of Chinese medicine.

Acknowledgements

I would like express my sincere thanks to all my teachers, who have enabled me to write this book. I would like to thank especially Dr. Nancy Zeng, who broadened my perspective of TCM and imparted her vast knowledge of herbal medicine, and Dr. Jake Fratkin, who provided the foundation for my love of Chinese herbal medicine. I thank Steve Swart for his patience, and for contributing his knowledge and efforts to Parts Two and Three.

Dagmar Ehling

My deepest thanks and appreciation to my teachers of Chinese herbal medicine, Drs. Daoshing and Maoshing Ni, who taught me so much by their example and by their patience with my endless questions. And, to Dr. Nancy Zeng who has enlarged my whole understanding of the art of prescribing Chinese herbs. A very special thanks to Li Hua Chuang, who patiently taught me to read Chinese herbal characters. Finally, my respect and admiration to my colleague, Dagmar Ehling, for inviting me to participate in this project and for her unfailing excellence and friendship.

Steve Swart

We are both grateful to Drs. Skya and Anthony Abbate, Dan and Barbara Raker, Ted Krueger, Caylor Wadlington, Rory Kerr, Kelly Corbet, Astrid Brouwer, Daniel Santos, and Dan Oldenburg.

Special appreciation goes to Suryadas, Henne, and Jakob.

Our Chinese technical editors, Dr. Li, Xiaorong and Dr. Chunyan Teng, deserve deep thanks for their careful, meticulous work consulting many direct Chinese texts relevant to Part 1 and Part 3. Thanks to Bruce Sturgeon for the painstaking editing of Part 4, the Cross Reference of Herb Names.

About the Authors

Dagmar Ehling, D.O.M., L.Ac., M.Ac., Dipl.Ac., is a graduate of Southwest Acupuncture College, Santa Fe, NM. She did post-graduate studies at the International Institute of Chinese Medicine, Santa Fe, NM, with Dr. Nancy Zeng. Raised in Germany in an atmosphere of Jungian psychology and bioenergetics, she came to the United States in 1984. Currently she has a private practice in Santa Fe, NM and is a faculty member of the International Institute of Chinese Medicine. She is a former editor of the quarterly "Acupuncture & Herbal Health Center Newsletter."

Steve Swart, D.O.M., L.Ac., Dipl.Ac., a graduate of the acupuncture program of Southwest Acupuncture College, Santa Fe, NM, began his formal study of traditional Chinese medicine with an interest in herbology in 1983 at the Oriental Healing Arts Institute in Los Angeles. Steve attended Emperor's College of Traditional Chinese Medicine in Santa Monica, CA, and also worked as an herbal pharmacist for Daoshing and Maoshing Ni, O.M.D.'s between 1987 and 1988. Steve is now in private practice in Santa Fe, NM.

About the Illustrations

The illustrations throughout Part 1 of this book are traditional Chinese folk designs from paper cut-out motifs. They are combined with Chinese calligraphy representing the various disharmony names in Part 1. Thanks go to Robert Zeng for his contribution of the calligraphy.

Future Editions

We have made every attempt to make this book accurate, complete, and user-friendly. We welcome your suggestions for improvement of future editions. Please contact the Project Editor at InWord Press with your comments.

InWord Press

InWord Press is dedicated to bringing information to light that facilitates personal healing. We publish resource books that integrate tradition with innovation for use in physical, emotional, and spiritual growth.

In addition to the authors who developed the material for this book, other members of the InWord Press team bring the book into your hands.

Thanks to Michelle Emmons, Barbara Raker, David Talbott, Carol Leyba, Lynne Egensteiner, Betsy Fogelman, Margaret Burns, Gary Cascio, Julie Mullen, Tierney Tully, Dennis Jarrett, and Dan Raker.

Table of Contents

Introduction

In China about 80% of all traditional Chinese medical patients are treated with herbs, while the remaining 20% are treated with acupuncture, Tui-na or Qi Gong. Loose herbs are very potent in treating a variety of medical disorders and they offer tremendous advantages to the practitioner who works in this modality.

The Chinese Herbalist's Handbook is a practical guide for the application of loose herbs in a Chinese medical practice. It aids the student or practitioner of Chinese herbal medicine in finding appropriate herbal formulas once a differential diagnosis has been established. It is intended to help demystify Chinese herbal medicine, and to assist practitioners in making the transition from textbook knowledge to effective clinical application.

Why This Book Was Written

This book has grown out of my personal experience as a Western student and practitioner of Chinese medicine. I recall the early days of an herbal clinic class I attended. A patient would be brought in and a student would present the case. We would discuss the patient's case in depth, taking into account symptoms, pulse, tongue, differential diagnosis and treatment principle. Then my teacher would ask us: "What formula would you use?" This usually provoked a long silence. Most students did not have the knowledge or the information readily at hand to prescribe formulas quickly.

Now, as a clinic supervisor and teacher, I still work with many students who are unable to integrate Chinese herbs into their treatment plans. I think the primary problem is fear that they do not have enough herbal knowledge. In most current Western training there is not enough hands-on clinical experience using herbs. Sometimes herbs are not learned by sight as thoroughly as they could be, so the student's knowledge is too abstract.

In China, herbal students memorize formulas by rote and they use rhymes to remember the exact ingredients of each formula. This process is not applied in the training of Western herbal students. Furthermore, a Western degree requires only three years of schooling, while in China 4 - 6 years of study are required.

For all these reasons, a good English-language reference guide is crucial to improving our working knowledge of herbs. *The Chinese Herbalist's Handbook* helps fill this need and assists practitioners in moving into the loose herb modality.

Cultural Context

In the Western world, holistic treatment modalities have gained more popularity in the past ten years and are growing steadily.

Much of the Western medical community is rethinking its approach, and Western health care professionals are increasingly accepting of Chinese medicine (I am now getting referrals from surgeons). Acupuncture is no longer considered Eastern voodoo, and today's patients are asking for more than the conventional Western medical approach. Many young Western practitioners now include bodywork, relaxation techniques, psychology, nutrition or homeopathy in their practices.

In this country, herbs are strange to us. In China, however, they are the norm. Chinese children grow up with herbs and Chinese people can buy prepared herbs in most stores. Taking herbs or even combining herbs with Western medical treatment is an integral part of Chinese culture.

In the West, we grow up with the quick-fix promise of pharmaceutical drugs. It takes a lot of re-education to change patterns so that herbal treatments can be accepted here as an effective modality. Many patients are tired of paying for expensive drugs with numerous undesirable side effects, and then taking other drugs to alleviate those side effects. More and more people are starting to realize that Western drugs, as beneficial and important as they may be in many cases, may also be detrimental.

Herbs vs. Pharmaceutical Drugs

It is crucial to understand the difference between the Chinese herbal approach (i.e., ingesting the whole plant/animal substance) versus the Western pharmacological approach (i.e. extracting the potent molecule). Western pharmacologists take a plant substance, find the most effective molecule for a certain disease, extract it, patent it and sell it in a very high concentration.

In contrast, an herb which is safe and effective in treating a variety of ailments is considered superior in China. The more illnesses it treats, the more precious it becomes. *Ren Shen / Ginseng* and *Ling Zhi / Ganoderma*, for instance, are thought to be very precious because they are tonics to many body systems.

What is considered a superior drug in Chinese medicine may be considered an inferior drug in Western medicine and vice versa. Chinese medicine follows nature's way, and seeks treatment success on a broader, more gradual path.

A good example is ephedrine. Derived from the Chinese herb *Ma Huang / Ephedra*, it was put into concentrated capsule form for the treatment of asthma in Western medicine. In its pharmaceutical form, ephedrine can overstimulate the heart, leading to high blood pressure, palpitations and increased nervousness. In Chinese medicine, however, *Ephedra* is used in its natural form, where the ephedrine has a concentration of less than 1% for the treatment of asthma. Although the beneficial effects are more gradual, there are far fewer negative side effects. *Ephedra* in its natural form is more suitable for gradual absorption into the metabolism of the body because the plant has other ingredients which offset many side effects.

Western culture fosters the quick-fix, pop-a-pill approach which can suppress symptoms immediately. Herbs are not a quick-fix like Western drugs, except in acute cases where the changes can be dramatic. But many patients who seek herbal treatments have chronic problems and it is important that they understand that herbs are slow and gradual in their efficacy. A practitioner needs to explain to the patient that changes are gradual because they are working on the root cause of the illness as well as treating the symptoms.

Patient Compliance

Patient education is the most effective tool for treatment success. Patient compliance is a pivotal issue in this country because people are used to pills and syrups which are easy to take.

When patients receive prescribed loose herbs, they will find themselves with bags of strange ingredients which they have to cook. The resulting herbal tea usually tastes and smells quite bitter and unfamiliar. Western patients are less likely to comply with prescriptions than Chinese people who grow up with this treatment modality.

Patients must be given written instructions on how to prepare herbs (see Appendix D). Explain thoroughly the decoction process, dosage and storage as there is much room for confusion. If your patient has never taken herbs before you may give him or her just one bag to see if they can handle preparing and taking the tea.

You will want to educate your patients on the efficacy and importance of herbal therapy. Prepare a pamphlet explaining the differences between loose herbs, patents, freeze-dried, and alcohol extracted herbal tinctures which can also serve as an introduction to general herbal therapy principles and the benefits of using herbs.

In my practice, 80 - 85 % of my patients are taking loose herbal decoctions. After I have explained the particular benefits of the herbs and given clear preparation instructions, the patient will usually take them for the required time.

I have found there are two kinds of patients. The first will refuse to make the effort to cook the teas or drink them. In my practice, those make up about 10 - 15 %. The other kind of patient will say something like, "It doesn't taste very good but, you know, I really felt something," or, the first week they might just say, "It really tastes bad." By the second week they may say, "It tastes bad but I actually crave it," or "It tastes bad but I'm willing to give it a chance," or "It really seems to make a difference in the way I feel." Those are the ones who follow through with herbal treatment. Generally those patients show marked acceleration in their response to treatment.

Patients need to understand, as well, that they are responsible for their own health and well-being. Life-style changes and taking care of bodily and psychological needs are key components of getting well. Patients should listen to their bodies and pay attention to symptoms, food, work situations and allergy-causing situations, in order to achieve well-being.

It is surprising how many patients are quite unaware of their own bodies. Part of Chinese medical therapy, the "Ten Questions," fosters bodily awareness. Normally, Western doctors do not ask these kinds of holistically-oriented, in-depth questions but rely mainly on objective information.

Herbal therapy makes patients feel more responsible for their well-being. They take an active role in the healing process by cooking herbs, storing them properly and self-administering them. Like deciding to eat well, exercise, breathe properly, or curb an addiction, herbs can be discussed as part of a general process of conscious life-style adjustment leading to better health.

About Prepared Medicines

Prepared medicines include patent medicines, tinctures, capsules, and freeze-dried herbs. Prepared medicines are adequate for patients who will not take herbal teas. However, the biggest problem with prepared medicines is that you can never tailor a formula for a specific differential syndrome or fine-tune to the patient's changing condition.

The beauty of prescribing loose herbs is that you can individually tailor each formula to the patient's needs, and as his/her condition improves you can change your emphasis. Patient compliance is sometimes easier with prepared herbal formulas, but even if you combine two prepared medicines together, they will usually still be less effective than loose herbal teas.

Some companies are now selling single herbs in a freeze-dried or tincture form. By using them, the practitioner can tailor a desired formula and achieve patient compliance at the same time. Another alternative is to powder loose herbs and have patients ingest them in powder form or as drafts, in which the powder is boiled for a short period of time in a small amount of water. The resulting tea is strained and consumed. Some practitioners also make personalized alcohol-extracted tinctures using various methods to extract the herbs. This is another approach to patient compliance issues.

It is sometimes useful to prescribe prepared medicines along with loose herbs, especially when using substances which are expensive, rare or derived from animals. Two good prepared medicine books are *Chinese Herbal Patent Formulas* by Jake Fratkin, and *Outline Guide to Chinese Herbal Patent Medicines In Pill Form* by Margaret Naeser.

Structure of *The Chinese Herbalist's Handbook*

I have structured this book with formulas in diagnostic categories according to their use in a clinical setting in order to create a system for prescribing Chinese herbs which is easily accessible.

In Part One, "Herbal Prescriptions According to Syndrome Differentiation," the formulas are arranged according to those that pertain to all Zang Fu syndromes. The Four Stages (Wen Bing), Six Divisions (Shang Han), Jin Ye (body fluid) disharmonies, selected internal medicine disorders, and miscellaneous syndromes are also included.

Formulas are organized alphabetically by Pinyin name under each diagnostic syndrome. Primary formulas for each syndrome are indicated with special symbols. Each formula listing includes indications, ingredients with recommended dosages, tongue and pulse readings, contraindications, and preparation methods. All listings include English names. Commercial extract formula names are given if available. Contraindications and cautions for pregnancy noted in this section are rather conservative and do not necessarily appear in the traditional literature. This is done to warn the less experienced practitioner of dangers which could result from the use of a particular prescription in pregnancy.

Part Two is the "Clinical Quick Reference to Single Herbs." It is a selected list of the most commonly used single herbs, broken down into traditional categories, and further divided into subcategories of specific herb functions. This is intended to help steer the practitioner in the right direction when making herb substitutions and modifications of a prescription.

Part Three is a "Table of Herbal Preparation Procedures" for single herbs. It is packed with specific information needed when mixing formulas, i.e., which herbs need to be powdered, cut in slices, cooked for longer or shorter time, etc. Toxic herbs and those contraindicated during pregnancy are noted. The standard dosage range for each herb is included.

Part Four is a listing of herbs with names sorted alphabetically four different ways. It cross-references single herbs according to different naming conventions: Pinyin, botanical, pharmaceutical, and common names.

The appendices include information for new practitioners, a suggested start-up pharmacy herb list, and a supplier source list.

Naming System

Standard Pinyin formula names are used throughout this book. English formula names have been included here for those who prefer them. Many were adapted from Bensky/Barolet's *Formulas & Strategies*. I feel it is important to standardize English translations for Chinese formulas, and *Formulas & Strategies* provides a high standard of excellence.

Chinese herbs are taught in a variety of ways in schools throughout this country. For single herbs, this book uses Pinyin and botanical names. For animal and mineral substances with no botanical name, either the zoological or the pharmaceutical name is substituted. This book uses a shortened version of the botanical/zoological names. If you are unsure about which herb or part of a specific substance is meant in a particular instance, please consult Part Four, the naming cross-reference, which details this information.

How To Use This Guide

Once you have arrived at a syndrome differentiation and treatment principle for your patient, turn to that particular heading in Part One and scan the formula indications in that section. There may be several formulas that appear to be possibilities for the patient.

Your next step is to compare the ingredients in the formulas, and then narrow down the possibilities until you arrive at the best formula for your patient. Depending on your experience, you may want to prepare a formula which is a combination of two or even three standard prescriptions. Part Two will help you to further modify your individual formula.

When ready to prepare your formula, you should check Part Three for preparation methods for individual herbs.

For example, let's say your patient has a differential diagnosis of damp and qi stagnation with Spleen and Stomach qi deficiency. The patient presents symptoms such as poor appetite, abdominal pain, fullness especially after eating, flatulence, belching, loose stools and low energy. His pulse is weak and slippery. His tongue is pale, swollen with teethmarks, and has a thick white coat.

Your treatment principle is to dispel damp, regulate qi in the middle jiao, and tonify Spleen and Stomach qi.

Go to Part One and look under "Accumulation of Tan Yin (Damp and Phlegm)" and look at the varying indications. You will find several formulas which might be possible for this patient:

1. Liu Jun Zi Tang - Six-Gentlemen Decoction treats Spleen qi deficiency with mild damp. Its ability to treat the damp accumulation is not strong enough and it does not address the qi stagnation adequately.

2. Ping Wei San - Calm the Stomach Powder treats Spleen qi deficiency with damp and qi stagnation causing fullness and distention. Look at the ingredients of Ping Wei San and you will find that the formula is very strong for drying damp but does not do enough for Spleen qi tonification and regulation which you desire. Continue your search.

3. Shen Ling Bai Zhu San - Ginseng, Poria and Atractylodes Powder addresses Spleen qi deficiency with damp but does not treat middle jiao qi stagnation sufficiently.

4. Xiang Sha Liu Jun Zi Tang - Six-Gentlemen Decoction with Aucklandia and Amomum treats Spleen qi deficiency, damp accumulation and middle jiao qi stagnation. You find that the ingredients in this formula address all three diagnostic factors.

Your patient at times has severe abdominal pain so you want to strengthen the qi regulating effect. Go to Part Two and look under "Herbs that Regulate Qi". The first subtitle discusses middle jiao qi regulators. The three most appropriate herbs listed are: *Zhi Shi / Citrus*, *Zhi Ke / Citrus*, and *Da Fu Pi / Areca*. Depending on your single herb knowledge (you may need to consult a materia medica), one of these herbs is added to Xiang Sha Liu Jun Zi Tang - Six-Gentlemen Decoction with Aucklandia and Amomum.

Next you should check each ingredient in Part Three to see whether there are special preparation instructions. *Ban Xia / Pinellia* comes prepared as *Fa Ban Xia* from your supplier but is still slightly toxic and should not be used during pregnancy. *Sha Ren / Amomum* should be crushed into small pieces when mixing the formula. *Mu Xiang / Saussurea* and *Sha Ren / Amomum* should be added during the last five minutes of the first boiling to optimize their aromatic properties. Because of this, both of these herbs should be put in a separate bag when mixing the formula. However, many practitioners will choose to put them right in with the other herbs in order to make the cooking process simpler for the patient.

This book does not cover prescriptions or herbs in depth or discuss the function of each herb in a given formula. Traditional modifications are generally not included. It is primarily designed to be a quick reference.

Knowing how to diagnose properly, form a treatment plan, and utilize single herbs are all prerequisites for using this guide. An in-depth discussion of diagnostic skills is beyond the scope of this book.

Should you choose to further research a prescription, we recommend the following comprehensive English language texts: *Chinese Herbal Medicine: Formulas & Strategies*, by Dan Bensky and Randall Barolet, and *Handbook Of Chinese Herbs And Formulas - Vol. 2*, by Him-che Yeung. For further research of single herbs we recommend *Chinese Herbal Medicine: Materia Medica*, by Dan Bensky and Andrew Gamble.

General Implications of Prescribing Herbs

As discussed above, in order to prescribe herbs effectively a correct diagnosis and treatment plan is essential. I am assuming the reader has proper knowledge of treatment principles and their application in prescribing herbs. There are many variables in Chinese medicine; always a delicate equilibrium needs to be found.

A few specific examples:

When nourishing yin, sticky or cloying herbs are primarily used, but may aggravate a pre-existing damp condition. The herbs for transforming damp are quite drying and may injure the yin causing more false heat.

General qi tonification formulas may cause heat because they usually include herbs which are warm in nature. If this effect is not desired, cool qi tonics should be used in place of warm qi tonics in such formulas.

Herbs which regulate qi and/or blood should not be used for long periods of time because they may deplete qi. The time period depends on the degree of qi deficiency for a particular patient. Herbs that save the qi should be added to such a formula if needed.

Herbs which tonify yang will eventually cause some heat. When this happens the yang tonification has to be decreased, or heat clearing or yin nourishing herbs need to be added to the yang nourishing formula.

In women, the menstrual cycle needs to be taken into account when prescribing. Usually, between the monthly menstruation and ovulation, deficiencies may show up more clearly. Between ovulation and the menstruation, problems of stagnation may be predominant.

During the course of treatment you may need to reevaluate your diagnosis and approach. Always pay close attention to the patient's symptom picture, pulse, tongue and any differences the patient may exhibit when reevaluating the treatment principle and formula. In my opinion, a reevaluation should be done about every two weeks. Make additions or deletions to your formula but also consider changing it completely. This is a skill which young practitioners develop with practice, both with regard to herbs and acupuncture.

Roughly 5 % of the population will not be able to handle herbs because of food allergies, odor sensitivities, or environmental illness - a disorder which is appearing with increasing frequency. With those patients, a more intensive acupuncture program is needed, or perhaps another treatment modality.

If herbs are not an option for a patient with a chronic condition, then 2 - 3 sessions a week of acupuncture are often suggested to achieve good results. However, using herbs with a once-a-week acupuncture treatment is generally more beneficial and also more cost-effective for the patient. Herbs will make a tremendous difference, especially in patients with either yin or blood deficiencies or damp accumulations (body fluid imbalances). Internal medical problems are also more successfully treated by combining acupuncture with herbs.

Summary

The Chinese herbal pharmacopeia is one of the most extensive in the world. Working within this tradition, one feels deeply the connection between natural substances and human health. Touching and smelling Chinese herbs is a soul-satisfying experience. I enjoy my herbal pharmacy immensely and feel that I have a relationship with the distinct personalities of each herb. There is a certain beauty involved in handling the herbs which goes beyond intellectual knowledge.

Different practitioners have favorite herbs which they use more frequently than others. This is related partly to subjective feeling and partly to their training. The same preferences are true for substitutions in formulas. In working with Chinese herbs, there is space for varying interpretations and intuition. Be open to experimenting and trusting your intuition.

The points discussed in this introduction are meant to clarify the implications of working within the Chinese herbal tradition and thereby empower the practitioner to move into this modality. Chinese herbal medicine can be a very enriching experience and is a never-ending learning process. When we prescribe herbs we are using a part of our Mother Earth as a medium through which we touch other people's lives. Finding balance between East and West, heaven and earth, inner and outer, body and spirit, yin and yang - is experiencing the Tao. I wish you well in your herbal endeavors.

Dagmar Ehling
February 1993

The Chinese Herbalist's Handbook

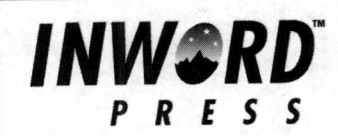

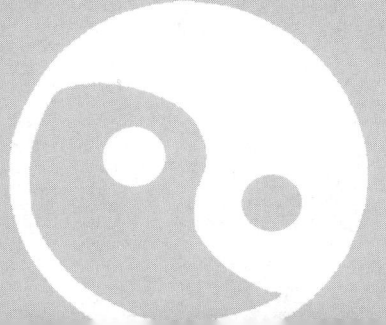

Part 1

Herbal Prescriptions According to Syndrome Differentiation

This chapter lists all prescriptions, with ingredients, dosages, tongue and pulse descriptions, preparation methods, and contraindications. Pinyin names are in the first column and botanical names are in the second. For each syndrome the prescriptions are arranged in alphabetical order according to the Chinese Pinyin name of each formula. Major formulas for each syndrome are indicated with a star ✪. Please note that all formulas should be decocted unless otherwise indicated. Herbs listed in brackets [...] are only sometimes included in the traditional formula. For animal and mineral substances with no botanical name, the zoological or the pharmaceutical name is used. The bold-faced paragraph next to each formula is a brief summary of indications and main symptoms.

For an in-depth understanding of each formula, I recommend the excellent *Formulas & Strategies* by Dan Bensky and Randall Barolet.

In this chapter, there are three prescriptions for which the exact English translations were unavailable. 1. 'Gui Xiong Si Wu Tang' is now translated as 'Altered Four-Substance Decoction', 2. 'Qing Gan Zhi Lin Tang' is 'Clear Liver and Stop Leukorrhea Decoction', and 3. 'Wu Bi Shan Yao Wan' is 'Dioscorea Pill'.

Summary of Symbols

T Tongue

P Pulse

✗ Contraindications

✪ **Major Formula** within Syndrome

☞ Special instructions

LUNG DISHARMONIES

WIND COLD INVASION

- chills greater than fever
- sneezing with clear watery nasal discharge
- body aches
- itchy throat

T thin white coat

P superficial, tight

Wind Cold

External wind cold entering the Stomach causing severe damp accumulation, which then leads to fever and chills, diarrhea, vomiting, fullness, or abdominal bloating.

T sticky white coat

P slippery, superficial

BU HUAN JING ZHENG QI SAN

Rectify the Qi Powder Worth More Than Gold

Extract Formula Name: Pinellia, Atractylodes, and Agastache Formula

Hou Po	Magnolia	9 - 12 g
Cang Zhu	Atractylodes	3 - 9 g
Huo Xiang	Agastache	6 - 9 g
Ban Xia	Pinellia	6 - 9 g
Chen Pi	Citrus	3 - 6 g
Gan Cao	Glycyrrhiza	3 - 6 g
[Sheng Jiang	Zingiber	3 - 6 g]
[Da Zao	Ziziphus	3 - 5 pc]

Exterior wind cold or heat with more internal heat which starts to go from the wei to the qi level into the yangming channel. Only mild exterior symptoms are present. Thirst, constipation, full and painful eye orbits, severe bodyaches, or restlessness are the main symptoms.

T   red, dry, thin yellow coat

P   superficial, slightly flooding, rapid

CHAI GE JIE JI TANG

Bupleurum and Kudzu Decoction to Release the Muscle Layer

Extract Formula Name: Bupleurum and Pueraria Combination

Chai Hu	Bupleurum	3 - 9 g
Ge Gen	Pueraria	9 - 12 g
Bai Zhi	Angelica	3 - 9 g
Shi Gao	Gypsum	6 - 15 g
Bai Shao Yao	Paeonia	6 - 9 g
Qiang Huo	Notopterygium	3 - 6 g
Huang Qin	Scutellaria	6 - 9 g
Jie Geng	Platycodon	3 - 6 g
Da Zao	Ziziphus	3 - 4 pc
Sheng Jiang	Zingiber	3 - 6 g
Gan Cao	Glycyrrhiza	3 - 6 g

Wind cold in the superficial and channel layer causing headaches and a common cold.

T   thin white coat

P   superficial

CHUAN XIONG CHA TIAO SAN

Ligusticum Chuanxiong Powder to be Taken with Green Tea

Extract Formula Name: Cnidium and Tea Formula

Chuan Xiong	Ligusticum	3 - 9 g
Bo He	Mentha	9 - 12 g
Jing Jie	Schizonepeta	3 - 9 g
Xi Xin	Asarum	1 - 4 g
Qiang Huo	Notopterygium	3 - 6 g
Fang Feng	Ledebouriella	3 - 6 g
Bai Zhi	Angelica	3 - 6 g
Gan Cao	Glycyrrhiza	3 - 6 g

Wind cold or heat in the early stage leading to a common cold. Symptoms include mild fever and chills, a slight headache and a stuffy nose.

T thin white coat

P superficial

CONG CHI TANG

Scallion and Prepared Soybean Decoction

Dan Dou Chi	Glycine	9 - 25 g
Cong Bai	Allium	9 - 12 g

Exterior wind cold damp with internal heat. The fever is greater than the chills. Symptoms also include thirst, restlessness, or headache.

T thin yellow coat

P rapid

DA QIANG HUO TANG

Major Notopterygium Decoction

Qiang Huo	Notopterygium	9 - 12 g
Fang Feng	Ledebouriella	9 - 12 g
Xi Xin	Asarum	3 - 6 g
Du Huo	Angelica	9 - 12 g
Guang Fang Ji	Aristolochia	9 - 12 g
Huang Lian	Coptis	3 - 9 g
Huang Qin	Scutellaria	6 - 12 g
Bai Zhi	Angelica	6 - 12 g
Cang Zhu	Atractylodes	6 - 12 g
Zhi Mu	Anemarrhena	9 - 15 g
Sheng Di Huang	Rehmannia	9 - 15 g
Chuan Xiong	Ligusticum	9 - 15 g
Zhi Gan Cao	Glycyrrhiza	3 - 9 g

Wind cold with internal heat manifesting especially in the upper jiao. There is lack of sweating or slight sweating due to the internal heat. The fever is greater than the chills.

T red, dry, thin white or yellow coat

P superficial, tight, rapid

DA QING LONG TANG

Major Bluegreen Dragon Decoction

Extract Formula Name: Major Blue Dragon Combination

Ma Huang	Ephedra	6 - 9 g
Xing Ren	Prunus	6 - 9 g
Shi Gao	Gypsum	15 - 20 g
Gui Zhi	Cinnamomum	6 g
Sheng Jiang	Zingiber	6 - 9 g
Da Zao	Ziziphus	3 - 12 pc
Gan Cao	Glycyrrhiza	3 - 6 g

Wind cold in the exterior with phlegm heat in the interior causing cough and wheezing. The phlegm expectoration is thick and yellow.

T sticky yellow coat

P slippery, rapid

DING CHUAN TANG

Arrest Wheezing Decoction

Extract Formula Name: Ma-Huang and Ginkgo Combination

Bai Guo	Gingko	6 - 9 g
Ma Huang	Ephedra	6 - 9 g
Kuan Dong Hua	Tussilago	6 - 9 g
Zi Su Zi	Perilla	3 - 6 g
Xing Ren	Prunus	3 - 6 g
Ban Xia	Pinellia	6 - 9 g
Sang Bai Pi	Morus	6 - 9 g
Huang Qin	Scutellaria	6 - 9 g
Gan Cao	Glycyrrhiza	3 - 6 g

Wind cold (common cold) without sweating leading to muscle aches and a stiff neck primarily.

T thin white coat

P superficial, tight

GE GEN TANG

Kudzu Decoction

Extract Formula Name: Pueraria Combination

Ge Gen	Pueraria	9 - 12 g
Ma Huang	Ephedra	6 - 9 g
Gui Zhi	Cinnamomum	3 - 6 g
Bai Shao Yao	Paeonia	6 g
Sheng Jiang	Zingiber	3 - 6 g
Da Zao	Ziziphus	3 - 4 pc
Gan Cao	Glycyrrhiza	3 - 6 g

Wind cold is lodged in the taiyang channels which leads to severe upper body muscle pain and spasms.

T   thin white coat

P   superficial

GUI ZHI JIA GE GEN TANG

Cinnamon Twig Decoction plus Kudzu

Extract Formula Name: Cinnamon and Pueraria Combination

Gui Zhi	Cinnamomum	6 - 9 g
Bai Shao Yao	Paeonia	6 - 9 g
Ge Gen	Pueraria	9 - 12 g
Sheng Jiang	Zingiber	3 - 6 g
Da Zao	Ziziphus	3 - 4 pc
Gan Cao	Glycyrrhiza	3 - 6 g

Wind cold lasting for eight to ten days causes the patient to develop mild heat symptoms such as itching, flushed face, and thirst.

T   red tip, thin white coat

P   slightly slow

GUI ZHI MA HUANG GE BAN TANG

Combined Cinnamon Twig and Ephedra Decoction

Extract Formula Name: Cinnamon and Ma-Huang Combination

Gui Zhi	Cinnamomum	3 - 6 g
Bai Shao Yao	Paeonia	3 - 6 g
Xing Ren	Prunus	3 - 6 g
Ma Huang	Ephedra	3 - 6 g
Sheng Jiang	Zingiber	3 - 6 g
Da Zao	Ziziphus	3 - 4 pc
Gan Cao	Glycyrrhiza	3 - 6 g

Wind cold with sticky or clear phlegm expectoration, or patient with pre-existing phlegm accumulation gets a wind cold invasion.

T thick white coat

P superficial, slippery

HUA GAI SAN

Canopy Powder

Extract Formula Name: Ma-Huang and Morus Formula

Ma Huang	Ephedra	6 - 9 g
Sang Bai Pi	Morus	6 - 9 g
Fu Ling	Poria	6 - 9 g
Zi Su Zi	Perilla	6 - 9 g
Chen Pi	Citrus	3 - 6 g
Xing Ren	Prunus	3 - 6 g
Gan Cao	Glycyrrhiza	3 - 6 g

Wind cold and damp accumulation, with qi stagnation in the middle jiao causing diarrhea, nausea, vomiting, headache, or fever and chills.

T white sticky coat

P soggy or slippery

☞ All ingredients should be ground into a powder. Take 6 g two to three times a day.

HUO XIANG ZHENG QI SAN

Agastache Powder to Rectify the Qi

Extract Formula Name: Agastache Formula

Huo Xiang	Agastache	9 g
Hou Po	Magnolia	6 - 9 g
Bai Zhi	Angelica	3 - 6 g
Zi Su Ye	Perilla	3 - 6 g
Chen Pi	Citrus	6 g
Bai Zhu	Atractylodes	6 g
Fu Ling	Poria	3 - 6 g
Ban Xia	Pinellia	6 g
Da Fu Pi	Areca	3 - 6 g
Jie Geng	Platycodon	6 g
Gan Cao	Glycyrrhiza	6 - 9 g
[Da Zao	Ziziphus	1 - 3 g]
[Sheng Jiang	Zingiber	3 - 6 g]

Wind cold invasion without sweating; milder than Ma Huang Tang - Ephedra Decoction. Symptoms include fever and chills, headache, body aches, and a runny nose with clear mucus.

T white coat

P superficial

JIA WEI XIANG SU SAN

Augmented Cyperus and Perilla Leaf Powder

Xiang Fu	Cyperus	6 - 9 g
Zi Su Ye	Perilla	6 g
Jing Jie	Schizonepeta	6 g
Qin Jiao	Gentiana	6 g
Fang Feng	Ledebouriella	6 g
Chuan Xiong	Ligusticum	3 - 6 g
Man Jing Zi	Vitex	6 g
Chen Pi	Citrus	3 - 6 g
Sheng Jiang	Zingiber	3 - 6 g
Gan Cao	Glycyrrhiza	3 - 6 g

Wind cold damp (excess type) changing to heat which causes a common cold. This formula is also useful for sores, furuncles, and pus.

T thin white coat

P superficial, tight

JING FANG BAI DU SAN

Schizonepeta and Ledebouriella Powder to Overcome Pathogenic Influences

Extract Formula Name: Schizonepeta and Siler Formula

Jing Jie	Schizonepeta	3 - 6 g
Fang Feng	Ledebouriellaa	3 - 6 g
Chuan Xiong	Ligusticum	3 - 6 g
Qiang Huo	Notopterygium	3 - 6 g
Du Huo	Angelica	3 - 6 g
Chai Hu	Bupleurum	3 - 6 g
Fu Ling	Poria	3 - 6 g
Qian Hu	Peucedanum	3 - 6 g
Zhi Ke	Citrus	3 - 6 g
Jie Geng	Platycodon	3 - 6 g
Sheng Jiang	Zingiber	3 - 6 g
Gan Cao	Glycyrrhiza	2 - 4 g
[Bo He	Mentha	3 g]

Wind cold damp with pre-existing internal damp causing muscle aches; or external wind damp cold and internal heat causing intolerance to wind and cold, joint or body aches, lack of sweating, or thirst.

T normal color, or red, thin yellowish coat

P superficial, rapid, maybe slippery

JIU WEI QIANG HUO TANG

Nine-Ingredient Decoction with Notopterygium

Extract Formula Name: Chianghuo Combination

Qiang Huo	Notopterygium	3 - 6 g
Cang Zhu	Atractylodes	3 - 6 g
Xi Xin	Asarum	1 - 3 g
Fang Feng	Ledebouriella	3 - 6 g
Chuan Xiong	Ligusticum	3 - 6 g
Huang Qin	Scutellaria	3 - 9 g
Bai Zhi	Angelica	3 - 6 g
Sheng Di Huang	Rehmannia	3 - 9 g
Gan Cao	Glycyrrhiza	3 - 6 g

Wind cold with pre-existing damp causing wind cold edema, and a headache which feels as if there is a belt around the head.

T white coat

P superficial, maybe slippery

MA HUANG JIA ZHU TANG

Ephedra Decoction plus Atractylodes

Ma Huang	Ephedra	6 - 9 g
Xing Ren	Prunus	6 - 9 g
Gui Zhi	Cinnamomum	3 - 6 g
Gan Cao	Glycyrrhiza	3 - 6 g
Bai Zhu	Atractylodes	6 - 9 g

Wind cold causes facial edema and scanty urination. This formula is also useful for jaundice accompanied by taiyang symptoms.

T thin white coat

P superficial, tight

MA HUANG LIAN QIAO CHI XIAO DOU TANG

Ephedra, Forsythia, and Aduki Bean Decoction

Ma Huang	Ephedra	3 - 9 g
Lian Qiao	Forsythia	6 - 9 g
Chi Xiao Dou	Phaseolus	6 - 9 g
Sang Bai Pi	Morus	6 - 9 g
Xing Ren	Prunus	6 - 9 g
Sheng Jiang	Zingiber	3 - 6 g
Da Zao	Ziziphus	3 - 4 pc
Gan Cao	Glycyrrhiza	3 - 6 g

Wind cold (excess type) without sweating causing asthma or a common cold.

T thin white coat

P superficial, tight

✪ **Major Formula**

MA HUANG TANG

Ephedra Decoction

Extract Formula Name: Ma-Huang Combination

Ma Huang	Ephedra	6 - 9 g
Xing Ren	Prunus	6 - 9 g
Gui Zhi	Cinnamomum	6 - 9 g
Gan Cao	Glycyrrhiza	3 - 6 g

Wind cold damp with slight heat symptoms and fullness, nausea, joint pain, and a light cough.

T red tip, thin white coat

P superficial, maybe slightly rapid, slippery

MA XING YI GAN TANG

Ephedra, Apricot Kernel, Coix, and Licorice Decoction

Extract Formula Name: Ma-Huang and Coix Combination

Ma Huang	Ephedra	6 - 9 g
Xing Ren	Prunus	6 - 9 g
Yi Yi Ren	Coix	12 g
Gan Cao	Glycyrrhiza	3 - 6 g

Wind cold cough (excess type) causing body aches or nasal congestion with profuse white phlegm discharge. May be used in combination with 'Zhi Sou San - Stop Coughing Powder' to treat cough.

T   thin white coat

P   superficial, tight

SAN NIU TANG

Three-Unbinding Decoction

Extract Formula Name: Ma-Huang, Licorice and Apricot Seed Combination

Ma Huang	Ephedra	6 - 9 g
Xing Ren	Prunus	6 - 9 g
Gan Cao	Glycyrrhiza	3 - 6 g

Wind cold asthma with pre-existing phlegm and water (excess type) producing mild exterior symptoms such as dyspnea, wheezing with mild fever and chills.

T   thick sticky white coat

P   superficial, tight

SHE GAN MA HUANG TANG

Belamcanda and Ephedra Decoction

She Gan	Belamcanda	6 - 9 g
Ma Huang	Ephedra	6 - 9 g
Ban Xia	Pinellia	6 - 9 g
Zi Wan	Aster	6 - 9 g
Kuan Dong Hua	Tussilago	6 - 9 g
Wu Wei Zi	Schisandra	3 - 6 g
Xi Xin	Asarum	6 - 9 g
Sheng Jiang	Zingiber	9 - 12 g
Da Zao	Ziziphus	7 - 9 pc

Wind cold causing wheezing, cough, dyspnea, and tightness in the chest.

T   thin white sticky coat

P   superficial

SHEN MI TANG

Mysterious Decoction

Ma Huang	Ephedra	6 - 9 g
Xing Ren	Prunus	6 - 9 g
Hou Po	Magnolia	6 - 12 g
Chai Hu	Bupleurum	3 - 6 g
Zi Su Ye	Perilla	3 - 6 g
Chen Pi	Citrus	3 - 6 g
Gan Cao	Glycyrrhiza	3 - 6 g

Wind cold with internal heat causing lack of sweating, delirious speech, fever and chills, insomnia, bleeding in the upper parts, or fullness type headache.

T red, dry, yellow coat

P flooding, rapid

SHI GAO TANG

Gypsum Decoction

Shi Gao	Gypsum	15 - 35 g
Ma Huang	Ephedra	6 - 9 g
Huang Lian	Coptis	3 - 6 g
Huang Qin	Scutellaria	6 - 9 g
Zhi Zi	Gardenia	6 - 9 g
Huang Bai	Phellodendron	6 - 9 g
Dan Dou Chi	Glycine	6 - 9 g

Summer damp cold with mild fever and chills and profuse sweating.

T sticky white coat

P superficial

SHI WEI XIANG RU YIN

Ten-Ingredient Decoction with Elsholtzia

Extract Formula Name: Elsholtiza Ten Combination

Xiang Ru	Elsholtzia	6 - 9 g
Ren Shen	Panax	6 - 9 g
Bai Zhu	Atractylodes	3 - 6 g
Huang Qi	Astragalus	6 - 12 g
Chen Pi	Citrus	3 - 6 g
Bian Dou	Dolichos	6 - 9 g
Hou Po	Magnolia	6 - 12 g
Mu Gua	Chaenomeles	6 g
Fu Ling	Poria	6 - 9 g
Gan Cao	Glycyrrhiza	3 - 6 g

Wind cold with internal cold and damp and food stagnation affecting the middle jiao. This formula also treats five kinds of stagnation: qi, damp, blood, food, and cold. Symptoms include fever and chills without sweating and body aches.

T   sticky white coat

P   superficial, slow, or choppy

WU JI SAN

Five-Accumulation Powder

Extract Formula Name: Tang-Kuei and Magnolia Formula

Ma Huang	Ephedra	3 - 6 g
Gan Jiang	Zingiber	3 - 6 g
Hou Po	Magnolia	6 - 9 g
Cang Zhu	Atractylodes	3 - 9 g
Bai Zhi	Angelica	3 - 6 g
Rou Gui	Cinnamomum	3 g
Chuan Xiong	Ligusticum	3 - 6 g
Bai Shao Yao	Paeonia	6 - 9 g
Zhi Ke	Citrus	3 - 6 g
Dang Gui	Angelica	3 - 9 g
Fu Ling	Poria	6 - 9 g
Ban Xia	Pinellia	6 - 9 g
Chen Pi	Citrus	3 - 6 g
Jie Geng	Platycodon	6 - 9 g
Zhi Gan Cao	Glycyrrhiza	3 - 6 g

Pronounced wind cold with mild qi stagnation, or wind cold invasion during pregnancy.

T   thin white coat

P   superficial, tight

XIANG SU CONG CHI TANG

Cyperus, Perilla Leaf, Scallion, and Prepared Soybean Decoction

Zi Su Ye	Perilla	6 - 9 g
Xiang Fu	Cyperus	6 - 9 g
Cong Bai	Allium	2 - 4 pc
Dan Dou Chi	Glycine	9 - 12 g
Chen Pi	Citrus	3 - 6 g
Zhi Gan Cao	Glycyrrhiza	3 - 6 g

Wind cold with internal qi stagnation causing belching, decreased appetite, fever and chills, headache, absence of sweating and middle jiao fullness.

T thin white coat

P superficial

XIANG SU SAN

Cyperus and Perilla Leaf Powder

Extract Formula Name: Cyperus and Perilla Formula

Xiang Fu	Cyperus	6 - 9 g
Zi Su Ye	Perilla	6 - 9 g
Chen Pi	Citrus	3 - 6 g
Zhi Gan Cao	Glycyrrhiza	3 - 6 g

Wind cold with internal water accumulation causing profuse phlegm expectoration, body aches, or superficial edema.

T moist white coat

P superficial, tight

XIAO QING LONG TANG

Minor Blue Dragon Decoction

Extract Formula Name: Minor Blue Dragon Combination

Ma Huang	Ephedra	6 - 9 g
Gui Zhi	Cinnamomum	6 - 9 g
Xi Xin	Asarum	3 g
Wu Wei Zi	Schisandra	6 - 9 g
Gan Jiang	Zingiber	3 g
Bai Shao Yao	Paeonia	6 - 9 g
Ban Xia	Pinellia	6 - 9 g
Gan Cao	Glycyrrhiza	3 - 6 g

Wind cold causing nasal obstruction with white or clear profuse discharge.

T thin moist white coat

P superficial

XIN YI SAN

Magnolia Flower Powder

Extract Formula Name: Magnolia Flower Formula

Xin Yi Hua	Magnolia	6 - 9 g
Mu Tong	Akebia	6 - 9 g
Chuan Xiong	Ligusticum	3 - 9 g
Qiang Huo	Notopterygium	3 - 6 g
Xi Xin	Asarum	3 g
Gao Ben	Ligusticum	6 - 9 g
Fang Feng	Ledebouriella	6 - 9 g
Sheng Ma	Cimicifuga	3 - 6 g
Bai Zhi	Angelica	3 - 6 g
Gan Cao	Glycyrrhiza	3 - 6 g

Wind edema with fever and chills, or decreased urination.

T thin white coat

P superficial, slippery, or deep

YUE BI JIA ZHU TANG

Maidservant from Yue Decoction plus Atractylodes

Extract Formula Name: Atractylodes Combination

Ma Huang	Ephedra	6 - 9 g
Shi Gao	Gypsum	9 - 20 g
Bai Zhu	Atractylodes	6 - 9 g
Sheng Jiang	Zingiber	3 - 9 g
Da Zao	Ziziphus	3 - 7 pc
Gan Cao	Glycyrrhiza	3 - 6 g

Whole body edema due to wind causing wind intolerance, scanty urination, possible sweating, possible fever, or thirst.

T thin white coat

P superficial

YUE BI TANG

Maidservant from Yue Decoction

Extract Formula Name: Ma-Huang and Gypsum Combination

Ma Huang	Ephedra	6 - 15 g
Sheng Jiang	Zingiber	3 - 9 g
Shi Gao	Gypsum	15 - 30 g
Da Zao	Ziziphus	6 - 12 pc
Gan Cao	Glycyrrhiza	3 - 6 g

Cough due to wind with sputum. Mild exterior symptoms with persisting cough.

T thin white coat

P superficial

ZHI SOU SAN

Stop Coughing Powder

Extract Formula Name: Platycodon and Schizonepeta Formula

Zi Wan	Aster	6 - 9 g
Jing Jie	Schizonepeta	6 - 9 g
Bai Qian	Cynanchum	6 - 9 g
Jie Geng	Platycodon	6 - 9 g
Bai Bu	Stemona	6 - 9 g
Chen Pi	Citrus	3 - 6 g
Gan Cao	Glycyrrhiza	3 - 6 g

Wind Cold with Underlying Deficiency

Qi deficient patient gets evil qi invading taiyang, shaoyang, and yangming channels. This causes irritability, constipation, full chest, or heaviness.

T   red, sticky coat

P   rapid, wiry

☞ Da Huang - Rheum should be added during the last 3 minutes of the decoction process.

✗ Qian Dan - Minium is toxic and should be substituted with Dai Zhe Shi - Haematitum or Sheng Tie Luo - Frusta Ferri. Caution during pregnancy.

CHAI HU JIA LONG GU MU LI TANG

Bupleurum plus Dragon Bone and Oyster Shell Decoction

Extract Formula Name: Bupleurum and D.B. Combination

Chai Hu	Bupleurum	9 - 12 g
Huang Qin	Scutellaria	6 g
Ren Shen	Panax	6 g
Gui Zhi	Cinnamomum	3 - 6 g
Ban Xia	Pinellia	6 g
Fu Ling	Poria	6 g
Da Huang	Rheum	6 g
Long Gu	Os Draconis	3 - 6 g
Mu Li	Ostrea	3 - 6 g
Sheng Jiang	Zingiber	3 - 6 g
Da Zao	Ziziphus	3 - 6 pc
Qian Dan	Minium	1 - 4 g

Yin or blood deficient patient gets a wind cold or wind heat invasion. Symptoms include mild chills, weakness, headaches, and fever.

T   pale or red, thin white coat

P   thin, weak, rapid

CONG BAI QI WEI YIN

Scallion Decoction with Seven-Ingredients

Cong Bai	Allium	9 - 12 g
Dan Dou Chi	Glycine	6 - 9 g
Ge Gen	Pueraria	9 - 12 g
Sheng Di Huang	Rehmannia	9 - 15 g
Mai Men Dong	Ophiopogon	9 - 12 g
Sheng Jiang	Zingiber	3 - 9 g

Wind edema or wind damp with Spleen and wei qi deficiency causing sweating, urinary difficulty, or edema in the superficial layer.

T pale, thin white coat

P superficial

FANG JI HUANG QI TANG

Stephania and Astragalus Decoction

Extract Formula Name: Stephania and Astragalus Combination

Han Fang Ji	Stephania	9 - 12 g
Huang Qi	Astragalus	9 - 15 g
Bai Zhu	Atractylodes	6 - 9 g
Sheng Jiang	Zingiber	3 - 6 g
Da Zao	Ziziphus	3 - 4 pc
Gan Cao	Glycyrrhiza	3 - 6 g

Wind cold (deficiency type) with slight sweating, and the patient starts to have internal heat. The fever is greater than the chills.

T red tip, thin white coat

P superficial, forceful

GUI ZHI ER YUE BI YI TANG

Two-parts Cinnamon Twig Decoction with One-part Maidservant from Yeu's Decoction

Gui Zhi	Cinnamomum	3 - 6 g
Bai Shao Yao	Paeonia	3 - 6 g
Ma Huang	Ephedra	3 - 6 g
Shi Gao	Gypsum	3 - 6 g
Sheng Jiang	Zingiber	3 - 6 g
Da Zao	Ziziphus	3 - 4 pc
Gan Cao	Glycyrrhiza	3 - 6 g

Wind cold (deficiency type) with sweating and underlying yang deficiency leading to a common cold. Symptoms include body aches and mild chills.

T pale, wet

P slow, tight

GUI ZHI JIA FU ZI TANG

Cinnamon Twig Decoction plus Aconite

Extract Formula Name: Cinnamon, Hoelen and Aconite Combination

Gui Zhi	Cinnamomum	6 - 9 g
Bai Shao Yao	Paeonia	6 - 9 g
Sheng Jiang	Zingiber	3 - 6 g
Da Zao	Ziziphus	3 - 4 pc
Gan Cao	Glycyrrhiza	3 - 6 g
Fu Zi	Aconitum	1 - 6 g

Wind cold is lodged in the taiyang channels which leads to severe upper body muscle pain and spasms.

T thin white coat

P superficial

GUI ZHI JIA GE GEN TANG

Cinnamon Twig Decoction plus Kudzu

Extract Formula Name: Cinnamon and Pueraria Combination

Gui Zhi	Cinnamomum	6 - 9 g
Bai Shao Yao	Paeonia	6 - 9 g
Ge Gen	Pueraria	9 - 12 g
Sheng Jiang	Zingiber	3 - 6 g
Da Zao	Ziziphus	3 - 4 pc
Gan Cao	Glycyrrhiza	3 - 6 g

Severe taiyin/taiyang disease with abdominal cramps as the main symptom.

T thin white coat

P superficial

GUI ZHI JIA SHAO YAO TANG

Cinnamon Twig Decoction plus Peony

Extract Formula Name: Cinnamon and Peony Combination

Gui Zhi	Cinnamomum	6 - 9 g
Bai Shao Yao	Paeonia	15 - 18 g
Sheng Jiang	Zingiber	3 - 6 g
Da Zao	Ziziphus	3 - 4 pc
Gan Cao	Glycyrrhiza	3 - 6 g

Mild taiyin with taiyang syndrome: wind cold with mild Spleen qi deficiency. The chills are predominant, and the patient experiences diarrhea with epigastric fullness.

T pale, thin white coat

P weak, may be superficial

GUI ZHI REN SHEN TANG

Cinnamon Twig and Ginseng Decoction

Extract Formula Name: Cinnamon and Ginseng Combination

Gui Zhi	Cinnamomum	9 - 12 g
Ren Shen	Panax	9 - 12 g
Gan Jiang	Zingiber	9 g
Bai Zhu	Atractylodes	9 g
Zhi Gan Cao	Glycyrrhiza	9 - 12 g

Wind cold (deficiency type) with sweating leading to a common cold.

T moist, thin white coat

P superficial, weak

✪ **Major Formula**

GUI ZHI TANG

Cinnamon Twig Decoction

Extract Formula Name: Cinnamon Combination

Gui Zhi	Cinnamomum	6 - 9 g
Bai Shao Yao	Paeonia	6 - 9 g
Sheng Jiang	Zingiber	3 - 6 g
Da Zao	Ziziphus	3 - 5 pc
Gan Cao	Glycyrrhiza	3 - 6 g

Wind cold (deficiency type) with internal fire: taiyang and yangming disorder. This causes sweating, chills, nasal congestion, and constipation with abdominal fullness.

T red, thin white or yellow coat

P superficial, rapid

✗ Caution during pregnancy.

HOU PO QI WU TANG

Seven-Substance Decoction with Magnolia Bark

Extract Formula Name: Magnolia 7 Combination

Hou Po	Magnolia	15 g
Da Huang	Rheum	9 g
Gui Zhi	Cinnamomum	6 g
Zhi Shi	Citrus	9 g
Sheng Jiang	Zingiber	12 g
Da Zao	Ziziphus	12 pc
Gan Cao	Glycyrrhiza	6 g

Mild yang deficiency with external wind cold without sweating. (shaoyin and taiyang disease). Symptoms include extreme chilliness with mild fever and severe fatigue.

T pale, white coat

P minute

MA HUANG FU ZI XI XIN TANG

Ephedra, Prepared Aconite, and Asarum Decoction

Extract Formula Name: Ma-Huang and Asarum Combination

Ma Huang	Ephedra	6 - 9 g
Fu Zi	Aconitum	3 - 6 g
Xi Xin	Asarum	3 - 6 g

Wind cold damp with pre-existing qi deficiency and mild heat which is just beginning. This causes high fever and chills, lack of sweating, tightness in the neck, or severe bodyaches.

T pale, swollen, teethmarks, sticky white coat

P slippery, superficial, slow, or soggy

REN SHEN BAI DU SAN

Ginseng Powder to Overcome Pathogenic Influences

Extract Formula Name: Ginseng and Mentha Formula

Chuan Xiong	Ligusticum	6 - 9 g
Du Huo	Angelica	6 - 9 g
Chai Hu	Bupleurum	6 - 9 g
Qiang Huo	Notopterygium	6 - 9 g
Qian Hu	Peucedanum	6 - 9 g
Ren Shen	Panax	6 - 9 g
Fu Ling	Poria	6 - 9 g
Zhi Ke	Citrus	6 - 9 g
Jie Geng	Platycodon	6 - 9 g
Gan Cao	Glycyrrhiza	3 - 6 g

Cold packs were used on a patient who had a common cold but also an underlying Spleen yang deficiency. Now the cold has moved into deeper layers and caused severe cold stagnation with water accumulation under the Heart. Symptoms include shortness of breath, watery sputum, angina, or stuffiness in the chest.

T pale, wet

P slow, slightly slippery

✗ Ba Dou - Croton is extremely toxic and should be used with caution. Do not use during pregnancy.

SAN WU BAI SAN

Three-White Herbs Powder

Jie Geng	Platycodon	3 - 6 g
Bei Mu	Fritillaria	6 - 12 g
Ba Dou	Croton	1 - 3 g

Wind cold with pre-existing qi and yang deficiency. Symptoms include fever and chills or cough with white and profuse phlegm expectoration.

T pale, swollen, teethmarks, white coat

P frail or superficial

SHEN SU YIN

Ginseng and Perilla Leaf Decoction

Extract Formula Name: Ginseng and Perilla Combination

Zhi Ke	Citrus	3 - 6 g
Ren Shen	Panax	6 - 9 g
Zi Su Ye	Perilla	6 - 9 g
Ge Gen	Pueraria	6 - 9 g
Qian Hu	Peucedanum	6 - 9 g
Fu Ling	Poria	6 - 9 g
Jie Geng	Platycodon	3 - 6 g
Mu Xiang	Saussurea	3 - 6 g
Ban Xia	Pinellia	6 - 9 g
Chen Pi	Citrus	3 - 6 g
Gan Cao	Glycyrrhiza	3 - 6 g
[Sheng Jiang	Zingiber	3 - 6 g]
[Da Zao	Ziziphus	3 - 6 pc]

Interior cold with yang deficiency and wind cold causing cold type hernia. Other symptoms include numb, cold hands and feet and body aches.

T   pale, moist, white coat

P   frail

✗   Do not take over a long period of time. Wu Tou - Aconitum is toxic.

WU TOU GUI ZHI TANG

Aconite and Cinnamon Twig Decoction

Extract Formula Name: Wu-tou and Cinnamon Combination

Gui Zhi	Cinnamomum	6 - 9 g
Wu Tou	Aconitum	3 - 6 g
Bai Shao Yao	Paeonia	6 - 9 g
Sheng Jiang	Zingiber	3 - 6 g
Da Zao	Ziziphus	3 - 5 pc
Gan Cao	Glycyrrhiza	3 - 6 g

Wind cold with internal damp causing a common cold without sweating, Stomach flu, heaviness in the head, cold intolerance, or nausea and vomiting.

T   white sticky coat

P   superficial

XIANG RU SAN

Elsholtzia Powder

Extract Formula Name: Elsholtzia Combination

Xiang Ru	Elsholtzia	9 - 12 g
Hou Po	Magnolia	9 - 12 g
Bian Dou	Dolichos	6 - 9 g

Qi/yang deficient patient with wind cold causing slight fever, lack of sweating, cold hands and feet, severe chills with a mild fever, and weakness.

T   pale, thin white coat

P   frail

ZAI ZAO SAN

Renewal Powder

Ren Shen	Panax	6 - 9 g
Huang Qi	Astragalus	6 - 12 g
Fu Zi	Aconitum	3 g
Xi Xin	Asarum	3 g
Gui Zhi	Cinnamomum	3 - 6 g
Chuan Xiong	Ligusticum	3 - 6 g
Qiang Huo	Notopterygium	3 - 6 g
Fang Feng	Ledebouriella	6 - 9 g
Sheng Jiang	Zingiber	3 - 6 g
Da Zao	Ziziphus	2 - 4 pc
Gan Cao	Glycyrrhiza	3 - 6 g

Lung

WIND HEAT INVASION

- fever greater than chills
- sore throat
- yellow nasal discharge
- body aches

T red tip, thin yellow or white coat

P superficial, rapid

Wind Heat

Wind heat causing thick nasal discharge with congestion, and frontal headache.

T yellow coat

P superficial, rapid

CANG ER ZI SAN

Xanthium Powder

Extract Formula Name: Xanthium Formula

Cang Er Zi	Xanthium	6 - 9 g
Xin Yi Hua	Magnolia	3 - 6 g
Bo He	Mentha	3 - 6 g
Bai Zhi	Angelica	6 - 9 g

Exterior wind cold or heat with internal heat which starts to go from the wei to the qi level into the yangming channel. Only mild exterior symptoms are present. Thirst, constipation, full and painful eye orbits, severe bodyaches, or restlessness are the main symptoms.

T red, dry, thin yellow coat

P superficial, slightly flooding, rapid

CHAI GE JIE JI TANG

Bupleurum and Kudzu Decoction to Release the Muscle Layer

Extract Formula Name: Bupleurum and Pueraria Combination

Chai Hu	Bupleurum	3 - 9 g
Ge Gen	Pueraria	9 - 12 g
Bai Zhi	Angelica	3 - 9 g
Shi Gao	Gypsum	6 - 15 g
Bai Shao Yao	Paeonia	6 - 9 g
Qiang Huo	Notopterygium	3 - 6 g
Huang Qin	Scutellaria	6 - 9 g
Jie Geng	Platycodon	3 - 6 g
Da Zao	Ziziphus	3 - 4 pc
Sheng Jiang	Zingiber	3 - 6 g
Gan Cao	Glycyrrhiza	3 - 6 g

Taiyang and shaoyang disease with joint congestion and intolerance to wind, or alternating fever and chills. Also useful for Liver overacting on Spleen.

T   thin white coat

P   possibly superficial

CHAI HU GUI ZHI TANG

Bupleurum and Cinnamon Twig Decoction

Extract Formula Name: Bupleurum and Cinnamon Combination

Gui Zhi	Cinnamomum	3 - 6 g
Chai Hu	Bupleurum	6 - 12 g
Ren Shen	Panax	3 - 6 g
Ban Xia	Pinellia	3 - 6 g
Huang Qin	Scutellaria	3 - 9 g
Bai Shao Yao	Paeonia	3 - 6 g
Sheng Jiang	Zingiber	3 - 6 g
Da Zao	Ziziphus	4 - 6 pc
Gan Cao	Glycyrrhiza	3 - 6 g

Wind heat with Lung heat leading to fever or soreness in the throat.

T   red tip, white coat

P   superficial, rapid

CONG BAI JIE GENG TANG

Scallion and Platycodon Decoction

Jie Geng	Platycodon	3 - 6 g
Cong Bai	Allium	9 - 12 g
Zhi Zi	Gardenia	6 - 9 g
Dan Dou Chi	Glycine	9 - 12 g
Lian Qiao	Forsythia	3 - 6 g
Bo He	Mentha	3 - 6 g
Dan Zhu Ye	Lophatherum	2 - 6 g
Gan Cao	Glycyrrhiza	3 - 6 g

Wind heat with internal heat: taiyang and yangming organ disease. The heat is severe. Symptoms include dark yellow urine, constipation, severe fever and chills, heat sensations in the body, sores and carbuncles, skin disorders, and a bitter taste.

T   bright or dark red, dry, yellow coat

P   flooding, rapid, wiry

☞ Ingredients should be ground into powder, then made into a pill with water. Take 6 g each time, twice a day.

✘ Do not use during pregnancy.

FANG FENG TONG SHENG SAN

Ledebouriella Powder that Sagely Unblocks

Extract Formula Name: Siler and Platycodon Formula

Fang Feng	Ledebouriella	9 - 15 g
Ma Huang	Ephedra	9 - 15 g
Da Huang	Rheum	9 - 15 g
Mang Xiao	Mirabilitum	9 - 15 g
Jing Jie	Schizonepeta	9 - 15 g
Bo He	Mentha	9 - 15 g
Zhi Zi	Gardenia	9 - 15 g
Hua Shi	Talcum	60 - 90 g
Shi Gao	Gypsum	15 - 30 g
Huang Qin	Scutellaria	15 - 30 g
Lian Qiao	Forsythia	9 - 15 g
Jie Geng	Platycodon	15 - 30 g
Dang Gui	Angelica	9 - 15 g
Bai Shao Yao	Paeonia	9 - 15 g
Chuan Xiong	Ligusticum	9 - 15 g
Bai Zhu	Atractylodes	9 - 15 g
Gan Cao	Glycyrrhiza	30 - 60 g

Wind heat with internal middle jiao heat and Large Intestine heat and damp causing dysentery: taiyang and yangming disease. Symptoms include fever, thirst, or burning anus.

T   red, yellow coat

P   rapid, slippery

GE GEN HUANG LIAN HUANG QIN TANG

Kudzu, Coptis, and Scutellaria Decoction

Extract Formula Name: Pueraria, Coptis and Scute Combination

Ge Gen	Pueraria	12 - 15 g
Huang Lian	Coptis	9 g
Huang Qin	Scutellaria	6 - 9 g
Gan Cao	Glycyrrhiza	3 - 6 g

Wind damp cold with damp heat causing epidemic influenza.

T pink or red, sticky white or yellow coat

P superficial, slippery

LIAN QIAO BAI DU SAN

Forsythia Powder to Overcome Pathogenic Influences

Lian Qiao	Forsythia	6 - 9 g
Jin Yin Hua	Lonicera	6 - 9 g
Fu Ling	Poria	6 - 9 g
Chuan Xiong	Ligusticum	3 - 9 g
Qiang Huo	Notopterygium	3 - 6 g
Du Huo	Angelica	6 - 9 g
Chai Hu	Bupleurum	6 - 9 g
Qian Hu	Peucedanum	6 - 9 g

Wind heat with fever, possible sweating, thirst, dyspnea, asthma: heat in the qi level.

T red tip or border, yellow coat

P rapid, flooding

MA XING SHI GAN TANG

Ephedra, Apricot Kernel, Gypsum, and Licorice Decoction

Extract Formula Name: Ma-Huang and Apricot Seed Combination

Ma Huang	Ephedra	6 - 15 g
Xing Ren	Prunus	6 - 9 g
Shi Gao	Gypsum	6 - 20 g
Gan Cao	Glycyrrhiza	3 - 6 g

Wind heat with toxin affecting the neck and head with swollen sore throat or glands, tonsillitis, or pharyngitis.

T red

P rapid

QIANG LAN TANG

Notopterygium and Isatis Root Decoction

Qiang Huo	Notopterygium	9 - 12 g
Ban Lan Gen	Isatis	12 - 20 g

Wind heat invasion leading to headaches.

T thin white coat
P superficial, rapid

QING KONG GAO

Clear Head Formula

Huang Qin	Scutellaria	6 - 9 g
Huang Lian	Coptis	6 - 9 g
Chuan Xiong	Ligusticum	12 - 15 g
Chai Hu	Bupleurum	6 - 9 g
Qiang Huo	Notopterygium	6 - 12 g
Fang Feng	Ledebouriella	6 - 12 g
Gan Cao	Glycyrrhiza	3 - 6 g
For frontal headaches add:		
Bai Zhi	Angelica	6 - 9 g
Ge Gen	Pueraria	6 - 9 g
Ma Huang	Ephedra	3 - 9 g
For occipital headaches add:		
Ma Huang	Ephedra	3 - 9 g
Qiang Huo	Notopterygium	6 - 9 g
For temple headaches add:		
Chai Hu	Bupleurum	6 - 9 g
Bai Shao Yao	Paeonia	6 - 9 g
For vertex headaches add:		
Man Jing Zi	Vitex	6 - 9 g
Gao Ben	Ligusticum	6 - 9 g

Wind heat with wind stroke causing paraplegia, or facial paralysis with severe heat symptoms.

T red, yellow coat

P rapid

✗ Caution during pregnancy.

QU FENG ZHI BAO DAN

Greatest Treasure Special Pill to Dispel Wind

Hua Shi	Talcum	12 - 15 g
Dang Gui	Angelica	9 - 12 g
Chuan Xiong	Ligusticum	9 g
Gan Cao	Glycyrrhiza	6 g
Fang Feng	Ledebouriella	6 - 9 g
Bai Shao Yao	Paeonia	6 - 9 g
Bai Zhu	Atractylodes	6 g
Du Huo	Angelica	6 g
Ren Shen	Panax	3 g
Qiang Huo	Notopterygium	3 - 6 g
Shu Di Huang	Rehmannia	6 g
Tian Ma	Gastrodia	6 g
Shi Gao	Gypsum	6 g
Huang Qin	Scutellaria	6 g
Jie Geng	Platycodon	3 g
Zhi Zi	Gardenia	1 - 3 g
Jing Jie	Schizonepeta	6 g
Bo He	Mentha	3 g
Da Huang	Rheum	6 g
Mang Xiao	Mirabilitum	6 g
Lian Qiao	Forsythia	3 - 6 g
Ma Huang	Ephedra	6 g
Huang Lian	Coptis	3 g
Huang Bai	Phellodendron	3 g
Xi Xin	Asarum	3 g
Quan Xie	Buthus	3 g

Wind heat causing coughing which is the first sign of the invasion. Symptoms include fever, thirst, or mild sweating.

T   red tip

P   superficial

SANG JU YIN

Mulberry Leaf and Chrysanthemum Decoction

Extract Formula Name: Morus and Chrysanthemum Combination

Sang Ye	Morus	6 - 9 g
Ju Hua	Chrysanthemum	3 g
Bo He	Mentha	3 g
Xing Ren	Prunus	6 - 9 g
Lu Gen	Phragmites	6 - 9 g
Jie Geng	Platycodon	3 - 6 g
Lian Qiao	Forsythia	3 - 6 g
Gan Cao	Glycyrrhiza	3 - 6 g

Wind heat and dryness attacks the Lungs. Symptoms include mild fever, dry or hacking cough with scanty sputum which is hard to expectorate.

T   dry, thin white coat

P   superficial, rapid

SANG XING TANG

Mulberry Leaf and Apricot Kernel Decoction

Extract Formula Name. Morus and Apricot Seed Combination

Sang Ye	Morus	3 - 6 g
Xing Ren	Prunus	4 - 6 g
Zhe Bei Mu	Fritillaria	3 - 6 g
Bei Sha Shen	Glehnia	6 - 9 g
Dan Dou Chi	Glycine	3 - 6 g
Zhi Zi	Gardenia	3 - 6 g
Li Pi	Pyrus	3 - 6 g

Wind heat causing measles and rashes. Symptoms include fever, chills, body aches, cough, or red eyes.

T red, dry

P superficial, rapid

SHENG MA GE GEN TANG

Cimicifuga and Kudzu Decoction

Extract Formula Name: Cimicifuga and Pueraria Combination

Sheng Ma	Cimicifuga	3 - 6 g
Chi Shao Yao	Paeonia	6 - 9 g
Ge Gen	Pueraria	3 - 6 g
Gan Cao	Glycyrrhiza	3 - 6 g

Wind heat and toxin causing measles, lack of sweating, cough, dark urine, or severe sore throat.

T red tip

P superficial, rapid

XUAN DU FA BIAO TANG

Dissipate Toxin and Release the Exterior Decoction

Sheng Ma	Cimicifuga	6 - 9 g
Ge Gen	Pueraria	6 - 9 g
Xing Ren	Prunus	6 - 9 g
Qian Hu	Peucedanum	6 - 9 g
Jie Geng	Platycodon	3 - 6 g
Bo He	Mentha	3 - 6 g
Fang Feng	Ledebouriella	3 - 6 g
Jing Jie	Schizonepeta	3 - 6 g
Lian Qiao	Forsythia	3 - 9 g
Niu Bang Zi	Arctium	3 - 6 g
Dan Zhu Ye	Lophatherum	3 - 6 g
Zhi Ke	Citrus	3 - 6 g
Mu Tong	Akebia	6 - 9 g
Gan Cao	Glycyrrhiza	3 - 6 g

Wind heat with strong internal heat causing fever or thirst.

T   red, thin yellow coat

P   rapid, superficial

YI WU CHAI GE JIE JI TANG

Bupleurum and Kudzu Decoction to Release the Muscle Layer from Medical Revelations

Chai Hu	Bupleurum	6 - 9 g
Ge Gen	Pueraria	6 - 9 g
Huang Qin	Scutellaria	6 - 9 g
Sheng Di Huang	Rehmannia	6 - 12 g
Mu Dan Pi	Paeonia	6 - 9 g
Zhe Bei Mu	Fritillaria	6 - 9 g
Chi Shao Yao	Paeonia	6 - 9 g
Zhi Mu	Anemarrhena	6 - 9 g
Gan Cao	Glycyrrhiza	3 - 6 g

Wind/toxic heat with damp and qi deficiency causing red, swollen sores or carbuncles.

T   thin sticky white coat

P   superficial

YIN QIAO BAI DU SAN

Honeysuckle and Forsythia Powder to Overcome Pathogenic Influences

Qiang Huo	Notopterygium	6 - 9 g
Chuan Xiong	Ligusticum	3 - 6 g
Du Huo	Angelica	3 - 6 g
Chai Hu	Bupleurum	6 - 9 g
Qian Hu	Peucedanum	6 - 9 g
Ren Shen	Panax	6 - 9 g
Jie Geng	Platycodon	3 - 6 g
Zhi Ke	Citrus	3 - 6 g
Fu Ling	Poria	3 - 6 g
Gan Cao	Glycyrrhiza	3 - 6 g
Jin Yin Hua	Lonicera	6 - 9 g
Lian Qiao	Forsythia	6 - 9 g

Wind/toxic heat causing a common cold, lack of sweating, rashes, sore throat, or throbbing headache.

T   normal color or red tip, thin yellow coat

P   superficial, rapid

✪ **Major Formula**

YIN QIAO SAN

Honeysuckle and Forsythia Powder

Extract Formula Name: Lonicera and Forsythia Formula

Jin Yin Hua	Lonicera	6 - 9 g
Lian Qiao	Forsythia	6 - 9 g
Niu Bang Zi	Arctium	6 - 9 g
Dan Dou Chi	Glycine	3 - 9 g
Bo He	Mentha	3 - 6 g
Jie Geng	Platycodon	3 - 6 g
Jing Jie	Schizonepeta	3 - 6 g
Dan Zhu Ye	Lophatherum	3 - 6 g
Lu Gen	Phragmites	3 - 9 g
Gan Cao	Glycyrrhiza	3 - 6 g

Cough due to wind with sputum. Mild exterior symptoms with persisting cough.

T   thin white coat

P   superficial

ZHI SOU SAN

Stop Coughing Powder

Extract Formula Name: Platycodon and Schizonepeta Formula

Zi Wan	Aster	6 - 9 g
Jing Jie	Schizonepeta	6 - 9 g
Bai Qian	Cynanchum	6 - 9 g
Jie Geng	Platycodon	6 - 9 g
Bai Bu	Stemona	6 - 9 g
Chen Pi	Citrus	3 - 6 g
Gan Cao	Glycyrrhiza	3 - 6 g

Wind Heat with Underlying Deficiency

Taiyang and shaoyang disease with joint congestion and intolerance to wind, or alternating fever and chills. Also useful for Liver overacting on Spleen.

T   thin white coat

P   possibly superficial

CHAI HU GUI ZHI TANG

Bupleurum and Cinnamon Twig Decoction

Extract Formula Name: Bupleurum and Cinnamon Combination

Gui Zhi	Cinnamomum	3 - 6 g
Chai Hu	Bupleurum	6 - 12 g
Ren Shen	Panax	3 - 6 g
Ban Xia	Pinellia	3 - 6 g
Huang Qin	Scutellaria	3 - 9 g
Bai Shao Yao	Paeonia	3 - 6 g
Sheng Jiang	Zingiber	3 - 6 g
Da Zao	Ziziphus	4 - 6 pc
Gan Cao	Glycyrrhiza	3 - 6 g

Wind heat common cold with pre-existing yin deficiency causing fever greater than chills, sore throat, dry mouth, night sweats, or bodyaches.

T   red, narrow and thin, scanty coat

P   rapid, thin

✪ **Major Formula**

JIA JIAN WEI ZHU TANG

Modified Polygonatum Odoratum Decoction

Yu Zhu	Polygonatum	6 - 9 g
Bai Wei	Cynanchum	3 - 6 g
Cong Bai	Allium	3 - 6 g
Dan Dou Chi	Glycine	9 - 12 g
Jie Geng	Platycodon	3 - 6 g
Da Zao	Ziziphus	2 - 5 pc
Gan Cao	Glycyrrhiza	3 - 6 g
Bo He	Mentha	3 - 6 g

Yin deficiency with wind cold which turns to heat and hides in the body, consuming more yin; or wind enters the body and consumes yin. Symptoms include night sweats, afternoon fever or heat, or blood-tinged sputum.

T red, dry, slight yellow coat

P weak, rapid

☞ Dissolve Bie Jia - Amyda first for about one hour, then decoct with the remaining herbs.

QIN JIAO BIE JIA SAN

Gentiana and Soft-shelled Turtle Shell Powder

Extract Formula Name: Chin-Chiu and T.S. Formula

Chai Hu	Bupleurum	6 - 9 g
Bie Jia	Amyda	6 - 12 g
Dang Gui	Angelica	6 - 9 g
Di Gu Pi	Lycium	6 - 9 g
Qin Jiao	Gentiana	6 - 9 g
Zhi Mu	Anemarrhena	6 - 12 g
[Wu Mei	Prunus	1 - 3 g]
[Qing Hao	Artemisia	1 - 3 g]

Wind heat with underlying mild yin deficiency. Symptoms include fever, sweating, five-palm heat, or night sweating.

T red

P superficial, slightly thin

WEI ZHU TANG

Polygonatum Odoratum Decoction

Yu Zhu	Polygonatum	6 - 9 g
Ma Huang	Ephedra	6 - 9 g
Cong Bai	Allium	3 - 6 g
Bai Wei	Cynanchum	6 - 9 g
Du Huo	Angelica	6 - 9 g
Chuan Xiong	Ligusticum	3 - 9 g
Xing Ren	Prunus	6 - 9 g
Shi Gao	Gypsum	12 - 15 g
Mu Xiang	Saussurea	3 - 6 g
Gan Cao	Glycyrrhiza	3 - 6 g

EXTERNAL DRYNESS ATTACKING THE LUNGS

- voice hoarseness
- dry skin and throat
- dry cough
- thirst with desire to drink

T dry

P empty

Lung heat with dryness and severe damage to the Lung yin as well as some wind symptoms. Manifestations include dry and itchy throat, full chest, or dry cough without phlegm.

T pink, dry, scanty coat

P weak or empty, rapid

☞ E Jiao - Equus should be dissolved at the end into the strained tea.

QING ZAO JIU FEI TANG

Eliminate Dryness and Rescue the Lungs Decoction

Extract Formula Name: Eriobotrya and Ophiopogon Combination

Sang Ye	Morus	6 - 9 g
Mai Men Dong	Ophiopogon	3 - 6 g
E Jiao	Equus	1 - 4 g
Ren Shen	Panax	6 - 9 g
Xing Ren	Prunus	3 - 6 g
Shi Gao	Gypsum	6 - 9 g
Pi Pa Ye	Eriobotrya	3 - 6 g
Gan Cao	Glycyrrhiza	3 - 6 g
Huo Ma Ren	Cannabis	3 - 6 g

Wind heat and dryness attacks the Lungs. Symptoms include mild fever, dry or hacking cough with scanty sputum which is hard to expectorate.

T dry, thin white coat

P superficial, rapid

SANG XING TANG

Mulberry Leaf and Apricot Kernel Decoction

Extract Formula Name: Morus and Apricot Seed Combination

Sang Ye	Morus	3 - 6 g
Xing Ren	Prunus	4 - 6 g
Zhe Bei Mu	Fritillaria	3 - 6 g
Bei Sha Shen	Glehnia	6 - 9 g
Dan Dou Chi	Glycine	3 - 6 g
Zhi Zi	Gardenia	3 - 6 g
Li Pi	Pyrus	3 - 6 g

Common cold with cold dryness affecting the Lungs. Symptoms include body aches, cough with white clear phlegm which is hard to expectorate, dryness but the patient has no desire to drink, and lack of sweating.

T dry white coat

P wiry

XING SU SAN

Apricot Kernel and Perilla Leaf Powder

Extract Formula Name: Apricot Seed and Perilla Formula

Zi Su Ye	Perilla	3 - 6 g
Xing Ren	Prunus	6 - 9 g
Qian Hu	Peucedanum	6 - 9 g
Zhi Ke	Citrus	3 - 6 g
Chen Pi	Citrus	3 - 6 g
Ban Xia	Pinellia	6 - 9 g
Fu Ling	Poria	6 - 9 g
Jie Geng	Platycodon	3 - 6 g
Sheng Jiang	Zingiber	3 - 6 g
Da Zao	Ziziphus	3 - 5 pc
Gan Cao	Glycyrrhiza	3 - 6 g

LUNG QI DEFICIENCY, WEI (DEFENSIVE) QI DEFICIENCY

- cough with watery expectoration
- frequent colds
- spontaneous day-time sweating
- weak cough

T pale

P weak

Lung qi deficiency without any heat symptoms causing cough, asthma, shortness of breath, or dyspnea.

T   pale, thin white coat

P   weak or frail

✪ **Major Formula**

BU FEI TANG

Tonify the Lungs Decoction

Extract Formula Name: Astragalus and Aster Combination

Huang Qi	Astragalus	12 - 20 g
Shu Di Huang	Rehmannia	12 - 20 g
Ren Shen	Panax	6 - 9 g
Zi Wan	Aster	6 - 9 g
Sang Bai Pi	Morus	6 - 12 g
Wu Wei Zi	Schisandra	6 - 9 g

Wind edema or wind damp with Spleen and wei qi deficiency causing sweating, urinary difficulty, or edema in the superficial layer.

T   pale, thin white coat

P   superficial

FANG JI HUANG QI TANG

Stephania and Astragalus Decoction

Extract Formula Name: Stephania and Astragalus Combination

Han Fang Ji	Stephania	9 - 12 g
Huang Qi	Astragalus	9 - 15 g
Bai Zhu	Atractylodes	6 - 9 g
Sheng Jiang	Zingiber	3 - 6 g
Da Zao	Ziziphus	3 - 4 pc
Gan Cao	Glycyrrhiza	3 - 6 g

Cold in the Lungs and Stomach causing Lung atrophy, cold extremities, or clear sputum.

T   pale, moist

P   weak, slow

GAN CAO GAN JIANG TANG

Licorice and Ginger Decoction

Extract Formula Name: Licorice and Ginger Combination

Zhi Gan Cao	Glycyrrhiza	9 - 12 g
Gan Jiang	Zingiber	6 - 9 g

Wei qi deficiency (defensive qi) due to Spleen qi/yang deficiency with qi stagnation symptoms. The patient experiences frequent colds or abdominal fullness.

T   pale, maybe light purple

P   weak

GUI ZHI LI ZHONG WAN

Cinnamon Twig with Regulate the Middle Pill

Gui Zhi	Cinnamomum	3 - 9 g
Gan Jiang	Zingiber	3 - 6 g
Bai Zhu	Atractylodes	6 - 9 g
Ren Shen	Panax	6 - 12 g
Gan Cao	Glycyrrhiza	3 - 6 g

Spleen/Stomach qi deficiency with cold and wei (defensive) qi deficiency; also useful for peptic ulcers and chronic allergies. Other symptoms include poor appetite or spontaneous sweating.

T   pale, thin white coat

P   weak, slow, thin, wiry

☞ Yi Tang - Saccharum Granorum should be added to the strained tea.

HUANG QI JIAN ZHONG TANG

Astragalus Decoction to Construct the Middle

Extract Formula Name: Astragalus Combination

Gui Zhi	Cinnamomum	9 g
Bai Shao Yao	Paeonia	18 g
Sheng Jiang	Zingiber	10 g
Da Zao	Ziziphus	3 - 6 pc
Gan Cao	Glycyrrhiza	6 g
Yi Tang	Saccharum Granorum	30 g
Huang Qi	Astragalus	9 g

Lung qi and yin deficiency resulting in cough and wheezing, and wei (defensive) qi deficiency.

T thin, scanty coat

P thin, rapid, weak

☞ E Jiao - Equus should be added at the end into the strained tea.

JIU XIAN SAN
Nine-Immortal Powder

Ren Shen	Panax	6 - 9 g
Wu Wei Zi	Schisandra	6 - 9 g
E Jiao	Equus	6 g
Bei Mu	Fritillaria	6 - 9 g
Kuan Dong Hua	Tussilago	6 - 9 g
Jie Geng	Platycodon	3 - 6 g
Ying Su Ke	Papaver	3 - 6 g
Wu Mei	Prunus	6 - 9 g
Sang Bai Pi	Morus	6 - 9 g
[Sheng Jiang	Zingiber	3 - 6 g]
[Da Zao	Ziziphus	3 g]

Qi and wei qi deficiency leading to spontaneous sweating which eventually injures the Heart yin. This leads to night sweating, insomnia, and palpitations.

T pale or red

P frail, thin

MU LI SAN
Oyster Shell Powder

Mu Li	Ostrea	15 - 30 g
Ma Huang Gen	Ephredra	3 - 9 g
Huang Qi	Astragalus	9 - 12 g
Fu Xiao Mai	Triticum	15 - 30 g

Lung qi deficiency damages Spleen qi which leads to damp accumulation with slight heat; or Lung qi deficiency with phlegm. Symptoms include wheezing, sticky yellow sputum, coughing of blood or pus, or heat in the chest.

T light purple, sticky white or yellow coat

P weak, superficial

REN SHEN GE JIE SAN
Ginseng and Gecko Powder

Ge Jie	Gekko	1 pair
Sang Bai Pi	Morus	6 - 9 g
Fu Ling	Poria	6 - 12 g
Xing Ren	Prunus	6 - 9 g
Chuan Bei Mu	Fritillaria	3 - 6 g
Ren Shen	Panax	6 - 12 g
Zhi Mu	Anemarrhena	6 - 9 g
Gan Cao	Glycyrrhiza	3 - 6 g

Lung/Kidney qi deficiency causing cough/asthma with wheezing. There are slightly more cold symptoms.

T   pale, thin sticky white coat

P   weak or frail

REN SHEN HU TAO TANG

Ginseng and Walnut Decoction

Extract Formula Name: Ginseng and Walnut Combination

Ren Shen	Panax	6 - 9 g
Hu Tao Ren	Juglans	3 - 6 pc
Sheng Jiang	Zingiber	3 - 6 pc
Da Zao	Ziziphus	3 pc

Spleen/Lung qi and blood deficiency with Heart yang deficiency, or ying level deficiency. The patient is easily startled, experiences shortness of breath, lack of taste sensation, insomnia, or palpitations. This formula is also useful for irregular periods or uterine bleeding.

T   pale, swollen

P   weak

REN SHEN YANG RONG WAN

Ginseng Decoction to Nourish the Nutritive Qi

Extract Formula Name: Ginseng Combination

Bai Shao Yao	Paeonia	9 - 15 g
Chen Pi	Citrus	3 - 6 g
Dang Gui	Angelica	3 - 9 g
Ren Shen	Panax	6 - 9 g
Huang Qi	Astragalus	6 - 12 g
Bai Zhu	Atractylodes	6 - 9 g
Shu Di Huang	Rehmannia	3 - 6 g
Wu Wei Zi	Schisandra	3 - 6 g
Fu Ling	Poria	3 - 6 g
Yuan Zhi	Polygala	2 - 6 g
Rou Gui	Cinnamomum	6 - 9 g
Gan Cao	Glycyrrhiza	3 - 6 g
[Da Zao	Ziziphus	2 pc]
[Gan Jiang	Zingiber	3 pc]

Lung/Kidney qi deficiency causing cough, asthma, and dyspnea.

T   pale

P   slow, weak

SHEN JIE SAN

Ginseng and Gecko Powder

Ren Shen	Panax	9 - 12 g
Ge Jie	Gekko	1 pair

Lung/Stomach qi deficiency with cough, expectoration of clear sputum, dry mouth, or thirst.

T pale, moist coat

P weak

SHENG JIANG GAN CAO TANG

Ginger and Licorice Decoction

Sheng Jiang	Zingiber	6 - 12 g
Ren Shen	Panax	6 - 9 g
Da Zao	Ziziphus	3 - 9 pc
Gan Cao	Glycyrrhiza	6 - 12 g

Lung qi/yin deficiency with sweating and chronic cough producing scanty sputum which is hard to expectorate. This formula is also useful for palpitations, collapse, insomnia, or irregular pulse.

T pale or red

P weak or frail, slightly rapid

SHENG MAI SAN

Generate the Pulse Powder

Ginseng and Ophiopogon Formula

Ren Shen	Panax	9 - 15 g
Mai Men Dong	Ophiopogon	12 - 18 g
Wu Wei Zi	Schisandra	6 - 9 g

Lung/Spleen qi deficiency with qi sinking in the chest causing shortness of breath, dyspnea, or loose stools.

T pale, thin white coat

P deep, weak

SHENG XIAN TANG

Raise the Sinking Decoction

Huang Qi	Astragalus	15 - 20 g
Sheng Ma	Cimicifuga	3 - 6 g
Zhi Mu	Anemarrhena	6 - 9 g
Chai Hu	Bupleurum	3 - 9 g
Jie Geng	Platycodon	3 - 6 g

Lung/wei qi deficiency with sweating, frequent colds, aversion to wind, and weakness.

T pale

P weak, frail, or superficial

✪ Major Formula

YU PING FENG SAN

Jade Windscreen Powder

Extract Formula Name: Siler and Astragalus Formula

Fang Feng	Ledebouriella	6 - 9 g
Bai Zhu	Atractylodes	9 - 15 g
Huang Qi	Astragalus	6 - 20 g

LUNG YIN DEFICIENCY

- dry cough with scanty yellowish sputum which is hard to expectorate
- afternoon heat or fever
- thirst with dryness in the throat
- malar flush

T red, scanty coat

P empty, rapid

Lung/Kidney yin deficiency with cough and asthma, hemoptysis, tidal fever, or night sweats. This formula is also known as 'Mai Wei Di Huang Wan.'

T red, slight coat

P rapid, thin

BA XIAN CHANG SHOU WAN

Eight-Immortal Pill for Longevity

Shan Zhu Yu	Cornus	6 - 9 g
Shan Yao	Dioscorea	6 - 9 g
Sheng Di Huang	Rehmannia	6 - 12 g
Mu Dan Pi	Paeonia	6 - 9 g
Ze Xie	Alisma	6 - 9 g
Fu Ling	Poria	6 - 9 g
Wu Wei Zi	Schisandra	6 - 9 g
Mai Men Dong	Ophiopogon	6 - 9 g

Lung/Kidney yin deficiency with bleeding in the upper parts due to false heat breaking the blood vessels; or chronic cough due to dryness in the throat.

T red, slight coat

P rapid, thin

✪ Major Formula

BAI HE GU JIN TANG

Lily Bulb Decoction to Preserve the Metal

Extract Formula Name: Lily Combination

Bai He	Lilium	3 - 12 g
Mai Men Dong	Ophiopogon	6 - 12 g
Sheng Di Huang	Rehmannia	6 - 12 g
Shu Di Huang	Rehmannia	6 - 12 g
Bei Mu	Fritillaria	3 - 6 g
Xuan Shen	Scrophularia	6 - 9 g
Dang Gui	Angelica	6 - 9 g
Bai Shao Yao	Paeonia	6 - 9 g
Jie Geng	Platycodon	3 - 6 g
Gan Cao	Glycyrrhiza	3 - 6 g

Upper jiao diabetes with heat: yangming channel syndrome with qi and yin deficiency causing severe sweating, fever, and thirst.

T red, dry yellow coat

P rapid, flooding, weak

☞ Decoct the first four herbs, then add the rice at the end. It will absorb the water to make a thick liquid.

BAI HU JIA REN SHEN TANG

White Tiger plus Ginseng Decoction

Extract Formula Name: Ginseng and Gypsum Combination

Shi Gao	Gypsum	15 - 20 g
Zhi Mu	Anemarrhena	9 - 12 g
Gan Cao	Glycyrrhiza	3 - 6 g
Ren Shen	Panax	3 - 9 g
Jing Mi	Oryza	9 - 12 g

Dryness in the Lungs with sticky phlegm and injury to the yin. The phlegm is very hard to expectorate. Other symptoms include wheezing and a very dry throat.

T red, dry, scanty coat

P empty, thin

BEI MU GUA LOU SAN

Fritillaria and Trichosanthes Fruit Powder

Chuan Bei Mu	Fritillaria	2 - 5 g
Gua Lou Ren	Trichosanthes	3 - 6 g
Fu Ling	Poria	6 - 9 g
Ju Hong	Citrus	3 - 6 g
Tian Hua Fen	Trichosanthes	3 - 6 g
Jie Geng	Platycodon	3 - 6 g

Lung yin deficiency produces false heat which burns the Lungs and causes dry cough with blood tinged sputum, tuberculosis, or bronchitis. There is wheezing, a scratchy throat, and slight thirst.

T red, slight, or no coat

P thin, rapid, or superficial

☞ E Jiao - Equus should be dissolved into the strained tea.

BU FEI E JIAO TANG

Tonify the Lungs Decoction with Ass-Hide Gelatin

E Jiao	Equus	6 - 9 g
Xing Ren	Prunus	6 - 9 g
Ma Dou Ling	Aristolochia	6 - 9 g
Jing Mi	Oryza	15 g
Niu Bang Zi	Arctium	6 - 9 g
Gan Cao	Glycyrrhiza	3 - 6 g

Lung/Kidney yin deficiency with bone steaming fever, cough with sticky phlegm, and five-palm heat.

T   red, scanty coat

P   thin, rapid

DA ZAO WAN

Great Creation Pill

Gui Ban	Chinemys	6 - 12 g
Huang Bai	Phellodendron	6 - 9 g
Zi He Che	Placenta Hominis	1 - 2 g
Huai Niu Xi	Achyranthes	6 - 9 g
Ren Shen	Panax	6 - 9 g
Du Zhong	Eucommia	6 - 9 g
Mai Men Dong	Ophiopogon	6 - 9 g
Tian Men Dong	Asparagus	6 - 9 g
Sheng Di Huang	Rehmannia	6 - 12 g

Lung yin deficiency with heat and bone-steaming fever, especially seen in children.

T   red, slight or no coat

P   rapid, thin

☞ Dissolve Bie Jia - Amyda first for about one hour, then decoct with the remaining herbs.

DI GU PI YIN

Lycium Root Bark Decoction

Di Gu Pi	Lycium	6 - 9 g
Zhi Mu	Anemarrhena	6 - 9 g
Bie Jia	Amyda	3 - 6 g
Ren Shen	Panax	3 - 9 g
Huang Qin	Scutellaria	6 - 9 g
Chai Hu	Bupleurum	6 - 9 g
Gan Cao	Glycyrrhiza	3 - 6 g
[Wu Mei	Prunus	1 - 3 g]
[Sheng Jiang	Zingiber	1 - 3 g]

Kidney/Lung qi/yin deficiency with wheezing, shortness of breath, or chronic cough. This formula is also known as 'Qi Wu Du Qi Wan'.

T red, slight coat

P thin, rapid

DU QI WAN

Capital Qi Pill

Extract Formula Name: Rehmannia and Schizandra Formula

Shan Zhu Yu	Cornus	6 - 9 g
Shan Yao	Dioscorea	6 - 9 g
Sheng Di Huang	Rehmannia	9 - 12 g
Fu Ling	Poria	6 - 9 g
Mu Dan Pi	Paeonia	6 - 9 g
Ze Xie	Alisma	6 - 9 g
Wu Wei Zi	Schisandra	6 - 9 g

Lung qi and yin deficiency with upper jiao diabetes. The main symptom is excessive thirst.

T red, thin yellow coat

P weak, thin, slightly rapid

ER DONG TANG

Ophiopogon and Asparagus Decoction

Mai Men Dong	Ophiopogon	12 - 15 g
Tian Men Dong	Asparagus	12 - 15 g
Tian Hua Fen	Trichosanthes	12 - 15 g
Huang Qin	Scutellaria	6 - 15 g
Zhi Mu	Anemarrhena	12 - 15 g
Gan Cao	Glycyrrhiza	3 - 6 g
Ren Shen	Panax	3 - 6 g

Lung/Kidney yin deficiency or jing deficiency with fire causing sweating, low back pain, slow mental and physical development in children, cough with scanty sticky blood-tinged phlegm, weight loss, or afternoon fever.

T red, slight yellow or no coat

P rapid, thin, or empty

HE CHE DA ZAO WAN

Pills of Human Placenta

Zi He Che	Placenta Hominis	9 - 30 g
Tian Men Dong	Asparagus	6 - 9 g
Mai Men Dong	Ophiopogon	6 - 9 g
Gui Ban	Chinemys	6 - 9 g
Shu Di Huang	Rehmannia	12 - 15 g
Huang Bai	Phellodendron	6 - 9 g
Du Zhong	Eucommia	6 - 9 g
Huai Niu Xi	Achyranthes	6 - 9 g

Kidney/Lung yin deficiency with Lung phlegm causing chronic bronchitis in the elderly, wheezing, or nausea.

T red, slight coat, or geographic

P thin, slightly rapid, slippery

JIN SHUI LIU JUN JIAN

Six-Gentlemen of Metal and Water Decoction

Chen Pi	Citrus	3 - 6 g
Ban Xia	Pinellia	6 - 9 g
Fu Ling	Poria	6 - 9 g
Gan Cao	Glycyrrhiza	3 - 6 g
Dang Gui	Angelica	6 - 9 g
Sheng Di Huang	Rehmannia	6 - 12 g
[Sheng Jiang	Zingiber	3 - 6 g]

Lung qi and yin deficiency resulting in cough and wheezing, and wei (defensive) qi deficiency.

T thin, scanty coat

P thin, rapid, weak

☞ E Jiao - Equus should be added at the end into the strained tea.

JIU XIAN SAN

Nine-Immortal Powder

Ren Shen	Panax	6 - 9 g
Wu Wei Zi	Schisandra	6 - 9 g
E Jiao	Equus	6 g
Bei Mu	Fritillaria	6 - 9 g
Kuan Dong Hua	Tussilago	6 - 9 g
Jie Geng	Platycodon	3 - 6 g
Ying Su Ke	Papaver	3 - 6 g
Wu Mei	Prunus	6 - 9 g
Sang Bai Pi	Morus	6 - 9 g
[Sheng Jiang	Zingiber	3 - 6 g]
[Da Zao	Ziziphus	3 g]

Liver fire attacking the Lung yin. This leads to thick blood-tinged phlegm, thirst, or bitter taste.

T red, cracked, sticky yellow coat

P wiry, rapid

KE XUE FANG

Coughing of Blood Formula

Zhi Zi	Gardenia	6 - 9 g
Gua Lou Ren	Trichosanthes	6 - 9 g
Qing Dai	Indigo	6 - 9 g
Fu Hai Shi	Pumice	6 - 9 g
He Zi	Terminalia	3 - 9 g

Stomach yin deficiency starts to produce heat which then burns Lung yin resulting in cough, wheezing, shortness of breath, or thirst.

T red, geographic spots, slight or no coat

P thin, rapid

MAI MEN DONG TANG

Ophiopogon Decoction

Extract Formula Name: Ophiopogon Combination

Mai Men Dong	Ophiopogon	6 - 12 g
Ren Shen	Panax	6 - 9 g
Ban Xia	Pinellia	6 - 9 g
Jing Mi	Oryza	9 - 12 g
Da Zao	Ziziphus	6 - 10 pc
Gan Cao	Glycyrrhiza	3 - 6 g

Yin deficiency with wind cold which turns to heat and hides in the body, consuming more yin; or wind enters the body and consumes yin. Symptoms include night sweats, afternoon fever or heat, or blood-tinged sputum.

T red, dry, slight yellow coat

P weak, rapid

☞ Dissolve Bie Jia - Amyda first for about one hour, then decoct with the remaining herbs.

QIN JIAO BIE JIA SAN

Gentiana and Soft-shelled Turtle Shell Powder

Extract Formula Name: Chin-Chiu and T.S. Formula

Chai Hu	Bupleurum	6 - 9 g
Bie Jia	Amyda	6 - 12 g
Dang Gui	Angelica	6 - 9 g
Di Gu Pi	Lycium	6 - 9 g
Qin Jiao	Gentiana	6 - 9 g
Zhi Mu	Anemarrhena	6 - 12 g
[Wu Mei	Prunus	1 - 3 g]
[Qing Hao	Artemisia	1 - 3 g]

Febrile disease causing low level chronic fever; or chronic disease damaged yin leading to later stages of febrile disease causing night sweats, AIDS, or tuberculosis.

T   red, dry, scanty coat

P   thin, rapid

☞ Bie Jia - Amyda should be soaked separately for 30 minutes to one hour, until it starts to dissolve; then soak the rest of the herbs. Qing Hao - Artemisia should be added at the end of the decoction process.

QING HAO BIE JIA TANG

Artemisia Annua and Soft-shelled Turtle Shell Decoction

Bie Jia	Amyda	9 - 12 g
Qing Hao	Artemisia	6 - 9 g
Mu Dan Pi	Paeonia	6 - 9 g
Sheng Di Huang	Rehmannia	6 - 12 g
Zhi Mu	Anemarrhena	6 - 9 g

Lung heat with dryness and severe damage to the Lung yin as well as some wind symptoms. Manifestations include dry and itchy throat, full chest, or dry cough without phlegm.

T   pink, dry, scanty coat

P   weak, or empty, rapid

☞ E Jiao - Equus should be dissolved at the end into the strained tea.

QING ZAO JIU FEI TANG

Eliminate Dryness and Rescue the Lungs Decoction

Extract Formula Name: Eriobotrya and Ophiopogon Combination

Sang Ye	Morus	6 - 9 g
Mai Men Dong	Ophiopogon	3 - 6 g
E Jiao	Equus	1 - 4 g
Ren Shen	Panax	6 - 9 g
Xing Ren	Prunus	3 - 6 g
Shi Gao	Gypsum	6 - 9 g
Pi Pa Ye	Eriobotrya	3 - 6 g
Gan Cao	Glycyrrhiza	3 - 6 g
Huo Ma Ren	Cannabis	3 - 6 g

Lung and Kidney yin deficiency with dryness in the Lungs causing chronic consumptive disease. Symptoms include thirst, night sweating, or scanty phlegm which is hard to expectorate.

T red, dry, scanty coat

P deep, thin, rapid

Lung yin deficiency with false heat and Spleen qi deficiency causing cough with scanty sputum and fatigue.

T red, cracked, slight coat

P thin, rapid

☞ Dissolve Bie Jia - Amyda first for about one hour, then decoct with the remaining herbs.

QONG YU SAN

Ginseng and Rehmannia Powder

Ren Shen	Panax	3 - 6 g
Sheng Di Huang	Rehmannia	15 - 30 g
Feng Mi	Mel	30 g
Fu Ling	Poria	15 - 30 g

REN SHEN HUANG QI SAN

Ginseng and Astragalus Powder

Ren Shen	Panax	6 - 12 g
Huang Qi	Astragalus	9 - 15 g
Fu Ling	Poria	6 - 9 g
Zhi Mu	Anemarrhena	6 - 9 g
Zi Wan	Aster	6 - 9 g
Sang Bai Pi	Morus	6 - 9 g
Qin Jiao	Gentiana	6 - 12 g
Jie Geng	Platycodon	3 - 6 g
Chai Hu	Bupleurum	6 - 9 g
Ban Xia	Pinellia	6 - 9 g
Di Gu Pi	Lycium	3 - 9 g
Sheng Di Huang	Rehmannia	6 - 15 g
Bie Jia	Amyda	6 - 12 g
Tian Men Dong	Asparagus	9 - 12 g
Chi Shao Yao	Paeonia	3 - 9 g
Gan Cao	Glycyrrhiza	3 - 6 g

Dryness damaged Lung and Stomach yin (wind is gone now) causing thirst, scanty sputum, and a persistent dry cough.

T   red, slight coat

P   rapid, weak

✪ Major Formula

SHA SHEN MAI MEN DONG TANG

Glehnia and Ophiopogon Decoction

Bei Sha Shen	Glehnia	6 - 15 g
Mai Men Dong	Ophiopogon	6 - 15 g
Sang Ye	Morus	3 - 9 g
Tian Hua Fen	Trichosanthes	6 - 9 g
Yu Zhu	Polygonatum	6 - 9 g
Bian Dou	Dolichos	3 - 9 g
Gan Cao	Glycyrrhiza	3 - 6 g

Lung qi/yin deficiency with sweating and chronic cough producing scanty sputum which is hard to expectorate. This formula is also useful for palpitations, collapse, insomnia, or irregular pulse.

T   pale or red

P   weak or frail, slightly rapid

SHENG MAI SAN

Generate the Pulse Powder

Ginseng and Ophiopogon Formula

Ren Shen	Panax	9 - 15 g
Mai Men Dong	Ophiopogon	12 - 18 g
Wu Wei Zi	Schisandra	6 - 9 g

Lung/Kidney yin deficiency with severe fire causing nosebleeds, or hemoptysis which occurs during or prior to the menses.

T   red, cracks

P   rapid, empty

SHUN JING TANG

Smooth the Menses Decoction

Shu Di Huang	Rehmannia	9 - 15 g
Mu Dan Pi	Paeonia	6 - 9 g
Dang Gui	Angelica	6 - 9 g
Bai Shao Yao	Paeonia	6 - 9 g
Bei Sha Shen	Glehnia	6 - 12 g
Jing Jie	Schizonepeta	6 - 9 g
Fu Ling	Poria	6 - 9 g

Diabetes manifesting mostly in the upper jiao. The main symptom is thirst.

T   thin and narrow, slightly red, less coat than normal

P   thin, slightly rapid

XIAO KE TANG

Wasting and Thirsting Decoction

Extract Formula Name: Rehmannia and Trichosanthes Formula

no pinyin name	Human milk	50 - 200 cc
Huang Lian	Coptis	9 - 12 g
Tian Hua Fen	Trichosanthes	15 - 20 g
Sheng Di Huang	Rehmannia	12 - 15 g
Ou Jie	Nelumbo	9 - 20 g
Feng Mi	Mel	15 - 20 g
Sheng Jiang	Zingiber	6 - 9 g

Heat in the Lungs injuring the Lung yin and qi causing afternoon fever, wheezing, cough, or sticky, scanty phlegm.

T   red, dry, yellow coat

P   thin, rapid

XIE BAI SAN

Drain the White Powder

Extract Formula Name: Morus and Lycium Formula

Di Gu Pi	Lycium	20 - 30 g
Sang Bai Pi	Morus	20 - 30 g
Jing Mi	Oryza	15 - 25 g
Zhi Gan Cao	Glycyrrhiza	3 - 6 g

Lung yin deficiency leading to dryness and soreness in the throat causing dry cough with little or no phlegm.

T   red, thin and narrow in size, less than normal coat

P   thin, slightly rapid

XUAN MAI GAN JIE TANG

Scrophularia, Ophiopogon, Platycodon, and Licorice Decoction

Xuan Shen	Scrophularia	9 - 12 g
Mai Men Dong	Ophiopogon	6 - 9 g
Jie Geng	Platycodon	3 - 6 g
Gan Cao	Glycyrrhiza	3 - 6 g

Lung/Kidney yin deficiency with toxin causing diptheria, laryngitis, coarse breathing, or dry hacking cough.

T red, dry, yellow coat

P thin, rapid, or empty

YANG YIN QING FEI TANG

Nourish the Yin and Clear the Lungs Decoction

Sheng Di Huang	Rehmannia	6 - 12 g
Xuan Shen	Scrophularia	6 - 9 g
Bai Shao Yao	Paeonia	6 - 9 g
Mai Men Dong	Ophiopogon	6 - 12 g
Bo He	Mentha	3 - 6 g
Chuan Bei Mu	Fritillaria	3 - 6 g
Mu Dan Pi	Paeonia	6 - 9 g
Gan Cao	Glycyrrhiza	3 - 6 g

Kidney/Lung yin deficiency with heat and Lung consumption resulting in shortness of breath, dry cough, dry stools, dark scanty urine, or heat in the five centers.

T red, slight yellow or no coat

P rapid, weak, thin

☞ E Jiao - Equus should be dissolved at the end into the strained tea.

YUE HUA WAN

Moonlight Pill

Mai Men Dong	Ophiopogon	6 - 12 g
Tian Men Dong	Asparagus	6 - 12 g
Shu Di Huang	Rehmannia	6 - 12 g
Sheng Di Huang	Rehmannia	6 - 12 g
Bei Sha Shen	Glehnia	6 - 15 g
Bai Bu	Stemona	6 - 9 g
Chuan Bei Mu	Fritillaria	3 - 6 g
Shan Yao	Dioscorea	6 - 9 g
Fu Ling	Poria	6 - 9 g
Ju Hua	Chrysanthemum	6 - 9 g
Sang Ye	Morus	6 - 9 g
San Qi	Panax	9 - 12 g
E Jiao	Equus	6 - 9 g
Ta Gan	Lutra	6 - 9 g

PHLEGM DAMP IN THE LUNGS

- cough with profuse white sputum
- stuffy sensation in the chest
- shortness of breath

T thick sticky white coat

P slippery

(Lung) phlegm damp with cough or coma causing wind phlegm, dizziness, or hypertension.

T thick sticky coat

P slippery

✗ Tian Nan Xing - Arisaema is slightly toxic.

DAO TAN TANG

Guide Out Phlegm Decoction

Ban Xia	Pinellia	6 - 9 g
Chen Pi	Citrus	3 - 6 g
Fu Ling	Poria	6 - 9 g
Gan Cao	Glycyrrhiza	3 - 6 g
Zhi Shi	Citrus	3 - 6 g
Tian Nan Xing	Arisaema	1 - 3 g
Sheng Jiang	Zingiber	3 g

Cold phlegm in the Lungs with underlying Kidney yang deficiency. This produces cough with clear watery fluids, or shortness of breath.

T pale, thick sticky white coat

P frail or slippery

GUI LING WU WEI GAN CAO TANG

Cinnamon Twig, Poria, Schisandra, and Licorice Decoction

Gui Zhi	Cinnamomum	6 - 12 g
Fu Ling	Poria	6 - 12 g
Wu Wei Zi	Schisandra	9 - 15 g
Gan Cao	Glycyrrhiza	6 - 9 g

Phlegm in the Lungs with underlying Kidney yang deficiency. The Kidneys are unable to grasp Lung qi, so qi ascends to the chest causing fullness in chest and epigastrium. This is known as running piglet disorder. Symptoms also include wheezing, spontaneous sweating, and cold hands and feet.

T   pale, sticky white coat

P   minute

☞ Hei Xi - Lead and Liu Huang - Sulphur should both be dry fried. The remaining herbs are ground and made into pills with wine. Adults take 6 - 9 g per day, children take 2-3 g per day.

✗ To prevent lead poisoning, do not take longer than 3 days. Do not use during pregnancy.

HEI XI DAN

Lead Special Pill

Hei Xi	Lead	60 g
Liu Huang	Sulphur	60 g
Fu Zi	Aconitum	30 g
Rou Gui	Cinnamomum	60 g
Xiao Hui Xiang	Foeniculum	30 g
Rou Dou Kou	Amomun	30 g
Chen Xiang	Aquilaria	30 g
Yang Qi Shi	Actinolitum	30 g
Bu Gu Zhi	Psoralea	30 g
Mu Xiang	Saussurea	30 g
Chuan Lian Zi	Melia	30 g
Hu Lu Ba	Trigonella	30 g

Watery fluids in the Lungs and Spleen yang deficiency causing cough, wheezing, and a stuffy sensation in the chest.

T   pale, sticky or slippery white coat

P   slippery, wiry

LING GAN WU WEI JIANG XIN TANG

Poria, Licorice, Schisandra, Ginger, and Asarum Decoction

Fu Ling	Poria	6 - 12 g
Gan Cao	Glycyrrhiza	3 - 9 g
Wu Wei Zi	Schisandra	6 - 9 g
Gan Jiang	Zingiber	3 - 9 g
Xi Xin	Asarum	6 - 9 g

Spleen/Stomach yang deficiency causing phlegm accumulation which affects the Lungs; or taiyang disease was mistreated and guided into the Spleen leading to water accumulation. Symptoms include dyspnea, clear phlegm expectoration, and fullness in the chest and flanks.

T pale, slippery white coat

P slippery, weak, deep

LING GUI ZHU GAN TANG

Poria, Cinnamon Twig, Atractylodes, and Licorice Decoction

Extract Formula Name: Hoelen and Atractylodes Combination

Fu Ling	Poria	6 - 12 g
Gui Zhi	Cinnamomum	3 - 9 g
Bai Zhu	Atractylodes	6 - 9 g
Gan Cao	Glycyrrhiza	3 - 6 g

Cough and wheezing with sticky phlegm which is hard to bring up after a mild wind cold invasion.

T sticky white coat

P slippery, superficial

LIU AN JIAN

Six-Serenity Decoction

Ban Xia	Pinellia	6 - 9 g
Fu Ling	Poria	6 - 9 g
Chen Pi	Citrus	3 - 6 g
Gan Cao	Glycyrrhiza	3 - 6 g
Bai Jie Zi	Brassica	1 - 3 g
Xing Ren	Prunus	3 - 6 g
[Sheng Jiang	Zingiber	3 - 6 g]

Phlegm damp with migrating body pains, chills, or fever.

T slippery or sticky white coat

P deep, slippery

✗ Tian Nan Xing - Arisaema is slightly toxic, and should only be used in small amounts.

QING SHI HUA TAN TANG

Clear Dampness and Transform Phlegm Decoction

Extract Formula Name: Pinellia and Arisaema Combination

Ban Xia	Pinellia	6 - 9 g
Chen Pi	Citrus	3 - 6 g
Fu Ling	Poria	6 - 9 g
Gan Cao	Glycyrrhiza	3 - 6 g
Cang Zhu	Atractylodes	3 - 6 g
Tian Nan Xing	Arisaema	1 - 3 g
Qiang Huo	Notopterygium	3 g
Huang Qin	Scutellaria	3 - 6 g
Bai Zhi	Angelica	3 - 6 g
Bai Jie Zi	Brassica	1 - 3 g
Gan Jiang	Zingiber	3 - 6 g
Sheng Jiang	Zingiber	3 - 6 g

Phlegm damp cough with cold in the Lungs, or food stagnation. Symptoms include dyspnea with profuse phlegm expectoration, and poor appetite.

T sticky white coat

P slippery

SAN ZI YANG QIN TANG

Three-Seed Decoction to Nourish One's Parents

Zi Su Zi	Perilla	6 - 9 g
Lai Fu Zi	Raphanus	6 - 9 g
Bai Jie Zi	Brassica	3 - 9 g

Wind cold asthma with pre-existing phlegm and water (excess type) producing mild exterior symptoms such as dyspnea, wheezing with mild fever and chills.

T   thick sticky white coat

P   superficial, tight

SHE GAN MA HUANG TANG

Belamcanda and Ephedra Decoction

She Gan	Belamcanda	6 - 9 g
Ma Huang	Ephedra	6 - 9 g
Ban Xia	Pinellia	6 - 9 g
Zi Wan	Aster	6 - 9 g
Kuan Dong Hua	Tussilago	6 - 9 g
Wu Wei Zi	Schisandra	3 - 6 g
Xi Xin	Asarum	6 - 9 g
Sheng Jiang	Zingiber	9 - 12 g
Da Zao	Ziziphus	7 - 9 pc

Lung phlegm damp with underlying Kidney qi deficiency causing wheezing with profuse phlegm.

T   sticky white coat

P   weak, slippery

✪ **Major Formula**

SU ZI JIANG QI TANG

Perilla Fruit Decoction for Directing Qi Downward

Extract Formula Name: Perilla Fruit Combination

Zhi Gan Cao	Glycyrrhiza	6 g
Ban Xia	Pinellia	6 - 9 g
Zi Su Zi	Perilla	6 - 12 g
Dang Gui	Angelica	6 - 9 g
Hou Po	Magnolia	6 - 12 g
Qian Hu	Peucedanum	6 - 9 g
Rou Gui	Cinnamomum	3 g
[Sheng Jiang	Zingiber	1 - 3 g]
[Zi Su Ye	Perilla	3 - 6 g]
[Da Zao	Ziziphus	3 g]

Lung phlegm fluid causing eye/facial edema, cough or asthma, or Lung abscess with phlegm.

T   sticky white coat

P   slippery

TING LI DA ZAO XIE FEI TANG

Lepidium and Jujube Decoction to Drain the Lungs

Extract Formula Name: Lepidium and Jujube Combination

Ting Li Zi	Lepidium	6 - 9 g
Da Zao	Ziziphus	6 - 12 pc

Qi and blood stagnation causing chest pain with water/damp accumulation: Liver affects the Lungs. Symptoms include hypochondriac pain, possible coughing, or raspy voice.

T   purple, thick sticky coat

P   wiry

☞ Xuan Fu Hua - Inula should be wrapped in a cheesecloth.

XIANG FU XUAN FU TANG

Cyperus and Inula Decoction

Xiang Fu	Cyperus	6 - 9 g
Xuan Fu Hua	Inula	6 - 9 g
Yi Yi Ren	Coix	9 - 15 g
Chen Pi	Citrus	3 - 6 g
Zi Su Zi	Perilla	6 - 9 g
Ban Xia	Pinellia	6 - 9 g
Fu Ling	Poria	6 - 9 g

Phlegm damp in the Lungs causing cough, wheezing, or shortness of breath. Phlegm expectoration may range from a clear to a thick white discharge.

T   thin or thick white coat

P   slippery

ZHI JIE ER CHEN TANG

Aurantium, Platycodon, and Two-Cured Decoction

Ban Xia	Pinellia	6 - 9 g
Chen Pi	Citrus	3 - 6 g
Fu Ling	Poria	6 - 9 g
Zhi Gan Cao	Glycyrrhiza	3 - 6 g
Zhi Ke	Citrus	3 - 9 g
Jie Geng	Platycodon	3 - 6 g

PHLEGM HEAT IN THE LUNGS

- barking cough with yellow or green expectoration
- shortness of breath
- heat sensation in the chest

T red, thick yellow sticky coat

P slippery, rapid

Water/heat accumulation in the chest and Lungs causing chest qi obstruction. Symptoms include stiff neck, and a full or suffocating sensation in the chest.

T red, sticky coat

P rapid, slippery

☞ Herbs should be made into 9 g pills with honey.

✗ Gan Sui - Euphorbia is toxic and should only be taken in small amounts. Do not use during pregnancy.

DA XIAN XIONG WAN

Major Sinking Into the Chest Pill

Da Huang	Rheum	25 g
Mang Xiao	Mirabilitum	17.5 g
Ting Li Zi	Lepidium	17.5 g
Xing Ren	Prunus	17.5 g
Gan Sui	Euphorbia	3 g

Wind cold in the exterior with phlegm heat in the interior causing cough and wheezing. The phlegm expectoration is thick and yellow.

T sticky yellow coat

P slippery, rapid

DING CHUAN TANG

Arrest Wheezing Decoction

Extract Formula Name: Ma-Huang and Ginkgo Combination

Bai Guo	Gingko	6 - 9 g
Ma Huang	Ephedra	6 - 9 g
Kuan Dong Hua	Tussilago	6 - 9 g
Zi Su Zi	Perilla	3 - 6 g
Xing Ren	Prunus	3 - 6 g
Ban Xia	Pinellia	6 - 9 g
Sang Bai Pi	Morus	6 - 9 g
Huang Qin	Scutellaria	6 - 9 g
Gan Cao	Glycyrrhiza	3 - 6 g

Phlegm heat in the Lungs; or dry cough with Kidney/Liver heat. The phlegm is hard to expectorate, or breathing is labored.

T red, sticky yellow coat

P rapid, slippery

GUA LOU ZHI SHI TANG

Trichosanthes Fruit and Immature Bitter Orange Decoction

Extract Formula Name: Trichosanthes and Chih-Shi Combination

Gua Lou Ren	Trichosanthes	3 - 6 g
Zhi Shi	Citrus	3 - 6 g
Zhe Bei Mu	Fritillaria	6 - 9 g
Fu Ling	Poria	6 - 9 g
Chen Pi	Citrus	3 - 6 g
Dang Gui	Angelica	3 - 9 g
Sha Ren	Amomum	3 - 6 g
Mu Xiang	Saussurea	3 - 6 g
Jie Geng	Platycodon	3 - 6 g
Zhi Zi	Gardenia	3 - 6 g
Huang Qin	Scutellaria	6 - 9 g
Zhu Ru	Bambusa	6 g
Gan Cao	Glycyrrhiza	3 - 6 g
Sheng Jiang	Zingiber	3 - 6 g
Zhu Li	Bambusa	1 - 3 g

Phlegm heat with damage to the Lung yin causing cough or asthma with thick yellow or green phlegm which is hard to expectorate, feelings of heat in the chest, tightness in the chest, or thirst without much desire to drink. This formula is useful for bronchitis.

T red, maybe geographic, dry, thick sticky yellow coat

P rapid, slippery, slightly thin

✪ **Major Formula**

QING JIN HUA TAN TANG

Clear Metal and Absorb Phlegm Decoction

Huang Qin	Scutellaria	6 - 12 g
Zhi Zi	Gardenia	3 - 6 g
Fu Ling	Poria	6 - 12 g
Zhe Bei Mu	Fritillaria	6 - 12 g
Jie Geng	Platycodon	3 - 6 g
Gua Lou	Trichosanthes	3 - 6 g
Zhi Mu	Anemarrhena	6 - 9 g
Sang Bei Pi	Morus	6 - 9 g
Mai Men Dong	Ophiopogon	6 - 9 g
Gan Cao	Glycyrrhiza	3 - 6 g

Phlegm heat cough causing yellow, sticky, phlegm expectoration or fullness in the chest. Symptoms include dyspnea, epigastric fullness, and nausea.

T   red, sticky yellow coat

P   rapid, slippery

✗   Dan Nan Xing - Arisaema is slightly toxic and should only be used in small amounts.

QING QI HUA TAN WAN

Clear the Qi and Transform Phlegm Pill

Ban Xia	Pinellia	6 - 9 g
Dan Nan Xing	Arisaema	1 - 3 g
Huang Qin	Scutellaria	6 - 9 g
Fu Ling	Poria	6 - 9 g
Gua Lou Ren	Trichosanthes	6 - 9 g
Chen Pi	Citrus	3 - 6 g
Zhi Shi	Citrus	3 - 6 g
Xing Ren	Prunus	3 - 9 g

Lung qi deficiency damages Spleen qi which leads to damp accumulation with slight heat; or Lung qi deficiency with phlegm. Symptoms include wheezing, sticky yellow sputum, coughing of blood or pus, or heat in the chest.

T   light purple, sticky white or yellow coat

P   weak, superficial

REN SHEN GE JIE SAN

Ginseng and Gecko Powder

Ge Jie	Gekko	1 pair
Sang Bai Pi	Morus	6 - 9 g
Fu Ling	Poria	6 - 12 g
Xing Ren	Prunus	6 - 9 g
Chuan Bei Mu	Fritillaria	3 - 6 g
Ren Shen	Panax	6 - 12 g
Zhi Mu	Anemarrhena	6 - 9 g
Gan Cao	Glycyrrhiza	3 - 6 g

Phlegm heat toxin and blood stagnation with pus causing Lung abscess, measles, whooping cough, cough with blood-streaked sputum, chest congestion, or low-grade fever.

T   red, sticky yellow coat

P   rapid, slippery

WEI JING TANG

Reed Decoction

Extract Formula Name: Phragmites Combination

Lu Gen	Phragmitis	40 - 60 g
Dong Gua Ren	Benincasa	15 - 25 g
Yi Yi Ren	Coix	15 - 20 g
Tao Ren	Prunus	6 - 9 g

Phlegm heat in the chest (Heart), or epigastrium (Stomach) leading to bronchitis, constipation, distending pain or pressure in the chest, numbness, or bitter taste.

T   red, sticky yellow coat

P   rapid, slippery

XIAO XIAN XIONG TANG

Minor Sinking Into the Chest Decoction

Extract Formula Name: Minor Trichosanthes Combination

Gua Lou	Trichosanthes	20 g
Huang Lian	Coptis	3 g
Ban Xia	Pinellia	6 - 9 g

HEART DISHARMONIES

Heart

HEART QI DEFICIENCY

- pale face
- shortness of breath
- palpitations
- spontaneous sweating

T pale or normal color

P weak, or empty

This formula treats insomnia due to Heart and Gallbladder qi deficiency. This is commonly seen in children causing them to appear timid and scared of everything, fear ghosts and burglars, or not want to sleep alone. They sweat easily, especially in the hands and soles.

T pale or normal color, slightly swollen

P weak, thready, deep

AN SHEN DING ZHI TANG

Calm Spirit and Stop Fear Decoction

Ren Shen	Panax	9 - 12 g
Fu Ling	Poria	6 - 9 g
Fu Shen	Poria	6 - 9 g
Shi Chang Pu	Acorus	3 - 9 g
Long Gu	Os Draconis	6 - 9 g
Yuan Zhi	Polygala	6 - 9 g

Heart qi deficiency with disturbed shen causing anxiety, palpitations, forgetfulness, or fright.

T pale

P weak

✪ Major Formula

✘ Zhu Sha - Cinnabaris is toxic, and should only be used short-term.

DING ZHI WAN

Settle the Emotions Pill

Ren Shen	Panax	12 - 15 g
Fu Ling	Poria	6 - 9 g
Shi Chang Pu	Acorus	6 - 9 g
Yuan Zhi	Polygala	6 - 9 g
Fu Shen	Poria	9 - 12 g
Zhu Sha	Cinnabaris	6 - 9 g

After taiyang disease the patient develops Heart qi and yang deficiency; deficient type angina.

T pale

P weak

GUI ZHI GAN CAO TANG

Cinnamon Twig and Licorice Decoction

Gui Zhi	Cinnamomum	3 - 9 g
Gan Cao	Glycyrrhiza	3 - 6 g

Heart yang is not warmed by the Kidneys leading to water accumulation which rises upwards causing abdominal pain, angina, Stomach cramping, tingling sensation in the abdomen, (ben ten qi - running piglet sensation), or scanty urine.

T pale, wet, sticky white coat

P deep, weak, slightly slow

LING GUI ZAO GAN TANG

Poria, Cinnamon Twig, Jujube, and Licorice Decoction

Fu Ling	Poria	9 - 12 g
Gui Zhi	Cinnamomum	3 - 9 g
Da Zao	Ziziphus	3 - 4 pc
Gan Cao	Glycyrrhiza	3 - 6 g

Heart

Heart qi deficiency with Spleen qi deficiency leading to anxiety, insomnia, spontaneous sweating, or palpitations.

T   pale, thin coating

P   weak

✗   Zhu Sha - Cinnabaris is toxic, and should only be used short-term.

MIAO XIANG SAN

Marvelously Fragrant Powder

Ren Shen	Panax	6 - 12 g
Fu Ling	Poria	9 - 12 g
Fu Shen	Poria	9 - 12 g
Yuan Zhi	Polygala	9 - 12 g
Huang Qi	Astragalus	9 - 15 g
Shan Yao	Dioscorea	9 - 12 g
Mu Xiang	Saussurea	12 - 15 g
Jie Geng	Platycodon	1 - 3 g
Zhu Sha	Cinnabaris	1 - 3 g
She Xiang	Moschus	0.3 - 0.5 g
Gan Cao	Glycyrrhiza	3 - 6 g

Heart/Kidney qi/yin deficiency causing incontinence, spermatorrhea, frequent urination, and forgetfulness.

T   pale or red

P   weak, thin

SANG PIAO XIAO SAN

Mantis Egg-Case Powder

Extract Formula Name: Mantis Formula

Sang Piao Xiao	Paratenodera	9 - 12 g
Long Gu	Os Draconis	12 - 25 g
Fu Shen	Poria	9 - 12 g
Ren Shen	Panax	9 - 12 g
Shi Chang Pu	Acorus	6 - 9 g
Dang Gui	Angelica	6 - 9 g
Gui Ban	Chinemys	9 - 15 g
Yuan Zhi	Polygala	9 - 15 g

Heart/Gallbladder qi deficiency with edema in the extremities, tight chest, palpitations, anxiety, or timidity.

T pale

P weak

SHI WEI WEN DAN TANG

Ten-Ingredient Decoction to Warm the Gallbladder

Ban Xia	Pinellia	6 - 9 g
Chen Pi	Citrus	3 - 6 g
Zhi Shi	Citrus	6 g
Fu Ling	Poria	6 g
Ren Shen	Panax	3 - 6 g
Suan Zao Ren	Ziziphus	3 - 6 g
Shu Di Huang	Rehmannia	3 - 9 g
Wu Wei Zi	Schisandra	3 - 6 g
Yuan Zhi	Polygala	3 - 6 g
Zhi Gan Cao	Glycyrrhiza	3 g
Da Zao	Ziziphus	2 pc
Sheng Jiang	Zingiber	5 pc

Heart qi blood deficiency causing insomnia, anxiety, restlessness, and poor memory.

T pale

P weak, thin

YANG XIN TANG

Nourish the Heart Decoction

Extract Formula Name: Astragalus and Zizyphus Combination

Sheng Di Huang	Rehmannia	6 - 12 g
Shu Di Huang	Rehmannia	6 - 12 g
Dang Gui	Angelica	6 - 9 g
Ren Shen	Panax	6 - 12 g
Mai Men Dong	Ophiopogon	6 - 9 g
Suan Zao Ren	Ziziphus	6 - 9 g
Fu Shen	Poria	6 - 9 g
Bai Zi Ren	Biota	6 - 9 g
Wu Wei Zi	Schisandra	6 - 9 g
Gan Cao	Glycyrrhiza	3 - 6 g
[Lian Zi	Nelumbo	3 - 6 g]
[Deng Xin Cao	Juncus	3 - 6 g]

Heart qi/blood or yin deficiency causing arrhythmia, insomnia, pressure in the chest, coronary Heart disease, and anxiety.

T   pale or red, thin white coat

P   weak

☞ E Jiao - Equus should be dissolved into the strained tea.

ZHI GAN CAO TANG

Honey-Fried Licorice Decoction

Extract Formula Name: Baked Licorice Combination

Zhi Gan Cao	Glycyrrhiza	12 - 15 g
Sheng Di Huang	Rehmannia	30 g
Ren Shen	Panax	6 - 9 g
Gui Zhi	Cinnamomum	6 - 9 g
Huo Ma Ren	Cannabis	6 - 9 g
Mai Men Dong	Ophiopogon	9 g
E Jiao	Equus	6 g
Da Zao	Ziziphus	6 - 9 pc
Sheng Jiang	Zingiber	6 - 9 g

HEART YANG DEFICIENCY

- tightness in the chest
- palpitations
- feeling of cold or cold hands
- fatigue

T   pale, light purple, swollen, moist

P   deep, weak

Chest Bi: chest yang deficiency with mild cold and phlegm accumulation causing tightness in the chest, shortness of breath, palpitations, cough, or asthma.

T   pale, light purple, wet, thick sticky white coat

P   slow, slippery, wiry

✪ **Major Formula**

GUA LOU XIE BAI BAI JIU TANG

Trichonsanthes Fruit, Chinese Chive, and Wine Decoction

Extract Formula Name: Trichosanthes, Bakeri and White Wine Combination

Gua Lou	Trichosanthes	9 - 12 g
Xie Bai	Allium	9 - 12 g
Bai Jiu	White Wine	30 - 60 cc

Taiyang disease or inappropriate warming therapy causing Heart yang deficiency with yin deficiency. This leads to disturbed shen, restlessness, mania, sweating, palpitations, or insomnia.

T pale or red, thin white or yellowish coat

P weak, thin

GUI ZHI GAN CAO LONG GU MU LI TANG

Cinnamon Twig, Licorice, Dragon Bone, and Oyster Shell Decoction

Gui Zhi	Cinnamomum	3 - 6 g
Zhi Gan Cao	Glycyrrhiza	6 g
Long Gu	Os Draconis	6 - 15 g
Mu Li	Ostrea	6 - 15 g

After taiyang disease the patient develops Heart qi and yang deficiency; deficient type angina.

T pale

P weak

GUI ZHI GAN CAO TANG

Cinnamon Twig and Licorice Decoction

Gui Zhi	Cinnamomum	3 - 9 g
Gan Cao	Glycyrrhiza	3 - 6 g

A wind cold invasion has gone internally due to incorrect warming needle technique. Wind cold has heated up and is now trapped inside with a complication of internal water accumulation. This causes unspecific abdominal pain which bothers the Heart (also known as 'running piglet sensation' = ben ten qi). This is an external pathogen with internal water stagnation and cold.

T pale, wet, white coat

P slow, slightly slippery

GUI ZHI JIA ROU GUI TANG

Cinnamon Twig Decoction plus Cinnamon Bark

Gui Zhi	Cinnamomum	6 - 9 g
Bai Shao Yao	Paeonia	6 - 9 g
Sheng Jiang	Zingiber	3 - 6 g
Da Zao	Ziziphus	3 - 4 pc
Gan Cao	Glycyrrhiza	3 - 6 g
Rou Gui	Cinnamomum	3 - 9 g

Heart and Kidneys are not communicating. Kidney yang deficiency leads to Heart yang deficiency causing palpitations, cool limbs, or insomnia.

T pale, swollen, thin moist white coat

P deep, weak

JIAO TAI WAN

Grand Communication Pill

Extract Formula Name: Coptis and Cinnamon Formula

Huang Lian	Coptis	18 - 20 g
Rou Gui	Cinnamomum	3 - 6 g

Heart yang is not warmed by the Kidneys leading to water accumulation which rises upwards causing abdominal pain, angina, Stomach cramping, tingling sensation in the abdomen, (ben ten qi - running piglet sensation), or scanty urine.

T   pale, wet, sticky white coat

P   deep, weak, slightly slow

✪ **Major Formula**

LING GUI ZAO GAN TANG

Poria, Cinnamon Twig, Jujube, and Licorice Decoction

Fu Ling	Poria	9 - 12 g
Gui Zhi	Cinnamomum	3 - 9 g
Da Zao	Ziziphus	3 - 4 pc
Gan Cao	Glycyrrhiza	3 - 6 g

Spleen/Lung qi and blood deficiency with Heart yang deficiency, or ying level deficiency. The patient is easily startled, experiences shortness of breath, lack of taste sensation, insomnia, or palpitations. This formula is also useful for irregular periods or uterine bleeding.

T   pale, swollen

P   weak

REN SHEN YANG RONG WAN

Ginseng Decoction to Nourish the Nutritive Qi

Extract Formula Name: Ginseng Combination

Bai Shao Yao	Paeonia	9 - 15 g
Chen Pi	Citrus	3 - 6 g
Dang Gui	Angelica	3 - 9 g
Ren Shen	Panax	6 - 9 g
Huang Qi	Astragalus	6 - 12 g
Bai Zhu	Atractylodes	6 - 9 g
Shu Di Huang	Rehmannia	3 - 6 g
Wu Wei Zi	Schisandra	3 - 6 g
Fu Ling	Poria	3 - 6 g
Yuan Zhi	Polygala	2 - 6 g
Rou Gui	Cinnamomum	6 - 9 g
Gan Cao	Glycyrrhiza	3 - 6 g
[Da Zao	Ziziphus	2 pc]
[Gan Jiang	Zingiber	3 pc]

HEART YIN DEFICIENCY

- insomnia with dream-disturbed sleep
- restlessness
- malarflush
- afternoon fever

T red, scanty coat, red tip

P thin, rapid, or empty

Kidney yin deficiency can't nourish the Heart which leads to Heart blood deficiency. Symptoms include insomnia, dizziness, poor memory, excessive dreaming, or night sweating.

T slightly red, or pale, scanty coat

P thin, rapid

BAI ZI YANG XIN WAN

Biota Seed Pill to Nourish the Heart

Bai Zi Ren	Biota	3 - 9 g
Mai Men Dong	Ophiopogon	6 - 9 g
Dang Gui	Angelica	6 - 12 g
Gou Qi Zi	Lycium	6 - 9 g
Xuan Shen	Scrophularia	6 - 12 g
Fu Shen	Poria	6 - 9 g
Shi Chang Pu	Acorus	6 - 9 g
Shu Di Huang	Rehmannia	12 - 15 g
Gan Cao	Glycyrrhiza	3 - 6 g

Mental disorder due to 1. Liver qi stagnation (use with Xiao Yao San); 2. Liver qi stagnation with fire burning the yin (use with Wen Dan Tang); 3. Yin deficiency with fire injuring the Heart.

T red, scanty coat

P thin, rapid

GAN MAI DA ZAO TANG

Licorice, Wheat, and Jujube Decoction

Extract Formula Name: Licorice and Jujube Combination

Gan Cao	Glycyrrhiza	9 - 12 g
Fu Xiao Mai	Triticum	9 - 15 g
Da Zao	Ziziphus	10 pc

Taiyang disease or inappropriate warming therapy causing Heart yang deficiency with yin deficiency. This leads to disturbed shen, restlessness, mania, sweating, palpitations, or insomnia.

T pale or red, thin white or yellowish coat

P weak, thin

GUI ZHI GAN CAO LONG GU MU LI TANG

Cinnamon Twig, Licorice, Dragon Bone, and Oyster Shell Decoction

Gui Zhi	Cinnamomum	3 - 6 g
Zhi Gan Cao	Glycyrrhiza	6 g
Long Gu	Os Draconis	6 - 15 g
Mu Li	Ostrea	6 - 15 g

Kidneys and Heart are not harmonizing accompanied with yin and yang deficiency. Symptoms include spermatorrhea, sexual dreams, or poor sleep.

T pale

P slow, hollow, weak

GUI ZHI JIA LONG GU MU LI TANG

Cinnamon Twig Decoction plus Dragon Bone and Oyster Shell

Extract Formula Name: Cinnamon and Dragon Bone Combination

Gui Zhi	Cinnamomum	6 - 9 g
Bai Shao Yao	Paeonia	6 - 9 g
Sheng Jiang	Zingiber	6 - 9 g
Da Zao	Ziziphus	4 - 12 pc
Mu Li	Ostrea	6 - 9 g
Long Gu	Os Draconis	6 - 9 g
Gan Cao	Glycyrrhiza	3 - 6 g

Heart/Kidney yin deficiency with fire after febrile disease leading to insomnia, palpitations, or tongue sores: shaoyin deficient heat syndrome.

T red, scanty coat

P rapid, thin

☞ E Jiao - Equus and egg yolks should be dissolved into the strained tea.

HUANG LIAN E JIAO TANG

Coptis and Ass-Hide Gelatin Decoction

Extract Formula Name: Coptis and Gelatin Combination

Huang Lian	Coptis	9 - 12 g
E Jiao	Equus	6 - 9 g
Huang Qin	Scutellaria	6 - 9 g
Bai Shao Yao	Paeonia	6 - 9 g
Ji Zi Huang	Egg yolks	2

1. Yin/blood deficiency with heat causing arrhythmia of the Heart. 2. High fever causing arrhythmia: yangming disease depleted yin which leads to an irregular Heart beat.

T red, scanty coat

P rapid, irregular

☞ E Jiao - Equus should be dissolved at the end into the strained tea.

JIA JIAN FU MAI TANG

Modified Restore-the-Pulse Decoction

Zhi Gan Cao	Glycyrrhiza	12 - 15 g
Bai Shao Yao	Paeonia	12 - 15 g
Mai Men Dong	Ophiopogon	9 - 12 g
Sheng Di Huang	Rehmannia	12 - 15 g
Huo Ma Ren	Cannabis	9 - 12 g
E Jiao	Equus	6 - 9 g

Qi and wei qi deficiency leading to spontaneous sweating which eventually injures the Heart yin. This leads to night sweating, insomnia, and palpitations.

T pale or red

P frail, thin

MU LI SAN

Oyster Shell Powder

Mu Li	Ostrea	15 - 30 g
Ma Huang Gen	Ephredra	3 - 9 g
Huang Qi	Astragalus	9 - 12 g
Fu Xiao Mai	Triticum	15 - 30 g

Heart yin/blood deficiency with false heat causing insomnia, poor memory, or restlessness.

T pale or red

P thin, rapid

✪ Major Formula

SUAN ZAO REN TANG

Sour Jujube Decoction

Extract Formula Name: Zizyphus Combination

Suan Zao Ren	Ziziphus	12 - 15 g
Fu Ling	Poria	6 - 9 g
Chuan Xiong	Ligusticum	3 - 9 g
Zhi Mu	Anemarrhena	6 - 12 g
Gan Cao	Glycyrrhiza	3 - 6 g

Heart/Kidney yin deficiency Heart blood deficiency and false heat where the Kidneys and Heart don't harmonize leading to insomnia, restlessness, palpitations, poor memory, or night sweats.

T red

P rapid, thin

✗ Zhu Sha - Cinnabaris is toxic and should only be used short-term.

✪ Major Formula

TIAN WANG BU XIN DAN

Emperor of Heaven's Special Pill to Tonify the Heart

Extract Formula Name: Ginseng and Zizyphus Formula

Ren Shen	Panax	9 - 12 g
Mai Men Dong	Ophiopogon	6 - 12 g
Tian Men Dong	Asparagus	6 - 9 g
Xuan Shen	Scrophularia	6 - 9 g
Dan Shen	Salvia	6 - 12 g
Sheng Di Huang	Rehmannia	15 - 30 g
Fu Ling	Poria	6 - 9 g
Wu Wei Zi	Schisandra	6 - 9 g
Jie Geng	Platycodon	3 - 6 g
Yuan Zhi	Polygala	6 - 9 g
Bai Zi Ren	Biota	6 - 9 g
Dang Gui	Angelica	6 - 9 g
Suan Zao Ren	Ziziphus	6 - 12 g
Zhu Sha	Cinnabaris	1 - 3 g

Kidney and Liver yin/blood deficiency with fire which bothers the Heart. This causes Heart and Liver fire or Liver yang excess leading to excessive dreaming, insomnia, or outbursts of anger.

T red, cracks, thin or thick yellow coat

P rapid, wiry, thin

☞ Ingredients should be powdered, made into 9 - 12 g pills and taken three times a day. Xi Jiao - Rhinoceros should be substituted with Shui Niu Jiao - Bubalus.

ZHEN ZHU MU WAN

Mother-Of-Pearl Pill

Zhen Zhu Mu	Pteria	15 - 20 g
Ren Shen	Panax	9 - 12 g
Dang Gui	Angelica	6 - 12 g
Shu Di Huang	Rehmannia	9 - 12 g
Suan Zao Ren	Ziziphus	6 - 9 g
Bai Zi Ren	Biota	6 - 9 g
Fu Shen	Poria	6 - 9 g
Chen Xiang	Aquilaria	6 - 9 g
Xi Jiao	Rhinoceros	1 - 3 g

Heart qi/blood or yin deficiency causing arrhythmia, insomnia, pressure in the chest, coronary Heart disease, and anxiety.

T   pale or red, thin white coat

P   weak

☞ E Jiao - Equus should be dissolved into the strained tea.

ZHI GAN CAO TANG

Honey-Fried Licorice Decoction

Extract Formula Name: Baked Licorice Combination

Zhi Gan Cao	Glycyrrhiza	12 - 15 g
Sheng Di Huang	Rehmannia	30 g
Ren Shen	Panax	6 - 9 g
Gui Zhi	Cinnamomum	6 - 9 g
Huo Ma Ren	Cannabis	6 - 9 g
Mai Men Dong	Ophiopogon	9 g
E Jiao	Equus	6 g
Da Zao	Ziziphus	6 - 9 pc
Sheng Jiang	Zingiber	6 - 9 g

Heart fire with qi/blood/yin deficiency causing mental depression, heat in the chest, excessive dreaming, or palpitations. This formula acts as a sedative.

T   red, thin coat

P   rapid, thin

☞ Either grind all herbs and take 6 - 9 g twice a day; or decoct and add Zhu Sha - Cinnabaris at the end of the decoction process.

✗ Zhu Sha - Cinnabaris is toxic and should not be used over a long period of time.

ZHU SHA AN SHEN WAN

Cinnabaris Pill to Calm the Spirit

Extract Formula Name: Cinnabaris Formula

Zhu Sha	Cinnabaris	3 - 9 g
Huang Lian	Coptis	6 - 12 g
Dang Gui	Angelica	3 - 6 g
Sheng Di Huang	Rehmannia	3 - 6 g
Zhi Gan Cao	Glycyrrhiza	6 - 9 g

HEART PHLEGM ACCUMULATION

- stuffiness in the chest
- mental disorientation, or mania
- lethargy
- rattling sound in the throat

T thick sticky coat

P slippery

Heart

Severe Heart phlegm accumulation and qi stagnation with yang deficiency. Angina can be severe, and the patient experiences numbness radiating down the arm, shortness of breath: chest bi-syndrome.

T pale, light purple, wet, thick sticky white coat

P slippery

⭐ **Major Formula**

GUA LOU XIE BAI BAN XIA TANG

Trichosanthes Fruit, Chinese Chive, and Pinellia Decoction

Extract Formula Name: Trichosanthes, Bakeri and Pinellia Combination

Gua Lou	Trichosanthes	9 - 12 g
Xie Bai	Allium	6 - 9 g
Ban Xia	Pinellia	9 - 12 g
Bai Jiu	White Wine	30 cc

Damp cold and phlegm causing sudden collapse, clenched jaw, or coma; or qi stagnation or damp cold leading to coldness in the chest and abdomen or chest pain, coma, or qi stagnation from an epidemic manifesting in fullness in the chest. The patient feels the urge to vomit or defecate but is unable to do so, which then leads to sudden loss of consciousness.

T pale

P slow, slippery

☞ The prescription is made into pills. Xi Jiao - Rhinoceros should be substituted with Shui Niu Jiao - Bubalus.

✘ Do not use during pregnancy. Zhu Sha - Cinnabaris is toxic, and should only be used short-term.

SU HE XIANG WAN

Liquid Styrax Pill

Extract Formula Name: Styrax Formula

Su He Xiang	Liquidambar	30 g
She Xiang	Moschus	60 g
Bing Pian	Dryobalanops	30 g
An Xi Xiang	Styrax	60 g
Ru Xiang	Boswellia	30 g
Tan Xiang	Santalum	60 g
Ding Xiang	Eugenia	60 g
Bi Ba	Piper	60 g
Xiang Fu	Cyperus	60 g
Xi Jiao	Rhinoceros	60 g
Bai Zhu	Atractylodes	60 g
He Zi	Terminalia	60 g
Zhu Sha	Cinnabaris	60 g
Mu Xiang	Saussurea	60 g
Chen Xiang	Aquilaria	60 g

Severe chest phlegm and qi stagnation leading to fullness, tightness, or cramping in the chest, with rebellious Stomach qi symptoms such as nausea and vomiting.

T purple, thick sticky white or yellowish coat

P slippery or wiry

ZHI SHI GUA LOU GUI ZHI TANG

Immature Bitter Orange, Trichosanthes Fruit, and Cinnamon Twig Decoction

Gua Lou Ren	Trichosanthes	6 - 12 g
Zhi Shi	Citrus	9 - 12 g
Xie Bai	Allium	9 - 12 g
Gui Zhi	Cinnamomum	3 - 6 g
Hou Po	Magnolia	12 - 15 g

HEART PHLEGM FIRE

- insomnia with dream-disturbed sleep
- mental restlessness
- muttering to oneself, or uncontrolled laughter
- speech impairment

T red, red tip, sticky yellow coat

P slippery, rapid

Phlegm fire obstructing the orifice causing mania, severe palpitations, cough with profuse phlegm, dizziness, wheezing, anxiety, bad dreams, or lumps in the neck.

T red, thick yellow sticky coat

P wiry, rapid, forceful

☞ Herbs should be made into 6 - 9 g pills. Adults take one pill one or two times a day.

✗ Do not use during pregnancy or post-partum.

GUN TAN WAN

Vaporize Phlegm Pill

Extract Formula Name: Lapis and Scute Formula

Da Huang	Rheum	200 - 240 g
Huang Qin	Scutellaria	200 - 240 g
Meng Shi	Lapis Micae Seu Chloriti	20 - 30 g
Chen Xiang	Aquilaria	9 - 15 g

Heart phlegm fire causing agitation, insomnia, mania, laughing or screaming without apparent reason, or severe head pain. There can be an underlying Liver qi stagnation and Spleen qi deficiency which further leads to phlegm stagnation..

T   red, sticky yellow coat

P   rapid, slippery, wiry

✗   Zhu Sha - Cinnabaris is toxic and should be used in small amounts. Do not use during pregnancy.

SHENG TIE LUO YIN

Iron Filings Decoction

Extract Formula Name: Iron Filings Combination

Sheng Tie Luo	Frusta Ferri	30 - 60 g
Dan Nan Xing	Arisaema	1 - 3 g
Zhe Bei Mu	Fritillaria	3 - 6 g
Mai Men Dong	Ophiopogon	6 - 9 g
Xuan Shen	Scrophularia	6 - 9 g
Tian Men Dong	Asparagus	6 - 9 g
Fu Shen	Poria	3 - 6 g
Fu Ling	Poria	3 - 6 g
Lian Qiao	Forsythia	3 - 6 g
Dan Shen	Salvia	3 - 6 g
Shi Chang Pu	Acorus	3 - 6 g
Gou Teng	Uncaria	3 - 6 g
Chen Pi	Citrus	3 - 6 g
Yuan Zhi	Polygala	3 - 6 g
Zhu Sha	Cinnabaris	0.5 g

HEART BLOOD DEFICIENCY

- pale face
- anxiety
- insomnia with dream-disturbed sleep
- dizziness

T pale, thin and narrow, dry

P thin

Heart

Heart blood and yin deficiency with Spleen qi deficiency leading to insomnia, decreased appetite, nightmares, irregular periods in women, or uterine bleeding which may manifest as ben lou - gushing or spotting; This formula is also useful for purpura due to Spleen qi/blood deficiency.

T pale, swollen, teethmarks, thin white coat

P weak, thin

✪ **Major Formula**

GUI PI TANG

Restore the Spleen Decoction

Extract Formula Name: Ginseng and Longan Combination

Ren Shen	Panax	6 - 9 g
Huang Qi	Astragalus	9 - 12 g
Fu Shen	Poria	6 - 9 g
Bai Zhu	Atractylodes	9 - 12 g
Long Yan Rou	Euphoria	9 - 12 g
Mu Xiang	Saussurea	3 - 6 g
Suan Zao Ren	Zizyphus	9 - 12 g
Dang Gui	Angelica	6 - 9 g
Yuan Zhi	Polygala	3 - 6 g
Gan Cao	Glycyrrhiza	3 - 6 g

---

1. Yin/blood deficiency with heat causing arrhythmia of the Heart. 2. High fever causing arrhythmia: yangming disease depleted yin which leads to an irregular Heart beat.

T red, scanty coat

P rapid, irregular

☞ E Jiao - Equus should be dissolved at the end into the strained tea.

JIA JIAN FU MAI TANG

Modified Restore-the-Pulse Decoction

Zhi Gan Cao	Glycyrrhiza	12 - 15 g
Bai Shao Yao	Paeonia	12 - 15 g
Mai Men Dong	Ophiopogon	9 - 12 g
Sheng Di Huang	Rehmannia	12 - 15 g
Huo Ma Ren	Cannabis	9 - 12 g
E Jiao	Equus	6 - 9 g

Heart qi blood deficiency causing insomnia, anxiety, restlessness, and poor memory.

T pale

P weak, thin

YANG XIN TANG

Nourish the Heart Decoction

Extract Formula Name: Astragalus and Zizyphus Combination

Sheng Di Huang	Rehmannia	6 - 12 g
Shu Di Huang	Rehmannia	6 - 12 g
Dang Gui	Angelica	6 - 9 g
Ren Shen	Panax	6 - 12 g
Mai Men Dong	Ophiopogon	6 - 9 g
Suan Zao Ren	Ziziphus	6 - 9 g
Fu Shen	Poria	6 - 9 g
Bai Zi Ren	Biota	6 - 9 g
Wu Wei Zi	Schisandra	6 - 9 g
Gan Cao	Glycyrrhiza	3 - 6 g
[Lian Zi	Nelumbo	3 - 6 g]
[Deng Xin Cao	Juncus	3 - 6 g]

Kidney and Liver yin/blood deficiency with fire which bothers the Heart. This causes Heart and Liver fire or Liver yang excess leading to excessive dreaming, insomnia, or outbursts of anger.

T red, cracks, thin or thick yellow coat

P rapid, wiry, thin

☞ Ingredients should be powdered, made into 9 - 12 g pills and taken three times a day. Xi Jiao - Rhinoceros should be substituted with Shui Niu Jiao - Bubalus.

ZHEN ZHU MU WAN

Mother-Of-Pearl Pill

Zhen Zhu Mu	Pteria	15 - 20 g
Ren Shen	Panax	9 - 12 g
Dang Gui	Angelica	6 - 12 g
Shu Di Huang	Rehmannia	9 - 12 g
Suan Zao Ren	Ziziphus	6 - 9 g
Bai Zi Ren	Biota	6 - 9 g
Fu Shen	Poria	6 - 9 g
Chen Xiang	Aquilaria	6 - 9 g
Xi Jiao	Rhinoceros	1 - 3 g

Heart

Heart qi/blood or yin deficiency causing arrhythmia, insomnia, pressure in the chest, coronary Heart disease, and anxiety.

T pale or red, thin white coat

P weak

☞ E Jiao - Equus should be dissolved into the strained tea.

ZHI GAN CAO TANG

Honey-Fried Licorice Decoction

Extract Formula Name: Baked Licorice Combination

Zhi Gan Cao	Glycyrrhiza	12 - 15 g
Sheng Di Huang	Rehmannia	30 g
Ren Shen	Panax	6 - 9 g
Gui Zhi	Cinnamomum	6 - 9 g
Huo Ma Ren	Cannabis	6 - 9 g
Mai Men Dong	Ophiopogon	9 g
E Jiao	Equus	6 g
Da Zao	Ziziphus	6 - 9 pc
Sheng Jiang	Zingiber	6 - 9 g

Heart fire with qi/blood/yin deficiency causing mental depression, heat in the chest, excessive dreaming, or palpitations. This formula acts as a sedative.

T red, thin coat

P rapid, thin

☞ Either grind all herbs and take 6 - 9 g twice a day; or decoct and add Zhu Sha - Cinnabaris at the end of the decoction process.

✗ Zhu Sha - Cinnabaris is toxic and should not be used over a long period of time.

ZHU SHA AN SHEN WAN

Cinnabaris Pill to Calm the Spirit

Extract Formula Name: Cinnabaris Formula

Zhu Sha	Cinnabaris	3 - 9 g
Huang Lian	Coptis	6 - 12 g
Dang Gui	Angelica	3 - 6 g
Sheng Di Huang	Rehmannia	3 - 6 g
Zhi Gan Cao	Glycyrrhiza	6 - 9 g

HEART BLOOD STAGNATION

- tightness in the chest
- pain in the chest which may radiate down the left arm
- cyanotic lips and nails
- cold extremities

T purple

P knotted

Qi stagnation in the upper and middle jiao with slow blood circulation causing intermittent chest pain, and epigastric or abdominal discomfort.

T purple

P choppy

DAN SHEN YIN

Salvia Decoction

Dan Shen	Salvia	30 g
Sha Ren	Amomum	5 g
Tan Xiang	Santalum	5 g

Severe Heart phlegm accumulation and qi stagnation with yang deficiency. Angina can be severe, and the patient experiences numbness radiating down the arm, shortness of breath: chest bi-syndrome.

T pale, light purple, wet, thick sticky white coat

P slippery

GUA LOU XIE BAI BAN XIA TANG

Trichosanthes Fruit, Chinese Chive, and Pinellia Decoction

Extract Formula Name: Trichosanthes, Bakeri and Pinellia Combination

Gua Lou	Trichosanthes	9 - 12 g
Xie Bai	Allium	6 - 9 g
Ban Xia	Pinellia	9 - 12 g
Bai Jiu	White Wine	30 cc

Blood stagnation in head, chest, and diaphragm causing angina, palpitations, insomnia, nightmares, or dysmenorrhea.

T purple or purple spots

P wiry

✘ Do not use during pregnancy.

✪ Major Formula

XUE FU ZHU YU TANG

Drive out Stasis in the Mansion of Blood Decoction

Extract Formula Name: Persica and Achyranthes Combination

Dang Gui	Angelica	6 - 9 g
Chuan Xiong	Ligusticum	3 - 9 g
Sheng Di Huang	Rehmannia	6 - 9 g
Chi Shao Yao	Paeonia	6 - 9 g
Tao Ren	Prunus	6 - 12 g
Hong Hua	Carthamus	6 - 9 g
Chuan Niu Xi	Cyathula	9 - 12 g
Jie Geng	Platycodon	3 - 6 g
Zhi Ke	Citrus	3 - 6 g
Chai Hu	Bupleurum	3 - 9 g
Gan Cao	Glycyrrhiza	3 - 6 g

Heart

HEART FIRE

- mental restlessness and agitation
- redness in the face
- mouth or tongue sores

T red, red tip, yellow coat

P forceful, rapid

Heart/Pericardium fire with toxic heat and fever which congeals into phlegm. This leads to delirium, coma, aphasia, or convulsions in children.

T dark red, sticky yellow coat

P rapid, forceful, wiry

☞ Herbs should be ground and made into 3 g pills. The adult dosage is one pill two to three times a day. Xi Jiao - Rhinoceros should be substituted with Shui Niu Jiao - Bubalus.

✗ Do not use during pregnancy. Do not take over a prolonged period of time. Note that Zhu Sha - Cinnabaris is toxic.

✪ Major Formula

AN GONG NIU HUANG WAN

Calm the Palace Pill with Cattle Gallstone

Extract Formula Name: Bos and Curcuma Formula

Niu Huang	Bos	25 - 30 g
Xi Jiao	Rhinoceros	25 - 30 g
She Xiang	Moschus	7.5 g
Huang Lian	Coptis	25 - 30 g
Zhi Zi	Gardenia	25 - 30 g
Huang Qin	Scutellaria	25 - 30 g
Bing Pian	Dryobalanops	7.5 g
Zhen Zhu Mu	Pteria	12 - 15 g
Yu Jin	Curcuma	25 - 30 g
Xiong Huang	Realgar	25 - 30 g
Zhu Sha	Cinnabaris	25 - 30 g

Heart fire and yang rising leading to severe insomnia, palpitations, hearing, or vision loss. The Kidneys and Heart don't harmonize.

T red, yellow coat

P rapid, maybe wiry

☞ Ingredients should be ground into powder, then made into pills with honey.

✗ Zhu Sha - Cinnabaris is toxic and should only be used short-term. Do not use during pregnancy.

CI ZHU WAN

Magnetite and Cinnabar Pill

Ci Shi	Magnetitum	60 g
Zhu Sha	Cinnabaris	30 g
Shen Qu	Massa Fermentata	120 g

Heart fire leading to Small Intestine fire, which in turn leads to Bladder damp heat causing hematuria, frequent urination, urinary retention, thirst, or tongue sores.

T bright red, sticky yellow coat

P rapid, wiry

DAO CHI SAN

Guide Out the Red Powder

Extract Formula Name: Rehmannia and Akebia Formula

Sheng Di Huang	Rehmannia	9 - 20 g
Dan Zhu Ye	Lophatherum	6 - 9 g
Mu Tong	Akebia	6 - 9 g
Gan Cao	Glycyrrhiza	3 - 6 g

Upper jiao heat with middle jiao cold usually caused by cold food which restricts Spleen qi. This leads to damp which then turns to heat. The heat rises upward and bothers the Heart causing thirst, restlessness, full/cold abdomen with pain, or nausea and vomiting.

T red or pale, red tip, thin sticky coat

P rapid, wiry

HUANG LIAN TANG

Coptis Decoction

Extract Formula Name: Coptis Combination

Huang Lian	Coptis	5 g
Gan Jiang	Zingiber	5 g
Gui Zhi	Cinnamomum	5 g
Ren Shen	Panax	3 g
Ban Xia	Pinellia	9 g
Da Zao	Ziziphus	9 - 12 pc
Gan Cao	Glycyrrhiza	6 g

Heart fire and excess heat leading to nose bleeding or premenstrual vomiting.

T red, yellow coat

P rapid, or empty

✗ Caution during pregnancy.

SAN HUANG SI WU TANG

Three-Yellow and Four-Substance Decoction

Shu Di Huang	Rehmannia	6 - 15 g
Bai Shao Yao	Paeonia	6 - 9 g
Chuan Xiong	Ligusticum	3 - 9 g
Dang Gui	Angelica	6 - 9 g
Huang Lian	Coptis	3 - 9 g
Da Huang	Rheum	6 - 12 g
Huang Qin	Scutellaria	6 - 9 g

Heart/Stomach fire with damp leading to fever, jaundice, fullness, alternating diarrhea or constipation, mouth and tongue sores, or carbuncles.

T   dark red, yellow coat

P   flooding, rapid

✗   Caution during pregnancy.

XIE XIN TANG

Drain the Epigastrium Decoction

Extract Formula Name: Coptis and Rhubarb Combination

Da Huang	Rheum	6 - 9 g
Huang Lian	Coptis	3 - 6 g
Huang Qin	Scutellaria	6 - 9 g

Heart fire with qi/blood/yin deficiency causing mental depression, heat in the chest, excessive dreaming, or palpitations. This formula acts as a sedative.

T   red, thin coat

P   rapid, thin

☞   Either grind all herbs and take 6 - 9 g twice a day; or decoct and add Zhu Sha - Cinnabaris at the end of the decoction process.

✗   Zhu Sha - Cinnabaris is toxic and should not be used over a long period of time.

ZHU SHA AN SHEN WAN

Cinnabaris Pill to Calm the Spirit

Extract Formula Name: Cinnabaris Formula

Zhu Sha	Cinnabaris	3 - 9 g
Huang Lian	Coptis	6 - 12 g
Dang Gui	Angelica	3 - 6 g
Sheng Di Huang	Rehmannia	3 - 6 g
Zhi Gan Cao	Glycyrrhiza	6 - 9 g

COLLAPSE OF YANG

- profuse and spontaneous sweating
- cyanotic lips
- shallow breathing
- palpitations

T purple or pale

P minute

Severe yang deficiency and cold causes the yang to be pushed superficially leading to superficial false yang symptoms. The patient gives the appearance that he/she will get better but in reality may die soon. Symptoms include diarrhea, low fever, or red face. Internal cold with superficial false heat: shaoyin syndrome.

T pale, red tip

P deep, faint

BAI TONG TANG

White Penetrating Decoction

Gan Jiang	Zingiber	3 - 6 g
Fu Zi	Aconitum	3 - 9 g
Cong Bai	Allium	3 - 6 g

Shock with severe sweating and qi loss after hemorrhaging or Heart failure.

T pale

P hollow or frail

DU SHEN TANG

Unaccompanied Ginseng Decoction

Ren Shen	Panax	30 g
[Da Zao	Ziziphus	3 - 6 g]

Kidney and Spleen yang deficiency with cold which has invaded all three yin channels (taiyin, shaoyin, and jueyin). Symptoms include shivering from cold, icy limbs and face, watery diarrhea, or cough with profuse saliva production.

T   pale, wet, thin white moist coat

P   minute or frail

☞ Remove She Xiang - Moschus, decoct the rest of the formula as usual, then add powdered Moschus to each dosage.

HUI YANG JIU JI TANG

Restore and Revive the Yang Decoction

Fu Zi	Aconitum	9 g
Rou Gui	Cinnamomum	3 - 6 g
Ren Shen	Panax	6 - 9 g
Gan Jiang	Zingiber	3 - 6 g
Fu Ling	Poria	6 - 9 g
Chen Pi	Citrus	3 - 6 g
Bai Zhu	Atractylodes	6 - 9 g
Wu Wei Zi	Schisandra	3 - 6 g
Ban Xia	Pinellia	6 - 9 g
Gan Cao	Glycyrrhiza	3 - 6 g
She Xiang	Moschus	0.3 g
[Sheng Jiang	Zingiber	1 - 3 g]

Severe yang and blood loss causing collapse and dehydration after sweating and diarrhea. The patient has cold extremities or chills.

T   pale

P   thin or hollow

SI NI JIA REN SHEN TANG

Frigid Extremities Decoction plus Ginseng

Extract Formula Name: G.L. and Aconite Combination with Ginseng

Fu Zi	Aconitum	6 - 9 g
Gan Jiang	Zingiber	3 - 6 g
Zhi Gan Cao	Glycyrrhiza	3 - 6 g
Ren Shen	Panax	6 - 9 g

Exterior cold has gone internally. qi and yang are very weak and Kidney/Spleen yang have been damaged. Symptoms include low blood pressure, cold limbs, shock, or sweating.

T   pale, or purple, moist white coat

P   minute

☞ The raw type of Aconite is used here since it is much warmer than the prepared kind. 6 - 12 g of honey are often added for detoxification. Fu Zi - Aconitum is soaked in 8 - 10 cups of boiling water for 30 minutes to one hour. The remaining herbs should be added during the last 25 minutes and decocted as usual.

✗ Fu Zi - Aconitum in its raw form is toxic and is intended for short-term use only.

❂ Major Formula

SI NI TANG

Frigid Extremities Decoction

Extract Formula Name: Aconite, Ginger and Licorice Combination

Fu Zi	Aconitum	9 - 15 g
Gan Jiang	Zingiber	6 - 12 g
Zhi Gan Cao	Glycyrrhiza	3 - 6 g

Shaoyin disease: severe yang deficiency with cold accumulation which causes false yang to be pushed to the exterior. The yang cannot stay in the interior causing icy limbs upon touch but no cold intolerance, flushed face, thirst without desire to drink, or a dry throat.

T   pale, light purple, teethmarks, thin white coat

P   slow, minute

TONG MAI SI NI TANG

Unblock the Pulse Decoction for Frigid Extremities

Extract Formula Name: Licorice, Aconite and Ginger Pulse Combination

Fu Zi	Aconitum	12 - 15 g
Gan Jiang	Zingiber	9 - 12 g
Gan Cao	Glycyrrhiza	3 - 6 g

SPLEEN DISHARMONIES

脾失调

SPLEEN QI DEFICIENCY

- fatigue, especially after eating
- decreased appetite and lassitude
- pale or sallow complexion
- abdominal distention or fullness
- loose stools

T pale, swollen, teethmarks

P weak

Spleen qi deficiency causing morning sickness, a restless fetus, loose stools, or poor appetite.

T pale, swollen, white coat

P weak

BAO TAI ZI SHENG WAN

Protect the Fetus and Aid Life Pill

Ren Shen	Panax	6 - 9 g
Fu Ling	Poria	6 - 9 g
Bai Zhu	Atractylodes	6 - 9 g
Gan Cao	Glycyrrhiza	3 - 6 g
Lian Zi	Nelumbo	6 - 9 g
Bian Dou	Dolichos	6 - 9 g
Huo Xiang	Agastache	6 - 9 g
Bai Dou Kou	Amomum	3 - 6 g
Chen Pi	Citrus	3 - 6 g
Jie Geng	Platycodon	3 - 6 g
Shan Yao	Dioscorea	6 - 9 g
Yi Yi Ren	Coix	6 - 12 g
Ze Xie	Alisma	6 - 9 g
Mai Ya	Hordeum	12 - 20 g
Qian Shi	Euryale	6 - 9 g
Shan Zha	Crataegus	6 - 12 g
Huang Lian	Coptis	3 g

Spleen/Source qi deficiency resulting in low-grade fever, fatigue, or loose stools. Purpura due to qi/yang deficiency. Pediatric department: measles, chickenpox, or smallpox which turn to purpura, and may result in shock.

T pale, white coat

P weak

BAO YUAN TANG

Preserve the Basal Decoction

Extract Formula Name: Astragalus, Ginseng, and Cinnamon Combination

Ren Shen	Panax	6 - 9 g
Huang Qi	Astragalus	6 - 12 g
Rou Gui	Cinnamomum	6 - 9 g
Gan Cao	Glycyrrhiza	3 - 6 g

Spleen/Stomach qi deficiency where the Spleen qi is sinking, or the Spleen is not governing the blood. qi deficiency can lead to (morning) fever, early periods, weakness, diarrhea, or pallor.

T pale, swollen, teethmarks, thin white coat

P weak

BU ZHONG YI QI TANG

Tonify the Middle and Augment the Qi Decoction

Extract Formula Name: Ginseng and Astragalus Combination

Ren Shen	Panax	6 - 12 g
Huang Qi	Astragalus	9 - 15 g
Dang Gui	Angelica	6 - 9 g
Chen Pi	Citrus	3 - 6 g
Sheng Ma	Cimicifuga	3 - 6 g
Chai Hu	Bupleurum	3 - 9 g
Bai Zhu	Atractylodes	3 - 9 g
Zhi Gan Cao	Glycyrrhiza	3 - 6 g

Heat and cold in the middle jiao with Spleen/Stomach qi deficiency, and cold predominance. The patient experiences mild middle jiao qi stagnation symptoms such as fullness or bloating.

T thin yellow coat

P weak, slightly wiry

GAN CAO XIE XIN TANG

Licorice Decoction to Drain the Epigastrium

Extract Formula Name: Pinellia and Licorice Combination

Ban Xia	Pinellia	6 - 9 g
Huang Qin	Scutellaria	9 - 12 g
Zhi Gan Cao	Glycyrrhiza	12 - 15 g
Gan Jiang	Zingiber	9 - 12 g
Ren Shen	Panax	9 - 12 g
Huang Lian	Coptis	3 - 6 g
Da Zao	Ziziphus	9 - 15 pc

Spleen/Stomach qi deficiency and cold causing vomiting during pregnancy.

T pale, thin white coat

P weak

GAN JIANG REN SHEN BAN XIA WAN

Ginger, Ginseng, and Pinellia Pill

Extract Formula Name: G.P. and Ginseng Formula

Gan Jiang	Zingiber	3 g
Ren Shen	Panax	3 g
Ban Xia	Pinellia	6 g
[Sheng Jiang	Zingiber	1 - 3 g]

Heart blood and yin deficiency with Spleen qi deficiency leading to insomnia, decreased appetite, nightmares, irregular periods in women, or uterine bleeding which may manifest as ben lou - gushing or spotting; This formula is also useful for purpura due to Spleen qi/blood deficiency.

T pale, swollen, teethmarks, thin white coat

P weak, thin

GUI PI TANG

Restore the Spleen Decoction

Extract Formula Name: Ginseng and Longan Combination

Ren Shen	Panax	6 - 9 g
Huang Qi	Astralagus	9 - 12 g
Fu Shen	Poria	6 - 9 g
Bai Zhu	Atractylodes	9 - 12 g
Long Yan Rou	Euphoria	9 - 12 g
Mu Xiang	Saussurea	3 - 6 g
Suan Zao Ren	Ziziphus	9 - 12 g
Dang Gui	Angelica	6 - 9 g
Yuan Zhi	Polygala	3 - 6 g
Gan Cao	Glycyrrhiza	3 - 6 g

Severe taiyin/taiyang disease with abdominal cramps as the main symptom.

T thin white coat

P superficial

GUI ZHI JIA SHAO YAO TANG

Cinnamon Twig Decoction plus Peony

Extract Formula Name: Cinnamon and Peony Combination

Gui Zhi	Cinnamomum	6 - 9 g
Bai Shao Yao	Paeonia	15 - 18 g
Sheng Jiang	Zingiber	3 - 6 g
Da Zao	Ziziphus	3 - 4 pc
Gan Cao	Glycyrrhiza	3 - 6 g

Mild taiyin with taiyang syndrome: wind cold with mild Spleen qi deficiency. The chills are predominant, and the patient experiences diarrhea with epigastric fullness.

T pale, thin white coat

P weak, maybe superficial

GUI ZHI REN SHEN TANG

Cinnamon Twig and Ginseng Decoction

Extract Formula Name: Cinnamon and Ginseng Combination

Gui Zhi	Cinnamomum	9 - 12 g
Ren Shen	Panax	9 - 12 g
Gan Jiang	Zingiber	9 g
Bai Zhu	Atractylodes	9 g
Zhi Gan Cao	Glycyrrhiza	9 - 12 g

Spleen qi deficiency with pre-existing taiyang syndrome but no direct exterior symptoms are present anymore. Symptoms include epigastric distention, vomiting, or poor appetite.

T pale, thin white coat

P weak

HOU PO SHENG JIANG BAN XIA TANG

Magnolia Bark, Ginger, and Pinellia Decoction

Extract Formula Name: Magnolia-Five Combination

Hou Po	Magnolia	6 - 12 g
Sheng Jiang	Zingiber	3 - 6 g
Ban Xia	Pinellia	6 - 9 g
Ren Shen	Panax	6 - 9 g
Gan Cao	Glycyrrhiza	3 - 6 g

Spleen/Stomach qi deficiency with cold and wei (defensive) qi deficiency; also useful for peptic ulcers and chronic allergies. Other symptoms include poor appetite or spontaneous sweating.

T pale, thin white coat

P weak, slow, thin, wiry

☞ Yi Tang - Saccharum Granorum is dissolved into the strained decoction.

HUANG QI JIAN ZHONG TANG

Astragalus Decoction to Construct the Middle

Extract Formula Name: Astragalus Combination

Gui Zhi	Cinnamomum	9 g
Bai Shao Yao	Paeonia	18 g
Sheng Jiang	Zingiber	10 g
Da Zao	Ziziphus	3 - 6 pc
Gan Cao	Glycyrrhiza	6 g
Yi Tang	Saccharum Granorum	30 g
Huang Qi	Astragalus	9 g

Spleen

Spleen qi deficiency during pregnancy with lethargy, spotting, or low back pain.

T   pale, swollen, teethmarks, thin white coat

P   weak, thin

☞ E Jiao - Equus should be added at the end to the strained tea.

JIA JIAN BU ZHONG YI QI TANG

Modified Tonify the Middle and Augment the Qi Decoction

Ren Shen	Panax	6 - 9 g
Huang Qi	Astragalus	6 - 12 g
Chen Pi	Citrus	3 - 6 g
Bai Zhu	Atractylodes	3 - 9 g
Sheng Ma	Cimicifuga	3 - 6 g
Chai Hu	Bupleurum	3 - 9 g
E Jiao	Equus	3 - 9 g
Ai Ye	Artemisia	3 - 9 g
Gan Cao	Glycyrrhiza	3 - 6 g

Spleen qi deficiency causing severe uterine bleeding which is pale in color, or early or irregular periods. The Spleen qi is sinking causing a restless fetus.

T   pale, swollen, teethmarks, thin white coat

P   weak

JU YUAN JIAN

Lift the Source Decoction

Ren Shen	Panax	6 - 9 g
Huang Qi	Astragalus	9 - 12 g
Sheng Ma	Cimicifuga	3 - 6 g
Bai Zhu	Atractylodes	3 - 6 g
Gan Cao	Glycyrrhiza	3 - 6 g

Spleen

Spleen/Stomach qi deficiency with mild damp symptoms including decreased appetite, middle jiao distention, or nausea and vomiting.

T pale, thin sticky coat

P weak, slightly slippery

LIU JUN ZI TANG

Six-Gentlemen Decoction

Extract Formula Name: Six Major Herbs Combination

Ren Shen	Panax	6 - 9 g
Bai Zhu	Atractylodes	6 - 9 g
Fu Ling	Poria	6 - 9 g
Chen Pi	Citrus	3 - 6 g
Ban Xia	Pinellia	6 - 9 g
Gan Cao	Glycyrrhiza	3 - 6 g

Heart qi deficiency with Spleen qi deficiency leading to anxiety, insomnia, spontaneous sweating, or palpitations.

T pale, thin coating

P weak

✗ Zhu Sha - Cinnabaris is toxic, and should only be used short-term.

MIAO XIANG SAN

Marvelously Fragrant Powder

Ren Shen	Panax	6 - 12 g
Fu Ling	Poria	9 - 12 g
Fu Shen	Poria	9 - 12 g
Yuan Zhi	Polygala	9 - 12 g
Huang Qi	Astragalus	9 - 15 g
Shan Yao	Dioscorea	9 - 12 g
Mu Xiang	Saussurea	12 - 15 g
Jie Geng	Platycodon	1 - 3 g
Zhu Sha	Cinnabaris	1 - 3 g
She Xiang	Moschus	0.3 - 0.5 g
Gan Cao	Glycyrrhiza	3 - 6 g

Spleen/Stomach qi deficiency causing diarrhea and vomiting with extreme thirst due to depletion of fluids. Commonly used in the pediatric department.

T   pale, swollen, teethmarks, thin white coat

P   weak

QI WEI BAI ZHU SAN

Seven-Ingredient Powder with Atractylodes Macrocephala

Ren Shen	Panax	6 - 9 g
Bai Zhu	Atractylodes	3 - 9 g
Mu Xiang	Saussurea	3 - 9 g
Fu Ling	Poria	6 - 9 g
Huo Xiang Ye	Agastache	9 - 15 g
Ge Gen	Pueraria	9 - 15 g
Gan Cao	Glycyrrhiza	3 - 6 g

Spleen qi deficiency causing thin, clear or reddish leukorrhea, with low back pain.

T   pale, thin white coat

P   deep, thin, slippery

QING DAI TANG

Clear Discharge Decoction

Shan Yao	Dioscorea	9 - 30 g
Mu Li	Ostrea	9 - 15 g
Long Gu	Os Draconis	9 - 15 g
Qian Cao Gen	Rubia	6 - 9 g
Hai Piao Xiao	Sepia	9 - 12 g

Lung yin deficiency with false heat and Spleen qi deficiency causing cough with scanty sputum and fatigue.

T red, cracked, slight coat

P thin, rapid

☞ Dissolve Bie Jia - Amyda for about one hour, then decoct with the remaining herbs.

REN SHEN HUANG QI SAN

Ginseng and Astragalus Powder

Ren Shen	Panax	6 - 12 g
Huang Qi	Astragalus	9 - 15 g
Fu Ling	Poria	6 - 9 g
Zhi Mu	Anemarrhena	6 - 9 g
Zi Wan	Aster	6 - 9 g
Sang Bai Pi	Morus	6 - 9 g
Qin Jiao	Gentiana	6 - 12 g
Jie Geng	Platycodon	3 - 6 g
Chai Hu	Bupleurum	6 - 9 g
Ban Xia	Pinellia	6 - 9 g
Di Gu Pi	Lycium	3 - 9 g
Sheng Di Huang	Rehmannia	6 - 15 g
Bie Jia	Amyda	6 - 12 g
Tian Men Dong	Asparagus	9 - 12 g
Chi Shao Yao	Paeonia	3 - 9 g
Gan Cao	Glycyrrhiza	3 - 6 g

Spleen qi deficiency with damp leading to diarrhea and irregular periods. Other symptoms include weight loss, fatigue, poor appetite, or pale face.

T pale, white coat

P weak or thin

SHEN LING BAI ZHU SAN

Ginseng, Poria, and Atractylodes Powder

Extract Formula Name: Ginseng and Atractylodes Formula

Ren Shen	Panax	9 - 15 g
Fu Ling	Poria	9 - 12 g
Bai Zhu	Atractylodes	3 - 9 g
Gan Cao	Glycyrrhiza	6 - 9 g
Lian Zi	Nelumbo	3 - 9 g
Yi Yi Ren	Coix	6 - 15 g
Shan Yao	Dioscorea	9 - 15 g
Bian Dou	Dolichos	6 - 9 g
Jie Geng	Platycodon	3 - 6 g
Sha Ren	Amomum	3 g

Spleen

Spleen/Kidney qi and yang deficiency causing edema which manifests mostly in the lower body. Other symptoms include cold limbs, poor appetite, decreased urination, or heaviness.

T   pale, sticky coat

P   deep, slow, maybe thin

SHI PI YIN

Bolster the Spleen Decoction

Extract Formula Name: Magnolia and Atractylodes Combination

Fu Zi	Aconitum	6 - 9 g
Bai Zhu	Atractylodes	6 - 9 g
Mu Gua	Chaenomeles	6 - 9 g
Hou Po	Magnolia	6 - 12 g
Gan Jiang	Zingiber	6 - 9 g
Mu Xiang	Saussurea	6 - 9 g
Fu Ling	Poria	6 - 9 g
Da Fu Pi	Areca	3 - 6 g
Cao Guo	Amomum	3 - 6 g
Zhi Gan Cao	Glycyrrhiza	3 - 6 g
[Da Zao	Ziziphus	1 - 3 pc]
[Sheng Jiang	Zingiber	3 - 6 g]

Stomach/Spleen qi deficiency. This is the basic prescription for building qi. Symptoms include poor appetite, loose bowel movements, or lethergy.

T   pale, thin white coat

P   weak, deep

✪ Major Formula

SI JUN ZI TANG

Four-Gentlemen Decoction

Extract Formula Name: Four Major Herbs Combination

Ren Shen	Panax	6 - 9 g
Bai Zhu	Atractylodes	3 - 9 g
Fu Ling	Poria	6 - 9 g
Gan Cao	Glycyrrhiza	3 - 6 g

Spleen qi deficiency with Liver qi stagnation causing leukorrhea. The discharge is thin, watery, or white. Other symptoms include loose stools, poor appetite, and possible irritability.

T pale, light purple, swollen, sticky white coat

P slippery, slow

WAN DAI TANG

End Discharge Decoction

Bai Zhu	Atractylodes	20 - 30 g
Cang Zhu	Atractylodes	3 - 6 g
Shan Yao	Dioscorea	20 - 30 g
Chen Pi	Citrus	3 - 6 g
Bai Shao Yao	Paeonia	6 - 12 g
Chai Hu	Bupleurum	3 - 6 g
Jing Jie	Schizonepeta	6 - 9 g
Che Qian Zi	Plantago	6 - 9 g
Ren Shen	Panax	6 - 9 g
Gan Cao	Glycyrrhiza	3 - 6 g

Spleen Qi deficiency with mild Qi stagnation and damp in the middle jiao. Symptoms include fullness in the epigastrium or abdomen, gas, loose stools, or epigastric pain.

T pale or light purple, swollen, teethmarks, white coat

P weak

WU WEI YI GONG SAN

Five-Herbs, an Exceptionally Effective Powder

Ren Shen	Panax	6 - 9 g
Fu Ling	Poria	6 - 9 g
Bai Zhu	Atractylodes	3 - 9 g
Gan Cao	Glycyrrhiza	3 - 6 g
Chen Pi	Citrus	3 - 6 g
[Da Zao	Ziziphus	3 - 6 g]
[Sheng Jiang	Zingiber	3 - 6 g]

Diarrhea due to Spleen qi deficiency with damp and Stomach heat causing dysentery with mucous and possible bleeding.

T sticky yellow coat

P slippery, rapid

XIANG LIAN WAN

Aucklandia and Coptis Pill

Extract Formula Name: Saussurea and Coptis Formula

Mu Xiang	Saussurea	6 - 9 g
Huang Lian	Coptis	3 - 6 g
Wu Zhu Yu	Evodia	3 - 12 g

1. Chronic Spleen qi deficiency with chronic cold evil qi leading to qi and blood deficiency. The main symptom is abdominal spasms. 2. Liver qi stagnation or Liver overacting on Spleen. In the latter two instances the dosage of 'Bai Shao Yao - Paeonia' should be increased.

T   pale or light purple, thin white coat

P   weak or slightly wiry

☞ Yi Tang - Saccharum Granorum should be added to the strained tea.

XIAO JIAN ZHONG TANG

Minor Construct the Middle Decoction

Extract Formula Name: Minor Cinnamon and Peony Combination

Yi Tang	Saccharum Granorum	15 - 30 g
Gui Zhi	Cinnamomum	3 - 9 g
Bai Shao Yao	Paeonia	6 - 9 g
Sheng Jiang	Zingiber	6 - 9 g
Da Zao	Ziziphus	3 - 5 pc
Zhi Gan Cao	Glycyrrhiza	3 - 6 g

Spleen qi with yin deficiency and heat accumulation causing constipation, or hardness and fullness in the abdomen.

T   cracked, thin dry yellowish coat

P   weak, thin, deep

XIN JIA HUANG LONG TANG

Newly-Augmented Yellow Dragon Decoction

Sheng Di Huang	Rehmannia	6 - 15 g
Ren Shen	Panax	6 - 9 g
Da Huang	Rheum	6 - 9 g
Mang Xiao	Mirabilitum	3 - 5 g
Mai Men Dong	Ophiopogon	9 - 15 g
Dang Gui	Angelica	6 - 9 g
Xuan Shen	Scrophularia	9 - 15 g
Gan Cao	Glycyrrhiza	3 - 6 g
Hai Shen	Strichopus	1 - 2 g

Spleen qi deficiency with middle jiao qi stagnation and diarrhea, or malnutrition in children.

T   pale, light purple, white coat

P   weak, thin

YI HUANG SAN

Benefit the Yellow Powder

Chen Pi	Citrus	30 g
Qing Pi	Citrus	15 g
Ding Xiang	Eugenia	3 - 6 g
He Zi	Terminalia	15 g
Zhi Gan Cao	Glycyrrhiza	15 g

Spleen qi deficiency causing damp which heats up. This leads to heat type leukorrhea with a fishy smell or delayed periods from qi and blood deficiency.

T   pale, thin sticky yellow or white coat

P   slippery, weak

YI HUANG TANG

Change Yellow (Discharge) Decoction

Shan Yao	Dioscorea	9 - 30 g
Huang Bai	Phellodendron	6 - 9 g
Qian Shi	Euryale	9 - 30 g
Bai Guo	Gingko	6 - 10 pc
Che Qian Zi	Plantago	3 - 6 g

Chronic middle jiao deficiency leading to visual disturbance and hearing loss or tinnitus.

T   pale, white coat

P   weak

YI QI CONG MING TANG

Augment the Qi and Increase Acuity Decoction

Extract Formula Name: Ginseng, Astragalus and Pueraria Combination

Ren Shen	Panax	6 - 12 g
Huang Qi	Astragalus	6 - 12 g
Zhi Gan Cao	Glycyrrhiza	6 - 12 g
Man Jing Zi	Vitex	6 - 9 g
Bai Shao Yao	Paeonia	3 - 9 g
Huang Bai	Phellodendron	3 - 9 g
Ge Gen	Pueraria	6 - 9 g
Sheng Ma	Cimicifuga	3 - 6 g

Spleen

Chronic Spleen qi deficiency causing qi stagnation. The qi stagnation gives rise to cold and heat symptoms in the middle jiao. This in turn damages the Spleen and Stomach again causing distention in the epigastrium and abdomen, or alternating constipation and diarrhea.

T   pale, thin yellowish coat

P   wiry

ZHI SHI XIAO PI WAN

Immature Bitter Orange Pill to Reduce Focal Distention

Zhi Shi	Citrus	6 - 12 g
Hou Po	Magnolia	6 - 15 g
Ban Xia	Pinellia	6 - 9 g
Huang Lian	Coptis	9 - 15 g
Fu Ling	Poria	6 - 9 g
Bai Zhu	Atractylodes	3 - 9 g
Ren Shen	Panax	6 - 9 g
Gan Jiang	Zingiber	3 - 6
Mai Ya	Hordeum	3 - 9 g
Zhi Gan Cao	Glycyrrhiza	3 - 6 g

1. Chronic food stagnation with severe Spleen qi deficiency.
2. Severe acute food stagnation with mild Spleen qi deficiency. Symptoms include epigastric and abdominal distention, loose stools, and poor appetite.

T   sticky coat

P   wiry

ZHI ZHU WAN

Immature Bitter Orange and Atractylodes Pill

Bai Zhu	Atractylodes	9 - 15 g
Zhi Shi	Citrus	6 - 12 g

Severe abdominal distention (pi man - fullness, firmness) due to Spleen qi deficiency, or qi stagnation with damp and heat. Symptoms include constipation, or odorous diarrhea, thirst, yellow urine, or fever.

T sticky yellow coat

P wiry, rapid

ZHONG MAN FEN XIAO WAN

Separate and Reduce Fullness in the Middle Pill

Hou Po	Magnolia	9 - 18 g
Jiang Huang	Curcuma	6 g
Zhi Shi	Citrus	9 - 12 g
Ban Xia	Pinellia	6 - 12 g
Ren Shen	Panax	3 g
Zhi Mu	Anemarrhena	6 - 9 g
Gan Jiang	Zingiber	3 - 6 g
Huang Lian	Coptis	3 - 9 g
Huang Qin	Scutellaria	9 - 15 g
Bai Zhu	Atractylodes	6 g
Ze Xie	Alisma	6 g
Sha Ren	Amomum	3 - 6 g
Chen Pi	Citrus	3 - 6 g
Fu Ling	Poria	6 - 9 g
Zhu Ling	Polyporus	3 - 6 g
Zhi Gan Cao	Glycyrrhiza	3 - 6 g

Spleen

SPLEEN QI AND BLOOD DEFICIENCY

- fatigue
- decreased appetite
- dizziness
- blurry vision
- loose stools

T pale

P weak, thin

Spleen qi and blood deficiency. Symptoms include dizziness, sallow complexion, chronic emaciation, mild fever, shortness of breath, or fatigue.

T pale, thin white coat

P thin, weak

✪ **Major Formula**

BA ZHEN TANG

Eight-Treasure Decoction

Extract Formula Name: Tang-kuei and Ginseng Eight Combination

Ren Shen	Panax	6 - 9 g
Bai Zhu	Atractylodes	3 - 9 g
Fu Ling	Poria	6 - 9 g
Gan Cao	Glycyrrhiza	3 - 6 g
Dang Gui	Angelica	6 - 12 g
Chuan Xiong	Ligusticum	3 - 6 g
Shu Di Huang	Rehmannia	6 - 15 g
Bai Shao Yao	Paeonia	6 - 9 g
[Da Zao	Ziziphus	2 - 3 pc]
[Sheng Jiang	Zingiber	2 - 6 g]

Qi and blood deficiency with blood stagnation. This formula is for a restless fetus, infertility, irregular periods, poor appetite, weakness, or fatigue.

T pale, thin white coat

P weak, maybe wiry

BA ZHEN YI MU WAN

Eight-Treasure Pill to Benefit Mothers

Shu Di Huang	Rehmannia	6 - 15 g
Chuan Xiong	Ligusticum	3 - 9 g
Dang Gui	Angelica	6 - 9 g
Bai Shao Yao	Paeonia	6 - 12 g
Ren Shen	Panax	6 - 12 g
Bai Zhu	Atractylodes	3 - 9 g
Fu Ling	Poria	6 - 9 g
Yi Mu Cao	Leonurus	6 - 18 g
Gan Cao	Glycyrrhiza	3 - 6 g

Spleen/Stomach qi deficiency where the Spleen qi is sinking, or the Spleen is not governing the blood. qi deficiency can lead to (morning) fever, early periods, weakness, diarrhea, or pallor.

T pale, swollen, teethmarks, thin white coat

P weak

BU ZHONG YI QI TANG

Tonify the Middle and Augment the Qi Decoction

Extract Formula Name: Ginseng and Astragalus Combination

Ren Shen	Panax	6 - 12 g
Huang Qi	Astragalus	9 - 15 g
Dang Gui	Angelica	6 - 9 g
Chen Pi	Citrus	3 - 6 g
Sheng Ma	Cimicifuga	3 - 6 g
Chai Hu	Bupleurum	3 - 9 g
Bai Zhu	Atractylodes	3 - 9 g
Zhi Gan Cao	Glycyrrhiza	3 - 6 g

Post-partum abdominal pain of the deficiency type after qi and blood loss from giving birth.

T pale

P frail

☞ E Jiao - Equus should be added to the strained tea.

CHANG NING TANG

Intestinal Serenity Decoction

Shu Di Huang	Rehmannia	6 - 12 g
Dang Gui	Angelica	6 - 12 g
Mai Men Dong	Ophiopogon	6 - 9 g
Ren Shen	Panax	6 - 9 g
Xu Duan	Dipsacus	6 - 9 g
Rou Gui	Cinnamomum	3 g
E Jiao	Equus	6 - 9 g
Shan Yao	Dioscorea	6 - 9 g
Gan Cao	Glycyrrhiza	3 - 6 g

Spleen

Kidney yin and Spleen qi/blood deficiency causing uterine prolapse with low back pain, night urination, or hearing loss and tinnitus.

T red or pale

P frail

DA BU YUAN JIAN

Great Tonify the Basal Decoction

Ren Shen	Panax	6 - 12 g
Shu Di Huang	Rehmannia	9 - 25 g
Shan Yao	Dioscorea	6 - 9 g
Shan Zhu Yu	Cornus	3 - 6 g
Gou Qi Zi	Lycium	6 - 9 g
Dang Gui	Angelica	6 - 9 g
Du Zhong	Eucommia	6 - 9 g
Gan Cao	Glycyrrhiza	3 - 6 g

Qi/blood deficiency with bleeding, fever, heat feelings in the muscles, thirst with a desire for warm liquids, or irregular periods.

T pale, thin coat

P empty

DANG GUI BU XUE TANG

Dang Gui Decoction to Tonify the Blood

Extract Formula Name: Tang-Kuei and Astragalus Combination

Huang Qi	Astragalus	30 g
Dang Gui	Angelica	6 g

Spleen qi and blood deficiency with slight cold leading to spasm pain or post-partum emaciation.

T pale, white coat

P weak

☞ Yi Tang - Saccharum Granorum should be added to the strained tea.

DANG GUI JIAN ZHONG TANG

Dang Gui Decoction to Construct the Middle

Extract Formula Name: Tang-Kuei, Cinnamon and Peony Combination

Yi Tang	Saccharum Granorum	6 - 20 g
Gui Zhi	Cinnamomum	3 - 9 g
Bai Shao Yao	Paeonia	6 - 9 g
Sheng Jiang	Zingiber	3 - 6 g
Da Zao	Ziziphus	3 - 6 pc
Gan Cao	Glycyrrhiza	3 - 6 g
Dang Gui	Angelica	6 - 9 g

Spleen qi and blood deficiency with yin deficiency and restless fetus. This prescription can be taken as a preventative during pregnancy.

T pale or red

P thin, weak

DANG GUI SAN

Dang Gui Powder

Extract Formula Name: Tang-Kuei Formula

Dang Gui	Angelica	6 - 12 g
Huang Qin	Scutellaria	6 - 12 g
Chuan Xiong	Ligusticum	3 g
Bai Zhu	Atractylodes	3 - 9 g
Bai Shao Yao	Paeonia	6 - 9 g

Liver overacting on Spleen causing mild cramping in the abdomen with Liver blood deficiency and some damp accumulation. Symptoms include urinary retention and lower body edema. This is often seen during pregnancy.

T pale, orange color on the sides

P weak, thin, or slightly wiry

DANG GUI SHAO YAO SAN

Dang Gui and Peony Powder

Extract Formula Name: Tang-Kuei and Peony Formula

Dang Gui	Angelica	6 - 9 g
Bai Shao Yao	Paeonia	3 - 9 g
Bai Zhu	Atractylodes	3 - 9 g
Fu Ling	Poria	6 - 9 g
Chuan Xiong	Ligusticum	3 - 6 g
Ze Xie	Alisma	6 - 9 g

Blood deficiency with external cold after childbirth. This leads to spasms or hernia pain which are both relieved by pressure.

T pale

P deep, wiry, weak

☞ This formula should be prepared as a stew with eight cups of water. Simmer until it is reduced to three to four cups.

DANG GUI SHENG JIANG YANG ROU TANG

Mutton Stew with Dang Gui and Fresh Ginger Decoction

Dang Gui	Angelica	9 - 12 g
Sheng Jiang	Zingiber	9 - 15 g
Yang Rou	Mutton	40 - 50 g

Spleen

Blood and yin deficient patient with cold evil qi which leads to obstruction of the channels which causes pain. This is known as jueyin syndrome in which the patient feels cold subjectively but not to the touch. Raynaud's disease.

T   pale, white coat

P   deep, thin, or minute

DANG GUI SI NI TANG

Dang Gui Decoction for Frigid Extremities

Extract Formula Name: Tang-Kuei and Jujube Combination

Dang Gui	Angelica	6 - 12 g
Gui Zhi	Cinnamomum	3 - 9 g
Bai Shao Yao	Paeonia	6 - 9 g
Mu Tong	Akebia	6 - 9 g
Xi Xin	Asarum	3 - 6 g
Da Zao	Ziziphus	3 - 5 pc
Gan Cao	Glycyrrhiza	3 - 6 g

Blood deficiency with yang deficiency and cold causing coldness in the uterus with dysmenorrhea. The blood is scanty, pale, and watery. The patient experiences severe cramping upon menstrual onset.

T   pale, light purple, some cracks, thin white coat

P   slow, thin, weak

GUI FU SI WU TANG

Cinnamon Bark, Aconite, and Four-Substance Decoction

Sheng Di Huang	Rehmannia	6 - 12 g
Dang Gui	Angelica	6 - 9 g
Chuan Xiong	Ligusticum	3 - 9 g
Bai Shao Yao	Paeonia	6 - 9 g
Rou Gui	Cinnamomum	3 - 9 g
Fu Zi	Aconitum	1 - 6 g

Heart blood and yin deficiency with Spleen qi deficiency leading to insomnia, decreased appetite, nightmares, irregular periods in women, or uterine bleeding which may manifest as ben lou - gushing or spotting; This formula is also useful for purpura due to Spleen qi/blood deficiency.

T pale, swollen, teethmarks, thin white coat

P weak, thin

GUI PI TANG

Restore the Spleen Decoction

Extract Formula Name: Ginseng and Longan Combination

Ren Shen	Panax	6 - 9 g
Huang Qi	Astralagus	9 - 12 g
Fu Shen	Poria	6 - 9 g
Bai Zhu	Atractylodes	9 - 12 g
Long Yan Rou	Euphoria	9 - 12 g
Mu Xiang	Saussurea	3 - 6 g
Suan Zao Ren	Ziziphus	9 - 12 g
Dang Gui	Angelica	6 - 9 g
Yuan Zhi	Polygala	3 - 6 g
Gan Cao	Glycyrrhiza	3 - 6 g

Blood deficiency giving rise to internal wind which then leads to tendon or muscle spasms, itchy skin rashes, or blurry vision.

T pale, quivery

P weak, maybe superficial

GUI XIONG SI WU TANG

Altered Four-Substance Decoction

Shu Di Huang	Rehmannia	9 - 15 g
Chuan Xiong	Ligusticum	3 - 9 g
Bai Shao Yao	Paeonia	6 - 9 g
Dang Gui	Angelica	6 - 9 g
Fang Feng	Ledebouriella	9 - 15 g
Bai Zhu	Atractylodes	6 - 9 g
Huai Niu Xi	Achyranthes	6 - 12 g
Tian Men Dong	Asparagus	9 - 12 g

Spleen

Chronic malaria has depleted Liver blood and Spleen qi and blood. The patient experiences alternating fever and chills which are aggravated with only mild stress.

T pale

P empty

HE REN YIN

Polygonum Multiflorum Root and Ginseng Decoction

He Shou Wu	Polygonum	9 - 20 g
Ren Shen	Panax	9 - 12 g
Chen Pi	Citrus	3 - 9 g
Dang Gui	Angelica	3 - 9 g
Wei Jiang	Zingiber	3 - 12 g

Yin/blood deficiency causing constipation with dry stools; or excess heat causing constipation.

T red, dry yellow coat

P rapid, thin, or empty

✗ Do not use during pregnancy.

MA ZI REN WAN

Hemp Seed Pill

Extract Formula Name: Apricot Seed and Linum Formula

Huo Ma Ren	Cannabis	6 - 12 g
Da Huang	Rheum	6 - 9 g
Xing Ren	Prunus	6 - 9 g
Zhi Shi	Citrus	3 - 6 g
Bai Shao Yao	Paeonia	6 - 9 g
Hou Po	Magnolia	6 - 12 g

Blood deficiency with deficient or excess heat causing purple menstrual blood, early periods, or thick leukorrhea with tidal fever.

T pale

P rapid, thin, weak

QIN LIAN SI WU TANG

Four-Substance Decoction with Scutellaria and Coptis

Huang Qin	Scutellaria	6 - 9 g
Huang Lian	Coptis	3 - 6 g
Chuan Xiong	Ligusticum	3 - 6 g
Bai Shao Yao	Paeonia	6 - 9 g
Dang Gui	Angelica	6 - 9 g
Mai Men Dong	Ophiopogon	6 - 9 g
Sheng Di Huang	Rehmannia	9 - 12 g

Spleen/Lung qi and blood deficiency with Heart yang deficiency, or ying level deficiency.
The patient is easily startled,
experiences shortness of
breath, lack of taste sensation,
insomnia, or palpitations. This
formula is also useful for irregular periods or uterine bleeding.

T pale, swollen

P weak

REN SHEN YANG RONG WAN

Ginseng Decoction to Nourish the Nutritive Qi

Extract Formula Name: Ginseng Combination

Bai Shao Yao	Paeonia	9 - 15 g
Chen Pi	Citrus	3 - 6 g
Dang Gui	Angelica	3 - 9 g
Ren Shen	Panax	6 - 9 g
Huang Qi	Astragalus	6 - 12 g
Bai Zhu	Atractylodes	6 - 9 g
Shu Di Huang	Rehmannia	3 - 6 g
Wu Wei Zi	Schisandra	3 - 6 g
Fu Ling	Poria	3 - 6 g
Yuan Zhi	Polygala	2 - 6 g
Rou Gui	Cinnamomum	6 - 9 g
Gan Cao	Glycyrrhiza	3 - 6 g
[Da Zao	Ziziphus	2 pc]
[Gan Jiang	Zingiber	3 pc]

Constipation due to yin/blood
deficiency. This is commonly
seen in the elderly, or after giving birth.

T red or pale, dry

P thin

RUN CHANG WAN I

Moisten the Intestines Pill from Master Shen's Book

Huo Ma Ren	Cannabis	9 - 15 g
Dang Gui	Angelica	9 - 12 g
Sheng Di Huang	Rehmannia	6 - 9 g
Tao Ren	Prunus	6 - 9 g
Zhi Ke	Citrus	6 - 9 g

Spleen

Wind heat invading the intestines and damaging the Spleen and Stomach qi. Severe constipation with blood deficiency which may lead to wind, or blood stagnation.

T   pale or purple

P   thin or choppy

RUN CHANG WAN II

Moisten the Intestines Pill from Discussion of the Spleen and Stomach

Da Huang	Rheum	9 - 12 g
Tao Ren	Prunus	15 - 25 g
Huo Ma Ren	Cannabis	15 - 30 g
Dang Gui Wei	Angelica	6 - 12 g
Qiang Huo	Notopterygium	6 - 9 g

Severe qi deficiency with yang and blood deficiency and cold symptoms. Irregular menstruation with a pale and watery flow, dizziness, pale or sallow face, cold limbs, or chills.

T   pale, wet, thin white coat

P   deep, weak, thready

SHAN HE YIN

Mountain and River Decoction

Shu Di Huang	Rehmannia	15 - 25 g
Dang Gui	Angelica	6 - 9 g
Bai Shao Yao	Paeonia	6 - 9 g
Chuan Xiong	Ligusticum	3 - 9 g
Rou Gui	Cinnamomum	3 - 9 g
Huang Qi	Astragalus	6 - 15 g

Spleen qi/blood deficiency causing slow blood circulation with deficiency type abdominal pain during menstruation, or bleeding sores.

T   pale, light purple, thin white coat

P   thin, weak

SHENG YU TANG

Sage-like Healing Decoction

Shu Di Huang	Rehmannia	15 - 25 g
Ren Shen	Panax	12 - 15 g
Dang Gui	Angelica	12 - 15 g
Huang Qi	Astragalus	15 - 20 g
Chuan Xiong	Ligusticum	6 - 9 g
Bai Shao Yao	Peonia	15 - 20 g

Qi/yang/blood deficiency. Symptoms include poor appetite, general malaise, mild cold symptoms, severe deficiency, rashes, dysmenorrhea, uterine bleeding, or post-partum deficiency.

T   pale, thin white coat

P   weak, thin, deep

SHI QUAN DA BU TANG

All-Inclusive Great Tonifying Decoction

Extract Formula Name: Ginseng and Tang-Kuei Ten Combination

Ren Shen	Panax	6 - 9 g
Fu Ling	Poria	9 - 12 g
Bai Zhu	Atractylodes	9 - 12 g
Gan Cao	Glycyrrhiza	3 - 6 g
Dang Gui	Angelica	12 - 15 g
Shu Di Huang	Rehmannia	15 - 20 g
Bai Shao Yao	Paeonia	12 - 15 g
Chuan Xiong	Ligusticum	3 - 9 g
Rou Gui	Cinnamomum	6 - 9 g
Huang Qi	Astragalus	15 - 20 g
[Da Zao	Ziziphus	1 - 3 g]
[Sheng Jiang	Zingiber	3 - 6 g]

Blood deficiency with blood stagnation. Symptoms include irregular menstruation, dysmenorrhea, dizziness, or pale or purple fingernails.

T   pale or purple

P   thin or choppy

✪ Major Formula

SI WU TANG

Four-Substance Decoction

Extract Formula Name: Tang-Kuei Four Combination

Shu Di Huang	Rehmannia	6 - 12 g
Chuan Xiong	Ligusticum	3 - 9 g
Dang Gui	Angelica	6 - 9 g
Bai Shao Yao	Paeonia	6 - 9 g

Spleen

Spleen qi/blood deficiency during pregnancy causing restless fetus, or use formula if the woman has a history of miscarriage or infertility.

T   pale, thin white coat

P   weak, thin, slippery

TAI SHAN PAN SHI WAN

Powder that Gives the Stability of Mount Tai

Ren Shen	Panax	6 - 9 g
Huang Qi	Astragalus	12 - 15 g
Shu Di Huang	Rehmannia	9 - 12 g
Chuan Xiong	Ligusticum	3 - 6 g
Bai Zhu	Atractylodes	9 - 12 g
Sha Ren	Amomum	1 - 3 g
Huang Qin	Scutellaria	6 - 9 g
Xu Duan	Dipsacus	3 - 6 g
Bai Shao Yao	Paeonia	6 - 9 g
Zhi Gan Cao	Glycyrrhiza	3 - 6 g
Nuo Mi	Glutinous Oryza	3 - 6 g

Mild blood deficiency with severe blood stagnation causing early periods or dysmenorrhea.

T   pale or purple

P   choppy or wiry

✗ Do not use during pregnancy.

TAO HONG SI WU TANG

Four-Substance Decoction with Safflower and Peach Pit

Shu Di Huang	Rehmannia	6 - 12 g
Bai Shao Yao	Paeonia	6 - 9 g
Chuan Xiong	Ligusticum	3 - 6 g
Dang Gui	Angelica	6 - 9 g
Tao Ren	Prunus	3 - 9 g
Hong Hua	Carthamus	3 - 6 g

Boils/carbuncles with pus and qi and blood deficiency. The pus stays trapped under the skin.

T   pale

P   weak

✗ Do not use during pregnancy.

TOU NONG SAN

Discharge Pus Powder

Huang Qi	Astragalus	15 g
Chuan Xiong	Ligusticum	3 - 9 g
Dang Gui	Angelica	6 - 9 g
Chuan Shan Jia	Manis	1 - 3 g
Zao Jiao Ci	Gleditsia	3 - 6 g

Blood deficiency causing constipation.

T   pale

P   weak, thin

WU REN WAN

Five-Seed Pill

Xing Ren	Prunus	9 - 20 g
Bai Zi Ren	Biota	3 - 6 g
Tao Ren	Prunus	9 - 15 g
Yu Li Ren	Prunus	3 - 6 g
Sha Ren	Amomum	3 - 6 g

Qi and blood deficiency with qi/blood and phlegm stagnation causing masses on the neck, breasts, or axilla areas.

T   pale or purple

P   weak or choppy

XIANG BEI YANG YING TANG

Cyperus and Fritillaria Decoction to Nourish the Nutritive Qi

Ren Shen	Panax	6 - 9 g
Bai Zhu	Atractylodes	3 - 6 g
Fu Ling	Poria	6 - 9 g
Chuan Xiong	Ligusticum	3 - 6 g
Chen Pi	Citrus	3 - 6 g
Dang Gui	Angelica	6 - 9 g
Xiang Fu	Cyperus	6 - 9 g
Shu Di Huang	Rehmannia	6 - 12 g
Bei Mu	Fritillaria	3 - 6 g
Bai Shao Yao	Paeonia	6 - 9 g
Jie Geng	Platycodon	3 - 6 g
Da Zao	Ziziphus	3 - 6 pc
Sheng Jiang	Zingiber	3 - 6 g
Gan Cao	Glycyrrhiza	1 - 3 g

Spleen

Blood deficiency with interior excess heat causing constipation; or blood stagnation with excess heat resulting in amenorrhea.

T   red or purple, yellow coat

P   rapid

✗   Do not use during pregnancy.

YU ZHU SAN

Jade Candle Powder

Chuan Xiong	Ligusticum	3 - 9 g
Shu Di Huang	Rehmannia	6 - 12 g
Dang Gui	Angelica	6 - 9 g
Bai Shao Yao	Paeonia	6 - 9 g
Da Huang	Rheum	6 - 9 g
Mang Xiao	Mirabilitum	3 - 6 g
Gan Cao	Glycyrrhiza	3 - 6 g

SPLEEN QI DEFICIENCY WITH DAMP

Please see under Jin Ye (Body Fluid) Disharmonies

SPLEEN YANG DEFICIENCY WITH COLD

- no appetite
- cold extremities
- sallow or pale complexion
- coldness and pain in the epigastrium
- watery stools with undigested food

T   pale, swollen, moist, teeth marks

P   deep, slow, weak

Spleen

Spleen yang deficiency with cold, qi, and blood stagnation causing epigastric or abdominal pain which is better with food.

T   pale, swollen, teethmarks, wet, light or dark purple

P   slow, frail

AN ZHONG SAN

Calm the Middle Powder

Extract Formula Name: Cardamon and Fennel Formula

Gui Zhi	Cinnamomum	3 - 9 g
Mu Li	Ostrea	3 - 9 g
Yan Hu Suo	Corydalis	6 - 9 g
Gao Liang Jiang	Alpinia	3 g
Xiao Hui Xiang	Foeniculum	3 - 9 g
Sha Ren	Amomum	3 g
Gan Cao	Glycyrrhiza	3 - 6 g
[Fu Ling	Poria	3-6 g]

Cold accumulation or yang deficiency in the abdomen leading to constipation with cramping pain. The qi stagnates and heats up which can cause a mild fever. Other symptoms include cold extremities and chills.

T   normal or pale, white coat

P   wiry or tight, deep

☞ Fu Zi - Aconitum should be powdered. Da Huang - Rheum should be added during the last 3 - 5 minutes of the decoction process.

✗ Do not use during pregnancy.

DA HUANG FU ZI TANG

Rhubarb and Aconite Decoction

Extract Formula Name: Rhubarb and Aconite Combination

Da Huang	Rheum	6 - 9 g
Fu Zi	Aconitum	6 g
Xi Xin	Asarum	3 - 6 g

Spleen yang deficiency with cold stagnation causing severe cramping pain, borborygmus, or possible vomiting.

T pale, light purple, swollen, moist white coat

P wiry or slow, deep

☞ Yi Tang - Saccharum Granorum is added to the strained tea.

DA JIAN ZHONG TANG

Major Construct the Middle Decoction

Extract Formula Name: Major Zanthoxylum Combination

Chuan Jiao	Zanthoxylum	3 - 6 g
Ren Shen	Panax	6 - 9 g
Gan Jiang	Zingiber	3 - 6 g
Yi Tang	Saccharum Granorum	20 g

Spleen/Kidney yang deficiency causing dawn diarrhea with middle jiao qi stagnation symptoms such as excruciating abdominal pain and severe fullness feelings.

T pale, swollen, teethmarks, light purple, white coat

P deep, weak, or slippery

DAN LIAO SI SHEN WAN

Four-Miracle Pill from the Tranquil Hut

Bu Gu Zhi	Psoralea	6 - 12 g
Xiao Hui Xiang	Foeniculum	3 - 9 g
Rou Dou Kou	Myristica	9 - 12 g
Mu Xiang	Saussurea	3 - 6 g

Spleen qi and blood deficiency with slight cold leading to spasm pain or post-partum emaciation.

T pale, white coat

P weak

☞ Yi Tang - Saccharum Granorum is added to the strained tea.

DANG GUI JIAN ZHONG TANG

Dang Gui Decoction to Construct the Middle

Extract Formula Name: Tang-Kuei, Cinnamon and Peony Combination

Yi Tang	Saccharum Granorum	6 - 20 g
Gui Zhi	Cinnamomum	3 - 9 g
Bai Shao Yao	Paeonia	6 - 9 g
Sheng Jiang	Zingiber	3 - 6 g
Da Zao	Ziziphus	3 - 6 pc
Gan Cao	Glycyrrhiza	3 - 6 g
Dang Gui	Angelica	6 - 9 g

Longstanding cold with blood and yang deficiency leading to diarrhea, nausea and vomiting, or abdominal cramps.

T pale, swollen, teethmarks, wet, white coat

P slow, frail

DANG GUI SI NI JIA WU ZHU YU SHENG JIANG TANG

Dang Gui Decoction for Frigid Extremities plus Evodia and Fresh Ginger

Extract Formula Name: Tang-Kuei, Evodia and Ginger Combination

Dang Gui	Angelica	6 - 9 g
Gui Zhi	Cinnamomum	3 - 9 g
Xi Xin	Asarum	3 - 6 g
Bai Shao Yao	Paeonia	6 - 9 g
Mu Tong	Akebia	6 - 9 g
Wu Zhu Yu	Evodia	3 - 6 g
Da Zao	Ziziphus	25 pc
Sheng Jiang	Zingiber	4 pc
Gan Cao	Glycyrrhiza	3 - 6 g

Blood and yin deficient patient with cold evil qi which leads to obstruction of the channels which causes pain. This is known as jueyin syndrome in which the patient feels cold subjectively but not to the touch. Raynaud's disease.

T pale, white coat

P deep, thin, or minute

DANG GUI SI NI TANG

Dang Gui Decoction for Frigid Extremities

Extract Formula Name: Tang-Kuei and Jujube Combination

Dang Gui	Angelica	6 - 12 g
Gui Zhi	Cinnamomum	3 - 9 g
Bai Shao Yao	Paeonia	6 - 9 g
Mu Tong	Akebia	6 - 9 g
Xi Xin	Asarum	3 - 6 g
Da Zao	Ziziphus	3 - 5 pc
Gan Cao	Glycyrrhiza	3 - 6 g

Spleen/Stomach qi yang deficiency resulting in hiccups, belching, and vomiting, and symptoms of coldness in the middle jiao.

T   pale, thin coat

P   weak, deep, maybe slow

✗   Contraindicated during pregnancy

DING XIANG SHI DI TANG

Clove and Kaki Decoction

Extract Formula Name: Clove and Kaki Combination

Ding Xiang	Eugenia	6 - 9 g
Shi Di	Diospyros	6 - 9 g
Ren Shen	Panax	3 - 9 g
Sheng Jiang	Zingiber	3 - 6 g

Spleen yang deficiency with a painful abdomen and watery vomiting.

T   pale, swollen, teethmarks, white coat

P   weak, deep, slow

DING YU LI ZHONG TANG

Clove and Evodia Decoction to Regulate the Middle

Ren Shen	Panax	6 - 9 g
Bai Zhu	Atractylodes	3 - 9 g
Gan Jiang	Zingiber	3 - 9 g
Wu Zhu Yu	Evodia	3 - 9 g
Ding Xiang	Eugenia	3 - 9 g
Zhi Gan Gao	Glycyrrhiza	3 - 6 g

Stomach/Spleen yang deficiency causing watery diarrhea and epigastric pain. Severe cold symptoms such as cold limbs and vomiting of clear fluids.

T   pale, swollen, teethmarks, white coat

P   minute

✪   Major Formula

FU ZI LI ZHONG WAN

Prepared Aconite Pill to Regulate the Middle

Extract Formula Name: Aconite, Ginseng, and Ginger Combination

Fu Zi	Aconitum	6 - 9 g
Ren Shen	Panax	3 - 9 g
Bai Zhu	Atractylodes	3 - 9 g
Gan Jiang	Zingiber	3 - 9 g
Zhi Gan Cao	Glycyrrhiza	3 - 6 g

Stomach and Spleen yang deficiency with wei qi deficiency
and internal heat and damp.
Symtoms include loose stools,
sweating, or cold hands and
feet.

T   pale or red, white or yellow
sticky coat

P   deep, weak, thin, or rapid

✗   Caution during pregnancy.

FU ZI XIE XIN TANG

Aconite Decoction to Drain the Epigastrium

Fu Zi	Aconitum	3 - 6 g
Da Huang	Rheum	6 - 9 g
Huang Qin	Scutellaria	3 - 6 g
Huang Lian	Coptis	3 - 6 g

Spleen/Stomach qi deficiency
and cold causing vomiting during pregnancy.

T   pale, thin white coat

P   weak

**GAN JIANG REN SHEN BAN XIA
WAN**

Ginger, Ginseng, and Pinellia Pill

Extract Formula Name: G.P. and Ginseng Formula

Gan Jiang	Zingiber	3 g
Ren Shen	Panax	3 g
Ban Xia	Pinellia	6 g
[Sheng Jiang	Zingiber	1 - 3 g]

Cold in the middle jiao resulting
in loose stools or watery non-
odorous diarrhea, cold extremities, or a desire for warm
drinks.

T   pale, light purple, thin white
or wet coat

P   slow, weak, or tight

GAO LIANG JIANG WAN

Galanga Pill

Gao Liang Jiang	Alpinia	3 - 6 g
Bi Ba	Piper	3 - 9 g

Spleen

Spleen/Kidney yang deficiency causing watery diarrhea with undigested food, spasms in hands and feet, fatigue, and spontanous severe sweating.

T pale, swollen, teethmarks, wet, white coat

P minute

GU ZHEN TANG

Stabilize the True Decoction

Fu Zi	Aconitum	6 - 9 g
Ren Shen	Panax	6 - 9 g
Bai Zhu	Atractylodes	6 - 9 g
Fu Ling	Poria	6 - 9 g
Huang Qi	Astragalus	6 - 15 g
Shan Yao	Dioscorea	6 - 9 g
Rou Gui	Cinnamomum	3 - 9 g
Gan Cao	Glycyrrhiza	3 - 6 g
[Sheng Jiang	Zingiber	3 - 6 g]
[Da Zao	Ziziphus	1 - 2 pc]

Severe cold stagnation with Spleen/Kidney yang deficiency causing coldness in the face, cramping pain in the center, or dawn diarrhea.

T pale, purple, wet coat

P slow, tight

GUI FU LI ZHONG WAN

Cinnamon and Prepared Aconite Decoction to Regulate the Middle

Ren Shen	Panax	10 - 15 g
Bai Zhu	Atractylodes	6 - 9 g
Gan Jiang	Zingiber	6 - 9 g
Gan Cao	Glycyrrhiza	3 - 6 g
Fu Zi	Aconitum	3 - 6 g
Gui Zhi	Cinnamomum	3 - 9 g

Spleen

Wei qi deficiency (defensive qi) due to Spleen qi/yang deficiency with qi stagnation symptoms. The patient experiences frequent colds or abdominal fullness.

T pale, maybe light purple

P weak

GUI ZHI LI ZHONG WAN

Cinnamon Twig with Regulate the Middle Pill

Gui Zhi	Cinnamomum	3 - 9 g
Gan Jiang	Zingiber	3 - 6 g
Bai Zhu	Atractylodes	6 - 9 g
Ren Shen	Panax	6 - 12 g
Gan Cao	Glycyrrhiza	3 - 6 g

Cold in the Spleen/Stomach after ingestion of cold food with damp and qi stagnation in the center. Symptoms include lack of appetite, loose stools, or nausea and vomiting.

T pale, sticky white coat

P weak, deep, or tight

HOU PO WEN ZHONG TANG

Magnolia Bark Decoction for Warming the Middle

Extract Formula Name: Magnolia and Saussurea Combination

Hou Po	Magnolia	30 g
Gan Jiang	Zingiber	2 g
Mu Xiang	Saussurea	15 g
Chen Pi	Citrus	30 g
Fu Ling	Poria	15 g
Cao Dou Kou	Alpinia	15 g
Zhi Gan Cao	Glycyrrhiza	15 g
[Sheng Jiang	Zingiber	3 g]

Upper jiao heat with middle jiao cold usually caused by cold food which restricts Spleen qi. This leads to damp which then turns to heat. The heat rises upward and bothers the Heart causing thirst, restlessness, full/cold abdomen with pain, or nausea and vomiting.

T red or pale, red tip, thin sticky coat

P rapid, wiry

HUANG LIAN TANG

Coptis Decoction

Extract Formula Name: Coptis Combination

Huang Lian	Coptis	5 g
Gan Jiang	Zingiber	5 g
Gui Zhi	Cinnamomum	5 g
Ren Shen	Panax	3 g
Ban Xia	Pinellia	9 g
Da Zao	Ziziphus	9 - 12 pc
Gan Cao	Glycyrrhiza	6 g

Qi/yang/blood deficiency with bleeding where the Spleen is not governing blood causing melena, hematemesis, or uterine bleeding which is pale in color.

T pale, thin white coat

P deep, thin, weak

☞ Fu Long Gan - Terra Flava Usta should be cooked 30 minutes prior to adding the remaining herbs. E Jiao - Equus should be added to the strained tea.

HUANG TU TANG

Yellow Earth Decoction

Extract Formula Name: Fu-lung-kan Combination

Fu Long Gan	Terra Flava Usta	30 g
E Jiao	Equus	9 g
Sheng Di Huang	Rehmannia	9 g
Fu Zi	Aconitum	9 g
Huang Qin	Scutellaria	9 g
Bai Zhu	Atractylodes	9 g
Gan Cao	Glycyrrhiza	9 g

Kidney and Spleen yang deficiency with cold which has invaded all three yin channels (taiyin, shaoyin, and jueyin). Symptoms include shivering from cold, icy limbs and face, watery diarrhea, or cough with profuse saliva production.

T   pale, wet, thin white moist coat

P   minute or frail

☞ Remove She Xiang - Moschus, decoct the rest of the formula as usual, then add powdered Moschus to each dosage.

HUI YANG JIU JI TANG

Restore and Revive the Yang Decoction

Fu Zi	Aconitum	9 g
Rou Gui	Cinnamomum	3 - 6 g
Ren Shen	Panax	6 - 9 g
Gan Jiang	Zingiber	3 - 6 g
Fu Ling	Poria	6 - 9 g
Chen Pi	Citrus	3 - 6 g
Bai Zhu	Atractylodes	6 - 9 g
Wu Wei Zi	Schisandra	3 - 6 g
Ban Xia	Pinellia	6 - 9 g
Gan Cao	Glycyrrhiza	3 - 6 g
She Xiang	Moschus	0.3 g
[Sheng Jiang	Zingiber	1 - 3 g]

Spleen yang deficiency with cold and phlegm. Cough or vomiting with clear sputum, and decreased appetite.

T   pale, moist white coat

P   deep, slow, slippery

LI ZHONG HUA TAN WAN

Regulate the Middle and Transform Phlegm Pill

Ren Shen	Panax	6 - 9 g
Fu Ling	Poria	6 - 9 g
Bai Zhu	Atractylodes	3 - 9 g
Gan Jiang	Zingiber	3 - 9 g
Ban Xia	Pinellia	6 - 9 g
Gan Cao	Glycyrrhiza	3 - 6 g

Middle jiao qi/yang deficiency resulting in loss of appetite, absence of thirst, watery diarrhea with undigested food, or cold or painful limbs.

T   pale, swollen, teethmarks, white coat

P   deep, weak

✪ **Major Formula**

LI ZHONG WAN

Regulate the Middle Pill

Extract Formula Name: Ginseng and Ginger Combination

Ren Shen	Panax	6 - 9 g
Gan Jiang	Zingiber	6 - 9 g
Bai Zhu	Atractylodes	6 - 9 g
Gan Cao	Glycyrrhiza	3 - 6 g

Liver qi stagnation with cold in the Stomach causing abdominal pain which is relieved by warmth. The Formula is also useful for dysmenorrhea.

T   pale, white coat

P   weak, slow, or wiry

LIANG FU WAN

Galanga and Cyperus Pill

Extract Formula Name: Galanga and Cyperus Formula

Gao Liang Jiang	Alpinia	6 - 9 g
Xiang Fu	Cyperus	6 - 9 g

Watery fluids in the Lungs and Spleen yang deficiency causing cough, wheezing, and a stuffy sensation in the chest.

T   pale, sticky or slippery white coat

P   slippery, wiry

LING GAN WU WEI JIANG XIN TANG

Poria, Licorice, Schisandra, Ginger, and Asarum Decoction

Fu Ling	Poria	6 - 12 g
Gan Cao	Glycyrrhiza	3 - 9 g
Wu Wei Zi	Schisandra	6 - 9 g
Gan Jiang	Zingiber	3 - 9 g
Xi Xin	Asarum	6 - 9 g

Spleen/Stomach yang defi-
ciency causing phlegm accumulation which affects the Lungs;
or taiyang disease was mistreated and guided into the
Spleen leading to water accumulation. Symptoms include
dyspnea, clear phlegm expectoration, and fullness in the chest
and flanks.

T pale, slippery white coat

P slippery, weak, deep

LING GUI ZHU GAN TANG

Poria, Cinnamon Twig, Atractylodes,
and Licorice Decoction

Extract Formula Name: Hoelen and
Atractylodes Combination

Fu Ling	Poria	6 - 12 g
Gui Zhi	Cinnamomum	3 - 9 g
Bai Zhu	Atractylodes	6 - 9 g
Gan Cao	Glycyrrhiza	3 - 6 g

Sudden cold stagnation and
cold food obstructing the Stomach and Large Intestines completely. This causes sudden,
severe pain and bowel obstruction.

T pale

P tight, deep

☞ The herbs should be powdered
and adults should take 1 g doses
with warm water.

✗ Ba Dou - Croton is a toxic herb
that should be used with extreme
caution. Do not use during pregnancy.

SAN WU BEI JI WAN

Three-Substance Pill for Emergencies

Extract Formula Name: Rhubarb, Ginger and Croton Formula

Da Huang	Rheum	30 g
Ba Dou	Croton	30 g
Gan Jiang	Zingiber	30 g

Severe qi deficiency with yang
and blood deficiency and cold
symptoms. Irregular menstruation with a pale and watery
flow, dizziness, pale or sallow
face, cold limbs, or chills.

T pale, wet, thin white coat

P deep, weak, thready

SHAN HE YIN

Mountain and River Decoction

Shu Di Huang	Rehmannia	15 - 25 g
Dang Gui	Angelica	6 - 9 g
Bai Shao Yao	Paeonia	6 - 9 g
Chuan Xiong	Ligusticum	3 - 9 g
Rou Gui	Cinnamomum	3 - 9 g
Huang Qi	Astragalus	6 - 15 g

Spleen/Kidney qi and yang deficiency causing edema which manifests mostly in the lower body. Other symptoms include cold limbs, poor appetite, decreased urination, or heaviness.

T   pale, sticky coat

P   deep, slow, maybe thin

SHI PI YIN

Bolster the Spleen Decoction

Extract Brion Name: Magnolia and Atractylodes Combination

Fu Zi	Aconitum	6 - 9 g
Bai Zhu	Atractylodes	6 - 9 g
Mu Gua	Chaenomeles	6 - 9 g
Hou Po	Magnolia	6 - 12 g
Gan Jiang	Zingiber	6 - 9 g
Mu Xiang	Saussurea	6 - 9 g
Fu Ling	Poria	6 - 9 g
Da Fu Pi	Areca	3 - 6 g
Cao Guo	Amomum	3 - 6 g
Zhi Gan Cao	Glycyrrhiza	3 - 6 g
[Da Zao	Ziziphus	1 - 3 pc]
[Sheng Jiang	Zingiber	3 - 6 g]

Exterior cold has gone internally. qi and yang are very weak and Kidney/Spleen yang have been damaged. Symptoms include low blood pressure, cold limbs, shock, or sweating.

T   pale, or purple, moist white coat

P   minute

☞ The raw type of Aconite is used here since it is much warmer than the prepared kind. 6 - 12 g of honey are often added for detoxification. Fu Zi - Aconitum is soaked in 8 - 10 cups of boiling water for 30 minutes to one hour. The remaining herbs should be added during the last 25 minutes and decocted as usual.

✗ Fu Zi - Aconitum in its raw form is toxic and is intended for short-term use only.

SI NI TANG

Frigid Extremities Decoction

Extract Formula Name: Aconite, Ginger and Licorice Combination

Fu Zi	Aconitum	9 - 15 g
Gan Jiang	Zingiber	6 - 12 g
Zhi Gan Cao	Glycyrrhiza	3 - 6 g

Spleen

Kidney/Spleen yang deficiency leading to dawn diarrhea.

T pale, white coat

P deep, weak, slow

SI SHEN WAN

Four-Miracle Pill

Extract Formula Name: Psoralea and Myristica Formula

Bu Gu Zhi	Psoralea	12 - 18 g
Rou Dou Kou	Myristica	6 - 9 g
Wu Zhu Yu	Evodia	3 - 6 g
Wu Wei Zi	Schisandra	6 - 9 g
[Sheng Jiang	Zingiber	3 - 6 g]
[Da Zao	Ziziphus	3 - 5 pc]

Kidney and Spleen yang deficiency which developed after a chronic damp heat dysentery causing damp cold. This obstructs the Large Intestines, manifesting as dark blood in the stools with pus.

T pale

P minute

☞ Ingredients should be ground into a powder.

TAO HUA TANG

Peach Blossom Decoction

Extract Formula Name: Kaolin and Oryza Combination

Chi Shi Zhi	Halloysitum Rubrum	20 - 30 g
Jing Mi	Oryza	20 - 30 g
Gan Jiang	Zingiber	6 - 9 g

Spleen yang deficiency causing constipation or diarrhea with pain. Dysentery with pus or blood.

T pale, swollen, teethmarks, white coat

P deep, weak, thin, or wiry

☞ Da Huang - Rheum should be added during the last 3 - 5 minutes of the decoction process.

✘ Do not use during pregnancy.

WEN PI TANG

Warm the Spleen Decoction

Da Huang	Rheum	6 - 12 g
Gan Jiang	Zingiber	3 - 9 g
Ren Shen	Panax	6 - 9 g
Fu Zi	Aconitum	6 - 9 g
Gan Cao	Glycyrrhiza	3 - 9 g

Spleen qi deficiency with cold which restricts the Liver and Stomach. This results in tight abdominal pain, cold in the middle and lower jiao, vomiting, or acid regurgitation; or cold causes vertex headaches via the Liver channel. This Liver qi stagnation is not due to emotional reasons but is caused by cold.

T pale, purplish, moist white coat

P slow, or wiry, thin

WU ZHU YU TANG

Evodia Decoction

Extract Formula Name: Evodia Combination

Wu Zhu Yu	Evodia	3 - 6 g
Ren Shen	Panax	6 - 9 g
Sheng Jiang	Zingiber	12 - 20 g
Da Zao	Ziziphus	6 - 12 pc

Spleen qi and yang deficiency with damp and water accumulation causing loose stools with undigested food.

T pale, swollen, teethmarks, white sticky coat

P weak, deep, or frail

XIAO BAN XIA TANG

Minor Pinellia Decoction

Ban Xia	Pinellia	6 - 9 g
Sheng Jiang	Zingiber	3 - 6 g

---

1. Chronic Spleen qi deficiency with chronic cold evil qi leading to qi and blood deficiency. The main symptom is abdominal spasms. 2. Liver qi stagnation or Liver overacting on Spleen. In the latter two instances the dosage of 'Bai Shao Yao - Paeonia' should be increased.

T pale or light purple, thin white coat

P weak or slightly wiry

☞ Yi Tang - Saccharum Granorum should be added to the strained tea.

XIAO JIAN ZHONG TANG

Minor Construct the Middle Decoction

Extract Formula Name: Minor Cinnamon and Peony Combination

Yi Tang	Saccharum Granorum	15 - 30 g
Gui Zhi	Cinnamomum	3 - 9 g
Bai Shao Yao	Paeonia	6 - 9 g
Sheng Jiang	Zingiber	6 - 9 g
Da Zao	Ziziphus	3 - 5 pc
Zhi Gan Cao	Glycyrrhiza	3 - 6 g

Cold damp has entered the Spleen leading to water accumulation and Spleen yang deficiency. This causes damp in the middle jiao which bothers the Gallbladder so the bile cannot circulate properly. This manifests as yin-type jaundice.

T   pale, white coat

P   weak, deep

YIN CHEN ZHU FU TANG

Artemisia Yinchenhao, Atractylodes and Prepared Aconite Decoction

Extract Formula Name: Capillaris, Atractylodes and Aconite Combination

Yin Chen Hao	Artemisia	3 - 6 g
Gan Jiang	Zingiber	3 - 6 g
Bai Zhu	Atractylodes	6 - 9 g
Rou Gui	Cinnamomum	1 - 3 g
Fu Zi	Aconitum	1 - 3 g
Zhi Gan Cao	Glycyrrhiza	3 - 6 g

Chronic diarrhea has depleted Spleen and Kidney yang causing prolapse of the rectum or bowel incontinence.

T   pale, white coat

P   deep, slow

ZHEN REN YANG ZANG TANG

True Man's Decoction to Nourish the Organs

Ren Shen	Panax	6 - 9 g
Rou Gui	Cinnamomum	3 g
Bai Zhu	Atractylodes	6 - 12 g
He Zi	Terminalia	6 - 9 g
Rou Dou Kou	Myristica	9 - 12 g
Ying Su Ke	Papaver	6 - 15 g
Mu Xiang	Saussurea	3 - 9 g
Dang Gui	Angelica	6 - 15 g
Bai Shao Yao	Paeonia	9 - 12 g
Zhi Gan Cao	Glycyrrhiza	3- 6 g

Spleen/Kidney qi and yang deficient patient suffers easily from wind cold with internal water accumulation, or experiences urinary difficulty, diarrhea, or edema.

T pale, swollen, teethmarks, moist, thin white coat

P frail or minute

ZHEN WU TANG

True Warrior Decoction

Extract Formula Name: Vitality Combination

Fu Zi	Aconitum	6 - 9 g
Bai Zhu	Atractylodes	6 - 9 g
Bai Shao Yao	Paeonia	6 - 9 g
Fu Ling	Poria	6 - 9 g
Sheng Jiang	Zingiber	6 - 9 g

Spleen yang deficiency with middle jiao qi stagnation causing fullness and distention.

T pale, light purple, swollen, teethmarks, white coat

P weak, deep

ZHI SHI LI ZHONG WAN

Immature Bitter Orange Pill to Regulate the Middle

Zhi Shi	Citrus	6 - 9 g
Ren Shen	Panax	6 - 9 g
Gan Jiang	Zingiber	3 - 9 g
Bai Zhu	Atractylodes	6 - 9 g
Fu Ling	Poria	6 - 9 g
Gan Cao	Glycyrrhiza	3 - 6 g

Joint pain due to cold damp and Spleen yang deficiency.

T pale, sticky white coat

P deep, slippery, thin

☞ Grind herbs into a powder and administer as a draft with 4 - 8 pieces of Sheng Jiang - Zingiber.

ZHU FU TANG

Atractylodes and Prepared Aconite Decoction

Bai Zhu	Atractylodes	90 - 120 g
Fu Zi	Aconitum	30 - 45 g
Gan Cao	Glycyrrhiza	30 - 45 g
[Sheng Jiang	Zingiber	4 - 8 pc]

SPLEEN QI SINKING

- bearing down sensation
- prolapses of any kind

T pale

P weak

Spleen/Stomach qi deficiency where the Spleen qi is sinking, or the Spleen is not governing the blood. qi deficiency can lead to (morning) fever, early periods, weakness, diarrhea, or pallor.

T pale, swollen, teethmarks, thin white coat

P weak

✪ **Major Formula**

BU ZHONG YI QI TANG

Tonify the Middle and Augment the Qi Decoction

Extract Formula Name: Ginseng and Astragalus Combination

Ren Shen	Panax	6 - 12 g
Huang Qi	Astragalus	9 - 15 g
Dang Gui	Angelica	6 - 9 g
Chen Pi	Citrus	3 - 6 g
Sheng Ma	Cimicifuga	3 - 6 g
Chai Hu	Bupleurum	3 - 9 g
Bai Zhu	Atractylodes	3 - 9 g
Zhi Gan Cao	Glycyrrhiza	3 - 6 g

Kidney yin and Spleen qi/blood deficiency causing uterine prolapse with low back pain, night urination, or hearing loss and tinnitus.

T red or pale

P frail

DA BU YUAN JIAN

Great Tonify the Basal Decoction

Ren Shen	Panax	6 - 12 g
Shu Di Huang	Rehmannia	9 - 25 g
Shan Yao	Dioscorea	6 - 9 g
Shan Zhu Yu	Cornus	3 - 6 g
Gou Qi Zi	Lycium	6 - 9 g
Dang Gui	Angelica	6 - 9 g
Du Zhong	Eucommia	6 - 9 g
Gan Cao	Glycyrrhiza	3 - 6 g

Spleen qi deficiency during pregnancy with lethargy, spotting, or low back pain.

T   pale, swollen, teethmarks, thin white coat

P   weak, thin

☞ E Jiao - Equus should be added at the end to the strained tea.

JIA JIAN BU ZHONG YI QI TANG

Modified Tonify the Middle and Augment the Qi Decoction

Ren Shen	Panax	6 - 9 g
Huang Qi	Astragalus	6 - 12 g
Chen Pi	Citrus	3 - 6 g
Bai Zhu	Atractylodes	3 - 9 g
Sheng Ma	Cimicifuga	3 - 6 g
Chai Hu	Bupleurum	3 - 9 g
E Jiao	Equus	3 - 9 g
Ai Ye	Artemisia	3 - 9 g
Gan Cao	Glycyrrhiza	3 - 6 g

Spleen qi deficiency causing severe uterine bleeding which is pale in color, or early or irregular periods. The Spleen qi is sinking causing a restless fetus.

T   pale, swollen, teethmarks, thin white coat

P   weak

JU YUAN JIAN

Lift the Source Decoction

Ren Shen	Panax	6 - 9 g
Huang Qi	Astragalus	9 - 12 g
Sheng Ma	Cimicifuga	3 - 6 g
Bai Zhu	Atractylodes	3 - 6 g
Gan Cao	Glycyrrhiza	3 - 6 g

Spleen qi deficiency with qi sinking in the chest causing shortness of breath, dyspnea, or loose stools.

T   pale, thin white coat

P   deep, weak

SHENG XIAN TANG

Raise the Sinking Decoction

Huang Qi	Astragalus	15 - 20 g
Sheng Ma	Cimicifuga	3 - 6 g
Zhi Mu	Anemarrhena	6 - 9 g
Chai Hu	Bupleurum	3 - 9 g
Jie Geng	Platycodon	3 - 6 g

Chronic diarrhea has depleted Spleen and Kidney yang causing prolapse of the rectum or bowel incontinence.

T   pale, white coat

P   deep, slow

ZHEN REN YANG ZANG TANG

True Man's Decoction to Nourish the Organs

Ren Shen	Panax	6 - 9 g
Rou Gui	Cinnamomum	3 g
Bai Zhu	Atractylodes	6 - 12 g
He Zi	Terminalia	6 - 9 g
Rou Dou Kou	Myristica	9 - 12 g
Ying Su Ke	Papaver	6 - 15 g
Mu Xiang	Saussurea	3 - 9 g
Dang Gui	Angelica	6 - 15 g
Bai Shao Yao	Paeonia	9 - 12 g
Zhi Gan Cao	Glycyrrhiza	3- 6 g

SPLEEN NOT CONTROLLING THE BLOOD

- bleeding under the skin (purpura)
- uterine bleeding
- bruising

T   pale

P   weak, thin

Spleen is cold and deficient, and fails to govern the blood. This leads to bleeding in the upper body. Liver yang rising symptoms usually accompany this symptom picture.

T   pale, thin white coat

P   slow, weak

BAI YE TANG

Biota Twig Decoction

Ce Bai Ye	Biota	6 - 9 g
Pao Jiang	Zingiber	6 - 9 g
Ai Ye	Artemisia	9 - 15 g

Spleen/Stomach qi deficiency where the Spleen qi is sinking, or the Spleen is not governing the blood. Qi deficiency can lead to (morning) fever, early periods, weakness, diarrhea, or pallor.

T pale, swollen, teethmarks, thin white coat

P weak

BU ZHONG YI QI TANG

Tonify the Middle and Augment the Qi Decoction

Extract Formula Name: Ginseng and Astragalus Combination

Ren Shen	Panax	6 - 12 g
Huang Qi	Astragalus	9 - 15 g
Dang Gui	Angelica	6 - 9 g
Chen Pi	Citrus	3 - 6 g
Sheng Ma	Cimicifuga	3 - 6 g
Chai Hu	Bupleurum	3 - 9 g
Bai Zhu	Atractylodes	3 - 9 g
Zhi Gan Cao	Glycyrrhiza	3 - 6 g

Qi/blood deficiency with bleeding, fever, heat feelings in the muscles, thirst with a desire for warm liquids, or irregular periods.

T pale, thin coat

P empty

DANG GUI BU XUE TANG

Dang Gui Decoction to Tonify the Blood

Extract Formula Name: Tang-Kuei and Astragalus Combination

Huang Qi	Astragalus	30 g
Dang Gui	Angelica	6 g

Spleen qi deficiency leading to uncontrolled menstrual bleeding which is pale and watery (ben lou syndrome).

T pale, swollen, teethmarks, thin coat

P hollow or thin, deep, weak

GU BEN ZHI BENG TANG

Stabilize the Root and Stop Excessive Uterine Bleeding Decoction

Shu Di Huang	Rehmannia	6 - 20 g
Bai Zhu	Atractylodes	6 - 15 g
Huang Qi	Astragalus	6 - 15 g
Dang Gui	Angelica	6 - 9 g
Ren Shen	Panax	6 - 9 g
Pao Jiang	Zingiber	3 - 6 g

Heart blood and yin deficiency with Spleen qi deficiency leading to insomnia, decreased appetite, nightmares, irregular periods in women, or uterine bleeding which may manifest as ben lou - gushing or spotting; This formula is also useful for purpura due to Spleen qi/blood deficiency.

T   pale, swollen, teethmarks, thin white coat

P   weak, thin

✪ Major Formula

GUI PI TANG

Restore the Spleen Decoction

Extract Formula Name: Ginseng and Longan Combination

Ren Shen	Panax	6 - 9 g
Huang Qi	Astralagus	9 - 12 g
Fu Shen	Poria	6 - 9 g
Bai Zhu	Atractylodes	9 - 12 g
Long Yan Rou	Euphoria	9 - 12 g
Mu Xiang	Saussurea	3 - 6 g
Suan Zao Ren	Zizyphus	9 - 12 g
Dang Gui	Angelica	6 - 9 g
Yuan Zhi	Polygala	3 - 6 g
Gan Cao	Glycyrrhiza	3 - 6 g

Qi/yang/blood deficiency with bleeding where the Spleen is not governing blood causing melena, hematemesis, or uterine bleeding which is pale in color.

T   pale, thin white coat

P   deep, thin, weak

☞ Fu Long Gan - Terra Flava Usta should be cooked 30 minutes prior to adding the remaining herbs. E Jiao - Equus should be added to the strained tea.

HUANG TU TANG

Yellow Earth Decoction

Extract Formula Name: Fu-lung-kan Combination

Fu Long Gan	Terra Flava Usta	30 g
E Jiao	Equus	9 g
Sheng Di Huang	Rehmannia	9 g
Fu Zi	Aconitum	9 g
Huang Qin	Scutellaria	9 g
Bai Zhu	Atractylodes	9 g
Gan Cao	Glycyrrhiza	9 g

Spleen qi deficiency during pregnancy with lethargy, spotting, or low back pain.

T pale, swollen, teethmarks, thin white coat

P weak, thin

☞ E Jiao - Equus should be added at the end to the strained tea.

JIA JIAN BU ZHONG YI QI TANG

Modified Tonify the Middle and Augment the Qi Decoction

Ren Shen	Panax	6 - 9 g
Huang Qi	Astragalus	6 - 12 g
Chen Pi	Citrus	3 - 6 g
Bai Zhu	Atractylodes	3 - 9 g
Sheng Ma	Cimicifuga	3 - 6 g
Chai Hu	Bupleurum	3 - 9 g
E Jiao	Equus	3 - 9 g
Ai Ye	Artemisia	3 - 9 g
Gan Cao	Glycyrrhiza	3 - 6 g

Spleen qi deficiency causing severe uterine bleeding which is pale in color, or early or irregular periods. The Spleen qi is sinking causing a restless fetus.

T pale, swollen, teethmarks, thin white coat

P weak

JU YUAN JIAN

Lift the Source Decoction

Ren Shen	Panax	6 - 9 g
Huang Qi	Astragalus	9 - 12 g
Sheng Ma	Cimicifuga	3 - 6 g
Bai Zhu	Atractylodes	3 - 6 g
Gan Cao	Glycyrrhiza	3 - 6 g

STOMACH DISHARMONIES

Stomach

STOMACH AND SPLEEN QI DEFICIENCY

- epigastric discomfort
- hiccups or nausea
- decreased appetite
- loose stools

T pale

P weak

Spleen/Stomach qi yang deficiency resulting in hiccups, belching, and vomiting, and symptoms of coldness in the middle jiao.

T pale, thin coat

P weak, deep, maybe slow

✗ Contraindicated during pregnancy

DING XIANG SHI DI TANG

Clove and Kaki Decoction

Extract Formula Name: Clove and Kaki Combination

Ding Xiang	Eugenia	6 - 9 g
Shi Di	Diospyros	6 - 9 g
Ren Shen	Panax	3 - 9 g
Sheng Jiang	Zingiber	3 - 6 g

Heat and cold in the middle jiao with Spleen/Stomach qi deficiency, and cold predominance. The patient experiences mild middle jiao qi stagnation symptoms such as fullness or bloating.

T   thin yellow coat

P   weak, slightly wiry

GAN CAO XIE XIN TANG

Licorice Decoction to Drain the Epigastrium

Extract Formula Name: Pinellia and Licorice Combination

Ban Xia	Pinellia	6 - 9 g
Huang Qin	Scutellaria	9 - 12 g
Zhi Gan Cao	Glycyrrhiza	12 - 15 g
Gan Jiang	Zingiber	9 - 12 g
Ren Shen	Panax	9 - 12 g
Huang Lian	Coptis	3 - 6 g
Da Zao	Ziziphus	9 - 15 pc

Spleen/Stomach qi deficiency and cold causing vomiting during pregnancy.

T   pale, thin white coat

P   weak

GAN JIANG REN SHEN BAN XIA WAN

Ginger, Ginseng, and Pinellia Pill

Extract Formula Name: G.P. and Ginseng Formula

Gan Jiang	Zingiber	3 g
Ren Shen	Panax	3 g
Ban Xia	Pinellia	6 g
[Sheng Jiang	Zingiber	1 - 3 g]

Spleen/Stomach qi deficiency with cold and wei (defensive) qi deficiency; also useful for peptic ulcers and chronic allergies. Other symptoms include poor appetite or spontaneous sweating.

T pale, thin white coat

P weak, slow, thin, wiry

☞ Yi Tang - Saccharum Granorum is added to the strained tea.

HUANG QI JIAN ZHONG TANG

Astragalus Decoction to Construct the Middle

Extract Formula Name: Astragalus Combination

Gui Zhi	Cinnamomum	9 g
Bai Shao Yao	Paeonia	18 g
Sheng Jiang	Zingiber	10 g
Da Zao	Ziziphus	3 - 6 pc
Gan Cao	Glycyrrhiza	6 g
Yi Tang	Saccharum Granorum	30 g
Huang Qi	Astragalus	9 g

Heat in the Stomach with qi and yin deficiency and rebellious Stomach qi causing thirst, vomiting, loss of appetite, nausea, or hiccups.

T red

P thin, rapid, weak

JU PI ZHU RU TANG I

Tangerine Peel and Bamboo Shaving Decoction

Extract Formula Name: Aurantium and Bamboo Combination

Chen Pi	Citrus	6 - 12 g
Ren Shen	Panax	6 - 9 g
Zhu Ru	Bambusa	6 - 12 g
Da Zao	Ziziphus	3 - 6 pc
Sheng Jiang	Zingiber	3 - 9 g
Gan Cao	Glycyrrhiza	3 - 6 g

Wind heat invading the intestines and damaging the Spleen and Stomach qi. Severe constipation with blood deficiency which may lead to wind, or blood stagnation.

T pale or purple

P thin or choppy

RUN CHANG WAN II

Moisten the Intestines Pill from Discussion of the Spleen and Stomach

Da Huang	Rheum	9 - 12 g
Tao Ren	Prunus	15 - 25 g
Huo Ma Ren	Cannabis	15 - 30 g
Dang Gui Wei	Angelica	6 - 12 g
Qiang Huo	Notopterygium	6 - 9 g

Lung/Stomach qi deficiency with cough, expectoration of clear sputum, dry mouth, or thirst.

T pale, moist coat

P weak

SHENG JIANG GAN CAO TANG

Ginger and Licorice Decoction

Sheng Jiang	Zingiber	6 - 12 g
Ren Shen	Panax	6 - 9 g
Da Zao	Ziziphus	3 - 9 pc
Gan Cao	Glycyrrhiza	6 - 12 g

Stomach/Spleen qi deficiency. This is the basic prescription for building qi. Symptoms include poor appetite, loose bowel movements, or lethergy.

T pale, thin white coat

P weak, deep

✪ Major Formula

SI JUN ZI TANG

Four-Gentlemen Decoction

Extract Formula Name: Four Major Herbs Combination

Ren Shen	Panax	6 - 9 g
Bai Zhu	Atractylodes	3 - 9 g
Fu Ling	Poria	6 - 9 g
Gan Cao	Glycyrrhiza	3 - 6 g

Phlegm accumulation with Stomach qi deficiency causing hiccups, fullness, or nausea and vomiting.

T pale, white sticky coat

P frail, slippery, or wiry

☞ Xuan Fu Hua - Inula should be wrapped in a cheese cloth for decoction.

XUAN FU DAI ZHE TANG

Inula and Hematite Decoction

Extract Formula Name: Inula and Hematite Combination

Xuan Fu Hua	Inula	6 - 9 g
Dai Zhe Shi	Haematitum	6 - 12 g
Ren Shen	Panax	6 - 9 g
Ban Xia	Pinellia	6 - 9 g
Da Zao	Ziziphus	3 - 6 pc
Sheng Jiang	Zingiber	6 - 9 g
Zhi Gan Cao	Glycyrrhiza	3 - 6 g

Stomach

Chronic Spleen qi deficiency causing qi stagnation. The qi stagnation gives rise to cold and heat symptoms in the middle jiao. This in turn damages the Spleen and Stomach again causing distention in the epigastrium and abdomen, or alternating constipation and diarrhea.

T pale, thin yellowish coat

P wiry

ZHI SHI XIAO PI WAN

Immature Bitter Orange Pill to Reduce Focal Distention

Zhi Shi	Citrus	6 - 12 g
Hou Po	Magnolia	6 - 15 g
Ban Xia	Pinellia	6 - 9 g
Huang Lian	Coptis	9 - 15 g
Fu Ling	Poria	6 - 9 g
Bai Zhu	Atractylodes	3 - 9 g
Ren Shen	Panax	6 - 9 g
Gan Jiang	Zingiber	3 - 6
Mai Ya	Hordeum	3 - 9 g
Zhi Gan Cao	Glycyrrhiza	3 - 6 g

QI AND BLOOD STAGNATION IN THE STOMACH

- stabbing pain which gets worse after eating
- melena
- hematemesis

T purple

P wiry or choppy

Intestinal abscess or acute appendicitis due to heat and blood stagnation causing mass formation in the lower right quadrant with pain.

T yellow sticky

P rapid, slippery

☞ Da Huang - Rheum should be added during the last 3 - 5 minutes of the decoction process. Mang Xiao - Mirabilitum should be added to the strained tea..

✗ Do not use with appendicitis during pregnancy.

DA HUANG MU DAN TANG

Rhubarb and Moutan Decoction

Extract Formula Name: Rhubarb and Moutan Combination

Da Huang	Rheum	6 - 12 g
Mang Xiao	Mirabilitum	6 - 12 g
Dong Gua Ren	Benincasa	12 - 20 g
Tao Ren	Prunus	9 - 12 g
Mu Dan Pi	Paeonia	6 - 9 g

Yin and blood deficiency with blood stagnation causing emaciation, no appetite, amenorrhea, tidal fever, or abdominal distention.

T red, pale, purple or purple spots

P thin, choppy

✗ Do not use during pregnancy.

DA HUANG ZHE CHONG WAN

Rhubarb and Eupolyphaga Pill

Da Huang	Rheum	12 - 18 g
Tu Bie Chong	Eupolyphaga	3 g
Xing Ren	Prunus	3 - 6 g
Gan Qi	Sinica	3 g
Sheng Di Huang	Rehmannia	12 - 18 g
Bai Shao Yao	Paeonia	6 - 12 g
Meng Chong	Tabanus	3 - 6 g
Qi Cao	Holotrichia	3 - 6 g
Tao Ren	Prunus	6 - 9 g
Shui Zhi	Hirudo	3 - 6 g
Huang Qin	Scutellaria	6 g
Gan Cao	Glycyrrhiza	3 - 6 g

Spleen/Kidney yang deficiency causing dawn diarrhea with middle jiao qi stagnation symptoms such as excruciating abdominal pain and severe fullness feelings.

T   pale, swollen, teethmarks, light purple, white coat

P   deep, weak, or slippery

DAN LIAO SI SHEN WAN

Four-Miracle Pill from the Tranquil Hut

Bu Gu Zhi	Psoralea	6 - 12 g
Xiao Hui Xiang	Foeniculum	3 - 9 g
Rou Dou Kou	Myristica	9 - 12 g
Mu Xiang	Saussurea	3 - 6 g

Qi stagnation in the upper and middle jiao with slow blood circulation causing intermittent chest pain, and epigastric or abdominal discomfort.

T   purple

P   choppy

DAN SHEN YIN

Salvia Decoction

Dan Shen	Salvia	30 g
Sha Ren	Amomum	5 g
Tan Xiang	Santalum	5 g

Heat and cold in the middle jiao with Spleen/Stomach qi deficiency, and cold predominance. The patient experiences mild middle jiao qi stagnation symptoms such as fullness or bloating.

T   thin yellow coat

P   weak, slightly wiry

GAN CAO XIE XIN TANG

Licorice Decoction to Drain the Epigastrium

Extract Formula Name: Pinellia and Licorice Combination

Ban Xia	Pinellia	6 - 9 g
Huang Qin	Scutellaria	9 - 12 g
Zhi Gan Cao	Glycyrrhiza	12 - 15 g
Gan Jiang	Zingiber	9 - 12 g
Ren Shen	Panax	9 - 12 g
Huang Lian	Coptis	3 - 6 g
Da Zao	Ziziphus	9 - 15 pc

Stomach

Qi/blood stagnation under the diaphragm and epigastrium, or masses in the abdomen or epigastrium.

T   purple

P   wiry or choppy

✗ Do not use during pregnancy.

✪ Major Formula

GE XIA ZHU YU TANG

Drive Out Blood Stasis Below the Diaphragm Decoction

Extract Formula Name: Persica and Carthamus Combination

Dang Gui	Angelica	6 - 9 g
Chuan Xiong	Ligusticum	6 - 9 g
Tao Ren	Prunus	6 - 9 g
Hong Hua	Carthamus	3 - 6 g
Mu Dan Pi	Paeonia	6 - 9 g
Chi Shao Yao	Paeonia	6 - 9 g
Yan Hu Suo	Corydalis	3 - 6 g
Xiang Fu	Cyperus	3 - 9 g
Zhi Ke	Citrus	3 - 6 g
Wu Ling Zhi	Trogopterus	6 - 9 g
Wu Yao	Lindera	3 - 6 g
Gan Cao	Glycyrrhiza	6 - 9 g

Cold in the Spleen/Stomach after ingestion of cold food with damp and qi stagnation in the center. Symptoms include lack of appetite, loose stools, or nausea and vomiting.

T   pale, sticky white coat

P   weak, deep, or tight

HOU PO WEN ZHONG TANG

Magnolia Bark Decoction for Warming the Middle

Extract Formula Name: Magnolia and Saussurea Combination

Hou Po	Magnolia	30 g
Gan Jiang	Zingiber	2 g
Mu Xiang	Saussurea	15 g
Chen Pi	Citrus	30 g
Fu Ling	Poria	15 g
Cao Dou Kou	Alpinia	15 g
Zhi Gan Cao	Glycyrrhiza	15 g
[Sheng Jiang	Zingiber	3 g]

Wind cold and damp accumulation, with qi stagnation in the middle jiao causing diarrhea, nausea, vomiting, headache, or fever and chills.

T white sticky coat

P soggy or slippery

☞ All ingredients should be ground into a powder. Take 6 g two to three times a day.

HUO XIANG ZHENG QI SAN

Agastache Powder to Rectify the Qi

Extract Formula Name: Agastache Formula

Huo Xiang	Agastache	9 g
Hou Po	Magnolia	6 - 9 g
Bai Zhi	Angelica	3 - 6 g
Zi Su Ye	Perilla	3 - 6 g
Chen Pi	Citrus	6 g
Bai Zhu	Atractylodes	6 g
Fu Ling	Poria	3 - 6 g
Ban Xia	Pinellia	6 g
Da Fu Pi	Areca	3 - 6 g
Jie Geng	Platycodon	6 g
Gan Cao	Glycyrrhiza	6 - 9 g
[Da Zao	Ziziphus	1 - 3 g]
[Sheng Jiang	Zingiber	3 - 6 g]

Stomach

Yangming organ syndrome in the abdomen (pi man zhao shi - firmness, fullness, dryness, excess) with blood stagnation causing acute yang jaundice, Gallbladder infection, intestinal obstruction, possible palpable mass, or nausea and vomiting.

T very red, maybe purplish, dry, rough surface, yellow/brown coat

P flooding, rapid

☞ Da Huang - Rheum should be added during the last 3 - 5 minutes of the decoction process. Mang Xiao - Mirabilitum should be dissolved into the strained tea.

✗ Do not use during pregnancy.

JIA JIAN CHENG QI TANG

Modified Order the Qi Decoction

Da Huang	Rheum	9 - 12 g
Mang Xiao	Mirabilitum	6 - 9 g
Hou Po	Magnolia	9 - 12 g
Zhi Shi	Citrus	6 g
Tao Ren	Prunus	9 - 15 g
Bai Shao Yao	Paeonia	9 - 15 g
Lai Fu Zi	Raphanus	6 - 12 g

Food stagnation with severe heat, qi, damp, and blood stagnation causing fullness, belching with sour taste, dysentery, or severe abdominal pain.

T forceful, rapid

P thick sticky yellow coat

✗ Do not use during pregnancy.

MU XIANG BING LANG WAN

Aucklandia and Betel Nut Pill

Mu Xiang	Saussurea	3 - 9 g
Bing Lang	Areca	3 - 9 g
Xiang Fu	Cyperus	3 - 9 g
Qing Pi	Citrus	3 - 6 g
Da Huang	Rheum	9 - 12 g
Qian Niu Zi	Pharbitis	9 - 18 g
E Zhu	Curcuma	3 - 9 g
Huang Bai	Phellodendron	6 - 12 g
Huang Lian	Coptis	3 - 9 g
[Sheng Jiang	Zingiber	3 - 6 g]

Stomach/Spleen deficiency with cold damp and middle jiao qi stagnation causing fullness and distention.

T thick sticky white coat

P slippery

PING WEI SAN

Calm the Stomach Powder

Extract Formula Name: Magnolia and Ginger Formula

Hou Po	Magnolia	6 - 12 g
Cang Zhu	Atractylodes	9 - 15 g
Chen Pi	Citrus	6 - 12 g
Gan Cao	Glycyrrhiza	3 - 6 g
[Da Zao	Ziziphus	3 - 6 pc]
[Sheng Jiang	Zingiber	3 - 6 g]

Stomach

Qi and blood stagnation with cold causing pain and discomfort in the Stomach and abdomen.

T dark purple

P wiry or choppy

✗ Do not use during pregnancy.

SHOU NIAN SAN

Pinch Powder

Wu Ling Zhi	Trogopterus	15 g
Yan Hu Suo	Corydalis	15 g
Mo Yao	Commiphora	15 g
Cao Guo	Amomum	15 g

Blood stagnation with fire in the lower jiao causing constipation, sudden abdominal pain, dysmenorrhea, intestinal obstruction, or melena. In severe cases this may lead to restlessness, or even delirium.

T purple

P choppy or forceful

☞ Da Huang - Rheum should be added during the last 3 - 5 minutes of the decoction process. Mang Xiao - Mirabilitum should be added to the strained tea.

✗ Do not use during pregnancy.

TAO HE CHENG QI TANG

Peach Pit Decoction to Order the Qi

Extract Formula Name: Prunus and Rhubarb Combination

Tao Ren	Prunus	9 - 15 g
Gui Zhi	Cinnamomum	6 - 9 g
Mang Xiao	Mirabilitum	3 - 6 g
Da Huang	Rheum	9 - 12 g
Gan Cao	Glycyrrhiza	3 - 6 g

Spleen/Stomach qi deficiency with qi stagnation and cold damp in the middle jiao causing abdominal fullness or morning sickness.

T pale, light purple, swollen, sticky white coat

P slippery, weak

XIANG SHA LIU JUN ZI TANG

Six-Gentlemen Decoction with Aucklandia and Amomum

Extract Formula Name: Saussurea and Cardamon Combination

Ren Shen	Panax	6 - 9 g
Fu Ling	Poria	6 - 9 g
Bai Zhu	Atractylodes	3 - 9 g
Chen Pi	Citrus	3 - 6 g
Ban Xia	Pinellia	6 - 9 g
Sha Ren	Amomum	3 g
Mu Xiang	Saussurea	3 - 6 g
Zhi Gan Cao	Glycyrrhiza	3 - 6 g

Excess fire with qi stagnation causing fullness, possible palpable mass, or constipation. This is a mild yangming organ disease.

T red, thin sticky yellow coat

P rapid, slightly forceful

✗ Do not use during pregnancy.

XIAO CHENG QI TANG

Minor Order the Qi Decoction

Extract Formula Name: Minor Rhubarb Combination

Da Huang	Rheum	9 - 12 g
Zhi Shi	Citrus	6 g
Hou Po	Magnolia	6 - 12 g

Spleen qi deficiency with middle jiao qi stagnation and diarrhea, or malnutrition in children.

T pale, light purple, white coat

P weak, thin

YI HUANG SAN

Benefit the Yellow Powder

Chen Pi	Citrus	30 g
Qing Pi	Citrus	15 g
Ding Xiang	Eugenia	3 - 6 g
He Zi	Terminalia	15 g
Zhi Gan Cao	Glycyrrhiza	15 g

Chronic Spleen qi deficiency causing qi stagnation. The qi stagnation gives rise to cold and heat symptoms in the middle jiao. This in turn damages the Spleen and Stomach again causing distention in the epigastrium and abdomen, or alternating constipation and diarrhea.

T   pale, thin yellowish coat

P   wiry

ZHI SHI XIAO PI WAN

Immature Bitter Orange Pill to Reduce Focal Distention

Zhi Shi	Citrus	6 - 12 g
Hou Po	Magnolia	6 - 15 g
Ban Xia	Pinellia	6 - 9 g
Huang Lian	Coptis	9 - 15 g
Fu Ling	Poria	6 - 9 g
Bai Zhu	Atractylodes	3 - 9 g
Ren Shen	Panax	6 - 9 g
Gan Jiang	Zingiber	3 - 6
Mai Ya	Hordeum	3 - 9 g
Zhi Gan Cao	Glycyrrhiza	3 - 6 g

Severe abdominal distention (pi man - fullness, firmness) due to Spleen qi deficiency, or qi stagnation with damp and heat. Symptoms include constipation, or odorous diarrhea, thirst, yellow urine, or fever.

T   sticky yellow coat

P   wiry, rapid

ZHONG MAN FEN XIAO WAN

Separate and Reduce Fullness in the Middle Pill

Hou Po	Magnolia	9 - 18 g
Jiang Huang	Curcuma	6 g
Zhi Shi	Citrus	9 - 12 g
Ban Xia	Pinellia	6 - 12 g
Ren Shen	Panax	3 g
Zhi Mu	Anemarrhena	6 - 9 g
Gan Jiang	Zingiber	3 - 6 g
Huang Lian	Coptis	3 - 9 g
Huang Qin	Scutellaria	9 - 15 g
Bai Zhu	Atractylodes	6 g
Ze Xie	Alisma	6 g
Sha Ren	Amomum	3 - 6 g
Chen Pi	Citrus	3 - 6 g
Fu Ling	Poria	6 - 9 g
Zhu Ling	Polyporus	3 - 6 g
Zhi Gan Cao	Glycyrrhiza	3 - 6 g

Stomach

FOOD OR PHLEGM STAGNATION IN THE STOMACH

- bad breath
- fullness and distention worse with eating and better with vomiting
- nausea
- sour regurgitation, or belching

T   thick sticky coat

P   forceful, slippery

Taiyang disease with high fever enters and damages the Stomach. It then fails to descend qi which leads to food, damp, or water accumulation (or heat and cold accumulation in the Stomach). This is known as firmness and fullness (pi man). Symptoms include epigastric fullness, gurgling, or loose stools.

T   yellow sticky coat

P   wiry, rapid

BAN XIA XIE XIN TANG

Pinellia Decoction to Drain the Epigastrium

Extract Formula Name: Pinellia Combination

Ban Xia	Pinellia	6 - 12 g
Huang Qin	Scutellaria	6 - 9 g
Huang Lian	Coptis	3 - 6 g
Gan Jiang	Zingiber	3 - 6 g
Ren Shen	Panax	6 - 9 g
Da Zao	Ziziphus	3 - 5 pc
Gan Cao	Glycyrrhiza	3 - 6 g

Food stagnation with indigestion, nausea and vomiting, fullness, diarrhea, foul belching, or no appetite.

T   white yellow or sticky yellow coat

P   slippery

✪ Major Formula

BAO HE WAN

Preserve Harmony Pill

Extract Formula Name: Citrus and Crataegus Formula

Lai Fu Zi	Raphanus	6 - 9 g
Lian Qiao	Forsythia	3 - 9 g
Shan Zha	Crataegus	6 - 12 g
Shen Qu	Massa Fermentata	6 - 12 g
Fu Ling	Poria	6 - 9 g
Ban Xia	Pinellia	6 - 9 g
Chen Pi	Citrus	3 - 6 g

Basic formula for phlegm amd damp accumulation from Stomach and Spleen qi deficiency. Symptoms include nausea and vomiting, or epigastric distention.

T sticky coat

P slippery

ER CHEN TANG

Two-Cured Decoction

Extract Formula Name: Citrus and Pinellia Combination

Ban Xia	Pinellia	6 - 9 g
Chen Pi	Citrus	3 - 6 g
Fu Ling	Poria	6 - 9 g
Gan Cao	Glycyrrhiza	3 - 6 g
[Sheng Jiang	Zingiber	3 - 6 g]
[Da Zao	Ziziphus	3 pc]

Damp/water accumulation in the middle jiao causing abdominal fullness, ascites, or scanty urination.

T sticky white coat

P slippery

FEN XIAO TANG

Separate and Reduce Decoction

Extract Formula Name: Hoelen and Alisma Combination

Cang Zhu	Atractylodes	3 - 6 g
Bai Zhu	Atractylodes	3 - 6 g
Hou Po	Magnolia	6 - 9 g
Fu Ling	Poria	6 - 9 g
Chen Pi	Citrus	3 - 6 g
Zhu Ling	Polyporus	3 - 6 g
Deng Xin Cao	Juncus	1 pc
Ze Xie	Alisma	3 - 6 g
Xiang Fu	Cyperus	3 - 6 g
Mu Xiang	Saussurea	3 - 6 g
Zhi Shi	Citrus	3 - 6 g
Sha Ren	Amomum	1 - 3 g
Da Fu Pi	Areca	3 - 6 g
Sheng Jiang	Zingiber	3 - 6 g

Stomach

1. Food stagnation, or overconsumption of alcohol has damaged the Spleen and now there is more cold stagnation in the middle jiao. The Spleen is very weak, and now produces more damp. 2. Alcohol poisoning with Spleen qi deficiency, damp and cold accumulation in the middle jiao. 3. Spleen qi deficiency with an abdominal mass or firmness (pi man).

T   pale, swollen, teethmarks, white sticky coat

P   deep, slippery, weak

GE HUA JIE XING TANG

Pueraria Flower Decoction

Ren Shen	Panax	6 - 9 g
Bai Zhu	Atractylodes	6 - 9 g
Fu Ling	Poria	9 - 12 g
Gan Cao	Glycyrrhiza	3 - 6 g
Chen Pi	Citrus	3 - 6 g
Mu Xiang	Saussurea	6 - 9 g
Sha Ren	Amomum	3 - 6 g
Ze Xie	Alisma	3 - 9 g
Zhu Ling	Polyporus	3 - 9 g
Qing Pi	Citrus	3 - 6 g
Shen Qu	Massa Fermentata	6 - 15 g
Ge Hua	Pueraria	6 - 15 g
Bai Dou Kou	Amomum	3 - 6 g

Phlegm or food stagnation in the chest/diaphragm/upper epigastrium area. This formula will relieve the stagnation by causing vomiting.

T   sticky coat

P   slippery, somewhat superficial in the first (cun) position.

☞ Decoct for only 5 - 10 minutes or make into a paste with 10 g of Dan Dou Chi - Glycine.

✘ This formula will cause vomiting. Do not use during pregnancy.

GUA DI SAN

Melon Pedicle Powder

Extract Formula Name: Melon Pedicle Formula

Gua Di	Cucumis	1 - 3 g
Chi Xiao Dou	Phaseolus	1 - 3 g

Food stagnation damaged the Spleen leading to qi/damp/food stagnation which starts to create some heat. Symptoms include indigestion or borborygmus.

T sticky yellow coat

P slippery, weak

JIAN PI WAN

Strengthen the Spleen Pill

Ren Shen	Panax	6 - 12 g
Bai Zhu	Atractylodes	9 - 15 g
Fu Ling	Poria	9 - 12 g
Shen Qu	Massa Fermentata	9 - 12 g
Shan Yao	Dioscorea	6 - 9 g
Shan Zha	Crataegus	6 - 9 g
Mu Xiang	Saussurea	3 g
Mai Ya	Hordeum	6 - 9 g
Huang Lian	Coptis	3 g
Rou Dou Kou	Myristica	3 - 9 g
Sha Ren	Amomum	3 - 6 g
Chen Pi	Citrus	3 - 6 g
Gan Cao	Glycyrrhiza	3 g

Stomach

Food stagnation with severe heat, qi, damp, and blood stagnation causing fullness, belching with sour taste, dysentery, or severe abdominal pain.

T forceful, rapid

P thick sticky yellow coat

✗ Do not use during pregnancy.

MU XIANG BING LANG WAN

Aucklandia and Betel Nut Pill

Mu Xiang	Saussurea	3 - 9 g
Bing Lang	Areca	3 - 9 g
Xiang Fu	Cyperus	3 - 9 g
Qing Pi	Citrus	3 - 6 g
Da Huang	Rheum	9 - 12 g
Qian Niu Zi	Pharbitis	9 - 18 g
E Zhu	Curcuma	3 - 9 g
Huang Bai	Phellodendron	6 - 12 g
Huang Lian	Coptis	3 - 9 g
[Sheng Jiang	Zingiber	3 - 6 g]

Food stagnation causing damp and heat. This leads to diarrhea which is usually incomplete, or tenesmus with a painful rectum.

T red, thick sticky coat

P slippery, rapid

✗ Do not use during pregnancy.

MU XIANG DAO ZHI WAN

Aucklandia to Guide Out Stagnation Pill

Zhi Shi	Citrus	6 - 15 g
Da Huang	Rheum	6 - 12 g
Huang Qin	Scutellaria	6 - 9 g
Huang Lian	Coptis	6 g
Fu Ling	Poria	6 - 9 g
Shen Qu	Massa Fermentata	6 - 15 g
Bai Zhu	Atractylodes	3 - 9 g
Ze Xie	Alisma	6 - 9 g
Mu Xiang	Saussurea	6 - 9 g
Bing Lang	Areca	6 - 9 g

Phlegm damp cough with cold in the Lungs or food stagnation. Symptoms include dyspnea with profuse phlegm expectoration, and poor appetite.

T sticky white coat

P slippery

SAN ZI YANG QIN TANG

Three-Seed Decoction to Nourish One's Parents

Zi Su Zi	Perilla	6 - 9 g
Lai Fu Zi	Raphanus	6 - 9 g
Bai Jie Zi	Brassica	3 - 9 g

Water accumulation with heat, damp and qi stagnation; or Stomach deficiency with food stagnation and water. Symptoms include diarrhea, borborygmus, or epigastric distention.

T   red, sticky yellow coat

P   slippery, rapid

SHENG JIANG XIE XIN TANG

Fresh Ginger Decoction to Drain the Epigastrium

Extract Formula Name: Pinellia and Ginger Combination

Sheng Jiang	Zingiber	9 - 12 g
Ban Xia	Pinellia	6 - 9 g
Ren Shen	Panax	6 - 12 g
Gan Jiang	Zingiber	3 - 6 g
Huang Qin	Scutellaria	6 - 9 g
Huang Lian	Coptis	3 - 6 g
Da Zao	Ziziphus	6 - 10 pc
Gan Cao	Glycyrrhiza	3 - 6 g

Stomach phlegm heat causing palpitations, insomnia, dizziness, bitter taste, or fullness in the chest.

T   sticky yellow coat

P   rapid, slippery

SHI YI WEI WEN DAN TANG

Eleven-Ingredient Decoction to Warm the Gallbladder

Chen Pi	Citrus	6 g
Ban Xia	Pinellia	6 - 9 g
Fu Ling	Poria	6 - 12 g
Gan Cao	Glycyrrhiza	3 - 6 g
Zhu Ru	Bambusa	6 - 12 g
Zhi Shi	Citrus	3 - 6 g
Shi Chang Pu	Acorus	6 - 9 g
Huang Lian	Coptis	3 - 6 g
Yuan Zhi	Polygala	3 - 6 g
Zhen Zhu Mu	Pteria	12 - 25 g
Ye Jiao Teng	Polygonum	12 - 25 g

Stomach

Chronic water accumulation in the chest and hypochondrium causing cough and shortness of breath.

T white sticky coat

P deep, wiry

☞ Grind ingredients into a powder and take in 0.7 g doses in the morning with a warm tea made from ten pieces of Da Zao - Ziziphus. Between five and six bowel movements are expected after each dose.

✗ Do not use during pregnancy or in weak patients. Gan Sui - Euphorbia is toxic.

SHI ZAO TANG

Ten-Jujube Decoction

Extract Formula Name: Jujube Combination

Gan Sui	Euphorbia	6 g
Yuan Hua	Daphne	6 g
Jing Da Ji	Euphorbia	6 g

Liver and Stomach imbalance with phlegm accumulation and Gallbladder heat. Symptoms include fullness in the chest, bitter taste, thirst without desire to drink, or vomiting. In severe cases, mental confusion or a rattly throat may be seen.

T red, sticky yellow coat

P rapid, slippery and/or wiry

WEN DAN TANG

Warm the Gallbladder Decoction

Extract Formula Name: Hoelen and Bamboo Combination

Ban Xia	Pinellia	6 - 9 g
Chen Pi	Citrus	9 - 12 g
Fu Ling	Poria	6 - 12 g
Zhi Shi	Citrus	3 - 6 g
Zhu Ru	Bambusa	6 g
Sheng Jiang	Zingiber	3 - 6 g
Gan Cao	Glycyrrhiza	3 - 6 g
Da Zao	Ziziphus	2 pc

Food stagnation with abdominal fullness, pain, or disgust at food.

T   thick sticky coat

P   slippery

XIANG SHA PING WEI SAN

Cyperus and Amomum Powder to Calm the Stomach

Xiang Fu	Cyperus	6 g
Sha Ren	Amomum	3 - 6 g
Cang Zhu	Atractylodes	6 - 12 g
Shan Zha	Crataegus	6 - 9 g
Chen Pi	Citrus	3 - 6 g
Bai Shao Yao	Paeonia	6 - 9 g
Zhi Ke	Citrus	3 - 6 g
Mai Ya	Hordeum	6 - 12 g
Sheng Jiang	Zingiber	3 - 6 g
Gan Cao	Glycyrrhiza	3 - 6 g

Stomach

Infant with food stagnation, vomiting, or poor digestion.

T   sticky coat

P   wiry

☞ Herbs should be powdered and mixed with glutinous rice.

XIAO RU WAN

Reduce Infantile Stagnation Pill

Xiang Fu	Cyperus	30 - 60 g
Shen Qu	Massa Fermentata	15 - 30 g
Mai Ya	Hordeum	15 - 30 g
Zhi Gan Cao	Glycyrrhiza	9 - 15 g
Chen Pi	Citrus	9 - 15 g
Sha Ren	Amomum	15 - 30 g

Phlegm accumulation with Stomach qi deficiency causing hiccups, fullness, or nausea and vomiting.

T   pale, white sticky coat

P   frail, slippery, or wiry

☞ Xuan Fu Hua - Inula should be wrapped in a cheese cloth for decoction.

XUAN FU DAI ZHE TANG

Inula and Hematite Decoction

Extract Formula Name: Inula and Hematite Combination

Xuan Fu Hua	Inula	6 - 9 g
Dai Zhe Shi	Haematitum	6 - 12 g
Ren Shen	Panax	6 - 9 g
Ban Xia	Pinellia	6 - 9 g
Da Zao	Ziziphus	3 - 6 pc
Sheng Jiang	Zingiber	6 - 9 g
Zhi Gan Cao	Glycyrrhiza	3 - 6 g

Stagnations of all kinds (qi, blood, food, damp, etc.). Symptoms include epigastric or chest fullness, nausea and vomiting, or poor appetite.

T   depends on particular syndrome involved

P   depends on particular syndrome involved

YUE JU WAN

Escape Restraint Pill

Chuan Xiong	Ligusticum	3 - 9 g
Cang Zhu	Atractylodes	3 - 9 g
Zhi Zi	Gardenia	3 - 9 g
Xiang Fu	Cyperus	3 - 9 g
Shen Qu	Massa Fermentata	3 - 9 g

Food stagnation in the middle jiao with damp and heat accumulation: cold and heat in the middle jiao with Spleen deficiency. Symptoms include fullness with pain, odorous diarrhea, mucus, tenesmus, gas, or constipation.

T   red, red sides, rough, thick sticky yellow coat

P   slippery, rapid, forceful

✗   Caution during pregnancy.

ZHI SHI DAO ZHI WAN

Immature Bitter Orange Pill to Guide Out Stagnation

Extract Formula Name: Chih-shih and Rhubarb Formula

Zhi Shi	Citrus	9 - 15 g
Shen Qu	Massa Fermentata	9 - 15 g
Da Huang	Rheum	15 - 25 g
Huang Qin	Scutellaria	6 - 9 g
Huang Lian	Coptis	6 - 9 g
Fu Ling	Poria	6 - 9 g
Ze Xie	Alisma	6 - 9 g
Bai Zhu	Atractylodes	6 - 9 g

Chronic Spleen qi deficiency causing qi stagnation. The qi stagnation gives rise to cold and heat symptoms in the middle jiao. This in turn damages the Spleen and Stomach again causing distention in the epigastrium and abdomen, or alternating constipation and diarrhea.

T   pale, thin yellowish coat

P   wiry

ZHI SHI XIAO PI WAN

Immature Bitter Orange Pill to Reduce Focal Distention

Zhi Shi	Citrus	6 - 12 g
Hou Po	Magnolia	6 - 15 g
Ban Xia	Pinellia	6 - 9 g
Huang Lian	Coptis	9 - 15 g
Fu Ling	Poria	6 - 9 g
Bai Zhu	Atractylodes	3 - 9 g
Ren Shen	Panax	6 - 9 g
Gan Jiang	Zingiber	3 - 6
Mai Ya	Hordeum	3 - 9 g
Zhi Gan Cao	Glycyrrhiza	3 - 6 g

1. **Chronic food stagnation with severe Spleen qi deficiency.**
2. **Severe acute food stagnation with mild Spleen qi deficiency. Symptoms include epigastric and abdominal distention, loose stools, and poor appetite.**

T   sticky coat

P   wiry

ZHI ZHU WAN

Immature Bitter Orange and Atractylodes Pill

Bai Zhu	Atractylodes	9 - 15 g
Zhi Shi	Citrus	6 - 12 g

Damp heat accumulation in the middle jiao. There is more damp than heat causing fullness in the abdomen, thirst without desire to drink, or immediate fullness upon eating or drinking. This formula is also useful for yang jaundice.

T   red, thick sticky coat

P   slippery, rapid

ZHONG JIAO XIAN BI TANG

Middle Jiao and Clear Damp Decoction

Xing Ren	Prunus	3 - 6 g
Yi Yi Ren	Coix	9 - 12 g
Hua Shi	Talcum	6 g
Dou Juan	Glycine	9 g
Zhi Zi	Gardenia	6 - 9 g
Lian Qiao	Forsythia	6 g
Ban Xia	Pinellia	6 - 9 g
Han Fang Ji	Stephania	6 - 9 g
Can Sha	Bombyx	3 - 6 g
Shan Zha	Crataegus	3 - 9 g
Bian Dou	Dolichos	6 - 9 g

COLD OR YANG DEFICIENCY IN THE STOMACH

- **if cold:** acute sharp pain in the epigastrium with a preference for warmth
- vomiting of clear fluid
- any cool fluid is immediately vomited
- **if yang deficiency:** the epigastric pain is better with eating, pressure, and/or warmth
- cold extremities

T   pale, moist, thick white coat

P   deep, slow, tight

Taiyang disease with high fever enters and damages the Stomach. It then fails to descend qi which leads to food, damp, or water accumulation (or heat and cold accumulation in the Stomach). This is known as firmness and fullness (pi man). Symptoms include epigastric fullness, gurgling, or loose stools.

T   yellow sticky coat

P   wiry, rapid

BAN XIA XIE XIN TANG

Pinellia Decoction to Drain the Epigastrium

Extract Formula Name: Pinellia Combination

Ban Xia	Pinellia	6 - 12 g
Huang Qin	Scutellaria	6 - 9 g
Huang Lian	Coptis	3 - 6 g
Gan Jiang	Zingiber	3 - 6 g
Ren Shen	Panax	6 - 9 g
Da Zao	Ziziphus	3 - 5 pc
Gan Cao	Glycyrrhiza	3 - 6 g

Cold accumulation or yang deficiency in the abdomen leading to constipation with cramping pain. The qi stagnates and heats up which can cause a mild fever. Other symptoms include cold extremities and chills.

T normal or pale, white coat

P wiry or tight, deep

☞ Fu Zi - Aconitum should be powdered. Da Huang - Rheum should be added during the last 3 - 5 minutes of the decoction process.

✗ Do not use during pregnancy.

DA HUANG FU ZI TANG

Rhubarb and Aconite Decoction

Extract Formula Name: Rhubarb and Aconite Combination

Da Huang	Rheum	6 - 9 g
Fu Zi	Aconitum	6 g
Xi Xin	Asarum	3 - 6 g

Spleen yang deficiency with cold stagnation causing severe cramping pain, borborygmus, or possible vomiting.

T pale, light purple, swollen, moist white coat

P wiry or slow, deep

☞ Yi Tang - Saccharum Granorum is added to the strained tea.

DA JIAN ZHONG TANG

Major Construct the Middle Decoction

Extract Formula Name: Major Zanthoxylum Combination

Chuan Jiao	Zanthoxylum	3 - 6 g
Ren Shen	Panax	6 - 9 g
Gan Jiang	Zingiber	3 - 6 g
Yi Tang	Saccharum Granorum	20 g

Spleen qi and blood deficiency with slight cold leading to spasm pain or post-partum emaciation.

T pale, white coat

P weak

☞ Yi Tang - Saccharum Granorum is added to the strained tea.

DANG GUI JIAN ZHONG TANG

Dang Gui Decoction to Construct the Middle

Extract Formula Name: Tang-Kuei, Cinnamon and Peony Combination

Yi Tang	Saccharum Granorum	6 - 20 g
Gui Zhi	Cinnamomum	3 - 9 g
Bai Shao Yao	Paeonia	6 - 9 g
Sheng Jiang	Zingiber	3 - 6 g
Da Zao	Ziziphus	3 - 6 pc
Gan Cao	Glycyrrhiza	3 - 6 g
Dang Gui	Angelica	6 - 9 g

Stomach

Longstanding cold with blood and yang deficiency leading to diarrhea, nausea and vomiting, or abdominal cramps.

T pale, swollen, teethmarks, wet, white coat

P slow, frail

DANG GUI SI NI JIA WU ZHU YU SHENG JIANG TANG

Dang Gui Decoction for Frigid Extremities plus Evodia and Fresh Ginger

Extract Formula Name: Tang-Kuei, Evodia and Ginger Combination

Dang Gui	Angelica	6 - 9 g
Gui Zhi	Cinnamomum	3 - 9 g
Xi Xin	Asarum	3 - 6 g
Bai Shao Yao	Paeonia	6 - 9 g
Mu Tong	Akebia	6 - 9 g
Wu Zhu Yu	Evodia	3 - 6 g
Da Zao	Ziziphus	25 pc
Sheng Jiang	Zingiber	4 pc
Gan Cao	Glycyrrhiza	3 - 6 g

Spleen/Stomach qi yang deficiency resulting in hiccups, belching, and vomiting, and symptoms of coldness in the middle jiao.

T pale, thin coat

P weak, deep, maybe slow

✗ Do not use during pregnancy

DING XIANG SHI DI TANG

Clove and Kaki Decoction

Extract Formula Name: Clove and Kaki Combination

Ding Xiang	Eugenia	6 - 9 g
Shi Di	Diospyros	6 - 9 g
Ren Shen	Panax	3 - 9 g
Sheng Jiang	Zingiber	3 - 6 g

Stomach/Spleen yang deficiency causing watery diarrhea and epigastric pain. Severe cold symptoms such as cold limbs and vomiting of clear fluids.

T pale, swollen, teethmarks, white coat

P minute

✪ Major Formula

FU ZI LI ZHONG WAN

Prepared Aconite Pill to Regulate the Middle

Extract Formula Name: Aconite, Ginseng, and Ginger Combination

Fu Zi	Aconitum	6 - 9 g
Ren Shen	Panax	3 - 9 g
Bai Zhu	Atractylodes	3 - 9 g
Gan Jiang	Zingiber	3 - 9 g
Zhi Gan Cao	Glycyrrhiza	3 - 6 g

Stomach and Spleen yang deficiency with wei qi deficiency and internal heat and damp. Symtoms include loose stools, sweating, or cold hands and feet.

T   pale or red, white or yellow sticky coat

P   deep, weak, thin, or rapid

✗   Caution during pregnancy.

FU ZI XIE XIN TANG

Aconite Decoction to Drain the Epigastrium

Fu Zi	Aconitum	3 - 6 g
Da Huang	Rheum	6 - 9 g
Huang Qin	Scutellaria	3 - 6 g
Huang Lian	Coptis	3 - 6 g

Cold in the Lungs and Stomach causing Lung atrophy, cold extremities, or clear sputum.

T   pale, moist

P   weak, slow

GAN CAO GAN JIANG TANG

Licorice and Ginger Decoction

Extract Formula Name: Licorice and Ginger Combination

Zhi Gan Cao	Glycyrrhiza	9 - 12 g
Gan Jiang	Zingiber	6 - 9 g

Heat and cold in the middle jiao with Spleen/Stomach qi deficiency, and cold predominance. The patient experiences mild middle jiao qi stagnation symptoms such as fullness or bloating.

T   thin yellow coat

P   weak, slightly wiry

GAN CAO XIE XIN TANG

Licorice Decoction to Drain the Epigastrium

Extract Formula Name: Pinellia and Licorice Combination

Ban Xia	Pinellia	6 - 9 g
Huang Qin	Scutellaria	9 - 12 g
Zhi Gan Cao	Glycyrrhiza	12 - 15 g
Gan Jiang	Zingiber	9 - 12 g
Ren Shen	Panax	9 - 12 g
Huang Lian	Coptis	3 - 6 g
Da Zao	Ziziphus	9 - 15 pc

Severe cold stagnation with Spleen/Kidney yang deficiency causing coldness in the face, cramping pain in the center, or dawn diarrhea.

T   pale, purple, wet coat

P   slow, tight

GUI FU LI ZHONG WAN

Cinnamon and Prepared Aconite Decoction to Regulate the Middle

Ren Shen	Panax	10 - 15 g
Bai Zhu	Atractylodes	6 - 9 g
Gan Jiang	Zingiber	6 - 9 g
Gan Cao	Glycyrrhiza	3 - 6 g
Fu Zi	Aconitum	3 - 6 g
Gui Zhi	Cinnamomum	3 - 9 g

Upper jiao heat with middle jiao cold usually caused by cold food which restricts Spleen qi. This leads to damp which then turns to heat. The heat rises upward and bothers the Heart causing thirst, restlessness, full/cold abdomen with pain, or nausea and vomiting.

T   red or pale, red tip, thin sticky coat

P   rapid, wiry

HUANG LIAN TANG

Coptis Decoction

Extract Formula Name: Coptis Combination

Huang Lian	Coptis	5 g
Gan Jiang	Zingiber	5 g
Gui Zhi	Cinnamomum	5 g
Ren Shen	Panax	3 g
Ban Xia	Pinellia	9 g
Da Zao	Ziziphus	9 - 12 pc
Gan Cao	Glycyrrhiza	6 g

Stomach

Wind cold and damp accumulation, with qi stagnation in the middle jiao causing diarrhea, nausea, vomiting, headache, or fever and chills.

T white sticky coat

P soggy or slippery

☞ All ingredients should be ground into a powder. Take 6 g two to three times a day.

HUO XIANG ZHENG QI SAN

Agastache Powder to Rectify the Qi

Extract Formula Name: Agastache Formula

Huo Xiang	Agastache	9 g
Hou Po	Magnolia	6 - 9 g
Bai Zhi	Angelica	3 - 6 g
Zi Su Ye	Perilla	3 - 6 g
Chen Pi	Citrus	6 g
Bai Zhu	Atractylodes	6 g
Fu Ling	Poria	3 - 6 g
Ban Xia	Pinellia	6 g
Da Fu Pi	Areca	3 - 6 g
Jie Geng	Platycodon	6 g
Gan Cao	Glycyrrhiza	6 - 9 g
[Da Zao	Ziziphus	1 - 3 g]
[Sheng Jiang	Zingiber	3 - 6 g]

Cold in the Stomach causing rebellious qi which leads to nausea, vomiting, or diarrhea.

T pale, white coat

P weak, slow

JU PI TANG

Tangerine Peel Decoction

Chen Pi	Citrus	9 - 12 g
Sheng Jiang	Zingiber	6 - 9 g

Middle jiao qi/yang deficiency resulting in loss of appetite, absence of thirst, watery diarrhea with undigested food, or cold or painful limbs.

T pale, swollen, teethmarks, white coat

P deep, weak

LI ZHONG WAN

Regulate the Middle Pill

Extract Formula Name: Ginseng and Ginger Combination

Ren Shen	Panax	6 - 9 g
Gan Jiang	Zingiber	6 - 9 g
Bai Zhu	Atractylodes	6 - 9 g
Gan Cao	Glycyrrhiza	3 - 6 g

Liver qi stagnation with cold in the Stomach causing abdominal pain which is relieved by warmth. The Formula is also useful for dysmenorrhea.

T   pale, white coat

P   weak, slow, or wiry

LIANG FU WAN

Galanga and Cyperus Pill

Extract Formula Name: Galanga and Cyperus Formula

Gao Liang Jiang	Alpinia	6 - 9 g
Xiang Fu	Cyperus	6 - 9 g

Sudden cold stagnation and cold food obstructing the Stomach and Large Intestines completely. This causes sudden, severe pain and bowel obstruction.

T   pale

P   tight, deep

☞ The herbs should be powdered and adults should take 1 g doses with warm water.

✗ Ba Dou - Croton is a toxic herb that should be used with extreme caution. Do not use during pregnancy.

SAN WU BEI JI WAN

Three-Substance Pill for Emergencies

Extract Formula Name: Rhubarb, Ginger and Croton Formula

Da Huang	Rheum	30 g
Ba Dou	Croton	30 g
Gan Jiang	Zingiber	30 g

Stomach deficiency with cold causing hiccups, vomiting, chronic belching, or fullness in the chest.

T   pale

P   weak

SHI DI TANG

Persimmon Calyx Decoction

Extract Formula Name: Kaki Combination

Shi Di	Diospyros	3 - 9 g
Ding Xiang	Eugenia	3 - 6 g
Sheng Jiang	Zingiber	3 - 9 g

Stomach

Spleen qi deficiency with cold which restricts the Liver and Stomach. This results in tight abdominal pain, cold in the middle and lower jiao, vomiting, or acid regurgitation; or cold causes vertex headaches via the Liver channel. This Liver qi stagnation is not due to emotional reasons but is caused by cold.

T pale, purplish, moist white coat

P slow, or wiry, thin

WU ZHU YU TANG

Evodia Decoction

Extract Formula Name: Evodia Combination

Wu Zhu Yu	Evodia	3 - 6 g
Ren Shen	Panax	6 - 9 g
Sheng Jiang	Zingiber	12 - 20 g
Da Zao	Ziziphus	6 - 12 pc

Wind cold with internal qi stagnation causing belching, decreased appetite fever and chills, headache, absence of sweating and middle jiao fullness.

T thin white coat

P superficial

XIANG SU SAN

Cyperus and Perilla Leaf Powder

Extract Formula Name: Cyperus and Perilla Formula

Xiang Fu	Cyperus	6 - 9 g
Zi Su Ye	Perilla	6 - 9 g
Chen Pi	Citrus	3 - 6 g
Zhi Gan Cao	Glycyrrhiza	3 - 6 g

---

1. Chronic Spleen qi deficiency with chronic cold evil qi leading to qi and blood deficiency. The main symptom is abdominal spasms. 2. Liver qi stagnation or Liver overacting on Spleen. In the latter two instances the dosage of 'Bai Shao Yao - Paeonia' should be increased.

T pale or light purple, thin white coat

P weak or slightly wiry

☞ Yi Tang - Saccharum Granorum should be added to the strained tea.

XIAO JIAN ZHONG TANG

Minor Construct the Middle Decoction

Extract Formula Name: Minor Cinnamon and Peony Combination

Yi Tang	Saccharum Granorum	15 - 30 g
Gui Zhi	Cinnamomum	3 - 9 g
Bai Shao Yao	Paeonia	6 - 9 g
Sheng Jiang	Zingiber	6 - 9 g
Da Zao	Ziziphus	3 - 5 pc
Zhi Gan Cao	Glycyrrhiza	3 - 6 g

STOMACH YIN DEFICIENCY

- constipation with dry stools
- afternoon heat
- thirst
- increased appetite

T red, geographic, scanty coat

P empty, or thin, rapid

Yangming channel disease, damp stagnation and yin deficiency leading to mouth sores, swollen, red gums with pus, bad breath, sore throat, or eye disorders.

T thick sticky yellow coat

P rapid, slippery, thin

GAN LU YIN

Sweet Dew Decoction

Extract Formula Name: Sweet Combination

Shu Di Huang	Rehmannia	6 - 9 g
Sheng Di Huang	Rehmannia	6 - 9 g
Huang Qin	Scutellaria	6 - 9 g
Zhi Ke	Citrus	3 - 6 g
Mai Men Dong	Ophiopogon	6 - 9 g
Tian Men Dong	Asparagus	6 - 9 g
Pi Pa Ye	Eriobotrya	12 - 18 g
Yin Chen Hao	Artemisia	6 - 9 g
Shi Hu	Dendrobium	6 - 9 g
Gan Cao	Glycyrrhiza	3 - 6 g

Epistaxis or hematemesis during menses due to Stomach deficiency and rebellious qi.

T pale

P weak, thin

JIA WEI MAI MEN DONG TANG

Augmented Ophiopogon Decoction

Mai Men Dong	Ophiopogon	9 - 15 g
Shan Yao	Dioscorea	9 - 12 g
Ren Shen	Panax	9 - 12 g
Dan Shen	Salvia	9 - 12 g
Ban Xia	Pinellia	6 - 9 g
Bai Shao Yao	Paeonia	6 - 9 g
Tao Ren	Prunus	3 - 6 g
Da Zao	Ziziphus	3 - 5 pc
Gan Cao	Glycyrrhiza	3 - 6 g

Heat in the Stomach with qi and yin deficiency and rebellious Stomach qi causing thirst, vomiting, loss of appetite, nausea, or hiccups.

T   red

P   thin, rapid, weak

JU PI ZHU RU TANG I

Tangerine Peel and Bamboo Shaving Decoction

Extract Formula Name: Aurantium and Bamboo Combination

Chen Pi	Citrus	6 - 12 g
Ren Shen	Panax	6 - 9 g
Zhu Ru	Bambusa	6 - 12 g
Da Zao	Ziziphus	3 - 6 pc
Sheng Jiang	Zingiber	3 - 9 g
Gan Cao	Glycyrrhiza	3 - 6 g

Stomach heat with qi and yin deficiency causing severe thirst, nausea and vomiting, or decreased appetite.

T   red, thin yellow coat

P   thin, weak, slightly rapid

JU PI ZHU RU TANG II

Tangerine Peel and Bamboo Shavings Decoction from Formulas to Aid the Living

Zhu Ru	Bambusa	6 - 9 g
Ban Xia	Pinellia	6 - 9 g
Chi Fu Ling	Poria	6 - 9 g
Ren Shen	Panax	3 - 6 g
Pi Pa Ye	Eriobotrya	6 - 9 g
Chen Pi	Citrus	3 - 6 g
Mai Men Dong	Ophiopogon	6 - 9 g
Zhi Gan Cao	Glycyrrhiza	3 - 6 g
[Sheng Jiang	Zingiber	3 - 6 pc]

Yin/blood deficiency causing constipation with dry stools; or excess heat causing constipation.

T red, dry yellow coat

P rapid, thin, or empty

✗ Do not use during pregnancy.

MA ZI REN WAN

Hemp Seed Pill

Extract Formula Name: Apricot Seed and Linum Formula

Huo Ma Ren	Cannabis	6 - 12 g
Da Huang	Rheum	6 - 9 g
Xing Ren	Prunus	6 - 9 g
Zhi Shi	Citrus	3 - 6 g
Bai Shao Yao	Paeonia	6 - 9 g
Hou Po	Magnolia	6 - 12 g

Stomach yin deficiency starts to produce heat which then burns Lung yin resulting in cough, wheezing, shortness of breath, or thirst.

T red, geographic spots, slight or no coat

P thin, rapid

MAI MEN DONG TANG

Ophiopogon Decoction

Extract Formula Name: Ophiopogon Combination

Mai Men Dong	Ophiopogon	6 - 12 g
Ren Shen	Panax	6 - 9 g
Ban Xia	Pinellia	6 - 9 g
Jing Mi	Oryza	9 - 12 g
Da Zao	Ziziphus	6 - 10 pc
Gan Cao	Glycyrrhiza	3 - 6 g

Blood deficiency causing constipation.

T pale

P weak, thin

WU REN WAN

Five-Seed Pill

Xing Ren	Prunus	9 - 20 g
Bai Zi Ren	Biota	3 - 6 g
Tao Ren	Prunus	9 - 15 g
Yu Li Ren	Prunus	3 - 6 g
Sha Ren	Amomum	3 - 6 g

Spleen qi with yin deficiency and heat accumulation causing constipation, or hardness and fullness in the abdomen.

T cracked, thin dry yellowish coat

P weak, thin, deep

XIN JIA HUANG LONG TANG

Newly-Augmented Yellow Dragon Decoction

Sheng Di Huang	Rehmannia	6 - 15 g
Ren Shen	Panax	6 - 9 g
Da Huang	Rheum	6 - 9 g
Mang Xiao	Mirabilitum	3 - 5 g
Mai Men Dong	Ophiopogon	9 - 15 g
Dang Gui	Angelica	6 - 9 g
Xuan Shen	Scrophularia	9 - 15 g
Gan Cao	Glycyrrhiza	3 - 6 g
Hai Shen	Strichopus	1 - 2 g

Stoamch heat causing hiccups.

T red

P rapid

☞ 6 - 9 g of ginger juice should be added to the tea.

XIN ZHI JU PI ZHU RU TANG

Newly-Formulated Tangerine Peel and Bamboo Shavings Decoction

Zhu Ru	Bambusa	6 - 9 g
Chen Pi	Citrus	3 - 9 g
Shi Di	Diospyros	6 - 9 g
Sheng Jiang Zhi	Zingiber	6 - 9 g

Stomach yin deficiency due to febrile disease or Liver fire. Symptoms include bleeding gums, increased appetite, and thirst.

T slightly red, dry, scanty yellowish coat

P thin

YI WEI TANG

Benefit the Stomach Decoction

Extract Formula Name: Glehnia and Ophiopogon Combination

Sheng Di Huang	Rehmannia	9 - 15 g
Mai Men Dong	Ophiopogon	9 - 15 g
Bei Sha Shen	Glehnia	6 - 12 g
Yu Zhu	Polygonatum	3 - 6 g
Bing Tang	Rock candy	1 - 3 g

Stomach fire has damaged Stomach yin causing bleeding gums, frontal headache, aching teeth, or excess hunger.

T   red, geographic, scanty yellow coat

P   rapid, empty, thin

✪ **Major Formula**

YU NU JIAN

Jade Woman Decoction

Extract Formula Name: Rehmannia and Gypsum Combination

Shi Gao	Gypsum	6 - 15 g
Zhi Mu	Anemarrhena	9 - 15 g
Mai Men Dong	Ophiopogon	6 - 15 g
Shu Di Huang	Rehmannia	12 - 15 g
Huai Niu Xi	Achyranthes	9 - 15 g

Middle jiao diabetes (xiao ke) leading to hunger as the key symptom due to Stomach yin deficiency.

T   red, scanty coat

P   thin, slightly rapid

YU QUAN WAN

Jade Spring Pill

Tian Hua Fen	Trichosanthes	6 - 9 g
Ren Shen	Panax	6 - 9 g
Fu Ling	Poria	6 - 9 g
Huang Qi	Astragalus	6 - 12 g
Zi Su Zi	Perilla	3 - 9 g
Mai Men Dong	Ophiopogon	6 - 12 g
Gan Cao	Glycyrrhiza	3 - 6 g

Diabetes due to Kidney and Stomach yin deficiency with qi deficiency causing thirst and frequent, profuse urination.

T   red, dry

P   weak, thin

YU YE TANG

Jade Fluid Decoction

Shan Yao	Dioscorea	15 - 30 g
Tian Hua Fen	Trichosanthes	6 - 9 g
Huang Qi	Astragalus	9 - 15 g
Ji Nei Jin	Gallus	3 - 6 g
Zhi Mu	Anemarrhena	12 - 18 g
Wu Wei Zi	Schisandra	6 - 9 g
Ge Gen	Pueraria	2 - 5 g

Fire in the yangming organ with yin deficiency causing constipation with very dry stools.

T   red, dry yellow coat

P   rapid, thin, wiry

☞ Da Huang - Rheum should be added during the last 3 minutes of the cooking process. Mang Xiao - Mirabilitum should be added to the strained tea.

✗ Do not use during pregnancy.

ZENG YE CHENG QI TANG

Increase the Fluids and Order the Qi Decoction

Xuan Shen	Scrophularia	15 - 25 g
Sheng Di Huang	Rehmannia	15 - 20 g
Mai Men Dong	Ophiopogon	15 - 20 g
Mang Xiao	Mirabilitum	3 - 6 g
Da Huang	Rheum	6 - 9 g

Yin deficiency with dryness and heat in the yangming leading to constipation.

T   red, dry, scanty yellow coat

P   thin, rapid, weak

ZENG YE TANG

Increase the Fluids Decoction

Extract Formula Name: Scrophularia and Ophiopogon Combination

Xuan Shen	Scrophularia	15 - 25 g
Sheng Di Huang	Rehmannia	15 - 20 g
Mai Men Dong	Ophiopogon	15 - 20 g

Qi level heat damaged the qi and yin. Now there is residual heat and a mild fever, dry mouth, and irritability.

T   red

P   rapid, weak, thin

ZHU YE SHI GAO TANG

Lophatherum and Gypsum Decoction

Extract Formula Name: Bamboo Leaves and Gypsum Combination

Dan Zhu Ye	Lophatherum	6 - 15 g
Shi Gao	Gypsum	20 - 30 g
Ban Xia	Pinellia	6 - 9 g
Ren Shen	Panax	3 - 6 g
Zhi Gan Cao	Glycyrrhiza	3 - 6 g
Jing Mi	Oryza	9 - 15 g
Mai Men Dong	Ophiopogon	12 - 15 g

STOMACH FIRE

- burning epigastric pain
- ravenous appetite
- gum bleeding
- mouth sores and bad breath

T red, thick yellow coat

P forceful, rapid

Toxic heat in the yangming channel causing dysentery, or pus or blood in the stools.

T red, yellow coat

P wiry, rapid, rolling

BAI TOU WENG TANG

Pulsatilla Decoction

Extract Formula Name: Anemone Combination

Bai Tou Weng	Pulsatilla	20 - 40 g
Huang Bai	Phellodendron	9 - 12 g
Qin Pi	Fraxinus	9 - 15 g
Huang Lian	Coptis	6 - 9 g

Intestinal abscess or acute appendicitis due to heat and blood stagnation causing mass formation in the lower right quadrant with pain.

T yellow sticky

P rapid, slippery

☞ Da Huang - Rheum should be added during the last 3 - 5 minutes of the decoction process. Mang Xiao - Mirabilitum should be added to the strained tea..

✗ Do not use with appendicitis during pregnancy.

DA HUANG MU DAN TANG

Rhubarb and Moutan Decoction

Extract Formula Name: Rhubarb and Moutan Combination

Da Huang	Rheum	6 - 12 g
Mang Xiao	Mirabilitum	6 - 12 g
Dong Gua Ren	Benincasa	12 - 20 g
Tao Ren	Prunus	9 - 12 g
Mu Dan Pi	Paeonia	6 - 9 g

Heat in the middle and upper jiao with fullness as the main symptom (pi-syndrome from pi man zhao shi - firmness, fullness, dryness, excess). Symptoms include nausea and vomiting, possible hematemesis, red face, palpitations, diarrhea, or bleeding in the upper body.

T red, yellow coat

P rapid

✗ Do not use during pregnancy.

DA HUANG XIE XIN TANG

Rhubarb to Drain the Epigastrium Decoction

Da Huang	Rheum	6 - 12 g
Huang Lian	Coptis	3 - 9 g

Wind heat with internal heat: taiyang and yangming organ disease. The heat is severe. Symptoms include dark yellow urine, constipation, severe fever and chills, heat sensations in the body, skin disorders, and a bitter taste.

T bright or dark red, dry, yellow coat

P flooding, rapid, wiry

☞ Ingredients should be ground into powder, then made into a pill with water. Take 6 g each time, twice a day.

✗ Do not use during pregnancy.

FANG FENG TONG SHENG SAN

Ledebouriella Powder that Sagely Unblocks

Extract Formula Name: Siler and Platycodon Formula

Fang Feng	Ledebouriella	9 - 15 g
Ma Huang	Ephedra	9 - 15 g
Da Huang	Rheum	9 - 15 g
Mang Xiao	Mirabilitum	9 - 15 g
Jing Jie	Schizonepeta	9 - 15 g
Bo He	Mentha	9 - 15 g
Zhi Zi	Gardenia	9 - 15 g
Hua Shi	Talcum	60 - 90 g
Shi Gao	Gypsum	15 - 30 g
Huang Qin	Scutellaria	15 - 30 g
Lian Qiao	Forsythia	9 - 15 g
Jie Geng	Platycodon	15 - 30 g
Dang Gui	Angelica	9 - 15 g
Bai Shao Yao	Paeonia	9 - 15 g
Chuan Xiong	Ligusticum	9 - 15 g
Bai Zhu	Atractylodes	9 - 15 g
Gan Cao	Glycyrrhiza	30 - 60 g

Stomach

Wind heat with internal middle jiao heat and Large Intestine heat and damp causing dysentery: taiyang and yangming disease. Symptoms include fever, thirst, or burning anus.

T red, yellow coat

P rapid, slippery

GE GEN HUANG LIAN HUANG QIN TANG

Kudzu, Coptis, and Scutellaria Decoction

Extract Formula Name: Pueraria, Coptis and Scute Combination

Ge Gen	Pueraria	12 - 15 g
Huang Lian	Coptis	9 g
Huang Qin	Scutellaria	6 - 9 g
Gan Cao	Glycyrrhiza	3 - 6 g

Fire in the upper/middle jiao (chest/diaphragm) causing thirst, red lips, epistaxis, redness in the face, dark yellow urine, constipation, or delirium.

T red, dry yellow coat

P rapid

✗ Do not use during pregnancy.

LIANG GE SAN

Cool the Diaphragm Powder

Extract Formula Name: Forsythia and Rhubarb Formula

Da Huang	Rheum	6 - 9 g
Mang Xiao	Mirabilitum	6 - 9 g
Zhi Zi	Gardenia	3 - 6 g
Huang Qin	Scutellaria	6 - 9 g
Bo He	Mentha	3 - 6 g
Lian Qiao	Forsythia	9 - 12 g
Gan Cao	Glycyrrhiza	3 - 6 g
[Dan Zhu Ye	Lophatherum	3 - 6 g]

Yin/blood deficiency causing constipation with dry stools; or excess heat causing constipation.

T red, dry yellow coat

P rapid, thin, or empty

✗ Do not use during pregnancy.

MA ZI REN WAN

Hemp Seed Pill

Extract Formula Name: Apricot Seed and Linum Formula

Huo Ma Ren	Cannabis	6 - 12 g
Da Huang	Rheum	6 - 9 g
Xing Ren	Prunus	6 - 9 g
Zhi Shi	Citrus	3 - 6 g
Bai Shao Yao	Paeonia	6 - 9 g
Hou Po	Magnolia	6 - 12 g

Liver and Stomach fire causing dizziness, bad breath, anger outbursts, oral sores or ulcers, or constipation.

T   red, sticky yellow coat

P   rapid, wiry, forceful

☞ Niu Huang - Bos should be added at the end of the decoction process. Bing Pian - Dryobalanops and Xiong Huang - Realgar should be powdered prior to the decoction. This prescription is available in prepared form.

✗   Do not use during pregnancy

NIU HUANG JIE DU PIEN

Antiphlogistic Pills with Bos Calculus

Niu Huang	Bos	3 - 6 g
Xiong Huang	Realgar	3 - 6 g
Da Huang	Rheum	6 - 9 g
Jie Geng	Platycodon	3 - 6 g
Bing Pian	Dryobalanops	3 - 6 g
Shi Gao	Gypsum	9 - 15 g
Huang Qin	Scutellaria	6 - 9 g
Gan Cao	Glycyrrhiza	3 - 6 g

Yangming channel disease/Stomach fire causing bleeding gums, toothache, soreness in the tongue, headaches, or red eyes.

T   red, dry

P   rapid, flooding

✪ **Major Formula**

QING WEI SAN

Clear the Stomach Powder

Extract Formula Name: Coptis and Rehmannia Formula

Huang Lian	Coptis	3 - 6 g
Sheng Di Huang	Rehmannia	9 - 12 g
Mu Dan Pi	Paeonia	9 - 12 g
Dang Gui Shen	Angelica	9 - 12 g
Sheng Ma	Cimicifuga	9 - 15 g

Severe Stomach fire causing gum problems, ravenous appetite, or foul breath.

T   red, sticky yellow coat

P   wiry, forceful, rapid

QING WEI TANG

Clear the Stomach Decoction

Shi Gao	Gypsum	12 - 15 g
Sheng Di Huang	Rehmannia	6 - 12 g
Huang Qin	Scutellaria	6 - 9 g
Huang Lian	Coptis	6 g
Mu Dan Pi	Paeonia	6 - 9 g
Sheng Ma	Cimicifuga	3 - 6 g

Qi stagnation with fire causing acute pancreatitis. The patient will vomit immediately after food or liquid intake, and experiences epigastric discomfort. Acute pancreatitis can cause shock or sudden death.

T red, thin yellow coat

P rapid, wiry

☞ Mu Xiang - Saussurea and Da Huang - Rheum should be added near the end of decoction process. Mang Xiao - Mirabilitum should be added to the strained tea.

✗ Do not use during pregnancy.

QING YI TANG

Clear the Pancreas Decoction

Chai Hu	Bupleurum	6 - 15 g
Bai Shao Yao	Paeonia	6 - 15 g
Huang Qin	Scutellaria	9 - 12 g
Yan Hu Suo	Corydalis	6 - 9 g
Da Huang	Rheum	9 - 15 g
Mu Xiang	Saussurea	6 - 9 g
Hu Huang Lian	Picrorhiza	6 - 9 g
Mang Xiao	Mirabilitum	6 - 9 g

Liver and Stomach fire causing any kind of sudden bleeding disorder. The fire heats up the blood leading to hematemesis, epistaxis, or hemoptysis.

T dark red, yellow coat

P rapid, forceful, wiry

☞ The herbs should be partially charred prior to the decoction process.

✗ Caution during pregnancy.

SHI HUI SAN

Ten Partially-Charred Substance Powder

Xiao Ji	Cephalanoplos	9 - 15 g
Da Ji	Cirsium	9 - 12 g
Ce Bai Ye	Biota	9 - 12 g
Qian Cao Gen	Rubia	9 - 12 g
Da Huang	Rheum	9 - 12 g
He Ye	Nelumbo	9 - 12 g
Zhi Zi	Gardenia	6 - 12 g
Bai Mao Gen	Imperata	9 - 12 g
Zong Lu Pi	Trachycarpus	6 - 9 g
Mu Dan Pi	Paeonia	6 - 9 g

Diarrhea due to Spleen qi deficiency with damp and Stomach heat causing dysentery with mucous and possible bleeding.

T sticky yellow coat

P slippery, rapid

XIANG LIAN WAN

Aucklandia and Coptis Pill

Extract Formula Name: Saussurea and Coptis Formula

Mu Xiang	Saussurea	6 - 9 g
Huang Lian	Coptis	3 - 6 g
Wu Zhu Yu	Evodia	3 - 12 g

Fire or heat hiding in the Spleen due to overeating leading to thirst, ravenous hunger, mouth sores, the tongues of infants hang out of the mouth, or drooling. Seen in the pediatric department.

T   red, dry, yellow coat

P   rapid

XIE HUANG SAN

Drain the Yellow Powder

Extract Formula Name: Siler and Licorice Formula

Shi Gao	Gypsum	12 - 15 g
Fang Feng	Ledebouriella	12 - 15 g
Huo Xiang	Agastache	3 - 6 g
Zhi Zi	Gardenia	1 - 3 g
Gan Cao	Glycyrrhiza	6 - 12 g

Heart/Stomach fire with damp leading to fever, jaundice, fullness, alternating diarrhea or constipation, mouth and tongue sores, or carbuncles.

T   dark red, yellow coat

P   flooding, rapid

✗   Caution during pregnancy.

XIE XIN TANG

Drain the Epigastrium Decoction

Extract Formula Name: Coptis and Rhubarb Combination

Da Huang	Rheum	6 - 9 g
Huang Lian	Coptis	3 - 6 g
Huang Qin	Scutellaria	6 - 9 g

Stomach fire has damaged Stomach yin causing bleeding gums, frontal headache, aching teeth, or excess hunger.

T   red, geographic, scanty yellow coat

P   rapid, empty, thin

✪   Major Formula

YU NU JIAN

Jade Woman Decoction

Extract Formula Name: Rehmannia and Gypsum Combination

Shi Gao	Gypsum	6 - 15 g
Zhi Mu	Anemarrhena	9 - 15 g
Mai Men Dong	Ophiopogon	6 - 15 g
Shu Di Huang	Rehmannia	12 - 15 g
Huai Niu Xi	Achyranthes	9 - 15 g

Heat in the center after incorrect purging therapy causing irritability, fever, or abdominal discomfort.

T   red

P   rapid, forceful

ZHI ZI GAN JIANG TANG

Gardenia and Ginger Decoction

Zhi Zi	Gardenia	3 - 9 g
Gan Jiang	Zingiber	3 - 6 g

Fullness or bloating in the epigastrium or abdomen with heat after strong purging therapy.

T red

P slightly rapid, weak

ZHI ZI HOU PO TANG

Gardenia and Magnolia Bark Decoction

Zhi Zi	Gardenia	6 - 12 g
Hou Po	Magnolia	6 - 12 g
Zhi Shi	Citrus	3 - 9 g

Liver qi stagnation causing Liver fire which burns the Stomach. This leads to vomiting or belching, ulcers due to heat, gas, sour or bitter regurgitation. This is a Liver/Stomach imbalance.

T red, dry, yellow coat

P rapid, wiry

☞ This formula may also be prepared as a powder with ten times the dosage.

ZUO JIN WAN

Left Metal Pill

Extract Formula Name: Coptis and Evodia Formula

Huang Lian	Coptis	12 - 18 g
Wu Zhu Yu	Evodia	1 - 4 g

PARASITES IN THE DIGESTIVE TRACT

- diarrhea
- occasional worms in the stools
- abdominal discomfort

T   unremarkable

P   unremarkable

Pediatric roundworms causing stagnation of qi/food in the middle jiao with Spleen deficiency and deficiency type heat. Symptoms include fever, vision disturbances, abdominal distention, or emaciation.

T   pale

P   frail

☞ Herbs should be ground into a fine powder and taken in the morning in 3 g doses together with pork broth.

BU DAI WAN

Cloth Sack Pill

Ye Ming Sha	Vespertilio	60 g
Wu Yi	Ulmus	60 g
Shi Jun Zi	Quisqualis	60 g
Lu Hui	Aloe	9 - 15 g
Ren Shen	Panax	9 - 15 g
Fu Ling	Poria	9 - 15 g
Bai Zhu	Atractylodes	9 - 15 g
Gan Cao	Glycyrrhiza	9 - 15 g

Upper right quadrant pain or mass due to roundworms in the biliary tract, also useful for tapeworms, pinworms, and fasciolopsis.

T   depends on syndrome involved

P   depends on syndrome involved

DAN DAO QU HUI TANG

Drive Roundworms from the Biliary Tract Decoction

Bing Lang	Areca	20 - 30 g
Ku Lian Gen Pi	Melia	9 - 15 g
Mu Xiang	Saussurea	6 - 9 g
Shi Jun Zi	Quisqualis	9 - 15 g
Zhi Ke	Citrus	3 - 6 g
Yu Jin	Curcuma	6 - 9 g

Worm infestation in the Large Intestines causing indigestion and Large Intestine function disorder with Spleen qi deficiency and Stomach heat. Symptoms include malnutrition in children, ascaris, tapeworms, nausea or vomiting after eating, or low grade fever.

T red

P weak, rapid

☞ Herbs should be powdered and made into pills with pig gall. Adults take 3 g doses on an empty stomach. The dosage is decreased in children.

FEI ER WAN

Fat Baby Pill

Huang Lian	Coptis	300 g
Shen Qu	Massa Fermentata	300 g
Shi Jun Zi	Quisqualis	150 g
Mai Ya	Hordeum	150 g
Rou Dou Kou	Myristica	150 g
Bing Lang	Areca	120 g
Mu Xiang	Saussurea	60 g

Stomach

Intestinal parasites with recurring abdominal pain (roundworms, pinworms, etc.).

T depends on syndrome involved

P depends on syndrome involved

☞ Powder herbs and make into pills with wheat dough. For adults the dosage should be 6 g daily in the morning. Small children should only take 1.5 g per day.

✗ Qian Dan - Minium is toxic, and should be administered with caution. Do not use during pregnancy.

HUA CHONG WAN I

Dissolve Parasites Pills

Bing Lang	Areca	1500 g
Qian Dan	Minium	1500 g
He Shi	Carpesium	1500 g
Ku Lian Gen Pi	Melia	1500 g
Ming Fan	Alumen	370 g

Intestinal parasites with recurring abdominal pain (roundworms, pinworms, etc.). This prescription is somewhat stronger than the previous formula.

T   depends on syndrome involved

P   depends on syndrome involved

✗   Qian Dan - Minium is toxic and should be administered with caution. Do not use during pregnancy.

HUA CHONG WAN II

Dissolve Parasites Pill from the Analytic Collection

Bing Lang	Areca	15 g
Qian Dan	Minium	15 g
He Shi	Carpesium	15 g
Ku Lian Gen Pi	Melia	15 g
Ming Fan	Alumen	3.5 g
Shi Jun Zi	Quisqualis	3.5 g
Wu Yi	Ulmus	3.5 g

Spleen/Stomach deficiency with cold and roundworms causing loose, watery stools.

T   pale, white coat

P   weak

LI ZHONG AN HUI TANG

Regulate the Middle and Calm Roundworms Decoction

Ren Shen	Panax	6 - 9 g
Fu Ling	Poria	6 - 9 g
Bai Zhu	Atractylodes	3 - 6 g
Gan Jiang	Zingiber	3 - 6 g
Chuan Jiao	Zanthoxylum	6 - 9 g
Wu Mei	Prunus	6 - 9 g

Roundworms with severe heat in the Liver and Stomach causing irritability.

T   red, yellow coat

P   rapid

LIAN MEI AN HUI TANG

Picrorhiza and Mume Decoction to Calm Roundworms

Chuan Jiao	Zanthoxylum	1 - 2 g
Hu Huang Lian	Picrorhiza	2 - 3 g
Wu Mei	Prunus	3 - 6 g
Bing Lang	Areca	6 - 9 g
Lei Wan	Omphalia	6 - 9 g
Huang Bai	Phellodendron	2 - 3 g

This prescription will cause diarrhea which contains tapeworms about five hours after ingestion.

T   depends on syndrome involved

P   depends on syndrome involved

☞ Nan Gua Zi - Cucurbita should be taken first. Take Bing Lang - Areca as a decocted tea about 2 hours later.

✗ Do not use during pregnancy.

QU TIAO TANG

Expel Tapeworms Decoction

Nan Gua Zi	Cucurbita	60 g
Bing Lang	Areca	30 g

Stomach

Trichomonas due to damp. External wash only!

T   not important

P   not important

☞ Herbs should be ground into a powder, then prepared as a draft.

✗ For external use only.

SHE CHUANG ZI SAN

Cnidium Powder

She Chuang Zi	Cnidium	9 - 15 g
Bai Bu	Stemona	9 - 15 g
Chuan Jiao	Zanthoxylum	9 - 15 g
Ming Fan	Alumen	9 - 15 g
Ku Shen	Sophora	9 - 15 g

---

1. Roundworms have migrated upward due to cold in the Large Intestines to the warmth of the epigastrium/chest. 2. Large Intestine cold and Stomach heat: mixed syndrome - jueyin syndrome.

T   pale

P   weak

☞ Wu Mei - Prunus should be soaked in vinegar for 12 hours.

WU MEI WAN

Mume Pill

Extract Formula Name: Mume Formula

Wu Mei	Prunus	20 - 25 g
Xi Xin	Asarum	1 - 3 g
Chuan Jiao	Zanthoxylum	1 - 3 g
Gan Jiang	Zingiber	12 - 15 g
Fu Zi	Aconitum	6 - 9 g
Huang Lian	Coptis	9 - 12 g
Huang Bai	Phellodendron	6 - 9 g
Gui Zhi	Cinnamomum	3 - 9 g
Dang Gui	Angelica	6 - 9 g
Ren Shen	Panax	6 - 9 g

EMETICS

- nausea and vomiting

T depends on the involved syndrome

P depends on the involved syndrome

Phlegm or food stagnation in the chest/diaphragm/upper epigastrium area. This formula will relieve the stagnation by causing vomiting.

T sticky coat

P slippery, somewhat superficial in the first (cun) position.

☞ Decoct for only 5 - 10 minutes or make into a paste with 10 g of Dan Dou Chi - Glycine.

✗ This formula will cause vomiting. Do not use during pregnancy.

GUA DI SAN

Melon Pedicle Powder

Extract Formula Name: Melon Pedicle Formula

Gua Di	Cucumis	1 - 3 g
Chi Xiao Dou	Phaseolus	1 - 3 g

Pre-existing phlegm or damp accumulation with shaoyang disease leading to malaria. There is a slight possibility that this formula can cause vomiting.

T thick sticky white coat

P superficial, slippery, wiry

✗ Note that Chang Shan - Dichroa is an emetic. The formula may cause vomiting.

JIE NUE QI BAO YIN

Seven-Treasure Decoction to Check Malarial Conditions

Chang Shan	Dichroa	3 - 5 g
Bing Lang	Areca	3 g
Chen Pi	Citrus	3 g
Hou Po	Magnolia	3 g
Cao Guo	Amomum	3 g
Qing Pi	Citrus	3 g
Gan Cao	Glycyrrhiza	3 g

Wind stroke with phlegm accumulation causing hemiplegia, facial paralysis, aphasia, or seizures from wind phlegm.

T sticky coat

P slippery, forceful

☞ Herbs should be ground into a powder and then taken as a draft. The actual dosage of Li Lu - Veratrum depends on the constitution of the patient.

✗ This formula causes vomiting.

SAN SHENG SAN

Three-Sage Powder

Gua Di	Cucumis	100 - 150 g
Li Lu	Veratrum	6 - 25 g
Fang Feng	Ledebouriella	100 - 150 g

Heat in the chest and Lungs due to taiyang disease; or lingering qi level heat manifesting in the yangming channel layer. In some patients this formula will induce vomiting, after which the symptoms will disappear.

T red, especially the tip, yellow coat

P rapid, forceful, superficial

✗ This prescription can cause vomiting.

ZHI ZI DOU CHI TANG

Gardenia and Prepared Soybean Decoction

Zhi Zi	Gardenia	6 - 9 g
Dan Dou Chi	Glycine	6 - 9 g

LIVER DISHARMONIES

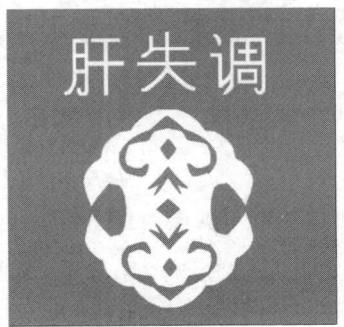

肝失调

LIVER QI STAGNATION

- irritability and sighing
- hypochondriac distention
- depression or moodswings
- belching and abdominal distention

T light purple

P wiry

Phlegm and Liver qi stagnation causing hysteria, plumpit qi, or depression.

T light purple, sticky white or yellowish coat

P slippery or wiry

✪ **Major Formula**

BAN XIA HOU PO TANG

Pinellia and Magnolia Bark Decoction

Extract Formula Name: Pinellia and Magnolia Combination

Ban Xia	Pinellia	6 - 9 g
Hou Po	Magnolia	6 - 15 g
Zi Su Ye	Perilla	3 - 6 g
Fu Ling	Poria	6 - 9 g
Sheng Jiang	Zingiber	9 - 12 g

Liver qi stagnation with false heat rising which affects the Heart and causes a tingling sensation in the epigastrium and chest (running piglet sensation).

T red sides, thin yellowish coat

P wiry, rapid

BEN TUN TANG

Running Piglet Decoction

Chuan Xiong	Ligusticum	6 g
Dang Gui	Angelica	6 - 9 g
Bai Shao Yao	Paeonia	6 - 12 g
Sheng Di Huang	Rehmannia	6 - 12 g
Huang Qin	Scutellaria	6 - 9 g
Ban Xia	Pinellia	9 - 12 g
Ge Gen	Pueraria	9 g
Sheng Jiang	Zingiber	3 - 6 g
Sang Bai Pi	Morus	6 - 9 g

Liver qi and mild blood stagnation causing dysmenorrhea or premenstrual syndrome.

T purple

P wiry

CHAI HU SU GAN SAN

Bupleurum Powder to Spread the Liver

Extract Formula Name: Bupleurum and Cyperus Combination

Chai Hu	Bupleurum	6 - 9 g
Chuan Xiong	Ligusticum	3 - 6 g
Xiang Fu	Cyperus	3 - 6 g
Bai Shao Yao	Paeonia	6 - 9 g
Zhi Ke	Citrus	3 - 6 g
Gan Cao	Glycyrrhiza	3 - 6 g
Chen Pi	Citrus	6 - 9 g

Early phase of appendicitis with Liver qi and blood stagnation symptoms.

T purple

P wiry

DAN HUANG SI NI SAN

Moutan and Phellodendron Powder for Frigid Extremitis

Chai Hu	Bupleurum	6 - 12 g
Bai Shao Yao	Paeonia	30 - 60 g
Huang Bai	Phellodendron	6 - 12 g
Mu Dan Pi	Paeonia	6 - 12 g
Zhi Shi	Citrus	3 - 12 g
Gan Cao	Glycyrrhiza	3 - 12 g

Liver/Spleen disharmony with heat. Symptoms include irregular menstruation, red or bloodshot eyes, or irritability.

T   red sides, light purple, thin white coat

P   wiry, rapid

DAN ZHI XIAO YAO SAN (JIA WEI XIAO YAO SAN)

Moutan, Gardenia, and Rambling Powder

Extract Formula Name: Bupleurum and Peony Formula

Mu Dan Pi	Paeonia	6 - 9 g
Zhi Zi	Gardenia	3 - 6 g
Chai Hu	Bupleurum	6 - 9 g
Bo He	Mentha	3 - 6 g
Dang Gui	Angelica	6 - 9 g
Bai Shao Yao	Paeonia	6 - 9 g
Bai Zhu	Atractylodes	3 - 9 g
Fu Ling	Poria	6 - 9 g
Gan Cao	Glycyrrhiza	3 - 6 g
[Sheng Jiang	Zingiber	3 - 6 g]

Liver qi stagnation with cold in the Liver channel causing a hernia.

T   pale, light purple

P   wiry

DAO QI TANG

Conduct the Qi Decoction

Mu Xiang	Saussurea	3 - 9 g
Chuan Lian Zi	Melia	9 - 12 g
Wu Zhu Yu	Evodia	3 - 6 g
Xiao Hui Xiang	Foeniculum	3 - 6 g

Mental disorder due to 1. Liver qi stagnation (use with Xiao Yao San); 2. Liver qi stagnation with fire burning the yin (use with Wen Dan Tang); 3. Yin deficiency with fire injuring the Heart.

T   red, scanty coat

P   thin, rapid

GAN MAI DA ZAO TANG

Licorice, Wheat, and Jujube Decoction

Extract Formula Name: Licorice and Jujube Combination

Gan Cao	Glycyrrhiza	9 - 12 g
Fu Xiao Mai	Triticum	9 - 15 g
Da Zao	Ziziphus	10 pc

Liver

Liver qi stagnation with blood deficiency causing delayed periods with clots.

T pale, purple

P choppy, wiry

GUO QI YIN

Delayed Menstruation Decoction

Shu Di Huang	Rehmannia	6 - 9 g
Dang Gui	Angelica	6 - 9 g
Bai Shao Yao	Paeonia	6 - 9 g
Chuan Xiong	Ligusticum	3 - 6 g
Hong Hua	Carthamus	3 - 6 g
Tao Ren	Prunus	3 - 6 g
Xiang Fu	Cyperus	3 - 6 g
Mu Tong	Akebia	3 - 6 g
E Zhu	Curcuma	3 - 6 g
Rou Gui	Cinnamomum	1 - 3 g
Gan Cao	Glycyrrhiza	3 - 6 g

Phlegm accumulation causing hardenings; or Liver qi stagnation leading to goiter or cancer.

T sticky coat

P slippery, wiry

HAI ZAO YU HU TANG

Sargassum Decoction for the Jade Flask

Hai Zao	Sargassum	3 - 6 g
Kun Bu	Laminaria	3 - 6 g
Hai Dai	Ecklonia	1.5 g
Du Huo	Angelica	3 - 6 g
Lian Qiao	Forsythia	3 - 6 g
Zhe Bei Mu	Fritillaria	3 - 6 g
Chuan Xiong	Ligusticum	3 - 6 g
Ban Xia	Pinellia	3 - 6 g
Dang Gui	Angelica	3 - 6 g
Chen Pi	Citrus	3 - 6 g
Qing Pi	Citrus	3 - 6 g
Gan Cao	Glycyrrhiza	3 - 6 g

Liver qi stagnation with heat causing hypochrondriac or abdominal pain and irritability.

T   red sides, yellow coat

P   wiry, rapid

☞ Grind into a powder and take 9 g each time.

JIN LING ZI SAN

Melia Toosandan Powder

Extract Formula Name: Melia and Corydalis Formula

Chuan Lian Zi	Melia	30 g
Yan Hu Suo	Corydalis	30 g

Liver qi stagnation with cold in the Stomach causing abdominal pain which is relieved by warmth. The formula is also useful for dysmenorrhea.

T   pale, white coat

P   weak, slow, or wiry

LIANG FU WAN

Galanga and Cyperus Pill

Extract Formula Name: Galanga and Cyperus Formula

Gao Liang Jiang	Alpinia	6 - 9 g
Xiang Fu	Cyperus	6 - 9 g

Kidney qi/yang deficiency causing qi/cold stagnation in the Liver channel. Symptoms include hernia, nodules in the lower jiao, impotence, or cold uterus with cramps prior to menses.

T   pale, purple

P   wiry or tight

NUAN GAN JIAN

Warm the Liver Decoction

Dang Gui	Angelica	6 - 9 g
Gou Qi Zi	Lycium	6 - 9 g
Wu Yao	Lindera	3 - 6 g
Chen Xiang	Aquilaria	3 - 6 g
Fu Ling	Poria	6 - 9 g
Rou Gui	Cinnamomum	3 - 6 g
Xiao Hui Xiang	Foeniculum	3 - 6 g
Sheng Jiang	Zingiber	3 - 6 g

Liver

Excess fire cholecystitis with Liver qi and damp stagnation causing alternating fever and chills or severe hypochondriac pain.

T   deep red, sticky yellow coat

P   wiry, slippery, rapid, or flooding

☞ Mang Xiao - Mirabilitum should be dissolved into the strained tea. Da Huang - Rheum should be added within the last 3 - 5 minutes of the decoction process.

✗ Do not use during pregnancy

QING DAN XIE HUO TANG

Clear the Gallbladder and Drain Fire Decoction

Chai Hu	Bupleurum	9 - 15 g
Ban Xia	Pinellia	6 - 9 g
Yin Chen Hao	Artemisia	15 - 25 g
Long Dan Cao	Gentiana	6 - 9 g
Yu Jin	Curcuma	6 - 9 g
Da Huang	Rheum	6 - 9 g
Huang Qin	Scutellaria	6 - 15 g
Zhi Zi	Gardenia	6 - 9 g
Mang Xiao	Mirabilitum	6 - 9 g
Mu Xiang	Saussurea	3 - 6 g

Qi stagnation with fire causing acute pancreatitis. The patient will vomit immediately after food or liquid intake, and experiences epigastric discomfort. Acute pancreatitis can cause shock or sudden death.

T   red, thin yellow coat

P   rapid, wiry

☞ Mu Xiang - Saussurea and Da Huang - Rheum should be added near the end of decoction process. Mang Xiao - Mirabilitum should be added to the strained tea.

✗ Do not use during pregnancy.

QING YI TANG

Clear the Pancreas Decoction

Chai Hu	Bupleurum	6 - 15 g
Bai Shao Yao	Paeonia	6 - 15 g
Huang Qin	Scutellaria	9 - 12 g
Yan Hu Suo	Corydalis	6 - 9 g
Da Huang	Rheum	9 - 15 g
Mu Xiang	Saussurea	6 - 9 g
Hu Huang Lian	Picrorhiza	6 - 9 g
Mang Xiao	Mirabilitum	6 - 9 g

Pain in the lower legs due to blood or yin deficiency, or spasmodic abdominal pain.

T   red or pale

P   weak, thin

SHAO YAO GAN CAO TANG

Peony and Licorice Decoction

Extract Formula Name: Peony and Licorice Combination

Bai Shao Yao	Paeonia	15 - 30 g
ZhiGan Cao	Glycyrrhiza	12 - 20 g

Liver overacting on the Lungs or Stomach leading to wheezing, shortness of breath, or epigastric distention respectively.

T light purple, thin coat

P wiry

SI MO TANG

Four-Milled Herb Decoction

Ren Shen	Panax	6 - 9 g
Chen Xiang	Aquilaria	3 - 6 g
Wu Yao	Lindera	3 - 6 g
Bing Lang	Areca	6 - 9 g

Liver overacting on Spleen with mild heat. This is the basic prescription for this syndrome.

T light purple, thin coat

P wiry, slightly wiry

✪ **Major Formula**

SI NI SAN

Frigid Extremities Powder

Extract Formula Name: Bupleurum and Chih-Shih Formula

Chai Hu	Bupleurum	6 - 9 g
Zhi Shi	Citrus	6 - 9 g
Bai Shao Yao	Paeonia	3 - 9 g
Zhi Gan Cao	Glycyrrhiza	3 - 6 g

Liver overacting on Stomach with pain, depression, fullness, regurgitation, and indigestion.

T white or yellow coat

P wiry

SU GAN WAN

Liver Soothing Pills

Chai Hu	Bupleurum	6 - 9 g
Bai Shao Yao	Paeonia	6 - 9 g
Fu Ling	Poria	6 - 9 g
Yan Hu Suo	Corydalis	3 - 6 g
Hou Po	Magnolia	6 - 12 g
Jiang Huang	Curcuma	6 - 9 g
Chen Xiang	Aquilaria	3 - 6 g
Chen Pi	Citrus	3 - 6 g
Zhi Ke	Citrus	3 - 6 g
Mu Xiang	Saussurea	3 - 6 g
Sha Ren	Amomum	3 - 6 g
Chuan Lian Zi	Melia	6 - 12 g
Bai Dou Kou	Amomum	3 - 6 g

Liver

External cold causing stagnation in the Liver channel. This leads to testicle pain and swelling in men, or to clear leukorrhea in women.

T pale, purple, thin white coat

P slow, wiry, or tight

☞ Ba Dou - Croton and Chuan Lian Zi - Melia should be dry fried for 5 - 10 minutes. Discard Ba Dou, then decoct as usual. This way the effect of Chuan Lian Zi is to actually warm the Liver channel.

TIAN TAI WU YAO SAN
Top-Quality Lindera Powder

Wu Yao	Lindera	6 - 9 g
Xiao Hui Xiang	Foeniculum	3 - 6 g
Gao Liang Jiang	Alpinia	3 - 6 g
Mu Xiang	Saussurea	3 - 6 g
Qing Pi	Citrus	3 - 6 g
Chuan Lian Zi	Melia	6 - 9 g
Bing Lang	Areca	6 - 9 g
Ba Dou	Croton	6 - 15 g

Liver qi stagnation causing severe acute hearing loss from emotional upset.

T light purple, thin white coat

P wiry

✗ Caution during pregnancy.

TONG QI SAN
Unblock the Qi Powder

Xiang Fu	Cyperus	6 - 9 g
Chai Hu	Bupleurum	6 - 9 g
Chuan Xiong	Ligusticum	3 - 9 g

Liver qi stagnation causes constipation. The bowel movements are often incomplete and have a thin and long shape. The person has an urge but can only discharge gas.

T light purple

P wiry

✗ Do not use during pregnancy.

WU MAO SAN
Five-Powder Formula

Wu Yao	Lindera	3 - 6 g
Mu Xiang	Saussurea	6 - 9 g
Zhi Shi	Prunus	6 - 9 g
Da Huang	Rheum	9 - 15 g
Chen Xiang	Aquilaria	6 - 9 g
Bing Lang	Areca	6 - 9 g

Liver qi stagnation causing late periods, irritability, premenstrual syndrome, or distention in the urinary tract.

T   light purple, thin coat

P   wiry

WU YAO TANG

Lindera Decoction

Wu Yao	Lindera	3 - 6 g
Dang Gui	Angelica	6 - 9 g
Xiang Fu	Cyperus	3 - 9 g
Mu Xiang	Saussurea	3 - 9 g
Gan Cao	Zingiber	3 - 6 g

Liver qi stagnation manifesting mostly as irregular periods. Menstruation is sometimes early or sometimes late, and the patient experiences severe premenstrual syndrome, cramping prior to the onset of bleeding, or breast distention.

T   light purple, thin coat

P   wiry

XIANG WU SAN

Cyperus and Lindera Powder

Xiang Fu	Cyperus	6 - 12 g
Wu Yao	Lindera	3 - 9 g
Chai Hu	Bupleurum	6 - 9 g
Bai Zhu	Atractylodes	3 - 9 g
Bai Shao Yao	Paeonia	6 - 9 g
Dang Gui	Angelica	6 - 9 g
Fu Ling	Poria	6 - 9 g

Liver

1. Chronic Spleen qi deficiency with chronic cold evil qi leading to qi and blood deficiency. The main symptom is abdominal spasms. 2. Liver qi stagnation or Liver overacting on Spleen. In the latter two instances the dosage of 'Bai Shao Yao - Paeonia' should be increased.

T   pale or light purple, thin white coat

P   weak or slightly wiry

☞ Yi Tang - Saccharum Granorum should be added to the strained tea.

XIAO JIAN ZHONG TANG

Minor Construct the Middle Decoction

Extract Formula Name: Minor Cinnamon and Peony Combination

Yi Tang	Saccharum Granorum	15 - 30 g
Gui Zhi	Cinnamomum	3 - 9 g
Bai Shao Yao	Paeonia	6 - 9 g
Sheng Jiang	Zingiber	6 - 9 g
Da Zao	Ziziphus	3 - 5 pc
Zhi Gan Cao	Glycyrrhiza	3 - 6 g

Liver/Spleen disharmony with blood deficiency: decreased appetite, irregular menstruation, pain in the flanks, or breast distention.

T light purple, pale, thin white coat

P wiry

✪ Major Formula

XIAO YAO SAN

Rambling Powder

Extract Formula Name: Bupleurum and Tang-Kuei Powder

Chai Hu	Bupleurum	6 - 9 g
Dang Gui	Angelica	6 - 9 g
Bai Zhu	Atractylodes	3 - 9 g
Bai Shao Yao	Paeonia	6 - 9 g
Fu Ling	Poria	6 - 9 g
Bo He	Mentha	3 - 6 g
Gan Cao	Glycyrrhiza	3 - 6 g
Sheng Jiang	Zingiber	3 - 6 g

Liver qi stagnation produces heat which consumes Kidney and Liver yin, or Liver overacts on the Spleen and Stomach causing emotional upset, nausea, belching with sour taste, hiatal hernia, or epigastric or abdominal pain; or Liver yin cannot nourish the tendons and ligaments producing heel or posterior hip pain.

T red, dry

P thin, wiry

YI GUAN JIAN

Linking Decoction

Extract Formula Name: Glehnia and Rehmannia Combination

Sheng Di Huang	Rehmannia	15 - 30 g
Gou Qi Zi	Lycium	6 - 15 g
Dang Gui	Angelica	6 - 12 g
Bei Sha Shen	Glehnia	6 - 9 g
Mai Men Dong	Ophiopogon	6 - 9 g
Chuan Lian Zi	Melia	3 - 6 g

Stagnations of all kinds (qi, blood, food, damp, etc.). Symptoms include epigastric or chest fullness, nausea and vomiting, or poor appetite.

T depends on particular syndrome involved

P depends on particular syndrome involved

YUE JU WAN

Escape Restraint Pill

Chuan Xiong	Ligusticum	3 - 9 g
Cang Zhu	Atractylodes	3 - 9 g
Zhi Zi	Gardenia	3 - 9 g
Xiang Fu	Cyperus	3 - 9 g
Shen Qu	Massa Fermentata	3 - 9 g

LIVER BLOOD STAGNATION

- menstrual clots
- dysmenorrhea with clots
- sharp localized pains

T   purple, or purple spots

P   wiry

Liver

Qi and blood deficiency with blood stagnation. This formula is for a restless fetus, infertility, irregular periods, poor appetite, weakness, or fatigue.

T   pale, thin white coat

P   weak, maybe wiry

BA ZHEN YI MU WAN

Eight-Treasure Pill to Benefit Mothers

Shu Di Huang	Rehmannia	6 - 15 g
Chuan Xiong	Ligusticum	3 - 9 g
Dang Gui	Angelica	6 - 9 g
Bai Shao Yao	Paeonia	6 - 12 g
Ren Shen	Panax	6 - 12 g
Bai Zhu	Atractylodes	3 - 9 g
Fu Ling	Poria	6 - 9 g
Yi Mu Cao	Leonurus	6 - 18 g
Gan Cao	Glycyrrhiza	3 - 6 g

Qi and blood stagnation with qi deficiency and blockage in the channels leading to wind stroke, hemiplegia, and atrophy in the lower limbs. The patient has difficulty walking.

T   purple, thin white coat

P   wiry, weak, slow

BU YANG HUAN WU TANG

Tonify the Yang to Restore Five-tenths Decoction

Extract Formula Name: Astragalus and Peony Combination

Huang Qi	Astragalus	60 - 120 g
Chuan Xiong	Ligusticum	3 - 6 g
Chi Shao Yao	Paeonia	3 - 6 g
Dang Gui Wei	Angelica	6 - 9 g
Hong Hua	Carthamus	3 - 6 g
Tao Ren	Prunus	3 - 6 g
Di Long	Pheretima	3 - 6 g

Liver qi and mild blood stagnation causing dysmenorrhea or premenstrual syndrome.

T   purple

P   wiry

✪ **Major Formula**

CHAI HU SU GAN SAN

Bupleurum Powder to Spread the Liver

Extrac Formula Name: Bupleurum and Cyperus Combination

Chai Hu	Bupleurum	6 - 9 g
Chuan Xiong	Ligusticum	3 - 6 g
Xiang Fu	Cyperus	3 - 6 g
Bai Shao Yao	Paeonia	6 - 9 g
Zhi Ke	Citrus	3 - 6 g
Gan Cao	Glycyrrhiza	3 - 6 g
Chen Pi	Citrus	6 - 9 g

Early phase of appendicitis with Liver qi and blood stagnation symptoms.

T   purple

P   wiry

DAN HUANG SI NI SAN

Moutan and Phellodendron Powder for Frigid Extremitis

Chai Hu	Bupleurum	6 - 12 g
Bai Shao Yao	Paeonia	30 - 60 g
Huang Bai	Phellodendron	6 - 12 g
Mu Dan Pi	Paeonia	6 - 12 g
Zhi Shi	Citrus	3 - 12 g
Gan Cao	Glycyrrhiza	3 - 12 g

Liver

Qi/blood stagnation under the diaphragm and epigastrium, or masses in the abdomen or epigastrium.

T   purple

P   wiry or choppy

✗   Do not use during pregnancy.

GE XIA ZHU YU TANG

Drive Out Blood Stasis Below the Diaphragm Decoction

Extract Formula Name: Persica and Carthamus Combination

Dang Gui	Angelica	6 - 9 g
Chuan Xiong	Ligusticum	6 - 9 g
Tao Ren	Prunus	6 - 9 g
Hong Hua	Carthamus	3 - 6 g
Mu Dan Pi	Paeonia	6 - 9 g
Chi Shao Yao	Paeonia	6 - 9 g
Yan Hu Suo	Corydalis	3 - 6 g
Xiang Fu	Cyperus	3 - 9 g
Zhi Ke	Citrus	3 - 6 g
Wu Ling Zhi	Trogopterus	6 - 9 g
Wu Yao	Lindera	3 - 6 g
Gan Cao	Glycyrrhiza	6 - 9 g

Blood and phlegm stagnation in the uterus leading to masses or lumps, amenorrhea, dysmenorrhea, or restless fetus.

T   purple, sticky coat

P   wiry, slippery, choppy

GUI ZHI FU LING WAN

Cinnamon Twig and Poria Pill

Extract Formula Name: Cinnamon and Hoelen Formula

Gui Zhi	Cinnamomum	6 - 12 g
Fu Ling	Poria	6 - 12 g
Mu Dan Pi	Paeonia	6 - 12 g
Tao Ren	Prunus	6 - 12 g
Chi Shao Yao	Paeonia	9 - 12 g

Qi and blood stagnation causing dysmenorrhea, clots, low back pain, or headaches prior to menses.

T purple

P wiry, choppy

✘ Do not use during pregnancy.

HONG HUA TAO REN JIAN

Carthamus and Peach Seed Decoction

Hong Hua	Carthamus	6 - 9 g
Tao Ren	Prunus	6 - 9 g
Chi Shao Yao	Paeonia	6 - 9 g
Dang Gui	Angelica	6 - 9 g
Chuan Xiong	Ligusticum	3 - 9 g
Sheng Di Huang	Rehmannia	6 - 12 g
Dan Shen	Salvia	6 - 9 g
Xiang Fu	Cyperus	6 - 9 g
Qing Pi	Citrus	3 - 6 g
Yan Hu Suo	Corydalis	6 - 9 g

Qi/blood stagnation causing delayed periods with clotty bleeding, and breast distention.

T normal, or purple

P wiry or choppy

JIA WEI WU YAO TANG

Augmented Lindera Decoction

Wu Yao	Lindera	10 g
Xiang Fu	Cyperus	10 g
Yan Hu Suo	Corydalis	10 g
Sha Ren	Amomum	10 g
Bing Lang	Areca	10 g
Mu Xiang	Saussurea	10 g
Gan Cao	Glycyrrhiza	10 g
[Sheng Jiang	Zingiber	1 - 3 g]

Qi/blood stagnation from external or internal injury of all kinds causing pain and bleeding.

T   purple

P   wiry or choppy

☞ Powder herbs and take in a 0.2 - 1.5 g dosage internally. For external use mix herbs with wine.

✗ Do not use during pregnancy. Zhu Sha - Cinnabaris is toxic, and should only be used short-term.

QI LI SAN

Seven-Thousandths of a Tael Powder

Extract Formula Name: Musk and Catechu Formula

Xue Jie	Dracaena	30 g
Ru Xiang	Boswellia	3 - 6 g
Hong Hua	Carthamus	3 - 6 g
Mo Yao	Commiphora	3 - 6 g
Er Cha	Acacia	6 - 9 g
Zhu Sha	Cinnabaris	3 - 5 g
She Xiang	Moschus	0.5 g
Bing Pian	Dryobalanops	0.5 g

Blood and cold stagnation in the lower jiao with mass formation, blood clots, and dysmenorrhea. This formula is also useful for liver cirrhosis.

T   pale, purple

P   wiry or choppy

✗ Do not use during pregnancy.

SHAO FU ZHU YU TANG

Drive Out Blood Stasis in the Lower Abdomen Decoction

Extract Formula Name: Cnidium and Bulrush Combination

Yan Hu Suo	Corydalis	3 - 6 g
Dang Gui	Angelica	6 - 9 g
Mo Yao	Commiphora	3 - 6 g
Rou Gui	Cinnamomum	3 - 6 g
Xiao Hui Xiang	Foeniculum	1.5 - 3 g
Gan Jiang	Zingiber	3 - 6 g
Pu Huang	Typha	6 - 9 g
Chi Shao Yao	Paeonia	6 - 9 g
Wu Ling Zhi	Trogopterus	6 - 9 g
Chuan Xiong	Ligusticum	3 - 9 g

Liver

Qi and blood stagnation in the channels causing pain in the extremities or muscles.

T   purple

P   wiry

SHEN TONG ZHU YU TANG

Drive Out Blood Stasis from a Painful Body Decoction

Chuan Xiong	Ligusticum	3 - 9 g
Tao Ren	Prunus	6 - 9 g
Hong Hua	Carthamus	6 - 9 g
Qin Jiao	Gentiana	6 - 9 g
Qiang Huo	Notopterygium	3 - 6 g
Dang Gui	Angelica	6 - 9 g
Chuan Niu Xi	Cyathula	6 - 12 g
Mo Yao	Commiphora	6 - 9 g
Wu Ling Zhi	Trogopterus	6 - 9 g
Di Long	Pheretima	6 - 9 g
Xiang Fu	Cyperus	3 - 6 g
Gan Cao	Glycyrrhiza	3 - 6 g

Post-partum retention of lochia due to blood and cold stagnation.

T   pale, purple

P   choppy

☞ Add yellow wine to the decoction.

SHENG HUA TANG

Generation and Transformation Decoction

Extract Formula Name: Tang-Kuei and Ginger Combination

Dang Gui	Angelica	15 - 28 g
Tao Ren	Prunus	6 - 9 g
Pao Jiang	Zingiber	3 - 6 g
Chuan Xiong	Ligusticum	6 - 9 g
Gan Cao	Glycyrrhiza	3 - 6 g

Post-partum blood (lochia) retention with dark clots and severe abdominal pain. The stagnation is in the Chong and Ren channels.

T   purple

P   wiry

✗ Do not use during pregnancy.

SHI XIAO SAN

Sudden Smile Powder

Extract Formula Name: Pteropus and Bulrush Formula

Pu Huang	Typha	6 - 12 g
Wu Ling Zhi	Trogopterus	6 - 9 g

Lower body wind cold damp bi-syndrome with blood stagnation causing low back pain, muscle aches, sciatica, or hemiplegia.

T purple

P wiry, slippery

✗ Do not use during pregnancy.

SHU JING HUO XUE TANG

Relax the Channels and Invigorate the Blood Decoction

Extract Formula Name: Clematis and Stephania Combination

Bai Shao Yao	Paeonia	6 - 9 g
Chuan Xiong	Ligusticum	3 - 9 g
Sheng Di Huang	Rehmannia	6 - 9 g
Dang Gui	Angelica	6 - 9 g
Cang Zhu	Atractylodes	3 - 6 g
Fu Ling	Poria	6 - 9 g
Long Dan Cao	Gentiana	6 - 9 g
Tao Ren	Prunus	3 - 6 g
Wei Ling Xian	Clematis	3 - 6 g
Huai Niu Xi	Achyranthes	6 - 9 g
Qiang Huo	Notopterygium	3 - 6 g
Chen Pi	Citrus	3 - 6 g
Fang Feng	Ledebouriella	6 - 9 g
Han Fang Ji	Stephania	6 - 9 g
Bai Zhi	Angelica	3 - 6 g
Sheng Jiang	Zingiber	3 - 6 g
Gan Cao	Glycyrrhiza	3 - 6 g

Liver

Blood deficiency with blood stagnation. Symptoms include irregular menstruation, dysmenorrhea, dizziness, or pale or purple fingernails.

T pale or purple

P thin or choppy

✪ Major Formula

SI WU TANG

Four-Substance Decoction

Extract Formula Name: Tang-Kuei Four Combination

Shu Di Huang	Rehmannia	6 - 12 g
Chuan Xiong	Ligusticum	3 - 9 g
Dang Gui	Angelica	6 - 9 g
Bai Shao Yao	Paeonia	6 - 9 g

Mild blood deficiency with severe blood stagnation causing early periods or dysmenorrhea.

T   pale or purple

P   choppy or wiry

✗   Do not use during pregnancy.

TAO HONG SI WU TANG

Four-Substance Decoction with Safflower and Peach Pit

Shu Di Huang	Rehmannia	6 - 12 g
Bai Shao Yao	Paeonia	6 - 9 g
Chuan Xiong	Ligusticum	3 - 6 g
Dang Gui	Angelica	6 - 9 g
Tao Ren	Prunus	3 - 9 g
Hong Hua	Carthamus	3 - 6 g

Blood stagnation in the head, face, and neck area leading to migraines or cyanotic lips.

T   purple or purple spots

P   wiry or choppy

☞ Decoct all herbs except She Xiang - Moschus for 15 minutes. Add 230 cc of rice wine and let cook for another 5 - 10 minutes, then add powdered She Xiang - Moschus and dissolve into the tea.

✗   Do not use during pregnancy.

TONG QIAO HUO XUE TANG

Unblock the Orifices and Invigorate the Blood Decoction

Extract Formula Name: Persica and Cnidium Combination

Hong Hua	Carthamus	6 - 9 g
Tao Ren	Prunus	6 - 9 g
Chuan Xiong	Ligusticum	3 - 9 g
Chi Shao Yao	Paeonia	6 - 9 g
Cong Bai	Allium	3 - 6 g
She Xiang	Moschus	0.1 - 0.3 g
Da Zao	Ziziphus	3 - 6 pc
Sheng Jiang	Zingiber	3 - 6 g

Qi and blood deficiency with qi/blood and phlegm stagnation causing masses on the neck, breasts, or axilla areas.

T pale or purple

P weak or choppy

XIANG BEI YANG YING TANG

Cyperus and Fritillaria Decoction to Nourish the Nutritive Qi

Ren Shen	Panax	6 - 9 g
Bai Zhu	Atractylodes	3 - 6 g
Fu Ling	Poria	6 - 9 g
Chuan Xiong	Ligusticum	3 - 6 g
Chen Pi	Citrus	3 - 6 g
Dang Gui	Angelica	6 - 9 g
Xiang Fu	Cyperus	6 - 9 g
Shu Di Huang	Rehmannia	6 - 12 g
Bei Mu	Fritillaria	3 - 6 g
Bai Shao Yao	Paeonia	6 - 9 g
Jie Geng	Platycodon	3 - 6 g
Da Zao	Ziziphus	3 - 6 pc
Sheng Jiang	Zingiber	3 - 6 g
Gan Cao	Glycyrrhiza	1 - 3 g

Qi and blood stagnation causing chest pain with water/damp accumulation: Liver affects the Lungs. Symptoms include hypochondriac pain, possible coughing, or raspy voice.

T purple, thick sticky coat

P wiry

☞ Xuan Fu Hua - Inula should be wrapped in a cheesecloth.

XIANG FU XUAN FU TANG

Cyperus and Inula Decoction

Xiang Fu	Cyperus	6 - 9 g
Xuan Fu Hua	Inula	6 - 9 g
Yi Yi Ren	Coix	9 - 15 g
Chen Pi	Citrus	3 - 6 g
Zi Su Zi	Perilla	6 - 9 g
Ban Xia	Pinellia	6 - 9 g
Fu Ling	Poria	6 - 9 g

Blood stagnation in head, chest, and diaphragm causing angina, palpitations, insomnia, nightmares, or dysmenorrhea.

T purple or purple spots

P wiry

✗ Do not use during pregnancy.

XUE FU ZHU YU TANG

Drive out Stasis in the Mansion of Blood Decoction

Extract Formula Name: Persica and Achyranthes Combination

Dang Gui	Angelica	6 - 9 g
Chuan Xiong	Ligusticum	3 - 9 g
Sheng Di Huang	Rehmannia	6 - 9 g
Chi Shao Yao	Paeonia	6 - 9 g
Tao Ren	Prunus	6 - 12 g
Hong Hua	Carthamus	6 - 9 g
Chuan Niu Xi	Cyathula	9 - 12 g
Jie Geng	Platycodon	3 - 6 g
Zhi Ke	Citrus	3 - 6 g
Chai Hu	Bupleurum	3 - 9 g
Gan Cao	Glycyrrhiza	3 - 6 g

Blood stagnation with abdominal pain, severe spasms, and irregular periods.

T purple, or purple spots

P choppy, wiry

✗ Do not use during pregnancy.

YAN HU SUO TANG

Corydalis Decoction

Yan Hu Suo	Corydalis	30 - 45 g
Chi Shao Yao	Paeonia	9 - 15 g
Rou Gui	Cinnamomum	9 - 15 g
Ru Xiang	Boswellia	60 - 90 g
Mo Yao	Commiphora	60 - 90 g
Jiang Huang	Curcuma	60 - 90 g
Dang Gui	Angelica	9 - 15 g
Mu Xiang	Saussurea	60 - 90 g
Pu Huang	Typha	9 - 15 g
Gan Cao	Glycyrrhiza	6 - 9 g
[Sheng Jiang	Zingiber	3 - 6 g]

Stagnations of all kinds (qi, blood, food, damp, etc.). Symptoms include epigastric or chest fullness, nausea and vomiting, or poor appetite.

T   depends on particular syndrome involved

P   depends on particular syndrome involved

YUE JU WAN

Escape Restraint Pill

Chuan Xiong	Ligusticum	3 - 9 g
Cang Zhu	Atractylodes	3 - 9 g
Zhi Zi	Gardenia	3 - 9 g
Xiang Fu	Cyperus	3 - 9 g
Shen Qu	Massa Fermentata	3 - 9 g

Deficient cold with blood stagnation causing uterine bleeding with pain which is better with the passage of clots.

T   pale, dark purple

P   choppy or wiry

☞ The first seven ingredients (which may be calcined) should be ground and made into 9 - 12 g pills with glutinous rice and water. The pills should be coated with Zhu Sha - Cinnabaris. One pill per day with wine is the recommeded dosage.

✗ Do not use during pregnancy. Zhu Sha - Cinnabaris is toxic and should therefore not be taken long-term.

ZHEN LING DAN

Rouse the Spirits Special Pill

Zi Shi Ying	Fluoritum	60 g
Yu Liang Shi	Limonite	60 g
Dai Zhe Shi	Haematitum	60 g
Wu Ling Zhi	Trogopterus	30 g
Ru Xiang	Boswellia	30 g
Chi Shi Zhi	Halloysitum Rubrum	60 g
Mo Yao	Commiphora	30 g
Zhu Sha	Cinnabaris	15 g

Liver

Localized swellings which are about to ulcerate with underlying qi deficiency and mild blood stagnation. Swellings are mildly painful and warm.

T   pale, light purple

P   weak

✗   Caution during pregnancy.

ZHONG HE TANG

Middle-Heartening Decoction

Ren Shen	Panax	6 - 9 g
Huang Qi	Astragalus	6 g
Dang Gui	Angelica	6 - 9 g
Fu Ling	Poria	6 - 9 g
Chuan Xiong	Ligusticum	3 - 6 g
Bai Zhu	Atractylodes	3 - 6 g
Bai Zhi	Angelica	3 - 6 g
Chen Pi	Citrus	6 g
Ru Xiang	Boswellia	3 - 6 g
Jin Yin Hua	Lonicera	3 - 6 g
Zao Jiao Ci	Gleditsia	3 g
Mo Yao	Commiphora	3 g
Gan Cao	Glycyrrhiza	3 g

LIVER OVERACTING ON SPLEEN OR STOMACH

- alternating diarrhea and constipation
- incomplete bowel movements
- gas and abdominal bloating
- belching or acid regurgitation
- irritability or emotional upset
- fatigue

T   pale, or light purple

P   wiry

Liver

Weak Spleen is overacted by the Liver, or congested Liver overacts on the Spleen. The qi deficiency is greater than the qi stagnation.

T   pale or light purple, thin white coat

P   weak or wiry

CHAI SHAO LIU JUN ZI TANG

Bupleurum, Peony, and Six-Gentlemen Decoction

Extract Formula Name: Bupleurum, Paeonia and Six Major Herbs Combination

Ren Shen	Panax	6 - 9 g
Fu Ling	Poria	6 - 9 g
Bai Zhu	Atractylodes	3 - 9 g
Chen Pi	Citrus	3 - 6 g
Ban Xia	Pinellia	6 - 9 g
Bai Shao Yao	Paeonia	6 - 9 g
Chai Hu	Bupleurum	6 - 9 g
Gan Cao	Glycyrrhiza	3 - 6 g

Liver/Spleen disharmony with heat. Symptoms include irregular menstruation, red or bloodshot eyes, or irritability.

T   red sides, light purple, thin white coat

P   wiry, rapid

DAN ZHI XIAO YAO SAN (JIA WEI XIAO YAO SAN)

Moutan, Gardenia, and Rambling Powder

Extract Formula Name: Bupleurum and Peony Formula

Mu Dan Pi	Paeonia	6 - 9 g
Zhi Zi	Gardenia	3 - 6 g
Chai Hu	Bupleurum	6 - 9 g
Bo He	Mentha	3 - 6 g
Dang Gui	Angelica	6 - 9 g
Bai Shao Yao	Paeonia	6 - 9 g
Bai Zhu	Atractylodes	3 - 9 g
Fu Ling	Poria	6 - 9 g
Gan Cao	Glycyrrhiza	3 - 6 g
[Sheng Jiang	Zingiber	3 - 6 g]

Liver overacting on Spleen causing mild cramping in the abdomen with Liver blood deficiency and some damp accumulation. Symptoms include urinary retention and lower body edema. This is often seen during pregnancy.

T   pale, orange color on the sides

P   weak, thin, or slightly wiry

DANG GUI SHAO YAO SAN

Dang Gui and Peony Powder

Extract Formula Name: Tang-Kuei and Peony Formula

Dang Gui	Angelica	6 - 9 g
Bai Shao Yao	Paeonia	3 - 9 g
Bai Zhu	Atractylodes	3 - 9 g
Fu Ling	Poria	6 - 9 g
Chuan Xiong	Ligusticum	3 - 6 g
Ze Xie	Alisma	6 - 9 g

Liver/Spleen disharmony with severe blood deficiency. This leads to dysmenorrhea and uterine bleeding.

T pale, thin white coat

P frail or wiry

HEI XIAO YAO SAN

Black Rambling Powder

Bai Zhu	Atractylodes	6 - 9 g
Di Huang	Rehmannia	6 - 15 g
Fu Ling	Poria	6 - 9 g
Chai Hu	Bupleurum	6 - 9 g
Bai Shao Yao	Paeonia	6 - 9 g
Dang Gui	Angelica	6 - 9 g
Gan Cao	Glycyrrhiza	3 - 6 g
[Bo He	Mentha	3 - 6 g]
[Sheng Jiang	Zingiber	3 - 6 g]

Liver overacting on the Stomach leading to constipation, belching, and abdominal pain.

T light purple, thin white coat

P wiry

✗ Caution during pregnancy

LIU MO TANG

Six-Milled Herb Decoction

Bing Lang	Areca	6 - 9 g
Wu Yao	Lindera	3 g
Chen Xiang	Aquilaria	3 - 6 g
Mu Xiang	Saussurea	3 - 6 g
Zhi Ke	Citrus	3 - 6 g
Da Huang	Rheum	6 - 9 g

Liver

Liver qi stagnation overacting on Spleen. This leads to damp which in turn heats up and then causes red leukorrhea. Or, the Liver fails to store the blood which also manifests as red leukorrhea.

T   purple or pale

P   wiry, or weak, thin

☞ E Jiao - Equus should be dissolved into the strained tea.

QING GAN ZHI LIN TANG

Clear Liver and Stop Leukorrhea Decoction

Bai Shao Yao	Paeonia	30 g
Dang Gui	Angelica	30 g
Shu Di Huang	Rehmannia	15 g
E Jiao	Equus	9 g
Mu Dan Pi	Paeonia	9 g
Huang Bai	Phellodendron	6 g
Huai Niu Xi	Achyranthes	6 g
Xiang Fu	Cyperus	3 g
Da Zao	Ziziphus	7 - 10 pc
no pinyin name	Small Black beans	30 g

Severe Liver qi/blood stagnation with Spleen qi/blood deficiency causing severe flank pain, and chronic hepatitis. The prescription also treats early stage liver cirrhosis.

T   purple, thin coat

P   wiry

SHU GAN LI PI TANG

Spread the Liver and Regulate the Spleen Decoction

Chai Hu	Bupleurum	9 - 12 g
Bai Zhu	Atractylodes	3 - 9 g
Dang Shen	Codonopsis	9 - 15 g
He Shou Wu	Polygonum	6 - 12 g
Dan Shen	Salvia	9 - 12 g
Xiang Fu	Cyperus	6 - 9 g
Ze Xie	Alisma	6 - 9 g
San Qi	Panax	3 g

Liver overacting on the Lungs or Stomach leading to wheezing, shortness of breath, or epigastric distention respectively.

T   light purple, thin coat

P   wiry

SI MO TANG

Four-Milled Herb Decoction

Ren Shen	Panax	6 - 9 g
Chen Xiang	Aquilaria	3 - 6 g
Wu Yao	Lindera	3 - 6 g
Bing Lang	Areca	6 - 9 g

Liver overacting on Spleen with mild heat. This is the basic prescription for this syndrome.

T light purple, thin coat

P wiry, slightly wiry

✪ **Major Formula**

SI NI SAN

Frigid Extremities Powder

Extract Formula Name: Bupleurum and Chih-Shih Formula

Chai Hu	Bupleurum	6 - 9 g
Zhi Shi	Citrus	6 - 9 g
Bai Shao Yao	Paeonia	3 - 9 g
Zhi Gan Cao	Glycyrrhiza	3 - 6 g

Liver overacting on Stomach with pain, depression, fullness, regurgitation, and indigestion.

T white or yellow coat

P wiry

SU GAN WAN

Liver Soothing Pills

Chai Hu	Bupleurum	6 - 9 g
Bai Shao Yao	Paeonia	6 - 9 g
Fu Ling	Poria	6 - 9 g
Yan Hu Suo	Corydalis	3 - 6 g
Hou Po	Magnolia	6 - 12 g
Jiang Huang	Curcuma	6 - 9 g
Chen Xiang	Aquilaria	3 - 6 g
Chen Pi	Citrus	3 - 6 g
Zhi Ke	Citrus	3 - 6 g
Mu Xiang	Saussurea	3 - 6 g
Sha Ren	Amomum	3 - 6 g
Chuan Lian Zi	Melia	6 - 12 g
Bai Dou Kou	Amomum	3 - 6 g

Liver/Spleen disharmony causing diarrhea and gurgling sounds in the abdomen.

T light purple, thin white coat

P wiry, thin, slow

TONG XIE YAO FANG

Important Formula for Painful Diarrhea

Extract Formula Name: Siler and Atractylodes Formula

Bai Shao Yao	Paeonia	9 - 12 g
Bai Zhu	Atractylodes	12 - 15 g
Fang Feng	Ledebouriella	6 - 9 g
Chen Pi	Citrus	6 - 9 g

Liver

Liver/Spleen disharmony leading to epigastric aches, acid regurgitation, diarrhea, or hot dysentery.

T light purple, thin coat

P wiry

☞ Herbs should be made into pills with flour.

WU JI WAN

Fifth and Sixth Heavenly Stem Pill

Huang Lian	Coptis	20 g
Bai Shao Yao	Paeonia	20 g
Wu Zhu Yu	Evodia	20 g

Wandering epigastric/abdominal pain after an attack of anger. There are no qi deficiency signs or symptoms.

T thin coat

P wiry

WU MO YIN ZI

Five-Milled Herb Decoction

Bing Lang	Areca	6 - 9 g
Zhi Shi	Citrus	6 - 9 g
Mu Xiang	Saussurea	6 - 9 g
Chen Xiang	Aquilaria	3 - 6 g
Wu Yao	Lindera	3 - 6 g

---

1. Chronic Spleen qi deficiency with chronic cold evil qi leading to qi and blood deficiency. The main symptom is abdominal spasms. 2. Liver qi stagnation or Liver overacting on Spleen. In the latter two instances the dosage of 'Bai Shao Yao - Paeonia' should be increased.

T pale or light purple, thin white coat

P weak or slightly wiry

☞ Yi Tang - Saccharum Granorum should be added to the strained tea.

XIAO JIAN ZHONG TANG

Minor Construct the Middle Decoction

Extract Formula Name: Minor Cinnamon and Peony Combination

Yi Tang	Saccharum Granorum	15 - 30 g
Gui Zhi	Cinnamomum	3 - 9 g
Bai Shao Yao	Paeonia	6 - 9 g
Sheng Jiang	Zingiber	6 - 9 g
Da Zao	Ziziphus	3 - 5 pc
Zhi Gan Cao	Glycyrrhiza	3 - 6 g

Liver/Spleen disharmony with blood deficiency: decreased appetite, irregular menstruation, pain in the flanks, or breast distention.

T light purple, pale, thin white coat

P wiry

✪ **Major Formula**

XIAO YAO SAN

Rambling Powder

Extract Formula Name: Bupleurum and Tang-Kuei Powder

Chai Hu	Bupleurum	6 - 9 g
Dang Gui	Angelica	6 - 9 g
Bai Zhu	Atractylodes	3 - 9 g
Bai Shao Yao	Paeonia	6 - 9 g
Fu Ling	Poria	6 - 9 g
Bo He	Mentha	3 - 6 g
Gan Cao	Glycyrrhiza	3 - 6 g
Sheng Jiang	Zingiber	3 - 6 g

Liver/Spleen disharmony with false heat due to Liver yin deficiency in children with chronic deficiency problems leading to spasms, seizures, hysteria, and being scared at night.

T red sides, light purple, thin yellowish coat

P wiry, slightly rapid, thin

YI GAN SAN

Restrain the Liver Powder

Extract Formula Name: Bupleurum Formula

Dang Gui	Angelica	6 - 9 g
Fu Ling	Poria	6 - 9 g
Bai Zhu	Atractylodes	6 - 9 g
Gou Teng	Uncaria	6 - 9 g
Chai Hu	Bupleurum	6 - 9 g
Chuan Xiong	Ligusticum	3 - 9 g
Gan Cao	Glycyrrhiza	3 - 6 g
[Chen Pi	Citrus	3 - 6 g]
[Ban Xia	Pinellia	6 - 9 g]

Liver

Liver qi stagnation causing Liver fire which burns the Stomach. This leads to vomiting or belching, ulcers due to heat, gas, sour or bitter regurgitation. This is a Liver/Stomach imbalance.

T red, dry, yellow coat

P rapid, wiry

☞ This formula may also be prepared as a powder with ten times the dosage.

ZUO JIN WAN

Left Metal Pill

Extract Formula Name: Coptis and Evodia Formula

Huang Lian	Coptis	12 - 18 g
Wu Zhu Yu	Evodia	1 - 4 g

LIVER YIN DEFICIENCY

- red, dry or blood shot eyes
- poor night vision
- malarflush and afternoon heat
- early but scanty menstruation

T red sides, scanty coat

P thin, rapid, wiry, or empty

Kidney/Liver yin deficiency with blood deficiency causing post-partum sweating, or night sweats.

T red, thin yellow coat

P thin, rapid

BA WEI DI HUANG WAN

Eight-Ingredient Pill with Rehmannia

Sheng Di Huang	Rehmannia	6 - 12 g
Shan Zhu Yu	Cornus	6 - 9 g
Shan Yao	Dioscorea	6 - 9 g
Fu Ling	Poria	6 - 9 g
Ze Xie	Alisma	6 - 9 g
Mu Dan Pi	Paeonia	6 - 9 g
Wu Wei Zi	Schisandra	6 - 9 g
Huang Qi	Astragalus	9 - 15 g

Liver blood/yin deficiency causing blurred vision, red and dry eyes, and muscle twitches.

T red, thin yellow coat

P thin, wiry, slightly rapid

BU GAN TANG

Tonify the Liver Decoction

Shu Di Huang	Rehmannia	9 - 20 g
Dang Gui	Angelica	6 - 12 g
Bai Shao Yao	Paeonia	6 - 12 g
Mu Gua	Chaenomeles	6 - 9 g
Suan Zao Ren	Ziziphus	6 - 9 g
Chuan Xiong	Ligusticum	3 - 9 g
Gan Cao	Glycyrrhiza	3 - 6 g
Mai Men Dong	Ophiopogon	6 - 9 g

Purpura due to yin deficiency with heat. Strong false fire due to Kidney and Liver yin deficiency which leads to tidal fever and night sweats.

T red, thin yellow coat or no coat

P rapid, thin, or empty

DA BU YIN WAN

Great Tonify the Yin Pill

Shu Di Huang	Rehmannia	6 - 12 g
Gui Ban	Chinemys	6 - 12 g
Huang Bai	Phellodendron	6 - 9 g
Zhi Mu	Anemarrhena	6 - 9 g

Liver wind due to Liver yin deficiency causing spasms and twitches.

T dark red, scanty yellow coat

P thin, wiry, rapid

☞ E Jiao - Equus should be added to the strained tea. Bie Jia - Amyda, Mu Li - Ostrea, and Gui Ban - Chinemys should all be crushed or powdered, and cooked 45 minutes prior to the other herbs. The egg-yolks are boiled hard, then made into a soft mass and mixed into the tea.

DA DING FENG ZHU

Major Arrest Wind Pearl

Ji Zi Huang	Egg Yolk	2
Wu Wei Zi	Schisandra	6 - 9 g
E Jiao	Equus	6 - 9 g
Bai Shao Yao	Paeonia	9 - 15 g
Mai Men Dong	Ophiopogon	9 - 15 g
Huo Ma Ren	Cannabis	3 - 6 g
Sheng Di Huang	Rehmannia	9 - 15 g
Bie Jia	Amyda	6 - 12 g
Gui Ban	Chinemys	6 - 12 g
Mu Li	Ostrea	6 - 12 g
Gan Cao	Glycyrrhiza	6 - 12 g

Kidney and Liver yin deficiency causing irregular menses a scanty menstrual flow, tinnitus, dizziness, or night sweating.

T   red, scanty coat

P   thin, rapid

DANG GUI DI HUANG YIN

Dang Gui and Rehmannia Decoction

Dang Gui	Angelica	6 - 9 g
Shu Di Huang	Rehmannia	6 - 12 g
Huai Niu Xi	Achyranthes	6 - 9 g
Shan Yao	Dioscorea	6 - 9 g
Du Zhong	Eucommia	6 - 9 g
Shan Zhu Yu	Cornus	6 - 9 g
Zhi Gan Cao	Glycyrrhiza	3 - 6 g

Liver/Kidney yin deficiency causing weakness in the low back and knees, or atrophy; or Liver cannot store the soul (hun) causing insomnia or bad dreams.

T   red, dry, scanty coat

P   thin, rapid

☞ Equal amounts of both herbs should be used.

ER ZHI WAN

Two-Ultimate Pill

Han Lian Cao	Eclipta	10 g
Nu Zhen Zi	Ligustrum	10 g

Liver qi stagnation with heat causing uterine bleeding which depletes yin (ben lou syndrome).

T   rapid, no coat

P   thin, rapid

GU JING WAN

Stabilize the Menses Pill

Extract Formula Name: Tortoise Shell and Scute Combination

Gui Ban	Chinemys	15 - 30 g
Chun Pi	Ailanthus	6 - 12 g
Bai Shao Yao	Paeonia	15 - 30 g
Huang Bai	Phellodendron	6 - 9 g
Huang Qin	Scutellaria	15 - 30 g
Xiang Fu	Cyperus	3 - 6 g

Kidney qi deficiency with Kidney/Liver yin deficiency causing amenorrhea, or back and knee pain.

T   pale or red, thin white or scanty coat

P   weak, maybe thin especially in the left chi (third) position

GUI SHEN TANG

Comeback Kidney Decoction

Shu Di Huang	Rehmannia	6 - 15 g
Shan Yao	Dioscorea	9 - 15 g
Shan Zhu Yu	Cornus	9 - 12 g
Gou Qi Zi	Lycium	9 - 15 g
Dang Gui	Angelica	9 - 12 g
Du Zhong	Eucommia	6 - 12 g
Fu Ling	Poria	6 - 12 g
Tu Si Zi	Cuscuta	9 - 12 g

Kidney and Liver yin deficiency causing bone bi-syndrome or wei syndrome. Deficient yin cannot nourish tendons and false heat burns tendons and muscles. This leads to atrophy, joint swelling, or deformities. The pain tends to be more fixed.

T   red, scanty coat

P   thin, rapid, weak

☞ All ingredients should be ground up as powder. Take 10 g each time, twice a day.

HU QIAN WAN

Hidden Tiger Pill

Extract Formula Name: Tiger Bone and Tortoise Shell Formula

Gui Ban	Chinemys	120 g
Huang Bai	Phellodendron	150 g
Shu Di Huang	Rehmannia	60 g
Zhi Mu	Anemarrhena	60 g
Bai Shao Yao	Paeonia	60 g
Suo Yang	Cynomorium	45 g
Hu Gu	Panthera	30 g
Chen Pi	Citrus	60 g
Gan Jiang	Zingiber	15 g

Liver yin deficiency with yang/wind rising causing palpitations, hypertension, or restlessness.

T   red, thin yellow coat

P   thin, rapid, slightly wiry

☞ Use iron water to cook these herbs.

JIAN LING TANG

Construct Roof Tiles Decoction

Huai Niu Xi	Achyranthes	30 g
Shan Yao	Dioscorea	30 g
Long Gu	Os Draconis	18 g
Mu Li	Ostrea	18 g
Dai Zhi Shi	Haematitum	24 g
Sheng Di Huang	Rehmannia	18 g
Bai Zi Ren	Biota	12 g
Bai Shao Yao	Paeonia	12 g

Kidney and Liver yin deficiency, yang deficiency, or jing deficiency causing spermatorrhea, tinnitus, or impotence.

T   pale or red, thin white coat

P   thin, weak

JIN SUO GU JING WAN

Metal Lock Pill to Stabilize the Essence

Extract Formula Name: Lotus Stamen Formula

Qian Shi	Euryale	6 - 12 g
Sha Yuan Ji Li	Astragalus	6 - 12 g
Long Gu	Os Draconis	6 - 9 g
Mu Li	Ostrea	6 - 9 g
Lian Xu	Nelumbo	6 - 9 g
Lian Zi	Nelumbo	9 - 15 g

Basic prescription for Kidney/Liver yin deficiency with mild damp. This can cause dry, flaky, pale red rashes, excess sexual activity, or sweating. In women it may lead to irregular menses or night sweating and afternoon heat.

T   red, thin yellow coat, or scanty coat

P   rapid, thin

✪ **Major Formula**

LIU WEI DI HUANG WAN

Six-Ingredient Pill with Rehmannia

Extract Formula Name: Rehmannia Six Formula

Shan Zhu Yu	Cornus	6 - 9 g
Shan Yao	Dioscorea	6 - 9 g
Sheng Di Huang	Rehmannia	6 - 12 g
Fu Ling	Poria	6 - 9 g
Ze Xie	Alisma	6 - 9 g
Mu Dan Pi	Paeonia	6 - 9 g

Kidney and Liver yin deficiency with yang rising causing vision disturbances, dry red eyes, or blurry vision.

T   red, scanty yellow coat

P   thin, rapid

MING MU DI HUANG WAN

Improve Vision Pill with Rehmannia

Shu Di Huang	Rehmannia	9 - 20 g
Sheng Di Huang	Rehmannia	9 - 15 g
Mu Dan Pi	Paeonia	6 - 9 g
Shan Yao	Dioscorea	6 - 9 g
Shan Zhu Yu	Cornus	6 - 9 g
Ze Xie	Alisma	6 - 9 g
Dang Gui	Angelica	6 - 9 g
Fu Shen	Poria	6 - 9 g
Chai Hu	Bupleurum	6 - 9 g
Wu Wei Zi	Schisandra	6 - 9 g

Hemorrhage in the eye due to trauma with underlying yin deficiency symptoms. Other symptoms include tinnitus, malar flush, or night sweating.

T   dark red, scanty yellow coat

P   thin, rapid, wiry

☞ Zhi Zi - Gardenia should be charcoaled to increase the stop bleeding effect. E Jiao - Equus should be added to the strained decoction.

NING XUE TANG

Quiet the Blood Decoction

Han Lian Cao	Eclipta	9 - 15 g
Xian He Cao	Agrimonia	9 - 15 g
Zhi Zi Tan	Gardenia	6 - 9 g
Sheng Di Huang	Rehmannia	9 - 15 g
Bai Lian	Ampelopsis	3 - 6 g
E Jiao	Equus	9 - 15 g
Bai Mao Gen	Imperata	9 - 15 g
Bai Shao Yao	Paeonia	9 - 15 g
Ce Bai Ye	Biota	9 - 15 g
Bai Ji	Bletilla	6 - 9 g

Liver

Liver blood/yin deficiency with Kidney qi deficiency causing early greying, hairloss, poor teeth, and seminal emissions.

T pale

P thin, weak

QI BAO MEI RAN DAN

Seven-Treasure Special Pill for Beautiful Whiskers

He Shou Wu	Polygonum	6 - 9 g
Huai Niu Xi	Achyranthes	6 - 12 g
Fu Ling	Poria	6 - 9 g
Tu Si Zi	Cuscuta	6 - 9 g
Gou Qi Zi	Lycium	6 - 9 g
Bu Gu Zhi	Psoralea	6 - 9 g
Dang Gui	Angelica	6 - 9 g

Kidney and Liver yin deficiency with eye disturbances.

T red, scanty yellow coat

P thin, rapid

QI JU DI HUANG WAN

Lycium Fruit, Chrysanthemum, and Rehmannia Pill

Extract Formula Name: Lycium, Chrysanthemum and Rehmannia Formula

Shu Di Huang	Rehmannia	6 - 12 g
Shan Yao	Dioscorea	6 - 9 g
Shan Zhu Yu	Cornus	6 - 9 g
Mu Dan Pi	Paeonia	6 - 9 g
Fu Ling	Poria	6 - 9 g
Ze Xie	Alisma	6 - 9 g
Gou Qi Zi	Lycium	6 - 12 g
Ju Hua	Chrysanthemum	6 - 9 g

Liver wind or yang rising due to yin or blood deficiency. Symptoms include spasms, vertigo, or heat in the palms, soles, and chest.

T dark red, dry, or geographic

P thin, rapid, wiry

☞ E Jiao - Equus should be dissoved at the end into the strained tea.

✗ Caution during pregnancy.

SAN JIA FU MAI TANG

Three-Shell Decoction to Restore the Pulse

Zhi Gan Cao	Glycyrrhiza	9 - 15 g
Bai Shao Yao	Paeonia	9 - 15 g
Sheng Di Huang	Rehmannia	9 - 15 g
E Jiao	Equus	6 - 9 g
Bie Jia	Amyda	9 - 20 g
Gui Ban	Chinemys	15 - 30 g
Huo Ma Ren	Cannabis	6 - 9 g
Mu Li	Ostrea	9 - 15 g
Mai Men Dong	Ophiopogon	9 - 15 g

Kidney and Liver yin deficiency with blood deficiency and wind damp. This leads to blurry vision, cough, constipation, or bi-syndrome.

T red, scanty yellow coat

P thin

☞ Herbs should be formed into 9 g pills. Adults take one pill two times a day.

SANG MA WAN

Mulberry Leaf and Sesame Seed Pill

Sang Ye	Morus	250 - 300 g
Hei Zhi Ma	Sesamum	100 - 120 g
Feng Mi	Mel	250 - 300 g

Kidney/Liver yin deficiency with yang rising causing blurry vision, photophobia, excessive tearing, poor night vision, early stage catarract, or blood-shot eyes.

T   red, thin and narrow in size, maybe cracked, scanty coat

P   thin, rapid

☞ Xi Jiao - Rhinoceros should be substituted with Shui Niu Jiao - Bubalus.

SHI HU YE GUANG WAN

Dendrobium Pill for Night Vision

Tian Men Dong	Asparagus	6- 9 g
Fu Ling	Poria	6 - 9 g
Ren Shen	Panax	6 - 9 g
Shu Di Huang	Rehmannia	12 - 15 g
Mai Men Dong	Ophiopogon	6 - 9 g
Tu Si Zi	Cuscuta	3 - 9 g
Ju Hua	Chrysanthemum	3 - 6 g
Xing Ren	Prunus	3 - 6 g
Jue Ming Zi	Cassia	6 - 9 g
Gou Qi Zi	Lycium	6 - 9 g
Shan Yao	Dioscorea	6 - 12 g
Wu Wei Zi	Schisandra	6 - 9 g
Huai Niu Xi	Achyranthes	6 - 12 g
Bai Ji Li	Tribulus	6 - 9 g
Chuan Xiong	Ligusticum	3 - 6 g
Rou Cong Rong	Cistanche	3 - 6 g
Shi Hu	Dendrobium	6 - 12 g
Zhi Ke	Citrus	3 - 6 g
Qing Xiang Zi	Celosia	3 - 9 g
Xi Jiao	Rhinoceros	1 - 3 g
Huang Lian	Coptis	3 - 6 g
Fang Feng	Ledebouriella	6 - 9 g
Ling Yang Jiao	Saiga	1 - 3 g
Gan Cao	Glycyrrhiza	3 - 6 g

Liver yin deficiency with yang or wind rising causing headaches, hypertension, tinnitus, or dizziness.

T   red

P   thin, rapid, wiry

TIAN MA GOU TENG YIN

Gastrodia and Uncaria Decoction

Extract Formula Name: Gastrodia and Uncaria Combination

Tian Ma	Gastrodia	9 - 12 g
Gou Teng	Uncaria	9 - 15 g
Chuan Niu Xi	Cyathula	9 - 12 g
Huang Qin	Scutellaria	6 - 9 g
Shi Jue Ming	Haliotis	15 - 25 g
Zhi Zi	Gardenia	3 - 6 g
Yi Mu Cao	Leonurus	6 - 12 g
Ye Jiao Teng	Polygonum	9 - 20 g
Du Zhong	Eucommia	6 - 12 g
Sang Ji Sheng	Loranthus	6 - 20 g
Fu Shen	Poria	6 - 12 g

Liver

Kidney and Liver yin deficiency causing amenorrhea, cold feeling in the abdomen, retarded growth in puberty, or clear leukorrhea.

T   pale or slightly red

P   weak, thin

☞ E Jiao - Equus should be added at the end to the strained tea.

TIAO GAN TANG

Regulating the Liver Decoction

Shan Yao	Dioscorea	9 - 12 g
E Jiao	Equus	6 - 12 g
Ba Ji Tian	Morinda	6 - 9 g
Dang Gui	Angelica	6 - 9 g
Ze Lan	Lycopus	6 - 12 g
Shan Zhu Yu	Cornus	6 - 9 g
Bai Shao Yao	Paeonia	6 - 9 g
Dan Shen	Salvia	6 - 9 g
Gan Cao	Glycyrrhiza	3 - 6 g

Liver qi stagnation produces heat which consumes Kidney and Liver yin, or Liver overacts on the Spleen and Stomach causing emotional upset, nausea, belching with sour taste, hiatal hernia, or epigastric or abdominal pain; or Liver yin cannot nourish the tendons and ligaments producing heel or posterior hip pain.

T red, dry

P thin, wiry

✪ **Major Formula**

YI GUAN JIAN

Linking Decoction

Extract Formula Name: Glehnia and Rehmannia Combination

Sheng Di Huang	Rehmannia	15 - 30 g
Gou Qi Zi	Lycium	6 - 15 g
Dang Gui	Angelica	6 - 12 g
Bei Sha Shen	Glehnia	6 - 9 g
Mai Men Dong	Ophiopogon	6 - 9 g
Chuan Lian Zi	Melia	3 - 6 g

Kidney and Liver yin/blood deficiency with fire which bothers the Heart. This causes Heart and Liver fire or Liver yang excess leading to excessive dreaming, insomnia, or outbursts of anger.

T red, cracks, thin or thick yellow coat

P rapid, wiry, thin

☞ Ingredients should be powdered, made into 9 - 12 g pills and taken three times a day. Xi Jiao - Rhinoceros should be substituted with Shui Niu Jiao - Bubalus.

ZHEN ZHU MU WAN

Mother-Of-Pearl Pill

Zhen Zhu Mu	Pteria	15 - 20 g
Ren Shen	Panax	9 - 12 g
Dang Gui	Angelica	6 - 12 g
Shu Di Huang	Rehmannia	9 - 12 g
Suan Zao Ren	Ziziphus	6 - 9 g
Bai Zi Ren	Biota	6 - 9 g
Fu Shen	Poria	6 - 9 g
Chen Xiang	Aquilaria	6 - 9 g
Xi Jiao	Rhinoceros	1 - 3 g

Kidney and Liver yin deficiency with damp stagnation. This causes poor vision, blurry vision, or dry eyes.

T red, sticky yellowish coat

P thin, weak

ZHU JING WAN

Preserve Vistas Pill

Tu Si Zi	Cuscuta	9 - 15 g
Shu Di Huang	Rehmannia	9 - 12 g
Che Qian Zi	Plantago	6 - 9 g

Kidney and Liver yin deficiency with false heat and bone steaming fever, lumbago, involuntary emissions, night sweats, or impotence. Stronger than 'Zuo Gui Yin'.

T red, scanty coat

P thin, rapid, or empty

ZUO GUI WAN

Restore the Left [Kidney] Pill

Extract Formula Name: Achyranthes and Rehmannia Formula

Shu Di Huang	Rehmannia	9 - 25 g
Gou Qi Zi	Lycium	9 - 12 g
Chuan Niu Xi	Cyathula	9 - 12 g
Shan Yao	Dioscorea	9 - 12 g
Shan Zhu Yu	Cornus	9 - 12 g
Lu Jiao Jiao	Cervus	9 - 12 g
Tu Si Zi	Cuscuta	9 - 12 g
Gui Ban	Chinemys	9 - 12 g

LIVER BLOOD DEFICIENCY

- blurry vision or spots in front of the eyes
- dizziness
- delayed, scanty and short menstruation
- soft or brittle nails

T pale, or orangy sides

P thin, weak, or choppy

Qi and blood deficiency with blood stagnation. This formula is for a restless fetus, infertility, irregular periods, poor appetite, weakness, or fatigue.

T pale, thin white coat

P weak, maybe wiry

BA ZHEN YI MU WAN

Eight-Treasure Pill to Benefit Mothers

Shu Di Huang	Rehmannia	6 - 15 g
Chuan Xiong	Ligusticum	3 - 9 g
Dang Gui	Angelica	6 - 9 g
Bai Shao Yao	Paeonia	6 - 12 g
Ren Shen	Panax	6 - 12 g
Bai Zhu	Atractylodes	3 - 9 g
Fu Ling	Poria	6 - 9 g
Yi Mu Cao	Leonurus	6 - 18 g
Gan Cao	Glycyrrhiza	3 - 6 g

Liver blood/yin deficiency causing blurred vision, red and dry eyes, and muscle twitches.

T red, thin yellow coat

P thin, wiry, slightly rapid

BU GAN TANG

Tonify the Liver Decoction

Shu Di Huang	Rehmannia	9 - 20 g
Dang Gui	Angelica	6 - 12 g
Bai Shao Yao	Paeonia	6 - 12 g
Mu Gua	Chaenomeles	6 - 9 g
Suan Zao Ren	Ziziphus	6 - 9 g
Chuan Xiong	Ligusticum	3 - 9 g
Gan Cao	Glycyrrhiza	3 - 6 g
Mai Men Dong	Ophiopogon	6 - 9 g

Kidney yin and Spleen qi/blood deficiency causing uterine prolapse with low back pain, night urination, or hearing loss and tinnitus.

T red or pale

P frail

DA BU YUAN JIAN

Great Tonify the Basal Decoction

Ren Shen	Panax	6 - 12 g
Shu Di Huang	Rehmannia	9 - 25 g
Shan Yao	Dioscorea	6 - 9 g
Shan Zhu Yu	Cornus	3 - 6 g
Gou Qi Zi	Lycium	6 - 9 g
Dang Gui	Angelica	6 - 9 g
Du Zhong	Eucommia	6 - 9 g
Gan Cao	Glycyrrhiza	3 - 6 g

Liver overacting on Spleen causing mild cramping in the abdomen with Liver blood deficiency and some damp accumulation. Symptoms include urinary retention and lower body edema. This is often seen during pregnancy.

T pale, orange color on the sides

P weak, thin, or slightly wiry

DANG GUI SHAO YAO SAN

Dang Gui and Peony Powder

Extract Formula Name: Tang-Kuei and Peony Formula

Dang Gui	Angelica	6 - 9 g
Bai Shao Yao	Paeonia	3 - 9 g
Bai Zhu	Atractylodes	3 - 9 g
Fu Ling	Poria	6 - 9 g
Chuan Xiong	Ligusticum	3 - 6 g
Ze Xie	Alisma	6 - 9 g

Blood deficiency with external cold after childbirth. This leads to spasms or hernia pain which are both relieved by pressure.

T pale

P deep, wiry, weak

☞ This formula should be prepared as a stew with eight cups of water. Simmer until it is reduced to three to four cups.

DANG GUI SHENG JIANG YANG ROU TANG

Mutton Stew with Dang Gui and Fresh Ginger Decoction

Dang Gui	Angelica	9 - 12 g
Sheng Jiang	Zingiber	9 - 15 g
Yang Rou	Mutton	40 - 50 g

Blood deficiency with yang deficiency and cold causing coldness in the uterus with dysmenorrhea. The blood is scanty, pale, and watery. The patient experiences severe cramping upon menstrual onset.

T pale, light purple, some cracks, thin white coat

P slow, thin, weak

GUI FU SI WU TANG

Cinnamon Bark, Aconite, and Four-Substance Decoction

Sheng Di Huang	Rehmannia	6 - 12 g
Dang Gui	Angelica	6 - 9 g
Chuan Xiong	Ligusticum	3 - 9 g
Bai Shao Yao	Paeonia	6 - 9 g
Rou Gui	Cinnamomum	3 - 9 g
Fu Zi	Aconitum	1 - 6 g

Weakness in the extremities with difficulty walking and muscle atrophy due to blood deficiency and damp stagnation.

T pale, sticky coat

P thin, slippery

JIA WEI SI WU TANG

Augmented Four-Substance Decoction

Dang Gui	Angelica	6 - 9 g
Huang Bai	Phellodendron	6 - 9 g
Mai Men Dong	Ophiopogon	6 - 9 g
Shu Di Huang	Rehmannia	9 - 12 g
Cang Zhu	Atractylodes	3 - 9 g
Du Zhong	Eucommia	3 - 6 g
Bai Shao Yao	Paeonia	3 - 9 g
Ren Shen	Panax	3 g
Wu Wei Zi	Schisandra	3 - 6 g
Zhi Mu	Anemarrhena	6 - 9 g
Huai Niu Xi	Achyranthes	3 - 9 g
Huang Lian	Coptis	3 g
Chuan Xiong	Ligusticum	3 - 6 g

Chong and Ren imbalance with blood deficiency causing restless fetus, pale post-partum bleeding, abdominal pain, a weak low back, or a cold uterus.

T pale

P frail, slow

☞ E Jiao - Equus should be dissolved at the end into the strained tea.

JIAO AI TANG

Ass-Hide Equus and Mugwort Decoction

Extract Formula Name: Tang-kuei and Equus Combination

E Jiao	Equus	6 - 9 g
Ai Ye	Artemisia	6 - 9 g
Dang Gui	Angelica	6 - 9 g
Sheng Di Huang	Rehmannia	18 g
Bai Shao Yao	Paeonia	12 g
Chuan Xiong	Ligusticum	6 g
Gan Cao	Glycyrrhiza	3 - 6 g

Liver blood/yin deficiency with Kidney qi deficiency causing early greying, hairloss, poor teeth, and seminal emissions.

T pale

P thin, weak

QI BAO MEI RAN DAN

Seven-Treasure Special Pill for Beautiful Whiskers

He Shou Wu	Polygonum	6 - 9 g
Huai Niu Xi	Achyranthes	6 - 12 g
Fu Ling	Poria	6 - 9 g
Tu Si Zi	Cuscuta	6 - 9 g
Gou Qi Zi	Lycium	6 - 9 g
Bu Gu Zhi	Psoralea	6 - 9 g
Dang Gui	Angelica	6 - 9 g

Liver wind or yang rising due to yin or blood deficiency. Symptoms include spasms, vertigo, or heat in the palms, soles, and chest.

T   dark red, dry, or geographic

P   thin, rapid, wiry

☞ E Jiao - Equus should be dissoved at the end into the strained tea.

✗ Caution during pregnancy.

SAN JIA FU MAI TANG

Three-Shell Decoction to Restore the Pulse

Zhi Gan Cao	Glycyrrhiza	9 - 15 g
Bai Shao Yao	Paeonia	9 - 15 g
Sheng Di Huang	Rehmannia	9 - 15 g
E Jiao	Equus	6 - 9 g
Bie Jia	Amyda	9 - 20 g
Gui Ban	Chinemys	15 - 30 g
Huo Ma Ren	Cannabis	6 - 9 g
Mu Li	Ostrea	9 - 15 g
Mai Men Dong	Ophiopogon	9 - 15 g

Qi/yang/blood deficiency. Symptoms include poor appetite, general malaise, mild cold symptoms, severe deficiency, rashes, dysmenorrhea, uterine bleeding, or post-partum deficiency.

T   pale, thin white coat

P   weak, thin, deep

SHI QUAN DA BU TANG

All-Inclusive Great Tonifying Decoction

Extract Formula Name: Ginseng and Tang-Kuei Ten Combination

Ren Shen	Panax	6 - 9 g
Fu Ling	Poria	9 - 12 g
Bai Zhu	Atractylodes	9 - 12 g
Gan Cao	Glycyrrhiza	3 - 6 g
Dang Gui	Angelica	12 - 15 g
Shu Di Huang	Rehmannia	15 - 20 g
Bai Shao Yao	Paeonia	12 - 15 g
Chuan Xiong	Ligusticum	3 - 9 g
Rou Gui	Cinnamomum	6 - 9 g
Huang Qi	Astragalus	15 - 20 g
[Da Zao	Ziziphus	1 - 3 g]
[Sheng Jiang	Zingiber	3 - 6 g]

Blood deficiency with blood stagnation. Symptoms include irregular menstruation, dysmenorrhea, dizziness, or pale or purple fingernails.

T pale or purple

P thin or choppy

❂ Major Formula

SI WU TANG

Four-Substance Decoction

Extract Formula Name: Tang-Kuei Four Combination

Shu Di Huang	Rehmannia	6 - 12 g
Chuan Xiong	Ligusticum	3 - 9 g
Dang Gui	Angelica	6 - 9 g
Bai Shao Yao	Paeonia	6 - 9 g

Blood deficiency which gives rise to wind. This causes an itchy rash which is dry and pale red.

T pale or purple

P thin

SI WU XIAO FENG SAN

Eliminate Wind Decoction with the Four-Substances

Sheng Di Huang	Rehmannia	6 - 9 g
Dang Gui	Angelica	6 - 9 g
Chi Shao Yao	Paeonia	3 - 6 g
Chuan Xiong	Ligusticum	3 - 6 g
Jing Jie	Schizonepeta	3 - 6 g
Fang Feng	Ledebouriella	3 - 6 g
Bai Xian Pi	Dictamnus	3 - 6 g
Bo He	Mentha	3 - 6 g
Chai Hu	Bupleurum	2 g
Du Huo	Angelica	3 g
Chan Tui	Cryptotympana	3 - 6 g
Da Zao	Ziziphus	2 - 3 pc

Blood deficiency causing wind which results in an itchy skin.

T pale

P thin, weak

XUE XU SHEN FENG

Blood Deficiency and Calm Wind Decoction

Gou Qi Zi	Lycium	6 - 12 g
He Shou Wu	Polygonum	6 - 9 g
Fang Feng	Ledebouriella	6 - 9 g
Chan Tui	Cryptotympana	6 - 9 g
Yu Zhu	Polygonatum	6 - 9 g

Liver

COLD IN THE LIVER CHANNEL

- testicular pain or pain in the scrotum
- contraction of the testis or shrinking sensation of the vagina
- ilioinguinal hernia

T pale, moist, thin white coat

P deep, slow, maybe wiry

Cold in the lower jiao causing a running piglet disorder. Symptoms include a tingling sensation around the umbilicus, abdomen, and sternum.

T pale, thin white coat

P wiry or tight

☞ Herbs should be cooked with a little sugar, then formed into 6 g pills. Adults take 2 - 3 pills a day with salt water.

BEN TUN WAN

Running Piglet Pill

Wu Zhu Yu	Evodia	3 - 6 g
Chuan Lian Zi	Melia	15 - 30 g
Ju He	Citrus	15 - 45 g
Fu Ling	Poria	15 - 45 g
Xiao Hui Xiang	Foeniculum	9 - 20 g
Mu Xiang	Saussurea	9 - 20 g
Li Zhi He	Litchi	15 - 25 g
Rou Gui	Cinnamomum	6 - 12 g
Fu Zi	Aconitum	6 - 12 g

Blood deficiency with external cold after childbirth. This leads to spasms or hernia pain which are both relieved by pressure.

T pale

P deep, wiry, weak

☞ This formula should be prepared as a stew with eight cups of water. Simmer until it is reduced to three to four cups.

DANG GUI SHENG JIANG YANG ROU TANG

Mutton Stew with Dang Gui and Fresh Ginger Decoction

Dang Gui	Angelica	9 - 12 g
Sheng Jiang	Zingiber	9 - 15 g
Yang Rou	Mutton	40 - 50 g

Liver qi stagnation with cold in the Liver channel causing a hernia.

T   pale, light purple

P   wiry

DAO QI TANG

Conduct the Qi Decoction

Mu Xiang	Saussurea	3 - 9 g
Chuan Lian Zi	Melia	9 - 12 g
Wu Zhu Yu	Evodia	3 - 6 g
Xiao Hui Xiang	Foeniculum	3 - 6 g

Cold damp stagnation in the lower jiao or cold and qi stagnation causing hard masses and nodules, testicular swelling, swelling of the scrotum, hernia, or fibroid tumors.

T   pale, thin sticky white coat

P   slow, wiry

JU HE WAN

Tangerine Seed Pill

Chuan Lian Zi	Melia	9 - 12 g
Ju He	Citrus	9 - 12 g
Tao Ren	Prunus	9 g
Rou Gui	Cinnamomum	3 - 6 g
Mu Tong	Akebia	6 g
Hai Dai	Laminaria	6 g
Hai Zao	Sargassum	6 g
Kun Bu	Laminaria	6 g
Mu Xiang	Saussurea	3 - 6 g
Yan Hu Suo	Corydalis	6 g
Hou Po	Magnolia	6 - 12 g
Zhi Shi	Citrus	3 - 6 g

Kidney qi/yang deficiency causing qi/cold stagnation in the Liver channel. Symptoms include hernia, nodules in the lower jiao, impotence, or cold uterus with cramps prior to menses.

T   pale, purple

P   wiry or tight

✪ Major Formula

NUAN GAN JIAN

Warm the Liver Decoction

Dang Gui	Angelica	6 - 9 g
Gou Qi Zi	Lycium	6 - 9 g
Wu Yao	Lindera	3 - 6 g
Chen Xiang	Aquilaria	3 - 6 g
Fu Ling	Poria	6 - 9 g
Rou Gui	Cinnamomum	3 - 6 g
Xiao Hui Xiang	Foeniculum	3 - 6 g
Sheng Jiang	Zingiber	3 - 6 g

Liver

Blood and cold stagnation in the lower jiao with mass formation, blood clots, and dysmenorrhea. This formula is also useful for liver cirrhosis.

T pale, purple

P wiry or choppy

✗ Do not use during pregnancy.

SHAO FU ZHU YU TANG

Drive Out Blood Stasis in the Lower Abdomen Decoction

Extract Formula Name: Cnidium and Bulrush Combination

Yan Hu Suo	Corydalis	3 - 6 g
Dang Gui	Angelica	6 - 9 g
Mo Yao	Commiphora	3 - 6 g
Rou Gui	Cinnamomum	3 - 6 g
Xiao Hui Xiang	Foeniculum	1.5 - 3 g
Gan Jiang	Zingiber	3 - 6 g
Pu Huang	Typha	6 - 9 g
Chi Shao Yao	Paeonia	6 - 9 g
Wu Ling Zhi	Trogopterus	6 - 9 g
Chuan Xiong	Ligusticum	3 - 9 g

Post-partum retention of lochia due to blood and cold stagnation.

T pale, purple

P choppy

☞ Add yellow wine to the decoction.

SHENG HUA TANG

Generation and Transformation Decoction

Extract Formula Name: Tang-Kuei and Ginger Combination

Dang Gui	Angelica	15 - 28 g
Tao Ren	Prunus	6 - 9 g
Pao Jiang	Zingiber	3 - 6 g
Chuan Xiong	Ligusticum	6 - 9 g
Gan Cao	Glycyrrhiza	3 - 6 g

External cold causing stagnation in the Liver channel. This leads to testicle pain and swelling in men, or to clear leukorrhea in women.

T   pale, purple, thin white coat

P   slow, wiry, or tight

☞ Ba Dou - Croton and Chuan Lian Zi - Melia should be dry fried for 5 - 10 minutes. Discard Ba Dou, then decoct as usual. This way the effect of Chuan Lian Zi is to actually warm the Liver channel.

TIAN TAI WU YAO SAN

Top-Quality Lindera Powder

Wu Yao	Lindera	6 - 9 g
Xiao Hui Xiang	Foeniculum	3 - 6 g
Gao Liang Jiang	Alpinia	3 - 6 g
Mu Xiang	Saussurea	3 - 6 g
Qing Pi	Citrus	3 - 6 g
Chuan Lian Zi	Melia	6 - 9 g
Bing Lang	Areca	6 - 9 g
Ba Dou	Croton	6 - 15 g

Deficient cold and blood stagnation causing menstrual irregularities, spotting between periods (lou syndrome), clots at the end of the period, coldness in the lower abdomen, or low-grade fever at night only.

T   pale, purple, dark purple spots

P   deep, slow, or tight

☞ E Jiao - Equus should be added at the end to the strained tea.

WEN JING TANG

Warm the Menses Decoction

Extract Formula Name: Tang-Kuei and Evodia Combination

Gui Zhi	Cinnamomum	6 - 9 g
Wu Zhu Yu	Evodia	6 - 9 g
Bai Shao Yao	Paeonia	6 - 9 g
Mai Men Dong	Ophiopogon	6 - 9 g
Mu Dan Pi	Paeonia	6 - 9 g
Ban Xia	Pinellia	6 - 9 g
Ren Shen	Panax	6 - 9 g
Dang Gui	Angelica	6 - 9 g
E Jiao	Equus	6 - 9 g
Chuan Xiong	Ligusticum	6 g
Sheng Jiang	Zingiber	3 - 6 g
Gan Cao	Glycyrrhiza	3 - 6 g

Liver

Spleen qi deficiency with cold which restricts the Liver and Stomach. This results in tight abdominal pain, cold in the middle and lower jiao, vomiting, or acid regurgitation; or cold causes vertex headaches via the Liver channel. This Liver qi stagnation is not due to emotional reasons but is caused by cold.

T   pale, purplish, moist white coat

P   slow, or wiry, thin

WU ZHU YU TANG

Evodia Decoction

Extract Formula Name: Evodia Combination

Wu Zhu Yu	Evodia	3 - 6 g
Ren Shen	Panax	6 - 9 g
Sheng Jiang	Zingiber	12 - 20 g
Da Zao	Ziziphus	6 - 12 pc

Cold causing severe abdominal distention with absence of bowel movements and urination, or vomiting right after meals. This formula is also for running piglet disorder (tingling sensation in the epigastrium or abdomen) or cold hernias.

T   pale

P   slow

☞ Herbs should be ground into a powder. Take as a draft in 3 - 9 g doses before meals.

ZHONG MAN FEN XIAO TANG

Separate and Reduce Fullness in the Middle Decoction

Chuan Wu	Aconitum	3 - 6 g
Huang Lian	Coptis	3 - 6 g
Qing Pi	Citrus	3 - 6 g
Ma Huang	Ephedra	3 - 6 g
Bi Cheng Qie	Litsea	3 - 6 g
Fu Ling	Poria	9 - 15 g
Ban Xia	Pinellia	9 - 15 g
Sheng Ma	Cimicifuga	9 - 15 g
Sheng Jiang	Zingiber	3 - 6 g
Gan Jiang	Zingiber	3 - 6 g
Wu Zhu Yu	Evodia	9 - 15 g
Cao Dou Kou	Alpinia	9 - 15 g
Ze Xie	Alisma	3 - 6 g
Yi Zhi Ren	Alpinia	9 - 15 g
Mu Xiang	Saussurea	9 - 15 g
Hou Po	Magnolia	9 - 15 g
Huang Bai	Phellodendron	9 - 15 g
Huang Qi	Astragalus	9 - 15 g
Ren Shen	Panax	3 - 6 g
Dang Gui	Angelica	3 - 6 g
Chai Hu	Bupleurum	3 - 6 g

DAMP HEAT IN THE LIVER AND LOWER JIAO

- fullness or pain in chest and hypochondriac region
- decreased appetite with nausea and vomiting
- vaginal itching or leukorrhea
- herpes lesions

T red, sticky yellow coat

P slippery, wiry, rapid

Herpes zoster around the waist. The cause is damp heat in the lower jiao.

T sticky yellow coat

P slippery

CHU SHI WEI LING TANG

Eliminate Dampness Decoction by Combining Calm the Stomach and Five-Ingredient Powder with Poria

Hou Po	Magnolia	6 - 12 g
Cang Zhu	Atractylodes	3 - 6 g
Zhu Ling	Polyporus	6 - 9 g
Chi Fu Ling	Poria	6 - 9 g
Ze Xie	Alisma	6 - 9 g
Chen Pi	Citrus	3 - 6 g
Bai Zhu	Atractylodes	3 - 6 g
Rou Gui	Cinnamomum	3 - 6 g
Hua Shi	Talcum	6 g
Zhi Zi	Gardenia	3 - 6 g
Fang Feng	Ledebouriella	6 - 9 g
Mu Tong	Akebia	6 - 9 g
Deng Xin Cao	Juncus	3 - 6 g
Gan Cao	Glycyrrhiza	3 - 6 g

Damp heat in the lower jiao causing low back pain, hot, swollen knees or feet, or odorous leukorrhea.

T sticky yellow coat

P slippery, rapid

ER MIAO SAN

Two-Marvel Powder

Cang Zhu	Atractylodes	15 g
Huang Bai	Phellodendron	15 g

Yang jaundice from damp heat lodged in the shaoyang level; or damp heat in the Gallbladder causing alternating fever and chills, bitter taste, or malaria.

T red, thick sticky yellow coat

P slippery, wiry, rapid

☞ Bi Yu San - Green Jade Powder consists of: Hua Shi - Talcum, 3 - 6 g; Gan Cao - Glycyrrhiza, 3 - 6 g; and Qing Dai - Indigo, 9 - 12 g. All three ingredients should be cooked separately in a cheesecloth, then decocted with the rest of the herbs.

HAO QIN QING DAN TANG

Artemisia Annua and Scutellaria Decoction to Clear the Gallbladder

Qing Hao	Artemisia	6 g
Zhu Ru	Bambusa	9 g
Huang Qin	Scutellaria	6 g
Zhi Ke	Citrus	5 g
Chi Fu Ling	Poria	9 g
Ban Xia	Pinellia	5 g
Chen Pi	Citrus	5 g
Bi Yu San	Green Jade Powder	9 g

Damp heat leukorrhea with low back pain, heat sensation along the leg, or eczema.

T red, sticky yellow coat

P wiry, rapid, slippery

JIA WEI ER MIAO SAN

Augmented Two-Marvel Powder

Huang Bai	Phellodendron	6 - 12 g
Cang Zhu	Atractylodes	9 - 15 g
Dang Gui Wei	Angelica	6 - 9 g
Bei Xie	Dioscorea	6 - 9 g
Han Fang Ji	Stephania	6 - 9 g
Chuan Niu Xi	Cyathula	6 - 9 g
Gui Ban	Chinemys	6 - 9 g

Damp heat in the lower jiao, or Liver fire. Symptoms include red and itchy eyes, temple headaches, odorous leukorrhea, or pruritus.

T red, sticky yellow coating

P wiry, rapid, slippery

✪ **Major Formula**

LONG DAN XIE GAN TANG

Gentiana Decoction to Drain the Liver

Extract Formula Name: Gentiana Combination

Long Dan Cao	Gentiana	6 - 9 g
Zhi Zi	Gardenia	3 - 9 g
Mu Tong	Akebia	6 - 9 g
Huang Qin	Scutellaria	6 - 9 g
Ze Xie	Alisma	6 - 9 g
Che Qian Zi	Plantago	6 - 9 g
Dang Gui	Angelica	6 - 9 g
Sheng Di Huang	Rehmannia	6 - 12 g
Chai Hu	Bupleurum	6 - 9 g
Gan Cao	Glycyrrhiza	3 - 6 g

Liver qi stagnation overacting on Spleen. This leads to damp which in turn heats up and then causes red leukorrhea. Or, the Liver fails to store the blood which also manifests as red leukorrhea.

T purple or pale

P wiry, or weak, thin

☞ E Jiao - Equus should be dissolved into the strained tea.

QING GAN ZHI LIN TANG

Clear Liver and Stop Leukorrhea Decoction

Bai Shao Yao	Paeonia	30 g
Dang Gui	Angelica	30 g
Shu Di Huang	Rehmannia	15 g
E Jiao	Equus	9 g
Mu Dan Pi	Paeonia	9 g
Huang Bai	Phellodendron	6 g
Huai Niu Xi	Achyranthes	6 g
Xiang Fu	Cyperus	3 g
Da Zao	Ziziphus	7 - 10 pc
no pinyin name	Small Black beans	30 g

Yellow leukorrhea with dark yellow urination from heat and damp in the lower jiao.

T red, sticky yellowish coat

P slippery, rapid

QING XIN LIAN ZI YIN

Clear the Heart with Lotus Seed Decoction

Extract Formula Name: Lotus Seed Combination

Huang Qin	Scutellaria	6 - 9 g
Mai Men Dong	Ophiopogon	6 - 9 g
Ren Shen	Panax	6 - 9 g
Huang Qi	Astragalus	6 - 15g
Di Gu Pi	Lycium	6 - 9 g
Che Qian Zi	Plantago	6 - 9 g
Lian Zi	Nelumbo	3 - 9 g
Chai Hu	Bupleurum	6 - 9 g
Fu Ling	Poria	6 - 9 g

Damp heat in the lower jiao with atrophy in the lower extremities, weakness and numbness, or swollen feet.

T red, sticky yellow coat

P rapid, slippery

SAN MIAO SAN

Three-Marvel Powder

Extract Formula Name: Phellodendron and Achyranthes Formula

Huai Niu Xi	Achyranthes	3 - 9 g
Huang Bai	Phellodendron	6 - 9 g
Cang Zhu	Atractylodes	6 - 12 g

Trichomonas due to damp. External wash only!

T not important

P not important

☞ Herbs should be ground into a powder, then prepared as a draft.

✘ For external use only.

SHE CHUANG ZI SAN

Cnidium Powder

She Chuang Zi	Cnidium	9 - 15 g
Bai Bu	Stemona	9 - 15 g
Chuan Jiao	Zanthoxylum	9 - 15 g
Ming Fan	Alumen	9 - 15 g
Ku Shen	Sophora	9 - 15 g

Damp heat in the lower jiao. Odorous leukorrhea, cloudy urine, and painful swollen feet.

T red, sticky yellow coat

P slippery, rapid

✪ Major Formula

SI MIAO SAN

Four-Marvel Powder

Cang Zhu	Atractylodes	6 - 9 g
Huang Bai	Phellodendron	6 - 9 g
Yi Yi Ren	Coix	6 - 12 g
Huai Niu Xi	Achyranthes	6 - 12 g

Trichomonas infection: damp heat causing yellow, odorous leukorrhea, and severe itching.

T red, sticky yellow coat

P rapid, slippery

WU MEI YIN CHEN TANG

Mume and Artemisia Yinchenhao Decoction

Wu Mei	Prunus	20 - 30 g
Yin Chen Hao	Artemisia	9 - 15 g
Hua Jiao	Zanthoxylum	6 - 9 g
Jin Yin Hua	Lonicera	6 - 12 g
Bian Xu	Polygonum	6 - 9 g
Bai Zhu	Atractylodes	6 - 9 g
Fu Ling	Poria	6 - 15 g
Long Dan Cao	Gentiana	6 - 9 g
Huang Bai	Phellodendron	6 - 9 g

Whole body yang jaundice due to damp heat in the Liver and Gallbladder.

T Red, thick sticky yellow coat

P slippery, rapid, forceful

✗ Do not use during pregnancy.

YIN CHEN HAO TANG

Artemisia Yinchenhao Decoction

Extract Formula Name: Capillaris Combination

Yin Chen Hao	Artemisia	15 - 30 g
Da Huang	Rheum	6 - 9 g
Zhi Zi	Gardenia	6 - 9 g

Liver

Damp heat accumulation in the middle jiao (Liver/Gallbladder) causing yang jaundice, dysurea, or hepatitis with mild fever.

T slightly red, thick sticky coat

P slippery, slightly rapid

YIN CHEN WU LING SAN

Artemisia Yinchenhao and Five-Ingredient Powder with Poria

Extract Formula Name: Capillaris and Hoelen Five Formula

Yin Chen Hao	Artemisia	10 - 20 g
Fu Ling	Poria	6 - 12 g
Zhu Ling	Polyporus	6 - 9 g
Bai Zhu	Atractylodes	3 - 9 g
Ze Xie	Alisma	6 - 9 g
Gui Zhi	Cinnamomum	3 - 9 g

Damp heat accumulation leading to leukorrhea. The discharge is very odorous, yellow, thick, and may be profuse.

T red, thick yellow sticky coat

P slippery, rapid

ZHI DAI TANG

Stop Leukorrhea Decoction

Fu Ling	Poria	6 - 9 g
Zhu Ling	Polyporus	6 - 9 g
Ze Xie	Alisma	6 - 9 g
Che Qian Zi	Plantago	3 - 9 g
Yin Chen Hao	Artemisia	15 g
Zhi Zi	Gardenia	3 - 6 g
Huang Bai	Phellodendron	3 - 9 g
Mu Dan Pi	Paeonia	6 - 12 g
Chi Shao Yao	Paeonia	6 - 9 g
Huai Niu Xi	Achyranthes	3 - 6 g

Yang jaundice due to damp heat in the interior. The heat is greater than the damp.

T red, sticky yellow coat

P slippery, rapid

ZHI ZI BAI PI TANG

Gardenia and Phellodendron Decoction

Extract Formula Name: Gardenia and Phellodendron Combination

Zhi Zi	Gardenia	9 - 15 g
Huang Bai	Phellodendron	6 - 9 g
Zhi Gan Cao	Glycyrrhiza	3 - 6 g

Damp heat accumulation in the middle jiao. There is more damp than heat causing fullness in the abdomen, thirst without desire to drink, or immediate fullness upon eating or drinking. This formula is also useful for yang jaundice.

T   red, thick sticky coat

P   slippery, rapid

ZHONG JIAO XIAN BI TANG

Middle Jiao and Clear Damp Decoction

Xing Ren	Prunus	3 - 6 g
Yi Yi Ren	Coix	9 - 12 g
Hua Shi	Talcum	6 g
Dou Juan	Glycine	9 g
Zhi Zi	Gardenia	6 - 9 g
Lian Qiao	Forsythia	6 g
Ban Xia	Pinellia	6 - 9 g
Han Fang Ji	Stephania	6 - 9 g
Can Sha	Bombyx	3 - 6 g
Shan Zha	Crataegus	3 - 9 g
Bian Dou	Dolichos	6 - 9 g

Damp heat in the lower jiao causing urinary difficulty and pain.

T   red, sticky coat

P   slippery

ZHU LING TANG II

Polyporus Decoction from Comprehensive Recordings

Zhu Ling	Polyporus	6 - 9 g
Mu Tong	Akebia	6 - 9 g
Sang Bai Pi	Morus	6 - 9 g
[Deng Xin Cao	Juncus	3 g]

Liver

LIVER FIRE

- uncontrolled anger outbursts
- bitter taste
- constipation and dark-yellow urine
- loud tinnitus
- bleeding in the upper parts like epistaxis, hemoptysis

T red, or red sides, yellow coat

P wiry, rapid, forceful

Liver fire causing sores on the head, severe headaches, bad breath, or hearing difficulty.

T red, yellow coat

P rapid, wiry

CHAI HU QING GAN TANG

Bupleurum Decoction to Clear the Liver

Extract Formula Name: Bupleurum and Rehmannia Combination

Chai Hu	Bupleurum	6 - 9 g
Chi Shao Yao	Paeonia	6 - 9 g
Lian Qiao	Forsythia	6 - 9 g
Chuan Xiong	Ligusticum	3 - 6 g
Dang Gui	Angelica	6 - 9 g
Sheng Di Huang	Rehmannia	6 - 9 g
Zhi Zi	Gardenia	3 - 6 g
Tian Hua Fen	Trichosanthes	6 - 9 g
Huang Qin	Scutellaria	3 - 9 g
Niu Bang Zi	Arctium	6 - 9 g
Fang Feng	Ledebouriella	3 - 6 g
Gan Cao	Glycyrrhiza	3 - 6 g

Liver/Spleen disharmony with heat. Symptoms include irregular menstruation, red or blood-shot eyes, or irritability.

T red sides, light purple, thin white coat

P wiry, rapid

DAN ZHI XIAO YAO SAN (JIA WEI XIAO YAO SAN)

Moutan, Gardenia, and Rambling Powder

Extract Formula Name: Bupleurum and Peony Formula

Mu Dan Pi	Paeonia	6 - 9 g
Zhi Zi	Gardenia	3 - 6 g
Chai Hu	Bupleurum	6 - 9 g
Bo He	Mentha	3 - 6 g
Dang Gui	Angelica	6 - 9 g
Bai Shao Yao	Paeonia	6 - 9 g
Bai Zhu	Atractylodes	3 - 9 g
Fu Ling	Poria	6 - 9 g
Gan Cao	Glycyrrhiza	3 - 6 g
[Sheng Jiang	Zingiber	3 - 6 g]

Liver/Gallbladder fire with headaches, mania, restlessness, bleeding gums, hypertension, purpura, otitis media, bitter taste, low-pitched tinnitus, melena, and possible coma.

T red, cracks, yellow coat

P rapid, wiry

☞ Herbs should be ground into a powder, then formed into pills with honey.

✘ Do not use during pregnancy.

✪ **Major Formula**

DANG GUI LONG HUI WAN

Dang Gui, Gentiana, and Aloe Decoction

Extract Formula Name: Tang-Kuei, Gentian and Aloe Formula

Dang Gui	Angelica	30 g
Long Dan Cao	Gentiana	15 g
Lu Hui	Aloe	15 g
Zhi Zi	Gardenia	30 g
Huang Lian	Coptis	30 g
Huang Qin	Scutellaria	30 g
Huang Bai	Phellodendron	6 - 9 g
Da Huang	Rheum	15 g
Mu Xiang	Saussurea	3 - 6 g
She Xiang	Moschus	1.5 g

Liver fire attacking the Lung yin. This leads to thick blood-tinged phlegm, thirst, or bitter taste.

T   red, cracked, sticky yellow coat

P   wiry, rapid

KE XUE FANG

Coughing of Blood Formula

Zhi Zi	Gardenia	6 - 9 g
Gua Lou Ren	Trichosanthes	6 - 9 g
Qing Dai	Indigo	6 - 9 g
Fu Hai Shi	Pumice	6 - 9 g
He Zi	Terminalia	3 - 9 g

Liver wind due to Liver fire causing hypertension, twitches, or headaches.

T   dark red, raw, dry

P   rapid, wiry

☞ Ling Yang Jiao - Saiga should be cooked one hour prior to adding the other herbs.

LING YANG GOU TENG YIN

Antelope Horn and Uncaria Decoction

Extract Formula Name: Antelope Horn and Uncaria Combination

Ling Yang Jiao	Saiga	3 - 6 g
Sang Ye	Morus	6 - 9 g
Sheng Di Huang	Rehmannia	9 - 15 g
Zhu Ru	Bambusa	9 - 15 g
Bai Shao Yao	Paeonia	6 - 9 g
Gou Teng	Uncaria	6 - 9 g
Chuan Bei Mu	Fritillaria	6 - 12 g
Ju Hua	Chrysanthemum	6 - 9 g
Fu Shen	Poria	6 - 9 g
Gan Cao	Glycyrrhiza	3 - 6 g

Damp heat in the lower jiao, or Liver fire. Symptoms include red and itchy eyes, temple headaches, odorous leukorrhea, or pruritus.

T red, sticky yellow coating

P wiry, rapid, slippery

✪ **Major Formula**

LONG DAN XIE GAN TANG

Gentiana Decoction to Drain the Liver

Extract Formula Name: Gentiana Combination

Long Dan Cao	Gentiana	6 - 9 g
Zhi Zi	Gardenia	3 - 9 g
Mu Tong	Akebia	6 - 9 g
Huang Qin	Scutellaria	6 - 9 g
Ze Xie	Alisma	6 - 9 g
Che Qian Zi	Plantago	6 - 9 g
Dang Gui	Angelica	6 - 9 g
Sheng Di Huang	Rehmannia	6 - 12 g
Chai Hu	Bupleurum	6 - 9 g
Gan Cao	Glycyrrhiza	3 - 6 g

Liver and Stomach fire causing dizziness, bad breath, anger outbursts, oral sores or ulcers, or constipation.

T red, sticky yellow coat

P rapid, wiry, forceful

☞ Niu Huang - Bos should be added at the end of the decoction process. Bing Pian - Dryobalanops and Xiong Huang - Realgar should be powdered prior to the decoction. This prescription is available in prepared form.

✗ Do not use during pregnancy

NIU HUANG JIE DU PIEN

Antiphlogistic Pills with Bos Calculus

Niu Huang	Bos	3 - 6 g
Xiong Huang	Realgar	3 - 6 g
Da Huang	Rheum	6 - 9 g
Jie Geng	Platycodon	3 - 6 g
Bing Pian	Dryobalanops	3 - 6 g
Shi Gao	Gypsum	9 - 15 g
Huang Qin	Scutellaria	6 - 9 g
Gan Cao	Glycyrrhiza	3 - 6 g

Liver

Qi stagnation with fire causing acute pancreatitis. The patient will vomit immediately after food or liquid intake, and experiences epigastric discomfort. Acute pancreatitis can cause shock or sudden death.

T   red, thin yellow coat

P   rapid, wiry

☞ Mu Xiang - Saussurea and Da Huang - Rheum should be added near the end of decoction process. Mang Xiao - Mirabilitum should be added to the strained tea.

✗ Do not use during pregnancy.

QING YI TANG

Clear the Pancreas Decoction

Chai Hu	Bupleurum	6 - 15 g
Bai Shao Yao	Paeonia	6 - 15 g
Huang Qin	Scutellaria	9 - 12 g
Yan Hu Suo	Corydalis	6 - 9 g
Da Huang	Rheum	9 - 15 g
Mu Xiang	Saussurea	6 - 9 g
Hu Huang Lian	Picrorhiza	6 - 9 g
Mang Xiao	Mirabilitum	6 - 9 g

Liver fire attacking the Lungs causing hemoptysis and pain in the chest.

T   red, sticky yellow coat

P   rapid, wiry

SANG DAN XIE BAI TANG

Mulberry Leaf and Paeonia Decoction to Drain the White

Sang Ye	Morus	6 - 9 g
Sang Bai Pi	Morus	6 - 12 g
Mu Dan Pi	Paeonia	3 - 9 g
Di Gu Pi	Lycium	6 - 12 g
Chuan Bei Mu	Fritillaria	6 - 9 g
Zhu Ru	Bambusa	3 - 6 g
Jing Mi	Oryza	6 - 9 g
Da Zao	Ziziphus	2 - 4 pc
Gan Cao	Glycyrrhiza	3 - 6 g

Liver and Stomach fire causing any kind of sudden bleeding disorder. The fire heats up the blood leading to hematemesis, epistaxis, or hemoptysis.

T dark red, yellow coat

P rapid, forceful, wiry

☞ The herbs should be partially charred prior to the decoction process.

✗ Caution during pregnancy.

SHI HUI SAN

Ten Partially-Charred Substance Powder

Xiao Ji	Cephalanoplos	9 - 15 g
Da Ji	Cirsium	9 - 12 g
Ce Bai Ye	Biota	9 - 12 g
Qian Cao Gen	Rubia	9 - 12 g
Da Huang	Rheum	9 - 12 g
He Ye	Nelumbo	9 - 12 g
Zhi Zi	Gardenia	6 - 12 g
Bai Mao Gen	Imperata	9 - 12 g
Zong Lu Pi	Trachycarpus	6 - 9 g
Mu Dan Pi	Paeonia	6 - 9 g

Liver heat/fire giving rise to wind causing itchy rash, hypertension, red eyes, high fever, or easily angered.

T red, dry, thin yellow coat

P rapid, wiry, or flooding

XIE QING WAN

Drain the Green Pill

Long Dan Cao	Gentiana	6 - 9 g
Zhi Zi	Gardenia	6 - 9 g
Chuan Xiong	Ligusticum	6 - 9 g
Qiang Huo	Notopterygium	6 - 9 g
Fang Feng	Ledebouriella	6 - 9 g
Dang Gui	Angelica	6 - 9 g
Da Huang	Rheum	6 - 9 g

Liver

Liver qi stagnation causing Liver fire which burns the Stomach. This leads to vomiting or belching, ulcers due to heat, gas, sour or bitter regurgitation. This is a Liver/Stomach imbalance.

T red, dry, yellow coat

P rapid, wiry

☞ This formula may also be prepared as a powder with ten times the dosage.

ZUO JIN WAN

Left Metal Pill

Extract Formula Name: Coptis and Evodia Formula

| Huang Lian | Coptis | 12 - 18 g |
| Wu Zhu Yu | Evodia | 1 - 4 g |

LIVER YANG RISING

- temple headaches
- tinnitus
- hearing impairment

T red sides

P wiry

Liver yin deficiency with yang/wind rising causing palpitations, hypertension, or restlessness.

T red, thin yellow coat

P thin, rapid, slightly wiry

☞ Use iron water to cook these herbs.

✪ **Major Formula**

JIAN LING TANG

Construct Roof Tiles Decoction

Huai Niu Xi	Achyranthes	30 g
Shan Yao	Dioscorea	30 g
Long Gu	Os Draconis	18 g
Mu Li	Ostrea	18 g
Dai Zhi Shi	Haematitum	24 g
Sheng Di Huang	Rehmannia	18 g
Bai Zi Ren	Biota	12 g
Bai Shao Yao	Paeonia	12 g

Kidney and Liver yin deficiency with yang rising causing vision disturbances, dry red eyes, or blurry vision.

T red, scanty yellow coat

P thin, rapid

MING MU DI HUANG WAN

Improve Vision Pill with Rehmannia

Shu Di Huang	Rehmannia	9 - 20 g
Sheng Di Huang	Rehmannia	9 - 15 g
Mu Dan Pi	Paeonia	6 - 9 g
Shan Yao	Dioscorea	6 - 9 g
Shan Zhu Yu	Cornus	6 - 9 g
Ze Xie	Alisma	6 - 9 g
Dang Gui	Angelica	6 - 9 g
Fu Shen	Poria	6 - 9 g
Chai Hu	Bupleurum	6 - 9 g
Wu Wei Zi	Schisandra	6 - 9 g

Liver wind or yang rising due to yin or blood deficiency. Symptoms include spasms, vertigo, or heat in the palms, soles, and chest.

T dark red, dry, or geographic

P thin, rapid, wiry

☞ E Jiao - Equus should be dissoved at the end into the strained tea.

✘ Caution during pregnancy.

SAN JIA FU MAI TANG

Three-Shell Decoction to Restore the Pulse

Zhi Gan Cao	Glycyrrhiza	9 - 15 g
Bai Shao Yao	Paeonia	9 - 15 g
Sheng Di Huang	Rehmannia	9 - 15 g
E Jiao	Equus	6 - 9 g
Bie Jia	Amyda	9 - 20 g
Gui Ban	Chinemys	15 - 30 g
Huo Ma Ren	Cannabis	6 - 9 g
Mu Li	Ostrea	9 - 15 g
Mai Men Dong	Ophiopogon	9 - 15 g

Liver

Kidney/Liver yin deficiency with yang rising causing blurry vision, photophobia, excessive tearing, poor night vision, early stage cataract, or blood-shot eyes.

T   red, thin and narrow in size, maybe cracked, scanty coat

P   thin, rapid

☞ Xi Jiao - Rhinoceros should be substituted with Shui Niu Jiao - Bubalus.

SHI HU YE GUANG WAN

Dendrobium Pill for Night Vision

Tian Men Dong	Asparagus	6- 9 g
Fu Ling	Poria	6 - 9 g
Ren Shen	Panax	6 - 9 g
Shu Di Huang	Rehmannia	12 - 15 g
Mai Men Dong	Ophiopogon	6 - 9 g
Tu Si Zi	Cuscuta	3 - 9 g
Ju Hua	Chrysanthemum	3 - 6 g
Xing Ren	Prunus	3 - 6 g
Jue Ming Zi	Cassia	6 - 9 g
Gou Qi Zi	Lycium	6 - 9 g
Shan Yao	Dioscorea	6 - 12 g
Wu Wei Zi	Schisandra	6 - 9 g
Huai Niu Xi	Achyranthes	6 - 12 g
Bai Ji Li	Tribulus	6 - 9 g
Chuan Xiong	Ligusticum	3 - 6 g
Rou Cong Rong	Cistanche	3 - 6 g
Shi Hu	Dendrobium	6 - 12 g
Zhi Ke	Citrus	3 - 6 g
Qing Xiang Zi	Celosia	3 - 9 g
Xi Jiao	Rhinoceros	1 - 3 g
Huang Lian	Coptis	3 - 6 g
Fang Feng	Ledebouriella	6 - 9 g
Ling Yang Jiao	Saiga	1 - 3 g
Gan Cao	Glycyrrhiza	3 - 6 g

Liver yin deficiency with yang or wind rising causing headaches, hypertension, tinnitus, or dizziness.

T red

P thin, rapid, wiry

⭐ Major Formula

TIAN MA GOU TENG YIN

Gastrodia and Uncaria Decoction

Extract Formula Name: Gastrodia and Uncaria Combination

Tian Ma	Gastrodia	9 - 12 g
Gou Teng	Uncaria	9 - 15 g
Chuan Niu Xi	Cyathula	9 - 12 g
Huang Qin	Scutellaria	6 - 9 g
Shi Jue Ming	Haliotis	15 - 25 g
Zhi Zi	Gardenia	3 - 6 g
Yi Mu Cao	Leonurus	6 - 12 g
Ye Jiao Teng	Polygonum	9 - 20 g
Du Zhong	Eucommia	6 - 12 g
Sang Ji Sheng	Loranthus	6 - 20 g
Fu Shen	Poria	6 - 12 g

Liver

Liver wind due to yang rising with underlying Kidney and Liver yin deficiency: headache, dizziness, restlessness, or belching due to Liver/Stomach disharmony, low-pitched tinnitus, wind stroke, or hypertension.

T red or light purple, trembling, yellow coat

P forceful, wiry

ZHEN GAN XI FENG TANG

Sedate the Liver and Extinguish Wind Decoction

Extract Formula Name: Dragon Bone and Two Shells Combination

Dai Zhe Shi	Haematitum	15 - 30 g
Huai Niu Xi	Achyranthes	15 - 30 g
Xuan Shen	Scrophularia	12 - 15 g
Bai Shao Yao	Paeonia	9 - 15 g
Tian Men Dong	Asparagus	9 - 15 g
Gui Ban	Chinemys	9 - 15 g
Long Gu	Os Draconis	9 - 15 g
Mu Li	Ostrea	9 - 15 g
Chuan Lian Zi	Melia	6 - 9 g
Mai Ya	Hordeum	6 - 9 g
Yin Chen Hao	Artemisia	6 - 9 g
Gan Cao	Glycyrrhiza	3 - 6 g

Kidney and Liver yin/blood deficiency with fire which bothers the Heart. This causes Heart and Liver fire or Liver yang excess leading to excessive dreaming, insomnia, or outbursts of anger.

T   red, cracks, thin or thick yellow coat

P   rapid, wiry, thin

☞ Ingredients should be powdered, made into 9 - 12 g pills and taken three times a day. Xi Jiao - Rhinoceros should be substituted with Shui Niu Jiao - Bubalus.

ZHEN ZHU MU WAN

Mother-Of-Pearl Pill

Zhen Zhu Mu	Pteria	15 - 20 g
Ren Shen	Panax	9 - 12 g
Dang Gui	Angelica	6 - 12 g
Shu Di Huang	Rehmannia	9 - 12 g
Suan Zao Ren	Ziziphus	6 - 9 g
Bai Zi Ren	Biota	6 - 9 g
Fu Shen	Poria	6 - 9 g
Chen Xiang	Aquilaria	6 - 9 g
Xi Jiao	Rhinoceros	1 - 3 g

LIVER WIND

- tremors, tics, convulsions, high fever
- hemiplegia, deviation of mouth or eye
- aphasia, numbness

T deviated, pale or red

P wiry, choppy

Liver wind due to Liver yin deficiency causing spasms and twitches.

T dark red, scanty yellow coat

P thin, wiry, rapid

☞ E Jiao - Equus should be added to the strained tea. Bie Jia - Amyda, Mu Li - Ostrea, and Gui Ban - Chinemys should all be crushed or powdered, and cooked 45 minutes prior to the other herbs. The egg-yolks are boiled hard, then made into a soft mass and mixed into the tea.

DA DING FENG ZHU

Major Arrest Wind Pearl

Ji Zi Huang	Egg Yolk	2
Wu Wei Zi	Schisandra	6 - 9 g
E Jiao	Equus	6 - 9 g
Bai Shao Yao	Paeonia	9 - 15 g
Mai Men Dong	Ophiopogon	9 - 15 g
Huo Ma Ren	Cannabis	3 - 6 g
Sheng Di Huang	Rehmannia	9 - 15 g
Bie Jia	Amyda	6 - 12 g
Gui Ban	Chinemys	6 - 12 g
Mu Li	Ostrea	6 - 12 g
Gan Cao	Glycyrrhiza	6 - 12 g

Liver

Liver wind and phlegm causing seizures, especially in children or from emotional upset. There may be loss of consciousness.

T   quivery, thick sticky white coat

P   slippery, wiry

☞ Form 6 g pills out of the powdered herbs with the liquid made from the herbs listed in brackets. Adults take one pill in the morning and one in the evening.

✗ Do not use during pregnancy. Zhu Sha - Cinnabaris is toxic and should only be used short-term.

DING XIAN WAN

Arrest Seizures Pill

Tian Ma	Gastrodia	20 - 30 g
Jiang Ban Xia	Pinellia	20 - 30 g
Dan Nan Xing	Arisaema	12 - 15 g
Chuan Bei Mu	Fritillaria	20 - 30 g
Fu Shen	Poria	20 - 30 g
Fu Ling	Poria	20 - 30 g
Jiang Can	Bombyx	12 - 15 g
Shi Chang Pu	Acorus	12 - 15 g
Deng Xin Cao	Juncus	12 - 15 g
Quan Xie	Buthus	12 - 15 g
Dan Shen	Salvia	40 - 60 g
Mai Men Dong	Ophiopogon	40 - 60 g
Hu Po	Succinum	12 - 15 g
Yuan Zhi	Polygala	15 - 20 g
Chen Pi	Citrus	15 - 20 g
Zhu Sha	Cinnabaris	9 g
[Gan Cao	Glycyrrhiza	120 g]
[Zhu Li	Bambusa	100 ml]
[Sheng Jiang Zhi	Zingiber juice	50 ml]

Blood/yin deficiency giving rise to wind. Symptoms include twitches, or rigidity in the extremities.

T red, scanty yellow coat

P thin, rapid

☞ The egg yolks and E Jiao - Equus should be added to the strained tea.

E JIAO JI ZI HUANG TANG

Ass-Hide Gelatin and Egg Yolk Decoction

E Jiao	Equus	6 - 9 g
Ji Zi Huang	Egg Yolks	2
Gou Teng	Uncaria	6 - 9 g
Mu Li	Ostrea	9 - 12 g
Shi Jue Ming	Haliotis	12 - 15 g
Bai Shao Yao	Paeonia	6 - 9 g
Sheng Di Huang	Rehmannia	9 - 12 g
Luo Shi Teng	Trachelospermum	6 - 9 g
Fu Shen	Poria	9 - 12 g
Zhi Gan Cao	Glycyrrhiza	3 g

Acute childhood convulsions due to severe heat with underlying qi deficiency causing wind. Symptoms include the eyes turning upward, drooling, fever, or rigidity in the jaw.

T red, yellow coat

P rapid, wiry

☞ Ling Yang Jiao - Saiga powder should be added to the strained tea.

GOU TENG YIN

Uncaria Decoction

Extract Formula Name: Gambir Formula

Gou Teng	Uncaria	9 - 12 g
Quan Xie	Buthus	.9 g
Ren Shen	Panax	3 - 6 g
Ling Yang Jiao	Saiga	0.5 g
Tian Ma	Gastrodia	6 - 9 g
Gan Cao	Glycyrrhiza	1 - 3 g

Blood deficiency giving rise to internal wind which then leads to tendon or muscle spasms, itchy skin rashes, or blurry vision.

T pale, quivery

P weak, maybe superficial

GUI XIONG SI WU TANG

Altered Four-Substance Decoction

Shu Di Huang	Rehmannia	9 - 15 g
Chuan Xiong	Ligusticum	3 - 9 g
Bai Shao Yao	Paeonia	6 - 9 g
Dang Gui	Angelica	6 - 9 g
Fang Feng	Ledebouriella	9 - 15 g
Bai Zhu	Atractylodes	6 - 9 g
Huai Niu Xi	Achyranthes	6 - 12 g
Tian Men Dong	Asparagus	9 - 12 g

Liver yin deficiency with yang/wind rising causing palpitations, hypertension, or restlessness.

T red, thin yellow coat

P thin, rapid, slightly wiry

☞ Use iron water to cook these herbs.

JIAN LING TANG

Construct Roof Tiles Decoction

Huai Niu Xi	Achyranthes	30 g
Shan Yao	Dioscorea	30 g
Long Gu	Os Draconis	18 g
Mu Li	Ostrea	18 g
Dai Zhi Shi	Haematitum	24 g
Sheng Di Huang	Rehmannia	18 g
Bai Zi Ren	Biota	12 g
Bai Shao Yao	Paeonia	12 g

Liver wind due to Liver fire causing hypertension, twitches, or headaches.

T   dark red, raw, dry

P   rapid, wiry

☞ Ling Yang Jiao - Saiga should be cooked one hour prior to adding the other herbs.

LING YANG GOU TENG YIN

Antelope Horn and Uncaria Decoction

Extract Formula Name: Antelope Horn and Uncaria Combination

Ling Yang Jiao	Saiga	3 - 6 g
Sang Ye	Morus	6 - 9 g
Sheng Di Huang	Rehmannia	9 - 15 g
Zhu Ru	Bambusa	9 - 15 g
Bai Shao Yao	Paeonia	6 - 9 g
Gou Teng	Uncaria	6 - 9 g
Chuan Bei Mu	Fritillaria	6 - 12 g
Ju Hua	Chrysanthemum	6 - 9 g
Fu Shen	Poria	6 - 9 g
Gan Cao	Glycyrrhiza	3 - 6 g

Liver wind or yang rising due to yin or blood deficiency. Symptoms include spasms, vertigo, or heat in the palms, soles, and chest.

T   dark red, dry, or geographic

P   thin, rapid, wiry

☞ E Jiao - Equus should be dissoved at the end into the strained tea.

✗ Caution during pregnancy.

SAN JIA FU MAI TANG

Three-Shell Decoction to Restore the Pulse

Zhi Gan Cao	Glycyrrhiza	9 - 15 g
Bai Shao Yao	Paeonia	9 - 15 g
Sheng Di Huang	Rehmannia	9 - 15 g
E Jiao	Equus	6 - 9 g
Bie Jia	Amyda	9 - 20 g
Gui Ban	Chinemys	15 - 30 g
Huo Ma Ren	Cannabis	6 - 9 g
Mu Li	Ostrea	9 - 15 g
Mai Men Dong	Ophiopogon	9 - 15 g

Liver

Liver yin deficiency with yang or wind rising causing headaches, hypertension, tinnitus, or dizziness.

T red

P thin, rapid, wiry

TIAN MA GOU TENG YIN

Gastrodia and Uncaria Decoction

Extract Formula Name: Gastrodia and Uncaria Combination

Tian Ma	Gastrodia	9 - 12 g
Gou Teng	Uncaria	9 - 15 g
Chuan Niu Xi	Cyathula	9 - 12 g
Huang Qin	Scutellaria	6 - 9 g
Shi Jue Ming	Haliotis	15 - 25 g
Zhi Zi	Gardenia	3 - 6 g
Yi Mu Cao	Leonurus	6 - 12 g
Ye Jiao Teng	Polygonum	9 - 20 g
Du Zhong	Eucommia	6 - 12 g
Sang Ji Sheng	Loranthus	6 - 20 g
Fu Shen	Poria	6 - 12 g

Liver wind or external wind with phlegm accumulation in the channels causing stroke, aphasia, cerebral hemorrhage, or numbness; or cold attacking the chest and axillae causing severe localized pain in the flanks.

T sticky white coat

P slippery or wiry

WU YAO SHUN QI SAN

Lindera Powder to Smooth the Flow of Qi

Extract Formula Name: Lindera Formula

Wu Yao	Lindera	9 - 15 g
Chen Pi	Citrus	9 - 15 g
Ma Huang	Ephedra	6 - 9 g
Bai Zhi	Angelica	3 - 9 g
Zhi Ke	Citrus	3 - 6 g
Jiang Can	Bombyx	3 g
Jie Geng	Platycodon	3 g
Chuan Xiong	Ligusticum	3 - 9 g
Pao Jiang	Zingiber	3 - 6 g
Gan Cao	Glycyrrhiza	3 - 6 g
[Da Zao	Ziziphus	3 - 8 pc]
[Sheng Jiang	Zingiber	3 - 6 g]

Liver heat/fire giving rise to wind causing itchy rash, hypertension, red eyes, high fever, or easily angered.

T red, dry, thin yellow coat

P rapid, wiry, or flooding

XIE QING WAN

Drain the Green Pill

Long Dan Cao	Gentiana	6 - 9 g
Zhi Zi	Gardenia	6 - 9 g
Chuan Xiong	Ligusticum	6 - 9 g
Qiang Huo	Notopterygium	6 - 9 g
Fang Feng	Ledebouriella	6 - 9 g
Dang Gui	Angelica	6 - 9 g
Da Huang	Rheum	6 - 9 g

External wind attacks the channels with pre-existing qi/Blood deficiency; or Liver wind with heat causing flaccid hemiplegia, aphasia, or mild fever. There may also be slight mental confusion.

T sticky yellow coat

P wiry, forceful, or rapid, slippery

XU MING TANG

Prolong Life Decoction

Extract Formula Name: Ma-Huang and Ginseng Combination

Gui Zhi	Cinnamomum	6 - 9 g
Ma Huang	Ephedra	6 - 9 g
Chuan Xiong	Ligusticum	3 - 6 g
Xing Ren	Prunus	6 - 9 g
Shi Gao	Gypsum	6 - 9 g
Ren Shen	Panax	6 - 9 g
Dang Gui	Angelica	6 - 9 g
Gan Jiang	Zingiber	6 - 9 g
Gan Cao	Glycyrrhiza	3 - 9 g

Liver

Liver wind due to yang rising with underlying Kidney and Liver yin deficiency: headache, dizziness, restlessness, or belching due to Liver/Stomach disharmony, low-pitched tinnitus, wind stroke, or hypertension.

T   red or light purple, trembling, yellow coat

P   forceful, wiry

❌ **Major Formula**

ZHEN GAN XI FENG TANG

Sedate the Liver and Extinguish Wind Decoction

Extract Formula Name: Dragon Bone and Two Shells Combination

Dai Zhe Shi	Haematitum	15 - 30 g
Huai Niu Xi	Achyranthes	15 - 30 g
Xuan Shen	Scrophularia	12 - 15 g
Bai Shao Yao	Paeonia	9 - 15 g
Tian Men Dong	Asparagus	9 - 15 g
Gui Ban	Chinemys	9 - 15 g
Long Gu	Os Draconis	9 - 15 g
Mu Li	Ostrea	9 - 15 g
Chuan Lian Zi	Melia	6 - 9 g
Mai Ya	Hordeum	6 - 9 g
Yin Chen Hao	Artemisia	6 - 9 g
Gan Cao	Glycyrrhiza	3 - 6 g

Liver wind due to fire in the pericardium, or phlegm heat obstructing the orifice causing stroke, high fever, irritability, loss of consciousness, or a raspy voice.

T dark red, sticky yellow grey coat

P rapid, slippery

☞ Herbs should be ground separately, then sifted together. Make into 3 g pills. Adults take one pill 2 - 3 times a day. Xi Jiao - Rhinoceros should be substituted with Shui Niu Jiao - Bubalus or 50 - 60 g of Bai Mao Gen - Imperata.

✗ Do not use during pregnancy. Zhu Sha - Cinnabaris is toxic and should not be used over a prolonged period of time.

ZHI BAO DAN

Greatest Treasure Special Pill

Extract Formula Name: Rhinoceros and Succinum Formula

Xi Jiao	Rhinoceros	20 - 30 g
Niu Huang	Bos	12 - 15 g
She Xiang	Moschus	0.1 - 0.3 g
Dai Mao	Eretmochelydis	20 - 30 g
An Xi Xiang	Styrax	30 - 45 g
Hu Po	Succinum	20 - 30 g
Xiong Huang	Realgar	20 - 30 g
Zhu Sha	Cinnabaris	20 - 30 g
Bing Pian	Dryobalanops	0.1 - 0.3 g

Severe heat causing Liver wind. This causes muscle twitches, convulsions, or spasms.

T red, deviated, yellow coat

P forceful

✗ Do not use during pregnancy. The formula is toxic and should not be taken over a prolonged period of time.

ZHI JING SAN

Stop Spasms Powder

Wu Gong	Scolopendra	10 g
Quan Xie	Buthus	10 g

GALLBLADDER DISHARMONIES

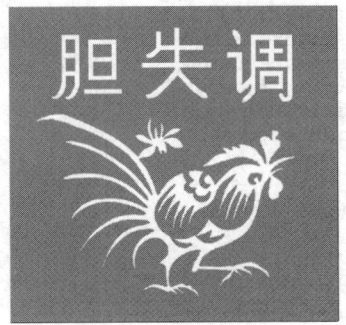

胆失调

DAMP HEAT IN THE GALLBLADDER

- costal pain and distention
- gallstones
- bitter taste
- nausea and vomiting
- fever and thirst

T thick sticky yellow coat

P wiry, slippery

Gall Bladder

1. Yangming organ disease (pi man zhao shi - fullness, firmness, dryness, excess) causing masses in the abdomen; or yang jaundice with gallstones where the heat is greater than damp. 2. Fire and toxin are severe, so the water parts extravasate causing watery dysentery with odorous stools, bowel incontinence while in a coma, mania, or convulsions with high fever.

T bright red, dry yellow or black coat

P rapid, forceful

☞ Da Huang - Rheum should be added during the last 3 - 5 minutes of the decoction process, and Mang Xiao - Mirabilite should be added into the strained tea.

✗ Do not use during pregnancy. The formula is very cold and can cause diarrhea and vomiting.

DA CHENG QI TANG

Major Order the Qi Decoction

Extract Formula Name: Major Rhubarb Combination

Da Huang	Rheum	6 - 12 g
Mang Xiao	Mirabilitum	6 - 12 g
Zhi Shi	Citrus	6 - 9 g
Hou Po	Magnolia	6 - 15 g

Damp heat with qi stagnation and pain causing gallstones.

T red, sticky yellow coat

P slippery, wiry, rapid

DAN DAO PAI SHI TANG

Biliary Lithagogue Decoction

Jin Qian Cao	Lysimachia	6 - 9 g
Yu Jin	Curcuma	6 - 9 g
Yin Chen Hao	Artemisia	6 - 9 g
Mu Xiang	Saussurea	3 - 6 g
Zhi Ke	Citrus	3 - 6 g
Da Huang	Rheum	6 - 9 g

Yang jaundice from damp heat lodged in the shaoyang level; or damp heat in the Gallbladder causing alternating fever and chills, bitter taste, or malaria.

T   red, thick sticky yellow coat

P   slippery, wiry, rapid

☞ Bi Yu San - Green Jade Powder consists of: Hua Shi - Talcum, 3 - 6 g; Gan Cao - Glycyrrhiza, 3 - 6 g; and Qing Dai - Indigo, 9 - 12 g. All three ingredients should be cooked separately in a cheese-cloth, then decocted with the rest of the herbs.

❂ **Major Formula**

HAO QIN QING DAN TANG

Artemisia Annua and Scutellaria Decoction to Clear the Gallbladder

Qing Hao	Artemisia	6 g
Zhu Ru	Bambusa	9 g
Huang Qin	Scutellaria	6 g
Zhi Ke	Citrus	5 g
Chi Fu Ling	Poria	9 g
Ban Xia	Pinellia	5 g
Chen Pi	Citrus	5 g
Bi Yu San	Green Jade Powder	9 g

Middle jiao phlegm heat with Gallbladder heat causing severe restlessness or bitter taste.

T   red, sticky yellow coat

P   rapid, slippery

HUANG LIAN WEN DAN TANG

Coptis Decoction to Warm the Gallbladder

Ban Xia	Pinellia	6 - 9 g
Chen Pi	Citrus	3 - 6 g
Fu Ling	Poria	6 - 9 g
Zhi Ke	Citrus	3 - 6 g
Zhu Ru	Bambusa	3 - 9 g
Huang Lian	Coptis	3 - 6 g
Sheng Jiang	Zingiber	3 - 6 g
Da Zao	Ziziphus	3 - 4 pc
Gan Cao	Glycyrrhiza	3 - 6 g

Gall Bladder

Wind cold causes facial edema and scanty urination. This formula is also useful for jaundice accompanied by taiyang symptoms.

T thin white coat

P superficial, tight

MA HUANG LIAN QIAO CHI XIAO DOU TANG

Ephedra, Forsythia, and Aduki Bean Decoction

Ma Huang	Ephedra	3 - 9 g
Lian Qiao	Forsythia	6 - 9 g
Chi Xiao Dou	Phaseolus	6 - 9 g
Sang Bai Pi	Morus	6 - 9 g
Xing Ren	Prunus	6 - 9 g
Sheng Jiang	Zingiber	3 - 6 g
Da Zao	Ziziphus	3 - 4 pc
Gan Cao	Glycyrrhiza	3 - 6 g

Excess fire cholecystitis with Liver qi and damp stagnation causing alternating fever and chills or severe hypochondriac pain.

T deep red, sticky yellow coat

P wiry, slippery, rapid, or flooding

☞ Mang Xiao - Mirabilitum should be dissolved into the strained tea. Da Huang - Rheum should be added within the last 3 - 5 minutes of the decoction process.

✗ Do not use during pregnancy

QING DAN XIE HUO TANG

Clear the Gallbladder and Drain Fire Decoction

Chai Hu	Bupleurum	9 - 15 g
Ban Xia	Pinellia	6 - 9 g
Yin Chen Hao	Artemisia	15 - 25 g
Long Dan Cao	Gentiana	6 - 9 g
Yu Jin	Curcuma	6 - 9 g
Da Huang	Rheum	6 - 9 g
Huang Qin	Scutellaria	6 - 15 g
Zhi Zi	Gardenia	6 - 9 g
Mang Xiao	Mirabilitum	6 - 9 g
Mu Xiang	Saussurea	3 - 6 g

Liver and Stomach imbalance with phlegm accumulation and Gallbladder heat. Symptoms include fullness in the chest, bitter taste, thirst without desire to drink, or vomiting. In severe cases, mental confusion or a rattly throat may be seen.

T   red, sticky yellow coat

P   rapid, slippery and/or wiry

WEN DAN TANG

Warm the Gallbladder Decoction

Extract Formula Name: Hoelen and Bamboo Combination

Ban Xia	Pinellia	6 - 9 g
Chen Pi	Citrus	9 - 12 g
Fu Ling	Poria	6 - 12 g
Zhi Shi	Citrus	3 - 6 g
Zhu Ru	Bambusa	6 g
Sheng Jiang	Zingiber	3 - 6 g
Gan Cao	Glycyrrhiza	3 - 6 g
Da Zao	Ziziphus	2 pc

Whole body yang jaundice due to damp heat in the Liver and Gallbladder.

T   Red, thick sticky yellow coat

P   slippery, rapid, forceful

✗   Do not use during pregnancy.

YIN CHEN HAO TANG

Artemisia Yinchenhao Decoction

Extract Formula Name: Capillaris Combination

Yin Chen Hao	Artemisia	15 - 30 g
Da Huang	Rheum	6 - 9 g
Zhi Zi	Gardenia	6 - 9 g

Damp heat accumulation in the middle jiao (Liver/Gallbladder) causing yang jaundice, dysurea, or hepatitis with mild fever.

T   slightly red, thick sticky coat

P   slippery, slightly rapid

YIN CHEN WU LING SAN

Artemisia Yinchenhao and Five-Ingredient Powder with Poria

Extract Formula Name: Capillaris and Hoelen Five Formula

Yin Chen Hao	Artemisia	10 - 20 g
Fu Ling	Poria	6 - 12 g
Zhu Ling	Polyporus	6 - 9 g
Bai Zhu	Atractylodes	3 - 9 g
Ze Xie	Alisma	6 - 9 g
Gui Zhi	Cinnamomum	3 - 9 g

Gall Bladder

Yang jaundice due to damp heat in the interior. The heat is greater than the damp.

T red, sticky yellow coat

P slippery, rapid

ZHI ZI BAI PI TANG

Gardenia and Phellodendron Decoction

Extract Formula Name: Gardenia and Phellodendron Combination

Zhi Zi	Gardenia	9 - 15 g
Huang Bai	Phellodendron	6 - 9 g
Zhi Gan Cao	Glycyrrhiza	3 - 6 g

Damp heat accumulation in the middle jiao. There is more damp than heat causing fullness in the abdomen, thirst without desire to drink, or immediate fullness upon eating or drinking. This formula is also useful for yang jaundice.

T red, thick sticky coat

P slippery, rapid

ZHONG JIAO XIAN BI TANG

Middle Jiao and Clear Damp Decoction

Xing Ren	Prunus	3 - 6 g
Yi Yi Ren	Coix	9 - 12 g
Hua Shi	Talcum	6 g
Dou Juan	Glycine	9 g
Zhi Zi	Gardenia	6 - 9 g
Lian Qiao	Forsythia	6 g
Ban Xia	Pinellia	6 - 9 g
Han Fang Ji	Stephania	6 - 9 g
Can Sha	Bombyx	3 - 6 g
Shan Zha	Crataegus	3 - 9 g
Bian Dou	Dolichos	6 - 9 g

DEFICIENCY IN THE GALLBLADDER

- lack of initiative
- timidity
- startled easily
- sighing

T pale

P weak

This formula treats insomnia due to Heart and Gallbladder qi deficiency. This is commonly seen in children causing them to appear timid and scared of everything, fear ghosts and burglars, or not want to sleep alone. They sweat easily, especially in the hands and soles.

T pale or normal color, slightly swollen

P weak, thready, deep

✪ **Major Formula**

AN SHEN DING ZHI TANG

Calm Spirit and Stop Fear Decoction

Ren Shen	Panax	9 - 12 g
Fu Ling	Poria	6 - 9 g
Fu Shen	Poria	6 - 9 g
Shi Chang Pu	Acorus	3 - 9 g
Long Gu	Os Draconis	6 - 9 g
Yuan Zhi	Polygala	6 - 9 g

Heart/Gallbladder qi deficiency with edema in the extremities, tight chest, palpitations, anxiety, or timidity.

T pale

P weak

SHI WEI WEN DAN TANG

Ten-Ingredient Decoction to Warm the Gallbladder

Ban Xia	Pinellia	6 - 9 g
Chen Pi	Citrus	3 - 6 g
Zhi Shi	Citrus	6 g
Fu Ling	Poria	6 g
Ren Shen	Panax	3 - 6 g
Suan Zao Ren	Ziziphus	3 - 6 g
Shu Di Huang	Rehmannia	3 - 9 g
Wu Wei Zi	Schisandra	3 - 6 g
Yuan Zhi	Polygala	3 - 6 g
Zhi Gan Cao	Glycyrrhiza	3 g
Da Zao	Ziziphus	2 pc
Sheng Jiang	Zingiber	5 pc

Gall Bladder

KIDNEY DISHARMONIES

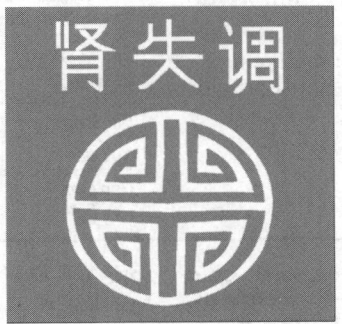

肾失调

KIDNEY QI DEFICIENCY

- sore and weak lower back and knees
- urinary incontinence, frequency, or dribbling
- spermatorrhea, or chronic leukorrhea

T pale, swollen

P deep, weak

Kidney qi/yin deficiency causing menorrhagia. Other symptoms may include low back pain, frequent urination, or weakness in the knees.

T   red or normal color, thin white coat

P   weak, especially in both chi (third) positions, slightly rapid

BAO YIN JIAN

Augment Yin Decoction

Huang Qin	Scutellaria	9 - 12 g
Huang Bai	Phellodendron	9 - 12 g
Sheng Di Huang	Rehmannia	9 - 15 g
Shu Di Huang	Rehmannia	9 - 15 g
Shan Yao	Dioscorea	6 - 9 g
Bai Shao Yao	Paeonia	6 - 12 g
Xu Duan	Dipsacus	6 - 9 g
Gan Cao	Glycyrrhiza	3 - 6 g

Kidney qi deficiency with cold and damp leading to frequent, or cloudy, painful urination.

T   pale

P   weak, or slippery

BEI XIE FEN QIN YIN I

Discorea Hypoglauca Decoction to Separate the Clear

Extract Formula Name: Tokoro Combination

Bei Xie	Dioscorea	6 - 12 g
Wu Yao	Lindera	6 - 9 g
Shi Chang Pu	Acorus	6 - 9 g
Yi Zhi Ren	Alpinia	6 - 9 g

Kidney/Lung qi/yin deficiency with wheezing, shortness of breath, or chronic cough. This formula is also known as 'Qi Wu Du Qi Wan'.

T   red, slight coat

P   thin, rapid

DU QI WAN

Capital Qi Pill

Extract Formula Name: Rehmannia and Schizandra Formula

Shan Zhu Yu	Cornus	6 - 9 g
Shan Yao	Dioscorea	6 - 9 g
Sheng Di Huang	Rehmannia	9 - 12 g
Fu Ling	Poria	6 - 9 g
Mu Dan Pi	Paeonia	6 - 9 g
Ze Xie	Alisma	6 - 9 g
Wu Wei Zi	Schisandra	6 - 9 g

Kidney qi and yang deficiency causing edema which manifests mostly in the superficial and muscle layers.

T pale, swollen, sticky white coat

P weak, deep, slippery

FANG JI FU LING TANG

Stephania and Poria Decoction

Extract Formula Name: Stephania and Hoelen Combination

Han Fang Ji	Stephania	9 - 12 g
Fu Ling	Poria	9 - 18 g
Gui Zhi	Cinnamomum	9 - 12 g
Huang Qi	Astragalus	9 - 12 g
Gan Cao	Glycyrrhiza	3 - 6 g

Turbid leukorrhea due to Kidney qi/yang deficiency. The Kidneys are unable to astringe.

T pale, swollen, slight teethmarks, wet, thin white coat

P minute or frail

FEN QING YIN

Separate Pure from Impure Powder

Bei Xie	Dioscorea	6 - 9 g
Yi Yi Ren	Coix	12 - 15 g
Wu Yao	Lindera	6 - 9 g
Shi Chang Pu	Acorus	6 - 9 g
Fu Ling	Poria	6 - 9 g
Chen Pi	Citrus	3 - 6 g
Gan Cao	Glycyrrhiza	3 - 6 g

Kidney

Spleen/Kidney qi deficiency resulting in spermatorrhea, no appetite, and weakness.

T pale, thin white coat

P deep, weak

✪ Major Formula

FU TU DAN

Poria and Cuscuta Special Pill

Extract Formula Name: Hoelen and Cuscuta Formula

Tu Si Zi	Cuscuta	6 - 9 g
Fu Ling	Poria	6 - 9 g
Wu Wei Zi	Schisandra	6 - 9 g
Lian Zi	Nelumbo	6 - 9 g
Shan Yao	Dioscorea	6 - 9 g

Kidney qi/yin deficiency causing irregular periods, leukorrhea, or a bearing-down sensation.

T red, thin white coat

P weak, especially the chi (third) positions

GU YIN JIAN

Stabilize the Yin Decoction

Shu Di Huang	Rehmannia	6 - 12 g
Shan Yao	Dioscorea	6 - 9 g
Wu Wei Zi	Schisandra	6 - 9 g
Shan Zhu Yu	Cornus	6 - 9 g
Tu Si Zi	Cuscuta	6 - 9 g
Ren Shen	Panax	6 - 9 g
Yuan Zhi	Polygala	3 g
Zhi Gan Cao	Glycyrrhiza	3 - 6 g

Kidney qi deficiency with Kidney/Liver yin deficiency causing amenorrhea, or back and knee pain.

T pale or red, thin white or scanty coat

P weak, maybe thin especially in the left chi (third) position

GUI SHEN TANG

Comeback Kidney Decoction

Shu Di Huang	Rehmannia	6 - 15 g
Shan Yao	Dioscorea	9 - 15 g
Shan Zhu Yu	Cornus	9 - 12 g
Gou Qi Zi	Lycium	9 - 15 g
Dang Gui	Angelica	9 - 12 g
Du Zhong	Eucommia	6 - 12 g
Fu Ling	Poria	6 - 12 g
Tu Si Zi	Cuscuta	9 - 12 g

Kidney qi and yang deficiency causing low back pain, coldness in the back, urinary difficulties, or pedal edema.

T pale, swollen, thin white coat

P frail

JIN GUI SHEN QI WAN

Kidney Qi Pill from the Golden Cabinet

Extract Formula Name: Rehmannia Eight Formula

Shu Di Huang	Rehmannia	24 g
Shan Zhu Yu	Cornus	12 g
Shan Yao	Dioscorea	12 g
Mu Dan Pi	Paeonia	9 g
Ze Xie	Alisma	9 g
Fu Ling	Poria	9 g
Rou Gui	Cinnamomum	3 g
Fu Zi	Aconitum	3 g

Kidney qi deficiency causing white leukorrhea.

T thin white coat

P weak

NEI BU WAN

Internal Tonification Pill

Lu Rong	Cervus	1 - 3 g
Rou Cong Rong	Cistanche	6 - 9 g
Tu Si Zi	Cuscuta	6 - 9 g
Huang Qi	Astralagus	6 - 15 g
Rou Gui	Cinnamomum	6 - 9 g
Fu Zi	Aconitum	3 - 6 g
Sha Yuan Ji Li	Astragalus	6 - 9 g
Zi Wan	Aster	6 - 9 g
Sang Piao Xiao	Paratenodera	6 - 9 g

Kidney

Liver blood/yin deficiency with Kidney qi deficiency causing early greying, hairloss, poor teeth, and seminal emissions.

T   pale

P   thin, weak

QI BAO MEI RAN DAN

Seven-Treasure Special Pill for Beautiful Whiskers

He Shou Wu	Polygonum	6 - 9 g
Huai Niu Xi	Achyranthes	6 - 12 g
Fu Ling	Poria	6 - 9 g
Tu Si Zi	Cuscuta	6 - 9 g
Gou Qi Zi	Lycium	6 - 9 g
Bu Gu Zhi	Psoralea	6 - 9 g
Dang Gui	Angelica	6 - 9 g

Lung/Kidney qi deficiency causing cough/asthma with wheezing. There are slightly more cold symptoms.

T   pale, thin sticky white coat

P   weak or frail

REN SHEN HU TAO TANG

Ginseng and Walnut Decoction

Extract Formula Name: Ginseng and Walnut Combination

Ren Shen	Panax	6 - 9 g
Hu Tao Ren	Juglans	3 - 6 pc
Sheng Jiang	Zingiber	3 - 6 pc
Da Zao	Ziziphus	3 pc

Heart/Kidney qi/yin deficiency causing incontinence, spermatorrhea, frequent urination, and forgetfulness.

T pale or red

P weak, thin

SANG PIAO XIAO SAN

Mantis Egg-Case Powder

Extract Formula Name: Mantis Formula

Sang Piao Xiao	Paratenodera	9 - 12 g
Long Gu	Os Draconis	12 - 25 g
Fu Shen	Poria	9 - 12 g
Ren Shen	Panax	9 - 12 g
Shi Chang Pu	Acorus	6 - 9 g
Dang Gui	Angelica	6 - 9 g
Gui Ban	Chinemys	9 - 15 g
Yuan Zhi	Polygala	9 - 15 g

Lung/Kidney qi deficiency causing cough, asthma, and dyspnea.

T pale

P slow, weak

SHEN JIE SAN

Ginseng and Gecko Powder

Ren Shen	Panax	9 - 12 g
Ge Jie	Gekko	1 pair

Spleen/Kidney qi and yang deficiency causing edema which manifests mostly in the lower body. Other symptoms include cold limbs, poor appetite, decreased urination, or heaviness.

T pale, sticky coat

P deep, slow, maybe thin

SHI PI YIN

Bolster the Spleen Decoction

Extract Formula Name: Magnolia and Atractylodes Combination

Fu Zi	Aconitum	6 - 9 g
Bai Zhu	Atractylodes	6 - 9 g
Mu Gua	Chaenomeles	6 - 9 g
Hou Po	Magnolia	6 - 12 g
Gan Jiang	Zingiber	6 - 9 g
Mu Xiang	Saussurea	6 - 9 g
Fu Ling	Poria	6 - 9 g
Da Fu Pi	Areca	3 - 6 g
Cao Guo	Amomum	3 - 6 g
Zhi Gan Cao	Glycyrrhiza	3 - 6 g
[Da Zao	Ziziphus	1 - 3 pc]
[Sheng Jiang	Zingiber	3 - 6 g]

Kidney

Kidney qi deficiency causing a restless fetus with spotting, threatened miscarriage, or frequent urination.

T   pale

P   frail

☞ E Jiao - Equus should be dissolved in water and used to form the other herbs into 6 g pills .

SHOU TAI WAN

Fetus Longevity Pill

Loranthus and Cuscuta Combination

E Jiao	Equus	30
Sang Ji Sheng	Loranthus	30 g
Tu Si Zi	Cuscuta	60 g
Xu Duan	Dipsacus	30 g

Lung phlegm damp with underlying Kidney qi deficiency causing wheezing with profuse phlegm.

T   sticky white coat

P   weak, slippery

SU ZI JIANG QI TANG

Perilla Fruit Decoction for Directing Qi Downward

Extract Formula Name: Perilla Fruit Combination

Zhi Gan Cao	Glycyrrhiza	6 g
Ban Xia	Pinellia	6 - 9 g
Zi Su Zi	Perilla	6 - 12 g
Dang Gui	Angelica	6 - 9 g
Hou Po	Magnolia	6 - 12 g
Qian Hu	Peucedanum	6 - 9 g
Rou Gui	Cinnamomum	3 g
[Sheng Jiang	Zingiber	1 - 3 g]
[Zi Su Ye	Perilla	3 - 6 g]
[Da Zao	Ziziphus	3 g]

Kidney qi/yang deficiency with enuresis or frequent, clear urination.

T   pale, swollen, teethmarks, white coat

P   minute

SUO QUAN WAN

Shut the Sluice Pill

Yi Zhi Ren	Alpinia	6 - 15 g
Shan Yao	Dioscorea	9 - 15 g
Wu Yao	Lindera	6 - 9 g

Chronic lin-syndrome due to Kidney qi deficiency causing urinary frequency with turbidity, incontinence, or enuresis.

T pale or normal color, thin white or yellowish coat

P weak, especially in the chi (third) positions

WU BI SHAN YAO WAN

Dioscorea Pill

Shu Di Huang	Rehmannia	12 - 15 g
Shan Yao	Dioscorea	12 - 15 g
Shan Zhu Yu	Cornus	6 - 9 g
Rou Cong Rong	Cistanche	6 - 9 g
Tu Si Zi	Cuscuta	6 - 9 g
Wu Wei Zi	Schisandra	6 - 12 g
Ze Xie	Alisma	6 - 9 g
Ba Ji Tian	Morinda	3 - 6 g
Du Zhong	Eucommia	9 - 12 g
Huai Niu Xi	Achyranthes	12 - 15 g
Fu Shen	Poria	9 - 12 g
Chi Shi Zhi	Halloysitum Rubrum	12 - 15 g

Kidney

Kidney qi deficiency causing infertility, urinary frequency, or incontinence.

T pale or normal color, thin white coat

P weak

☞ For infertility and a stronger qi and blood tonifying effect add 'Dang Gui Bu Xue Tang - Dang Gui Decoction to Tonify the Blood' and 'Si Jun Zi Tang - Four-Gentlemen Decoction.'

WU ZI YAN ZONG WAN

Five-Seeds Normalizing Pill

Wu Wei Zi	Schisandra	6 - 12 g
Fu Pen Zi	Rubus	6 - 9 g
Tu Si Zi	Cuscuta	6 - 9 g
Che Qian Zi	Plantago	6 - 9 g
Gou Qi Zi	Lycium	6 - 12 g

Kidney qi deficiency leading to spermatorrhea, or white leukorrhea in women.

T pale or normal color, thin white coat

P weak

YI YUAN JIAN

Benefit the Source Decoction

Yuan Zhi	Polygala	3 g
Shan Yao	Dioscorea	6 g
Qian Shi	Euryale	6 g
Suan Zao Ren	Ziziphus	6 g
Bai Zhu	Atractylodes	4.5 g
Fu Ling	Poria	4.5 g
Ren Shen	Panax	3 - 6 g
Wu Wei Zi	Schisandra	14 pc
Jin Ying Zi	Rosa	6 g
Gan Cao	Glycyrrhiza	3 g

Infertility due to Kidney qi deficiency.

T normal color or pale, thin white coat

P weak, especially in both chi (third) positions

YU LIN WAN

Nourish Cute Animal Pill

Lu Jiao Shuang	Cervus	6 - 9 g
Tu Si Zi	Cuscuta	6 - 9 g
Du Zhong	Eucommia	6 - 12 g
Chuan Jiao	Zanthoxylum	3 - 6 g
Zi He Che	Placenta Hominis	3 - 9 g
Xiang Fu	Cyperus	6 - 9 g

KIDNEY YANG DEFICIENCY

- cold and sore knees and lower back
- frequent, clear and profuse or scanty urination
- infertility, impotence

T pale, swollen, teethmarks, moist

P deep, weak

Cold accumulation or yang deficiency in the abdomen leading to constipation with cramping pain. The qi stagnates and heats up which can cause a mild fever. Other symptoms include cold extremities and chills.

T normal or pale, white coat

P wiry or tight, deep

☞ Fu Zi - Aconitum should be powdered. Da Huang - Rheum should be added during the last 3 - 5 minutes of the decoction process.

✗ Do not use during pregnancy.

DA HUANG FU ZI TANG

Rhubarb and Aconite Decoction

Extract Formula Name: Rhubarb and Aconite Combination

Da Huang	Rheum	6 - 9 g
Fu Zi	Aconitum	6 g
Xi Xin	Asarum	3 - 6 g

Spleen/Kidney yang deficiency causing dawn diarrhea with middle jiao qi stagnation symptoms such as excruciating abdominal pain and severe fullness feelings.

T pale, swollen, teethmarks, light purple, white coat

P deep, weak, or slippery

DAN LIAO SI SHEN WAN

Four-Miracle Pill from the Tranquil Hut

Bu Gu Zhi	Psoralea	6 - 12 g
Xiao Hui Xiang	Foeniculum	3 - 9 g
Rou Dou Kou	Myristica	9 - 12 g
Mu Xiang	Saussurea	3 - 6 g

Kidney

Bone bi-syndrome: wind cold damp with Kidney yang deficiency and yin and blood deficiency. Symptoms include chronic joint pain, cold knees, joint deformities, or stiffness or weakness in the joints.

T   pale, thin white coat

P   frail

DU HUO JI SHENG TANG

Angelica Pubescens and Sangjisheng Decoction

Extract Formula Name: Tuhuo and Loranthus Combination

Du Huo	Angelica	6 - 9 g
Sang Ji Sheng	Loranthus	6 - 12 g
Qin Jiao	Gentiana	6 - 9 g
Fang Feng	Ledebouriella	6 - 9 g
Dang Gui	Angelica	6 - 9 g
Rou Gui	Cinnamomum	6 g
Ren Shen	Panax	6 - 9 g
Huai Niu Xi	Achyranthes	6 - 9 g
Du Zhong	Eucommia	6 - 9 g
Sheng Di Huang	Rehmannia	6 - 9 g
Fu Ling	Poria	6 - 9 g
Chuan Xiong	Ligusticum	3 - 6 g
Bai Shao Yao	Paeonia	6 - 9 g
Xi Xin	Asarum	3 - 6 g
Gan Cao	Glycyrrhiza	3 - 6 g

Kidney yin and yang deficiency with fire causing menopause, hot flashes, or urinary frequency.

T   red

P   rapid or normal rate, thin

ER XIAN TANG

Two-Immortal Decoction

Extract Formula Name: Curculigo and Epimedium Combination

Yin Yang Huo	Epimedium	9 - 15 g
Xian Mao	Curculigo	9 - 15 g
Dang Gui	Angelica	6 - 9 g
Huang Bai	Phellodendron	6 - 9 g
Zhi Mu	Anemarrhena	6 - 9 g
Ba Ji Tian	Morinda	6 - 9 g

Kidney qi and yang deficiency causing edema which manifests mostly in the superficial and muscle layers.

T   pale, swollen, sticky white coat

P   weak, deep, slippery

FANG JI FU LING TANG

Stephania and Poria Decoction

Extract Formula Name: Stephania and Hoelen Combination

Han Fang Ji	Stephania	9 - 12 g
Fu Ling	Poria	9 - 18 g
Gui Zhi	Cinnamomum	9 - 12 g
Huang Qi	Astragalus	9 - 12 g
Gan Cao	Glycyrrhiza	3 - 6 g

Turbid leukorrhea due to Kidney qi/yang deficiency. The Kidneys are unable to astringe.

T   pale, swollen, slight teethmarks, wet, thin white coat

P   minute or frail

FEN QING YIN

Separate Pure from Impure Powder

Bei Xie	Dioscorea	6 - 9 g
Yi Yi Ren	Coix	12 - 15 g
Wu Yao	Lindera	6 - 9 g
Shi Chang Pu	Acorus	6 - 9 g
Fu Ling	Poria	6 - 9 g
Chen Pi	Citrus	3 - 6 g
Gan Cao	Glycyrrhiza	3 - 6 g

Severe Kidney yang deficiency where the yang is unable to nourish the limbs leading to edema, and severe body aches with cold and damp symptoms: cold bi-syndrome.

T   pale, moist white coat

P   deep, minute, or choppy

FU ZI TANG

Prepared Aconite Decoction

Extract Formula Name: Aconite Combination

Fu Zi	Aconitum	9 - 15 g
Ren Shen	Panax	3 - 6 g
Fu Ling	Poria	9 - 12 g
Bai Zhu	Atractylodes	3 - 12 g
Bai Shao Yao	Paeonia	6 - 9 g

Spleen/Kidney yang deficiency causing watery diarrhea with undigested food, spasms in hands and feet, fatigue, and spontanous severe sweating.

T pale, swollen, teethmarks, wet, white coat

P minute

GU ZHEN TANG

Stabilize the True Decoction

Fu Zi	Aconitum	6 - 9 g
Ren Shen	Panax	6 - 9 g
Bai Zhu	Atractylodes	6 - 9 g
Fu Ling	Poria	6 - 9 g
Huang Qi	Astragalus	6 - 15 g
Shan Yao	Dioscorea	6 - 9 g
Rou Gui	Cinnamomum	3 - 9 g
Gan Cao	Glycyrrhiza	3 - 6 g
[Sheng Jiang	Zingiber	3 - 6 g]
[Da Zao	Ziziphus	1 - 2 pc]

Severe cold stagnation with Spleen/Kidney yang deficiency causing coldness in the face, cramping pain in the center, or dawn diarrhea.

T pale, purple, wet coat

P slow, tight

GUI FU LI ZHONG WAN

Cinnamon and Prepared Aconite Decoction to Regulate the Middle

Ren Shen	Panax	10 - 15 g
Bai Zhu	Atractylodes	6 - 9 g
Gan Jiang	Zingiber	6 - 9 g
Gan Cao	Glycyrrhiza	3 - 6 g
Fu Zi	Aconitum	3 - 6 g
Gui Zhi	Cinnamomum	3 - 9 g

Cold phlegm in the Lungs with underlying Kidney yang deficiency. This produces cough with clear watery fluids, or shortness of breath.

T pale, thick sticky white coat

P frail or slippery

GUI LING WU WEI GAN CAO TANG

Cinnamon Twig, Poria, Schisandra, and Licorice Decoction

Gui Zhi	Cinnamomum	6 - 12 g
Fu Ling	Poria	6 - 12 g
Wu Wei Zi	Schisandra	9 - 15 g
Gan Cao	Glycyrrhiza	6 - 9 g

Kidney yin and yang deficiency with qi and blood deficiency causing impotence, low back and knee pain, or weight loss. The deficiency is very severe, and the formula is deep-acting.

T pale, thin white coat

P frail, or rapid

☞ Ingredients should be prepared as a syrup. Herbs should be decocted and cane sugar then added to the tea. Doses of about 6 g should be taken with salt water.

GUI LU ER XIAN JIAO

Tortoise Shell and Deer Antler Syrup

Lu Jiao	Cervus	500 g
Ren Shen	Panax	45 g
Gou Qi Zi	Lycium	250 g
Gui Ban	Chinemys	150 g

Kidneys and Heart are not harmonizing accompanied with yin and yang deficiency. Symptoms include spermatorrhea, sexual dreams, or poor sleep.

T pale

P slow, hollow, weak

GUI ZHI JIA LONG GU MU LI TANG

Cinnamon Twig Decoction plus Dragon Bone and Oyster Shell

Extract Formula Name: Cinnamon and Dragon Bone Combination

Gui Zhi	Cinnamomum	6 - 9 g
Bai Shao Yao	Paeonia	6 - 9 g
Sheng Jiang	Zingiber	6 - 9 g
Da Zao	Ziziphus	4 - 12 pc
Mu Li	Ostrea	6 - 9 g
Long Gu	Os Draconis	6 - 9 g
Gan Cao	Glycyrrhiza	3 - 6 g

Kidney

Phlegm in the Lungs with underlying Kidney yang deficiency. The Kidneys are unable to grasp Lung qi, so qi ascends to the chest causing fullness in chest and epigastrium. This is known as running piglet disorder. Symptoms also include wheezing, spontaneous sweating, and cold hands and feet.

T   pale, sticky white coat

P   minute

☞ Hei Xi - Lead and Liu Huang - Sulphur should both be dry fried. The remaining herbs are ground and made into pills with wine. Adults take 6 - 9 g per day, children take 2-3 g per day.

✗ To prevent lead poisoning, do not take longer than 3 days. Do not use during pregnancy.

HEI XI DAN
Lead Special Pill

Hei Xi	Lead	60 g
Liu Huang	Sulphur	60 g
Fu Zi	Aconitum	30 g
Rou Gui	Cinnamomum	60 g
Xiao Hui Xiang	Foeniculum	30 g
Rou Dou Kou	Amomun	30 g
Chen Xiang	Aquilaria	30 g
Yang Qi Shi	Actinolitum	30 g
Bu Gu Zhi	Psoralea	30 g
Mu Xiang	Saussurea	30 g
Chuan Lian Zi	Melia	30 g
Hu Lu Ba	Trigonella	30 g

Kidney and Spleen yang deficiency with cold which has invaded all three yin channels (taiyin, shaoyin, and jueyin). Symptoms include shivering from cold, icy limbs and face, watery diarrhea, or cough with profuse saliva production.

T   pale, wet, thin white moist coat

P   minute or frail

☞ Remove She Xiang - Moschus, decoct the rest of the formula as usual, then add powdered Moschus to each dosage.

HUI YANG JIU JI TANG
Restore and Revive the Yang Decoction

Fu Zi	Aconitum	9 g
Rou Gui	Cinnamomum	3 - 6 g
Ren Shen	Panax	6 - 9 g
Gan Jiang	Zingiber	3 - 6 g
Fu Ling	Poria	6 - 9 g
Chen Pi	Citrus	3 - 6 g
Bai Zhu	Atractylodes	6 - 9 g
Wu Wei Zi	Schisandra	3 - 6 g
Ban Xia	Pinellia	6 - 9 g
Gan Cao	Glycyrrhiza	3 - 6 g
She Xiang	Moschus	0.3 g
[Sheng Jiang	Zingiber	1 - 3 g]

Kidney qi/yang deficiency resulting in constipation.

T pale, white coat

P weak, deep, or minute

JI CHUAN JIAN

Benefit the River Decoction

Dang Gui	Angelica	9 - 15 g
Rou Cong Rong	Cistanche	6 - 9 g
Huai Niu Xi	Achyranthes	6 g
Zhi Ke	Citrus	3 g
Ze Xie	Alisma	4.5 g
Sheng Ma	Cimicifuga	2 - 3 g

Kidney yang deficiency causing edema, scanty urination, or benign prostate hypertrophy.

T pale, swollen, teethmarks, white sticky coat

P deep, wiry, slippery, thin

JI SHENG SHEN QI WAN

Kidney Qi Pill from Formulas to Aid the Living

Shu Di Huang	Rehmannia	6 - 12 g
Shan Yao	Dioscorea	6 - 12 g
Shan Zhu Yu	Cornus	6 - 9 g
Mu Dan Pi	Paeonia	6 - 12 g
Ze Xie	Alisma	6 - 9 g
Fu Ling	Poria	6 - 9 g
Fu Zi	Aconitum	6 - 9 g
Rou Gui	Cinnamomum	3 - 9 g
Che Qian Zi	Plantago	6 - 9 g
Chuan Niu Xi	Cyathula	6 - 9 g

Kidney

Heart and Kidneys are not communicating. Kidney yang deficiency leads to Heart yang deficiency causing palpitations, cool limbs, or insomnia.

T pale, swollen, thin moist white coat

P deep, weak

JIAO TAI WAN

Grand Communication Pill

Extract Formula Name: Coptis and Cinnamon Formula

Huang Lian	Coptis	18 - 20 g
Rou Gui	Cinnamomum	3 - 6 g

Kidney qi and yang deficiency causing low back pain, coldness in the back, urinary difficulties, or pedal edema.

T   pale, swollen, thin white coat

P   frail

✪ Major Formula

JIN GUI SHEN QI WAN

Kidney Qi Pill from the Golden Cabinet

Extract Formula Name: Rehmannia Eight Formula

Shu Di Huang	Rehmannia	24 g
Shan Zhu Yu	Cornus	12 g
Shan Yao	Dioscorea	12 g
Mu Dan Pi	Paeonia	9 g
Ze Xie	Alisma	9 g
Fu Ling	Poria	9 g
Rou Gui	Cinnamomum	3 g
Fu Zi	Aconitum	3 g

Kidney and Liver yin deficiency, yang deficiency, or jing deficiency causing spermatorrhea, tinnitus, or impotence.

T   pale or red, thin white coat

P   thin, weak

JIN SUO GU JING WAN

Metal Lock Pill to Stabilize the Essence

Extract Formula Name: Lotus Stamen Formula

Qian Shi	Euryale	6 - 12 g
Sha Yuan Ji Li	Astragalus	6 - 12 g
Long Gu	Os Draconis	6 - 9 g
Mu Li	Ostrea	6 - 9 g
Lian Xu	Nelumbo	6 - 9 g
Lian Zi	Nelumbo	9 - 15 g

Kidney yang deficiency causing pronounced low back pain with severe immobility of the back, and weak legs.

T   pale

P   deep, weak, thin

☞ Herbs should be made into 3 g pills with honey. Du Zhong - Eucommia should be fried in ginger juice. Bu Gu Zhi - Psoralea should be fried with wine.

QING E WAN

Young Maiden Pill

Du Zhong	Eucommia	200 g
Hu Tao Ren	Juglans	6 g
Bu Gu Zhi	Psoralea	100 g
Da Suan	Allium	20 g

Kidney yang deficiency causing pedal edema, dark face, and low back pain, dribbling urination, or chronic deafness.

T   pale, swollen, teethmarks, white coat

P   frail

SHI BU WAN

Ten-Tonic Pill

Fu Zi	Aconitum	6 - 12 g
Rou Gui	Cinnamomum	3 - 6 g
Wu Wei Zi	Schisandra	6 - 12 g
Shan Yao	Dioscorea	6 - 12 g
Lu Rong	Cervus	3 - 6 g
Mu Dan Pi	Paeonia	3 - 6 g
Shan Zhu Yu	Cornus	3 - 6 g
Fu Ling	Poria	3 - 6 g
Ze Xie	Alisma	3 - 6 g
Shu Di Huang	Rehmannia	3 - 6 g

Leukorrhea or cloudy spermatorrhea due to Kidney yang deficiency.

T   pale

P   frail

SHUI LU ER XIAN DAN

Water and Earth Immortals Special Pill

Qian Shi	Euryale	10 g
Jin Ying Zi	Rosa	10 g

Kidney/Spleen yang deficiency leading to dawn diarrhea.

T   pale, white coat

P   deep, weak, slow

SI SHEN WAN

Four-Miracle Pill

Extract Formula Name: Psoralea and Myristica Formula

Bu Gu Zhi	Psoralea	12 - 18 g
Rou Dou Kou	Myristica	6 - 9 g
Wu Zhu Yu	Evodia	3 - 6 g
Wu Wei Zi	Schisandra	6 - 9 g
[Sheng Jiang	Zingiber	3 - 6 g]
[Da Zao	Ziziphus	3 - 5 pc]

Kidney

Kidney and Spleen yang deficiency which developed after a chronic damp heat dysentery causing damp cold. This obstructs the Large Intestines, manifesting as dark blood in the stools with pus.

T pale

P minute

☞ Ingredients should be ground into a powder.

TAO HUA TANG

Peach Blossom Decoction

Extract Formula Name: Kaolin and Oryza Combination

Chi Shi Zhi	Halloysitum Rubrum	20 - 30 g
Jing Mi	Oryza	20 - 30 g
Gan Jiang	Zingiber	6 - 9 g

Kidney qi and yang deficiency with severe urinary incontinence and frequency or low back pain.

T pale

P frail

TU SI ZI WAN

Cuscuta Seed Pill

Tu Si Zi	Cuscuta	6 - 12 g
Rou Cong Rong	Cistanche	6 - 12 g
Wu Wei Zi	Schisandra	6 - 9 g
Lu Rong	Cervus	6 - 9 g
Shan Yao	Dioscorea	6 - 9 g
Sang Piao Xiao	Paratenodera	6 - 9 g
Wu Yao	Lindera	6 - 9 g
Yi Zhi Ren	Alpinia	6 - 9 g
Fu Zi	Aconitum	6 - 9 g
Mu Li	Ostrea	6 - 12 g
Ji Nei Jin	Gallus	3 g

Yin jaundice due to Kidney yang deficiency.

T pale, swollen, teethmarks, moist white coat

P deep, weak, thin

YIN CHEN SI NI TANG

Artemisia Yinchenhao Decoction for Frigid Extremities

Yin Chen Hao	Artemisia	3 - 9 g
Fu Zi	Aconitum	3 - 6 g
Pao Jiang	Zingiber	3 - 6 g
Gan Cao	Glycyrrhiza	3 - 6 g

Kidney yang and essence deficiency causing amenorrhea, infertility, cold back or knees, pedal edema, or impotence.

T   pale, swollen, teethmarks, thin white coat

P   minute

YOU GUI WAN

Restore the Right Pill

Extract Formula Name: Eucommia and Rehmannia Formula

Rou Gui	Cinnamomum	6 - 9 g
Fu Zi	Aconitum	3 - 6 g
Gou Qi Zi	Lycium	6 - 9 g
Shan Yao	Dioscorea	6 - 9 g
Shu Di Huang	Rehmannia	12 - 20 g
Shan Zhu Yu	Cornus	6 - 9 g
Du Zhong	Eucommia	6 - 9 g
Dang Gui	Angelica	6 - 9 g
Tu Si Zi	Cuscuta	6 - 9 g
Lu Jiao Jiao	Cervus	6 - 9 g

Kidney yang deficiency causing cold extremities, frequent urination, incontinence, decreased sexual function, or cold uterus. If the yang deficiency is chronic there will be heat symptoms: true yang deficiency with false heat symptoms such as redness in the face or thirst.

T   pale, swollen, teethmarks, white coat

P   frail or minute

YOU GUI YIN

Restore the Right Decoction

Shu Di Huang	Rehmannia	9 - 20 g
Gou Qi Zi	Lycium	6 - 9 g
Shan Zhu Yu	Cornus	6 g
Du Zhong	Eucommia	6 - 9 g
Fu Zi	Aconitum	6 - 9 g
Shan Yao	Dioscorea	6 - 9 g
Rou Gui	Cinnamomum	3 - 6 g
Zhi Gan Cao	Glycyrrhiza	3 - 6 g

Kidney

Impotence or infertility due to Kidney yang deficiency with simultaneous qi and blood deficiency. Symptoms include blurry vision, low back pain, and poor memory.

T   pale, thin white coat

P   frail

ZAN YU DAN

Special Pill to Aid Fertility

Rou Cong Rong	Cistanche	6 - 12 g
Fu Zi	Aconitum	6 g
Ba Ji Tian	Morinda	6 - 12 g
Rou Gui	Cinnamomum	6 g
She Chuang Zi	Cnidium	6 g
Xian Mao	Curculigo	6 - 12 g
Dang Gui	Angelica	9 - 15 g
Bai Zhu	Atractylodes	12 - 18 g
Gou Qi Zi	Lycium	9 - 15 g
Yin Yang Huo	Epimedium	6 - 12 g
Shan Zhu Yu	Cornus	6 - 12 g
Shu Di Huang	Rehmannia	6 - 12 g
Jiu Zi	Allium	6 - 12 g
Du Zhong	Eucommia	6 - 12 g

Spleen/Kidney qi and yang deficient patient suffers easily from wind cold with internal water accumulation, or experiences urinary difficulty, diarrhea, or edema.

T   pale, swollen, teethmarks, moist, thin white coat

P   frail or minute

ZHEN WU TANG

True Warrior Decoction

Extract Formula Name: Vitality Combination

Fu Zi	Aconitum	6 - 9 g
Bai Zhu	Atractylodes	6 - 9 g
Bai Shao Yao	Paeonia	6 - 9 g
Fu Ling	Poria	6 - 9 g
Sheng Jiang	Zingiber	6 - 9 g

KIDNEY JING DEFICIENCY

- weak or brittle bones
- premature greying of hair or hair loss
- decreased sexual desire
- in children: slow bone development, mental slowness or retardation

T red, peeled

P empty

Lung/Kidney yin deficiency or jing deficiency with fire causing sweating, low back pain, slow mental and physical development in children, cough with scanty sticky blood-tinged phlegm, weight loss, or afternoon fever.

T red, slight yellow or no coat

P rapid, thin, or empty

HE CHE DA ZAO WAN

Pills of Human Placenta

Zi He Che	Placenta Hominis	9 - 30 g
Tian Men Dong	Asparagus	6 - 9 g
Mai Men Dong	Ophiopogon	6 - 9 g
Gui Ban	Chinemys	6 - 9 g
Shu Di Huang	Rehmannia	12 - 15 g
Huang Bai	Phellodendron	6 - 9 g
Du Zhong	Eucommia	6 - 9 g
Huai Niu Xi	Achyranthes	6 - 9 g

Kidney qi/yin deficiency causing slow mental development in children or low energy.

T pale, scanty coat

P thin

JIA WEI LIU WEI DI HUANG WAN

Augmented Six-Ingredient Pill with Rehmannia

Shu Di Huang	Rehmannia	6 - 12 g
Shan Yao	Dioscorea	6 - 9 g
Shan Zhu Yu	Cornus	6 - 9 g
Fu Ling	Poria	6 - 9 g
Ze Xie	Alisma	6 - 9 g
Mu Dan Pi	Paeonia	6 - 9 g
Lu Rong	Cervus	3 - 9 g
She Xiang	Moschus	1 - 2 g
Wu Jia Pi	Acanthopanax	6 - 12 g

Kidney

Kidney and Liver yin deficiency, yang deficiency, or jing deficiency causing spermatorrhea, tinnitus, or impotence.

T pale or red, thin white coat

P thin, weak

JIN SUO GU JING WAN

Metal Lock Pill to Stabilize the Essence

Extract Formula Name: Lotus Stamen Formula

Qian Shi	Euryale	6 - 12 g
Sha Yuan Ji Li	Astragalus	6 - 12 g
Long Gu	Os Draconis	6 - 9 g
Mu Li	Ostrea	6 - 9 g
Lian Xu	Nelumbo	6 - 9 g
Lian Zi	Nelumbo	9 - 15 g

Liver blood/yin deficiency with Kidney qi deficiency causing early greying, hairloss, poor teeth, and seminal emissions.

T pale

P thin, weak

QI BAO MEI RAN DAN

Seven-Treasure Special Pill for Beautiful Whiskers

He Shou Wu	Polygonum	6 - 9 g
Huai Niu Xi	Achyranthes	6 - 12 g
Fu Ling	Poria	6 - 9 g
Tu Si Zi	Cuscuta	6 - 9 g
Gou Qi Zi	Lycium	6 - 9 g
Bu Gu Zhi	Psoralea	6 - 9 g
Dang Gui	Angelica	6 - 9 g

Liver/Kidney yin and jing (essence) deficiency causing slow development in children; or premature aging in adults, in addition to common yin deficiency signs and symptoms. The formula is also for early menopause, spermatorrhea, low sex drive, infertility, or low sperm count.

T red, scanty coat

P thin, rapid

✪ Major Formula

ZUO GUI YIN

Restore the Left [Kidney] Decoction

Shu Di Huang	Rehmannia	6 - 15 g
Shan Zhu Yu	Cornus	6 - 9 g
Shan Yao	Dioscorea	6 - 9 g
Gou Qi Zi	Lycium	6 - 9 g
Fu Ling	Poria	6 - 9 g
Zhi Gan Cao	Glycyrrhiza	3 - 6 g

KIDNEY YIN DEFICIENCY

- nightsweats, or five-palm heat
- thirst and dry mouth, especially at night
- dizziness, tinnitus

T red, peeled, scanty coat, cracks

P thin, rapid, or empty

Kidney/Liver yin deficiency with blood deficiency causing post-partum sweating, or night sweats.

T red, thin yellow coat

P thin, rapid

BA WEI DI HUANG WAN

Eight-Ingredient Pill with Rehmannia

Sheng Di Huang	Rehmannia	6 - 12 g
Shan Zhu Yu	Cornus	6 - 9 g
Shan Yao	Dioscorea	6 - 9 g
Fu Ling	Poria	6 - 9 g
Ze Xie	Alisma	6 - 9 g
Mu Dan Pi	Paeonia	6 - 9 g
Wu Wei Zi	Schisandra	6 - 9 g
Huang Qi	Astragalus	9 - 15 g

Lung/Kidney yin deficiency with cough and asthma, hemoptysis, tidal fever, or night sweats. This formula is also known as 'Mai Wei Di Huang Wan'.

T red, slight coat

P rapid, thin

BA XIAN CHANG SHOU WAN

Eight-Immortal Pill for Longevity

Shan Zhu Yu	Cornus	6 - 9 g
Shan Yao	Dioscorea	6 - 9 g
Sheng Di Huang	Rehmannia	6 - 12 g
Mu Dan Pi	Paeonia	6 - 9 g
Ze Xie	Alisma	6 - 9 g
Fu Ling	Poria	6 - 9 g
Wu Wei Zi	Schisandra	6 - 9 g
Mai Men Dong	Ophiopogon	6 - 9 g

Kidney

Lung/Kidney yin deficiency with bleeding in the upper parts due to false heat breaking the blood vessels; or chronic cough due to dryness in the throat.

T   red, slight coat

P   rapid, thin

BAI HE GU JIN TANG

Lily Bulb Decoction to Preserve the Metal

Extract Formula Name: Lily Combination

Bai He	Lilium	3 - 12 g
Mai Men Dong	Ophiopogon	6 - 12 g
Sheng Di Huang	Rehmannia	6 - 12 g
Shu Di Huang	Rehmannia	6 - 12 g
Bei Mu	Fritillaria	3 - 6 g
Xuan Shen	Scrophularia	6 - 9 g
Dang Gui	Angelica	6 - 9 g
Bai Shao Yao	Paeonia	6 - 9 g
Jie Geng	Platycodon	3 - 6 g
Gan Cao	Glycyrrhiza	3 - 6 g

Kidney yin deficiency can't nourish the Heart which leads to Heart blood deficiency. Symptoms include insomnia, dizziness, poor memory, excessive dreaming, or night sweating.

T   slightly red, or pale, scanty coat

P   thin, rapid

BAI ZI YANG XIN WAN

Biota Seed Pill to Nourish the Heart

Bai Zi Ren	Biota	3 - 9 g
Mai Men Dong	Ophiopogon	6 - 9 g
Dang Gui	Angelica	6 - 12 g
Gou Qi Zi	Lycium	6 - 9 g
Xuan Shen	Scrophularia	6 - 12 g
Fu Shen	Poria	6 - 9 g
Shi Chang Pu	Acorus	6 - 9 g
Shu Di Huang	Rehmannia	12 - 15 g
Gan Cao	Glycyrrhiza	3 - 6 g

Kidney qi/yin deficiency causing menorrhagia. Other symptoms may include low back pain, frequent urination, or weakness in the knees.

T   red or normal color, thin white coat

P   weak, especially in both chi (third) positions, slightly rapid

BAO YIN JIAN

Augment Yin Decoction

Huang Qin	Scutellaria	9 - 12 g
Huang Bai	Phellodendron	9 - 12 g
Sheng Di Huang	Rehmannia	9 - 15 g
Shu Di Huang	Rehmannia	9 - 15 g
Shan Yao	Dioscorea	6 - 9 g
Bai Shao Yao	Paeonia	6 - 12 g
Xu Duan	Dipsacus	6 - 9 g
Gan Cao	Glycyrrhiza	3 - 6 g

Purpura due to yin deficiency with heat. Strong false fire due to Kidney and Liver yin deficiency which leads to tidal fever and night sweats.

T   red, thin yellow coat or no coat

P   rapid, thin, or empty

DA BU YIN WAN

Great Tonify the Yin Pill

Shu Di Huang	Rehmannia	6 - 12 g
Gui Ban	Chinemys	6 - 12 g
Huang Bai	Phellodendron	6 - 9 g
Zhi Mu	Anemarrhena	6 - 9 g

Kidney yin and Spleen qi/blood deficiency causing uterine prolapse with low back pain, night urination, or hearing loss and tinnitus.

T   red or pale

P   frail

DA BU YUAN JIAN

Great Tonify the Basal Decoction

Ren Shen	Panax	6 - 12 g
Shu Di Huang	Rehmannia	9 - 25 g
Shan Yao	Dioscorea	6 - 9 g
Shan Zhu Yu	Cornus	3 - 6 g
Gou Qi Zi	Lycium	6 - 9 g
Dang Gui	Angelica	6 - 9 g
Du Zhong	Eucommia	6 - 9 g
Gan Cao	Glycyrrhiza	3 - 6 g

Kidney

Lung/Kidney yin deficiency with bone steaming fever, cough with sticky phlegm, and five-palm heat.

T   red, scanty coat

P   thin, rapid

DA ZAO WAN

Great Creation Pill

Gui Ban	Chinemys	6 - 12 g
Huang Bai	Phellodendron	6 - 9 g
Zi He Che	Placenta Hominis	1 - 2 g
Huai Niu Xi	Achyranthes	6 - 9 g
Ren Shen	Panax	6 - 9 g
Du Zhong	Eucommia	6 - 9 g
Mai Men Dong	Ophiopogon	6 - 9 g
Tian Men Dong	Asparagus	6 - 9 g
Sheng Di Huang	Rehmannia	6 - 12 g

Kidney and Liver yin deficiency causing irregular menses, a scanty menstrual flow, tinnitus, dizziness, or night sweating.

T   red, scanty coat

P   thin, rapid

DANG GUI DI HUANG YIN

Dang Gui and Rehmannia Decoction

Dang Gui	Angelica	6 - 9 g
Shu Di Huang	Rehmannia	6 - 12 g
Huai Niu Xi	Achyranthes	6 - 9 g
Shan Yao	Dioscorea	6 - 9 g
Du Zhong	Eucommia	6 - 9 g
Shan Zhu Yu	Cornus	6 - 9 g
Zhi Gan Cao	Glycyrrhiza	3 - 6 g

Yin deficient patient has very high fever, profuse sweating, thirst, or yellow, scanty urine.

T   red, cracked, slight coat

P   rapid, thin

DANG GUI LIU HUANG TANG

Dang Gui and Six-Yellow Decoction

Extract Formula Name: Tang-Kuei and Six-Yellows Combination

Dang Gui	Angelica	6 - 9 g
Shu Di Huang	Rehmannia	6 - 9 g
Sheng Di Huang	Rehmannia	6 - 12 g
Huang Qi	Astralagus	12 - 15 g
Huang Qin	Scutellaria	6 - 12 g
Huang Lian	Coptis	3 - 6 g
Huang Bai	Phellodendron	6 - 12 g

Kidney/Lung qi/yin deficiency with wheezing, shortness of breath, or chronic cough. This formula is also known as 'Qi Wu Du Qi Wan'.

T red, slight coat

P thin, rapid

DU QI WAN

Capital Qi Pill

Extract Formula Name: Rehmannia and Schizandra Formula

Shan Zhu Yu	Cornus	6 - 9 g
Shan Yao	Dioscorea	6 - 9 g
Sheng Di Huang	Rehmannia	9 - 12 g
Fu Ling	Poria	6 - 9 g
Mu Dan Pi	Paeonia	6 - 9 g
Ze Xie	Alisma	6 - 9 g
Wu Wei Zi	Schisandra	6 - 9 g

Kidney yin deficiency with hearing problems, high-pitched tinnitus, dizziness, or hearing loss in the elderly.

T red, scanty yellow coat

P thin, rapid

ER LONG ZUO CI WAN

Pill for Deafness that is Kind to the Left [Kidney]

Shu Di Huang	Rehmannia	6 - 12 g
Shan Yao	Dioscorea	6 - 9 g
Shan Zhu Yu	Cornus	6 - 9 g
Mu Dan Pi	Paeonia	6 - 9 g
Fu Ling	Poria	6 - 9 g
Ze Xie	Alisma	6 - 9 g
Ci Shi	Magnetitum	6 - 9 g
Wu Wei Zi	Schisandra	6 - 9 g
Shi Chang Pu	Acorus	6 - 9 g

Kidney

Kidney yin and yang deficiency with fire causing menopause, hot flashes, or urinary frequency.

T red

P rapid or normal rate, thin

ER XIAN TANG

Two-Immortal Decoction

Extract Formula Name: Curculigo and Epimedium Combination

Yin Yang Huo	Epimedium	9 - 15 g
Xian Mao	Curculigo	9 - 15 g
Dang Gui	Angelica	6 - 9 g
Huang Bai	Phellodendron	6 - 9 g
Zhi Mu	Anemarrhena	6 - 9 g
Ba Ji Tian	Morinda	6 - 9 g

Liver/Kidney yin deficiency causing weakness in the low back and knees, or atrophy; or Liver cannot store the soul (hun) causing insomnia or bad dreams.

T red, dry, scanty coat

P thin, rapid

☞ Equal amounts of both herbs should be used.

ER ZHI WAN

Two-Ultimate Pill

Han Lian Cao	Eclipta	10 g
Nu Zhen Zi	Ligustrum	10 g

Kidney qi/yin deficiency causing irregular periods, leukorrhea, or a bearing-down sensation.

T red, thin white coat

P weak, especially the chi (third) positions

GU YIN JIAN

Stabilize the Yin Decoction

Shu Di Huang	Rehmannia	6 - 12 g
Shan Yao	Dioscorea	6 - 9 g
Wu Wei Zi	Schisandra	6 - 9 g
Shan Zhu Yu	Cornus	6 - 9 g
Tu Si Zi	Cuscuta	6 - 9 g
Ren Shen	Panax	6 - 9 g
Yuan Zhi	Polygala	3 g
Zhi Gan Cao	Glycyrrhiza	3 - 6 g

Kidney yin and yang deficiency with qi and blood deficiency causing impotence, low back and knee pain, or weight loss. The deficiency is very severe, and the formula is deep-acting.

T pale, thin white coat

P frail, or rapid

☞ Ingredients should be prepared as a syrup. Herbs should be decocted and cane sugar then added to the tea. Doses of about 6 g should be taken with salt water.

GUI LU ER XIAN JIAO

Tortoise Shell and Deer Antler Syrup

Lu Jiao	Cervus	500 g
Ren Shen	Panax	45 g
Gou Qi Zi	Lycium	250 g
Gui Ban	Chinemys	150 g

Kidney qi deficiency with Kidney/Liver yin deficiency causing amenorrhea, or back and knee pain.

T pale or red, thin white or scanty coat

P weak, maybe thin especially in the left chi (third) position

GUI SHEN TANG

Comeback Kidney Decoction

Shu Di Huang	Rehmannia	6 - 15 g
Shan Yao	Dioscorea	9 - 15 g
Shan Zhu Yu	Cornus	9 - 12 g
Gou Qi Zi	Lycium	9 - 15 g
Dang Gui	Angelica	9 - 12 g
Du Zhong	Eucommia	6 - 12 g
Fu Ling	Poria	6 - 12 g
Tu Si Zi	Cuscuta	9 - 12 g

Kidney

Lung/Kidney yin deficiency or jing deficiency with fire causing sweating, low back pain, slow mental and physical development in children, cough with scanty sticky blood-tinged phlegm, weight loss, or afternoon fever.

T   red, slight yellow or no coat

P   rapid, thin, or empty

HE CHE DA ZAO WAN

Pills of Human Placenta

Zi He Che	Placenta Hominis	9 - 30 g
Tian Men Dong	Asparagus	6 - 9 g
Mai Men Dong	Ophiopogon	6 - 9 g
Gui Ban	Chinemys	6 - 9 g
Shu Di Huang	Rehmannia	12 - 15 g
Huang Bai	Phellodendron	6 - 9 g
Du Zhong	Eucommia	6 - 9 g
Huai Niu Xi	Achyranthes	6 - 9 g

Kidney and Liver yin deficiency causing bone bi-syndrome or wei syndrome. Deficient yin cannot nourish tendons and false heat burns tendons and muscles. This leads to atrophy, joint swelling, or deformities. The pain tends to be more fixed.

T   red, scanty coat

P   thin, rapid, weak

☞ All ingredients should be ground up as powder. Take 10 g each time, twice a day.

HU QIAN WAN

Hidden Tiger Pill

Extract Formula Name: Tiger Bone and Tortoise Shell Formula

Gui Ban	Chinemys	120 g
Huang Bai	Phellodendron	150 g
Shu Di Huang	Rehmannia	60 g
Zhi Mu	Anemarrhena	60 g
Bai Shao Yao	Paeonia	60 g
Suo Yang	Cynomorium	45 g
Hu Gu	Panthera	30 g
Chen Pi	Citrus	60 g
Gan Jiang	Zingiber	15 g

Heart/Kidney yin deficiency with fire after febrile disease leading to insomnia, palpitations, or tongue sores: shaoyin deficient heat syndrome.

T red, scanty coat

P rapid, thin

☞ E Jiao - Equus and egg yolks should be dissolved into the strained tea.

HUANG LIAN E JIAO TANG

Coptis and Ass-Hide Gelatin Decoction

Extract Formula Name: Coptis and Gelatin Combination

Huang Lian	Coptis	9 - 12 g
E Jiao	Equus	6 - 9 g
Huang Qin	Scutellaria	6 - 9 g
Bai Shao Yao	Paeonia	6 - 9 g
Ji Zi Huang	Egg yolks	2

1. Yin/blood deficiency with heat causing arrhythmia of the Heart. 2. High fever causing arrhythmia: yangming disease depleted yin which leads to an irregular Heart beat.

T red, scanty coat

P rapid, irregular

☞ E Jiao - Equus should be dissolved at the end into the strained tea.

JIA JIAN FU MAI TANG

Modified Restore-the-Pulse Decoction

Zhi Gan Cao	Glycyrrhiza	12 - 15 g
Bai Shao Yao	Paeonia	12 - 15 g
Mai Men Dong	Ophiopogon	9 - 12 g
Sheng Di Huang	Rehmannia	12 - 15 g
Huo Ma Ren	Cannabis	9 - 12 g
E Jiao	Equus	6 - 9 g

Kidney qi/yin deficiency causing slow mental development in children or low energy.

T pale, scanty coat

P thin

JIA WEI LIU WEI DI HUANG WAN

Augmented Six-Ingredient Pill with Rehmannia

Shu Di Huang	Rehmannia	6 - 12 g
Shan Yao	Dioscorea	6 - 9 g
Shan Zhu Yu	Cornus	6 - 9 g
Fu Ling	Poria	6 - 9 g
Ze Xie	Alisma	6 - 9 g
Mu Dan Pi	Paeonia	6 - 9 g
Lu Rong	Cervus	3 - 9 g
She Xiang	Moschus	1 - 2 g
Wu Jia Pi	Acanthopanax	6 - 12 g

Kidney

Kidney/Lung yin deficiency with Lung phlegm causing chronic bronchitis in the elderly, wheezing, or nausea.

T   red, slight coat, or geographic

P   thin, slightly rapid, slippery

JIN SHUI LIU JUN JIAN

Six-Gentlemen of Metal and Water Decoction

Chen Pi	Citrus	3 - 6 g
Ban Xia	Pinellia	6 - 9 g
Fu Ling	Poria	6 - 9 g
Gan Cao	Glycyrrhiza	3 - 6 g
Dang Gui	Angelica	6 - 9 g
Sheng Di Huang	Rehmannia	6 - 12 g
[Sheng Jiang	Zingiber	3 - 6 g]

Kidney and Liver yin deficiency, yang deficiency, or jing deficiency causing spermatorrhea, tinnitus, or impotence.

T   pale or red, thin white coat

P   thin, weak

JIN SUO GU JING WAN

Metal Lock Pill to Stabilize the Essence

Extract Formula Name: Lotus Stamen Formula

Qian Shi	Euryale	6 - 12 g
Sha Yuan Ji Li	Astragalus	6 - 12 g
Long Gu	Os Draconis	6 - 9 g
Mu Li	Ostrea	6 - 9 g
Lian Xu	Nelumbo	6 - 9 g
Lian Zi	Nelumbo	9 - 15 g

Basic prescription for Kidney/Liver yin deficiency with mild damp. This can cause dry, flaky, pale red rashes, excess sexual activity, or sweating. In women it may lead to irregular menses or night sweating and afternoon heat.

T   red, thin yellow coat, or scanty coat

P   rapid, thin

✪ Major Formula

LIU WEI DI HUANG WAN

Six-Ingredient Pill with Rehmannia

Extract Formula Name: Rehmannia Six Formula

Shan Zhu Yu	Cornus	6 - 9 g
Shan Yao	Dioscorea	6 - 9 g
Sheng Di Huang	Rehmannia	6 - 12 g
Fu Ling	Poria	6 - 9 g
Ze Xie	Alisma	6 - 9 g
Mu Dan Pi	Paeonia	6 - 9 g

Kidney and Liver yin deficiency with yang rising causing vision disturbances, dry red eyes, or blurry vision.

T red, scanty yellow coat

P thin, rapid

MING MU DI HUANG WAN

Improve Vision Pill with Rehmannia

Shu Di Huang	Rehmannia	9 - 20 g
Sheng Di Huang	Rehmannia	9 - 15 g
Mu Dan Pi	Paeonia	6 - 9 g
Shan Yao	Dioscorea	6 - 9 g
Shan Zhu Yu	Cornus	6 - 9 g
Ze Xie	Alisma	6 - 9 g
Dang Gui	Angelica	6 - 9 g
Fu Shen	Poria	6 - 9 g
Chai Hu	Bupleurum	6 - 9 g
Wu Wei Zi	Schisandra	6 - 9 g

Liver blood/yin deficiency with Kidney qi deficiency causing early greying, hairloss, poor teeth, and seminal emissions.

T pale

P thin, weak

QI BAO MEI RAN DAN

Seven-Treasure Special Pill for Beautiful Whiskers

He Shou Wu	Polygonum	6 - 9 g
Huai Niu Xi	Achyranthes	6 - 12 g
Fu Ling	Poria	6 - 9 g
Tu Si Zi	Cuscuta	6 - 9 g
Gou Qi Zi	Lycium	6 - 9 g
Bu Gu Zhi	Psoralea	6 - 9 g
Dang Gui	Angelica	6 - 9 g

Kidney

Kidney and Liver yin deficiency with eye disturbances.

T red, scanty yellow coat

P thin, rapid

QI JU DI HUANG WAN

Lycium Fruit, Chrysanthemum, and Rehmannia Pill

Extract Formula Name: Lycium, Chrysanthemum and Rehmannia Formula

Shu Di Huang	Rehmannia	6 - 12 g
Shan Yao	Dioscorea	6 - 9 g
Shan Zhu Yu	Cornus	6 - 9 g
Mu Dan Pi	Paeonia	6 - 9 g
Fu Ling	Poria	6 - 9 g
Ze Xie	Alisma	6 - 9 g
Gou Qi Zi	Lycium	6 - 12 g
Ju Hua	Chrysanthemum	6 - 9 g

Purpura due to yin deficiency with false heat. This prescription should be used with 'Da Bu Yin Wan' to strengthen the yin tonifying effect.

T red, dry, cracked, thin scanty yellow coat

P thin, rapid

☞ E Jiao - Equus should be dissolved at the end into the strained tea.

QIAN CAO GEN WAN

Rubia Pill

Qian Cao Gen	Rubia	6 - 9 g
Huang Qin	Scutellaria	6 - 9 g
E Jiao	Equus	9 - 15 g
Ce Bai Ye	Biota	12 - 20 g
Sheng Di Huang	Rehmannia	9 - 15 g
Gan Cao	Glycyrrhiza	3 - 6 g

Yin deficiency with severe false heat or tidal/bone steaming fever causing red lips, heat sensation in the bones, five-palm heat, night sweats, or delirium.

T red, slight yellow coat or no coat

P rapid, thin, weak, or empty

P Dissolve Bie Jia - Amyda first for about one hour, then decoct with the remaining herbs.

QING GU SAN

Cool the Bones Powder

Yin Chai Hu	Stellaria	6 - 12 g
Hu Huang Lian	Picrorhiza	6 - 9 g
Di Gu Pi	Lycium	6 - 9 g
Qing Hao	Artemisia	6 - 9 g
Bie Jia	Amyda	6 - 9 g
Qin Jiao	Gentiana	3 - 9 g
Zhi Mu	Anemarrhena	6 - 12 g
Gan Cao	Glycyrrhiza	3 - 6 g

Febrile disease causing low level chronic fever; or chronic disease damaged yin leading to later stages of febrile disease causing night sweats, AIDS, or tuberculosis.

T   red, dry, scanty coat

P   thin, rapid

☞ Bie Jia - Amyda should be soaked separately for 30 minutes to one hour, until it starts to dissolve; then soak the rest of the herbs. Qing Hao - Artemisia should be added at the end of the decoction process.

QING HAO BIE JIA TANG

Artemisia Annua and Soft-shelled Turtle Shell Decoction

Bie Jia	Amyda	9 - 12 g
Qing Hao	Artemisia	6 - 9 g
Mu Dan Pi	Paeonia	6 - 9 g
Sheng Di Huang	Rehmannia	6 - 12 g
Zhi Mu	Anemarrhena	6 - 9 g

Yin deficiency with false heat causing early periods or constipation.

T   red, scanty yellowish coat

P   thin, rapid

QING JING SAN

Clear the Menses Powder

Shu Di Huang	Rehmannia	6 - 12 g
Mu Dan Pi	Paeonia	6 - 9 g
Di Gu Pi	Lycium	6 - 9 g
Qing Hao	Artemisia	3 - 6 g
Bai Shao Yao	Paeonia	6 - 9 g
Fu Ling	Poria	6 g
Huang Bai	Phellodendron	3 g

Kidney

Heat in the ying level with yin deficiency causing high fever which is worse at night, delirious speech, or mild purpura.

T   dark red and dry

P   rapid, thin

☞ Xi Jiao - Rhinoceros should be substituted with 9 g of Shui Niu Jiao - Bubalus or 30 g of Bai Mao Gen - Imperata.

QING YING TANG

Clear the Nutritive Level Decoction

Extract Formula Name: Rhinoceros and Scrophularia Combination

Xi Jiao	Rhinoceros	3 - 6 g
Sheng Di Huang	Rehmannia	9 - 12 g
Mai Men Dong	Ophiopogon	6 - 9 g
Huang Lian	Coptis	3 - 6 g
Xuan Shen	Scrophularia	6 - 9 g
Dan Zhu Ye	Lophatherum	6 g
Lian Qiao	Forsythia	6 g
Dan Shen	Salvia	6 - 9 g
Jin Yin Hua	Lonicera	6 - 9 g

Lung and Kidney yin deficiency with dryness in the Lungs causing chronic consumptive disease. Symptoms include thirst, night sweating, or scanty phlegm which is hard to expectorate.

T   red, dry, scanty coat

P   deep, thin, rapid

QONG YU SAN

Ginseng and Rehmannia Powder

Ren Shen	Panax	3 - 6 g
Sheng Di Huang	Rehmannia	15 - 30 g
Feng Mi	Mel	30 g
Fu Ling	Poria	15 - 30 g

Kidney and Liver yin deficiency with blood deficiency and wind damp. This leads to blurry vision, cough, constipation, or bi-syndrome.

T   red, scanty yellow coat

P   thin

☞ Herbs should be formed into 9 g pills. Adults take one pill two times a day.

SANG MA WAN

Mulberry Leaf and Sesame Seed Pill

Sang Ye	Morus	250 - 300 g
Hei Zhi Ma	Sesamum	100 - 120 g
Feng Mi	Mel	250 - 300 g

Kidney/Liver yin deficiency with yang rising causing blurry vision, photophobia, excessive tearing, poor night vision, early stage catarract, or blood-shot eyes.

T red, thin and narrow in size, maybe cracked, scanty coat

P thin, rapid

☞ Xi Jiao - Rhinoceros should be substituted with Shui Niu Jiao - Bubalus.

SHI HU YE GUANG WAN

Dendrobium Pill for Night Vision

Tian Men Dong	Asparagus	6- 9 g
Fu Ling	Poria	6 - 9 g
Ren Shen	Panax	6 - 9 g
Shu Di Huang	Rehmannia	12 - 15 g
Mai Men Dong	Ophiopogon	6 - 9 g
Tu Si Zi	Cuscuta	3 - 9 g
Ju Hua	Chrysanthemum	3 - 6 g
Xing Ren	Prunus	3 - 6 g
Jue Ming Zi	Cassia	6 - 9 g
Gou Qi Zi	Lycium	6 - 9 g
Shan Yao	Dioscorea	6 - 12 g
Wu Wei Zi	Schisandra	6 - 9 g
Huai Niu Xi	Achyranthes	6 - 12 g
Bai Ji Li	Tribulus	6 - 9 g
Chuan Xiong	Ligusticum	3 - 6 g
Rou Cong Rong	Cistanche	3 - 6 g
Shi Hu	Dendrobium	6 - 12 g
Zhi Ke	Citrus	3 - 6 g
Qing Xiang Zi	Celosia	3 - 9 g
Xi Jiao	Rhinoceros	1 - 3 g
Huang Lian	Coptis	3 - 6 g
Fang Feng	Ledebouriella	6 - 9 g
Ling Yang Jiao	Saiga	1 - 3 g
Gan Cao	Glycyrrhiza	3 - 6 g

Kidney

Lung/Kidney yin deficiency with severe fire causing nosebleeds, or hemoptysis which occurs during or prior to the menses.

T red, cracks

P rapid, empty

SHUN JING TANG

Smooth the Menses Decoction

Shu Di Huang	Rehmannia	9 - 15 g
Mu Dan Pi	Paeonia	6 - 9 g
Dang Gui	Angelica	6 - 9 g
Bai Shao Yao	Paeonia	6 - 9 g
Bei Sha Shen	Glehnia	6 - 12 g
Jing Jie	Schizonepeta	6 - 9 g
Fu Ling	Poria	6 - 9 g

Heart/Kidney yin deficiency, Heart blood deficiency, and false heat where the Kidneys and Heart don't harmonize leading to insomnia, restlessness, palpitations, poor memory, or night sweats.

T red

P rapid, thin

✗ Zhu Sha - Cinnabaris is toxic and should only be used short-term.

TIAN WANG BU XIN DAN

Emperor of Heaven's Special Pill to Tonify the Heart

Extract Formula Name: Ginseng and Zizyphus Formula

Ren Shen	Panax	9 - 12 g
Mai Men Dong	Ophiopogon	6 - 12 g
Tian Men Dong	Asparagus	6 - 9 g
Xuan Shen	Scrophularia	6 - 9 g
Dan Shen	Salvia	6 - 12 g
Sheng Di Huang	Rehmannia	15 - 30 g
Fu Ling	Poria	6 - 9 g
Wu Wei Zi	Schisandra	6 - 9 g
Jie Geng	Platycodon	3 - 6 g
Yuan Zhi	Polygala	6 - 9 g
Bai Zi Ren	Biota	6 - 9 g
Dang Gui	Angelica	6 - 9 g
Suan Zao Ren	Ziziphus	6 - 12 g
Zhu Sha	Cinnabaris	1 - 3 g

Kidney and Liver yin deficiency causing amenorrhea, cold feeling in the abdomen, retarded growth in puberty, or clear leukorrhea.

T pale or slightly red

P weak, thin

☞ E Jiao - Equus should be added at the end to the strained tea.

TIAO GAN TANG

Regulating the Liver Decoction

Shan Yao	Dioscorea	9 - 12 g
E Jiao	Equus	6 - 12 g
Ba Ji Tian	Morinda	6 - 9 g
Dang Gui	Angelica	6 - 9 g
Ze Lan	Lycopus	6 - 12 g
Shan Zhu Yu	Cornus	6 - 9 g
Bai Shao Yao	Paeonia	6 - 9 g
Dan Shen	Salvia	6 - 9 g
Gan Cao	Glycyrrhiza	3 - 6 g

Lung/Kidney yin deficiency with toxin causing diptheria, laryngitis, coarse breathing, or dry hacking cough.

T red, dry, yellow coat

P thin, rapid, or empty

YANG YIN QING FEI TANG

Nourish the Yin and Clear the Lungs Decoction

Sheng Di Huang	Rehmannia	6 - 12 g
Xuan Shen	Scrophularia	6 - 9 g
Bai Shao Yao	Paeonia	6 - 9 g
Mai Men Dong	Ophiopogon	6 - 12 g
Bo He	Mentha	3 - 6 g
Chuan Bei Mu	Fritillaria	3 - 6 g
Mu Dan Pi	Paeonia	6 - 9 g
Gan Cao	Glycyrrhiza	3 - 6 g

Liver qi stagnation produces heat which consumes Kidney and Liver yin, or Liver overacts on the Spleen and Stomach causing emotional upset, nausea, belching with sour taste, hiatal hernia, or epigastric or abdominal pain; or Liver yin cannot nourish the tendons and ligaments producing heel or posterior hip pain.

T red, dry

P thin, wiry

YI GUAN JIAN

Linking Decoction

Extract Formula Name: Glehnia and Rehmannia Combination

Sheng Di Huang	Rehmannia	15 - 30 g
Gou Qi Zi	Lycium	6 - 15 g
Dang Gui	Angelica	6 - 12 g
Bei Sha Shen	Glehnia	6 - 9 g
Mai Men Dong	Ophiopogon	6 - 9 g
Chuan Lian Zi	Melia	3 - 6 g

Kidney yin deficiency leading to lower jiao diabetes (xiao ke). Frequent urination is the main symptom.

T red, scanty coat

P thin, slightly rapid

YI YIN TANG

Benefit-Yin Decoction

Shu Di Huang	Rehmannia	15 g
Sheng Di Huang	Rehmannia	15 g
Bai Shao Yao	Paeonia	9 - 15 g
Mai Men Dong	Ophiopogon	9 - 15 g
Huai Niu Xi	Achyranthes	6 - 15 g
Dan Shen	Salvia	12 - 15 g
Gan Cao	Glycyrrhiza	3 - 6 g

Kidney and Liver yin/blood deficiency with fire which bothers the Heart. This causes Heart and Liver fire or Liver yang excess leading to excessive dreaming, insomnia, or outbursts of anger.

T red, cracks, thin or thick yellow coat

P rapid, wiry, thin

☞ Ingredients should be powdered, made into 9 - 12 g pills and taken three times a day. Xi Jiao - Rhinoceros should be substituted with Shui Niu Jiao - Bubalus.

ZHEN ZHU MU WAN

Mother-Of-Pearl Pill

Zhen Zhu Mu	Pteria	15 - 20 g
Ren Shen	Panax	9 - 12 g
Dang Gui	Angelica	6 - 12 g
Shu Di Huang	Rehmannia	9 - 12 g
Suan Zao Ren	Ziziphus	6 - 9 g
Bai Zi Ren	Biota	6 - 9 g
Fu Shen	Poria	6 - 9 g
Chen Xiang	Aquilaria	6 - 9 g
Xi Jiao	Rhinoceros	1 - 3 g

Kidney yin deficiency with heat and mild damp causing afternoon fever, night sweats, spermatorrhea, or malarflush.

T   red, scanty coat

P   thin, rapid

ZHI BAI DI HUANG WAN

Anemarrhena, Phellodendron, and Rehmannia Pill

Extract Formula Name: Anemarrhena, Phellodendron and Rehmannia Formula

Huang Bai	Phellodendron	3 - 9 g
Zhi Mu	Anemarrhena	6 - 9 g
Sheng Di Huang	Rehmannia	15 - 25 g
Shan Yao	Dioscorea	9 - 12 g
Shan Zhu Yu	Cornus	9 - 12 g
Mu Dan Pi	Paeonia	6 - 9 g
Ze Xie	Alisma	6 - 9 g
Fu Ling	Poria	6 - 9 g

Kidney and Liver yin deficiency with damp stagnation. This causes poor vision, blurry vision, or dry eyes.

T   red, sticky yellowish coat

P   thin, weak

ZHU JING WAN

Preserve Vistas Pill

Tu Si Zi	Cuscuta	9 - 15 g
Shu Di Huang	Rehmannia	9 - 12 g
Che Qian Zi	Plantago	6 - 9 g

Kidney and Liver yin deficiency with false heat and bone steaming fever, lumbago, involuntary emissions, night sweats, or impotence. Stronger than 'Zuo Gui Yin'.

T   red, scanty coat

P   thin, rapid, or empty

ZUO GUI WAN

Restore the Left [Kidney] Pill

Extract Formula Name: Achyranthes and Rehmannia Formula

Shu Di Huang	Rehmannia	9 - 25 g
Gou Qi Zi	Lycium	9 - 12 g
Chuan Niu Xi	Cyathula	9 - 12 g
Shan Yao	Dioscorea	9 - 12 g
Shan Zhu Yu	Cornus	9 - 12 g
Lu Jiao Jiao	Cervus	9 - 12 g
Tu Si Zi	Cuscuta	9 - 12 g
Gui Ban	Chinemys	9 - 12 g

Liver/Kidney yin and jing (essence) deficiency causing slow development in children; or premature aging in adults, in addition to common yin deficiency signs and symptoms. The formula is also for early menopause, spermatorrhea, low sex drive, infertility, or low sperm count.

T red, scanty coat

P thin, rapid

ZUO GUI YIN

Restore the Left [Kidney] Decoction

Shu Di Huang	Rehmannia	6 - 15 g
Shan Zhu Yu	Cornus	6 - 9 g
Shan Yao	Dioscorea	6 - 9 g
Gou Qi Zi	Lycium	6 - 9 g
Fu Ling	Poria	6 - 9 g
Zhi Gan Cao	Glycyrrhiza	3 - 6 g

BLADDER DISHARMONIES

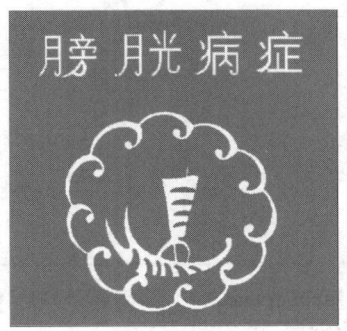

膀 胱 病 症

LIN SYNDROME — DISORDERS OF THE BLADDER

- urinary frequency, urgency
- burning or pale turbid urine
- gravel or calculi in urine, or hematurea

T depends on involved syndrome

P depends on involved syndrome

Bladder

Bladder damp heat: heat lin-syndrome causing burning urination, scanty yellow urine, urgency and frequency.

T red, sticky yellow coat

P wiry, rapid, slippery, forceful

✪ **Major Formula**

BA ZHENG SAN

Eight-Herb Powder for Rectification

Extract Formula Name: Dianthus Formula

Mu Tong	Akebia	6 - 9 g
Qu Mai	Dianthus	9 - 12 g
Zhi Zi	Gardenia	3 - 6 g
Da Huang	Rheum	3 - 9 g
Hua Shi	Talcum	9 - 20 g
Bian Xu	Polygonum	9 - 12 g
Che Qian Zi	Plantago	6 - 12 g
Deng Xin Cao	Juncus	6 g
Gan Cao	Glycyrrhiza	3 - 6 g

Kidney qi deficiency with cold and damp leading to frequent, or cloudy, painful urination.

T pale

P weak, or slippery

BEI XIE FEN QIN YIN I

Dioscorea Hypoglauca Decoction to Separate the Clear

Extract Formula Name: Tokoro Combination

Bei Xie	Dioscorea	6 - 12 g
Wu Yao	Lindera	6 - 9 g
Shi Chang Pu	Acorus	6 - 9 g
Yi Zhi Ren	Alpinia	6 - 9 g

Damp heat in the Bladder causing cloudy and painful urination, urinary retention, or urgency.

T red, sticky yellow coat

P rapid, wiry, slippery

BEI XIE FEN QIN YIN II

Dioscorea Hypoglauca Decoction to Separate the Clear from Medical Revelations

Bei Xie	Dioscorea	6 - 9 g
Dan Shen	Salvia	3 - 9 g
Huang Bai	Phellodendron	6 - 9 g
Che Qian Zi	Plantago	3 - 6 g
Shi Chang Pu	Acorus	3 - 6 g
Bai Zhu	Atractylodes	3 - 9 g
Fu Ling	Poria	6 - 9 g
Lian Xin	Nelumbo	4 g

Lin-syndrome: urinary disten-tion caused by qi lin-syndrome, which is essentially caused by Liver qi stagnation. Acute type: urinary problems after emo-tional upset.

T   possibly red sides

P   wiry

CHEN XIANG SAN

Aquilaria Wood Powder

Chen Xiang	Aquilaria	9 - 12 g
Shi Wei	Pyrrosia	6 - 9 g
Hua Shi	Talcum	3 - 12 g
Bai Shao Yao	Paeonia	6 - 9 g
Dang Gui	Angelica	6 - 12 g
Dong Kui Zi	Malva	6 - 9 g
Wang Bu Liu Xing	Vaccaria	3 - 9 g
Gan Cao	Glycyrrhiza	3 - 6 g

Heart fire leading to Small In-testine fire, which in turn leads to Bladder damp heat causing hematuria, frequent urination, urinary retention, thirst, or tongue sores.

T   bright red, sticky yellow coat

P   rapid, wiry

✪ **Major Formula**

DAO CHI SAN

Guide Out the Red Powder

Extract Formula Name: Rehmannia and Akebia Formula

Sheng Di Huang	Rehmannia	9 - 20 g
Dan Zhu Ye	Lophatherum	6 - 9 g
Mu Tong	Akebia	6 - 9 g
Gan Cao	Glycyrrhiza	3 - 6 g

Damp heat in the Bladder caus-ing frequent and burning urina-tion. This may be seen during pregnancy.

T   red, sticky yellow coat

P   rapid, slippery

JIA WEI WU LIN SAN

Augmented Five-Ingredient Powder for Painful Urinary Dysfunction

Chi Fu Ling	Poria	6 - 12 g
Chi Shao Yao	Paeonia	6 - 15 g
Dang Gui	Angelica	6 - 9 g
Zhi Zi	Gardenia	6 - 15 g
Ze Xie	Alisma	6 - 9 g
Mu Tong	Akebia	6 - 9 g
Che Qian Zi	Plantago	6 - 9 g
Hua Shi	Talcum	9 - 15 g
Sheng Di Huang	Rehmannia	6 - 12 g
Gan Cao	Glycyrrhiza	3 - 6 g

Bladder

Bladder damp heat with calculi.

T red, sticky yellow coat

P slippery, rapid

SAN JIN TANG

Three-Gold Decoction

Jin Qian Cao	Lysimachia	6 - 45 g
Jin Sha Teng	Lygodium	9 - 25 g
Dong Kui Zi	Malva	6 - 9 g
Ji Nei Jin	Gallus	6 - 9 g
Shi Wei	Pyrrosia	6 - 9 g
Qu Mai	Dianthus	9 - 12 g

Bladder damp heat with calculi or gravel. Stone lin syndrome manifesting as severe heat and mild damp.

T sticky coat

P wiry, rapid

SHI WEI SAN

Pyrrosia Leaf Powder

Shi Wei	Pyrrosia	6 - 9 g
Dong Kui Zi	Malva	3 - 6 g
Mu Tong	Akebia	3 - 6 g
Qu Mai	Dianthus	6 g
Hua Shi	Talcum	6 - 12 g
Che Qian Zi	Plantago	6 - 9 g
Gan Cao	Glycyrrhiza	3 = 6 g

Kidney qi/yang deficiency with enuresis or frequent, clear urination.

T pale, swollen, teethmarks, white coat

P minute

SUO QUAN WAN

Shut the Sluice Pill

Yi Zhi Ren	Alpinia	6 - 15 g
Shan Yao	Dioscorea	9 - 15 g
Wu Yao	Lindera	6 - 9 g

Chronic lin-syndrome due to Kidney qi deficiency causing urinary frequency with turbidity, incontinence, or enuresis.

T pale or normal color, thin white or yellowish coat

P weak, especially in the chi (third) positions

WU BI SHAN YAO WAN

Dioscorea Pill

Shu Di Huang	Rehmannia	12 - 15 g
Shan Yao	Dioscorea	12 - 15 g
Shan Zhu Yu	Cornus	6 - 9 g
Rou Cong Rong	Cistanche	6 - 9 g
Tu Si Zi	Cuscuta	6 - 9 g
Wu Wei Zi	Schisandra	6 - 12 g
Ze Xie	Alisma	6 - 9 g
Ba Ji Tian	Morinda	3 - 6 g
Du Zhong	Eucommia	9 - 12 g
Huai Niu Xi	Achyranthes	12 - 15 g
Fu Shen	Poria	9 - 12 g
Chi Shi Zhi	Halloysitum Rubrum	12 - 15 g

Bladder damp heat with underlying Kidney qi deficiency causing urgent, painful, or scanty urination.

T red, sticky yellow coat

P rapid, thin, or slippery

WU LIN SAN

Five-Ingredient Powder for Painful Urinary Dysfunction

Extract Formula Name: Gardenia and Hoelen Formula

Zhi Zi	Gardenia	6 - 9 g
Chi Fu Ling	Poria	6 - 9 g
Dang Gui	Angelica	6 - 9 g
Chi Shao Yao	Paeonia	6 - 9 g
Gan Cao	Glycyrrhiza	3 - 6 g

Bladder

Heat and water accumulation in the lower jiao (Bladder) with slight taiyang symptoms (wind cold); or Spleen qi deficiency with damp and water causing edema in the skin or muscle layer.

T sticky white or yellow coat

P slippery or superficial

⭐ **Major Formula**

WU LING SAN

Five-Ingredient Powder with Poria

Extract Formula Name: Hoelen Five Herbs Formula

Fu Ling	Poria	6 - 9 g
Zhu Ling	Polyporus	6 - 9 g
Ze Xie	Alisma	6 - 9 g
Gui Zhi	Cinnamomum	3 - 9 g
Bai Zhu	Atractylodes	6 - 9 g

Liver qi stagnation causing late periods, irritability, premenstrual syndrome, or distention in the urinary tract.

T light purple, thin coat

P wiry

WU YAO TANG

Lindera Decoction

Wu Yao	Lindera	3 - 6 g
Dang Gui	Angelica	6 - 9 g
Xiang Fu	Cyperus	3 - 9 g
Mu Xiang	Saussurea	3 - 9 g
Gan Cao	Zingiber	3 - 6 g

Blood lin-syndrome causing urinary bleeding with pain, burning urination, frequency, urgency, scanty urination, lower abdominal pain, or Kidney pain.

T red and thin, or red and swollen, yellow coat

P rapid

XIAO JI YIN ZI

Cephalanoplos Decoction

Extract Formula Name: Cephalanoplos Combination

Sheng Di Huang	Rehmannia	15 50 g
Dan Zhu Ye	Lophatherum	6 - 9 g
Mu Tong	Akebia	9 - 15 g
Gan Cao	Glycyrrhiza	3 - 6 g
Ou Jie	Nelumbo	6 - 9 g
Zhi Zi	Gardenia	3 - 6 g
Hua Shi	Talcum	9 - 15 g
Pu Huang	Typha	3 - 6 g
Dang Gui	Angelica	6 - 15 g
Xiao Ji	Cephalanoplos	9 - 15 g

Yangming channel syndrome affecting the lower jiao; or wind cold causing heat in the Spleen/Stomach which burns the yin. This leads to water dysfunction and stagnation which heats up leading to Lin-syndrome: Heat Lin or damp heat edema.

T red, sticky yellow coat

P rapid

☞ E Jiao - Equus should be added to the strained tea.

ZHU LING TANG I

Polyporus Decoction

Extract Formula Name: Polyporus Combination

Zhu Ling	Polyporus	6 - 9 g
Fu Ling	Poria	6 - 9 g
Hua Shi	Talcum	6 - 9 g
Ze Xie	Alisma	6 - 9 g
E Jiao	Equus	6 - 9 g

Damp heat in the lower jiao causing urinary difficulty and pain.

T red, sticky coat

P slippery

ZHU LING TANG II

Polyporus Decoction from Comprehensive Recordings

Zhu Ling	Polyporus	6 - 9 g
Mu Tong	Akebia	6 - 9 g
Sang Bai Pi	Morus	6 - 9 g
[Deng Xin Cao	Juncus	3 g]

Bladder

LARGE INTESTINE DISHARMONIES

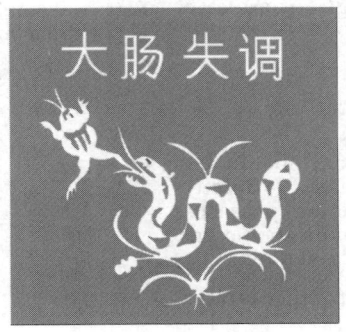

LARGE INTESTINE DISORDERS

- constipation, burning anus
- diarrhea with odorous stools
- abdominal distention or pain

T depends on involved syndrome

P depends on involved syndrome

Toxic heat in the yangming channel causing dysentery, or pus or blood in the stools.

T red, yellow coat

P wiry, rapid, rolling

BAI TOU WENG TANG

Pulsatilla Decoction

Extract Formula Name: Anemone Combination

Bai Tou Weng	Pulsatilla	20 - 40 g
Huang Bai	Phellodendron	9 - 12 g
Qin Pi	Fraxinus	9 - 15 g
Huang Lian	Coptis	6 - 9 g

Intestinal abscess or acute appendicitis due to heat and blood stagnation causing mass formation in the lower right quadrant with pain.

T yellow sticky

P rapid, slippery

☞ Da Huang - Rheum should be added during the last 3 - 5 minutes of the decoction process. Mang Xiao - Mirabilitum should be added to the strained tea.

✗ Do not use with appendicitis during pregnancy.

DA HUANG MU DAN TANG

Rhubarb and Moutan Decoction

Extract Formula Name: Rhubarb and Moutan Combination

Da Huang	Rheum	6 - 12 g
Mang Xiao	Mirabilitum	6 - 12 g
Dong Gua Ren	Benincasa	12 - 20 g
Tao Ren	Prunus	9 - 12 g
Mu Dan Pi	Paeonia	6 - 9 g

Water/heat accumulation in the chest and abdomen causing qi obstruction which leads to pancreatitis with edema, intestinal obstruction, or lumps.

T red, sticky coat

P rapid, slippery

☞ Soak and cook Gan Sui - Euphorbia, add Da Huang - Rheum during the last 3 - 5 minutes, then dissolve Mang Xiao - Mirabilitum into the strained tea.

✗ Gan Sui - Euphorbia is toxic, and should only be taken in small amounts. Do not use during pregnancy.

DA XIAN XIONG TANG

Major Sinking Into the Chest Decoction

Extract Formula Name: Rhubarb and Kansui Combination

Da Huang	Rheum	9 - 15 g
Mang Xiao	Mirabilitum	9 - 12 g
Gan Sui	Euphorbia	0.6 - 1 g

Heat in the yangming channel with pre-existing severe blood stagnation in the lower jiao which affects the uterus and the intestines. Symptoms include jaundice, mania, fever, melena with dry stools which are relatively easy to discharge, dysmenorrhea, amenorrhea, abdominal fullness, or bleeding in the stomach. This formula is stronger than 'Di Dang Wan - Resistance Pill.'

T red, dark purple

P wiry, rapid

✗ Do not use during pregnancy. Use only for a short duration.

DI DANG TANG

Resistance Decoction

Da Huang	Rheum	6 - 12 g
Tao Ren	Prunus	6 - 9 g
Shui Zhi	Hirudo	1 - 3 g
Meng Chong	Tabanus	1 - 3 g

Heat in the yangming channel with pre-existing severe blood stagnation in the lower jiao which affects the uterus and the intestines. Symptoms include jaundice, mania, fever, melena with dry stools which are relatively easy to discharge, dysmenorrhea, amenorrhea, abdominal fullness, or bleeding in the stomach. This formula is somewhat milder than 'Di Dang Tang - Resistance Decoction.'

T red, purple

P wiry, rapid

☞ Ingredients should all be ground up, then formed into pills.

✗ Caution during pregnancy.

DI DANG WAN

Resistance Pill

Da Huang	Rheum	12 g
Shui Zhi	Hirudo	20 - 30 g
Meng Chong	Tabanus	20 - 30 g
Tao Ren	Prunus	9 - 12 g

Large Intestine

Severe damp heat causing bright red blood in stools, bitter taste, or constipation.

T red, sticky yellow coat

P rapid, slippery

DI YU SAN

Sanguisorba Powder

Di Yu	Sanguisorba	6 - 9 g
Zhi Zi	Gardenia	6 - 9 g
Qian Cao Gen	Rubia	6 - 9 g
Huang Lian	Coptis	6 - 9 g
Fu Ling	Poria	6 - 9 g
Huang Qin	Scutellaria	6 - 9 g

Qi and blood stagnation with water accumulation causing intestinal obstruction, lack of gas or bowel movements.

T purple, sticky white or yellow coat

P slippery, rapid

☞ All herbs except Gan Sui - Euphorbia should be decocted. Soak and decoct Gan Sui separately and add at the end.

✘ Gan Sui - Euphorbia is extremely toxic and should be taken with caution. Do not use during pregnancy.

GAN SUI TONG JIE TANG

Euphorbia for Intestinal Obstruction Decoction

Gan Sui	Euphorbia	0.5 - 1 g
Tao Ren	Prunus	6 - 9 g
Chuan Niu Xi	Cyathula	6 - 9 g
Hou Po	Magnolia	9 - 30 g
Da Huang	Rheum	12 - 25 g
Chi Shao Yao	Paeonia	9 - 15 g
Mu Xiang	Saussurea	3 - 9 g

Wind heat with internal middle jiao heat and Large Intestine heat and damp causing dysentery: taiyang and yangming disease. Symptoms include fever, thirst, or burning anus.

T red, yellow coat

P rapid, slippery

GE GEN HUANG LIAN HUANG QIN TANG

Kudzu, Coptis, and Scutellaria Decoction

Extract Formula Name: Pueraria, Coptis and Scute Combination

Ge Gen	Pueraria	12 - 15 g
Huang Lian	Coptis	6 - 9 g
Huang Qin	Scutellaria	6 - 9 g
Gan Cao	Glycyrrhiza	3 - 6 g

Dry heat accumulation in the Large Intestines with shen (spirit) disturbance causing insomnia, irritability, or constipation.

T red, dry, thin yellow coat

P rapid

☞ Herbs should be ground and formed into 3 g pills.

✗ Do not use during pregnancy. This is a very strong purgative and should only be used once or twice.

GENG YI WAN

Pill Requiring a Change of Clothes

Zhu Sha	Cinnabaris	12 - 18 g
Lu Hui	Aloe	18 - 25 g

Wind heat enters the Large Intestines; or damp toxin (food) obstructs the intestines. This leads to bleeding which is bright red, lack of pain, or internal hemorrhoids.

T red, yellow coat

P rapid, wiry

HUAI HUA SAN

Sophora Japonica Flower Powder

Extract Formula Name: Sophora Formula

Huai Hua Mi	Sophora	12 - 15 g
Jing Jie	Schizonepeta	3 - 6 g
Ce Bai Ye	Biota	9 - 12 g
Zhi Ke	Citrus	3 - 6 g

Bleeding hemorrhoids caused by wind heat, toxic heat, or damp heat in the intestines. This formula is also for prolapse of the rectum.

T red, thin sticky yellow coat

P rapid

☞ All ingredients should be ground into a powder. Take 9 g each time, twice a day.

HUAI JIAO WAN

Sophora Japonica Fruit Pill

Huai Jiao	Sophora	500 g
Di Yu	Sanguisorba	250 g
Huang Qin	Scutellaria	250 g
Fang Feng	Ledebouriella	250 g
Zhi Ke	Citrus	250 g
Dang Gui	Angelica	250 g

Large Intestine

Yangming organ heat with qi/blood deficiency causing odorous urgent dysentery with abdominal pain which is worse with pressure, fatigue, or possible hallucinations.

T   dry yellow coat

P   weak

✗   Do not use during pregnancy.

HUANG LONG TANG

Yellow Dragon Decoction

Da Huang	Rheum	12 g
Mang Xiao	Mirabilitum	9 g
Hou Po	Magnolia	12 g
Zhi Shi	Citrus	9 g
Dang Gui	Angelica	9 g
Ren Shen	Panax	6 g
Jie Geng	Platycodon	3 - 6 g
Sheng Jiang	Zingiber	3 - 6 g
Da Zao	Ziziphus	1 - 3 pc
Gan Cao	Glycyrrhiza	3 g

Heat entering the intestines leading to damp heat dysentery. Symptoms include fever, bitter taste, or odorous diarrhea.

T   red, yellow coat

P   rapid

HUANG QIN TANG

Scutellaria Decoction

Extract Formula Name: Scute and Licorice Combination

Huang Qin	Scutellaria	9 g
Bai Shao Yao	Paeonia	9 g
Da Zao	Ziziphus	4 - 5 pc
Gan Cao	Glycyrrhiza	3 g

Externally contracted damp heat dysentery causing explosive, odorous, watery diarrhea, tenesmus, or burning anus.

T   sticky yellow coat

P   rapid, slippery

JIA WEI BAI TOU WENG TANG

Augmented Pulsatilla Decoction

Bai Tou Weng	Pulsatilla	6 - 9 g
Qin Pi	Fraxinus	3 - 6 g
Huang Lian	Coptis	3 - 6 g
Huang Qin	Scutellaria	6 - 9 g
Huang Bai	Phellodendron	6 - 9 g
Bai Shao Yao	Paeonia	6 - 9 g

Yin/blood deficiency causing constipation with dry stools; or excess heat causing constipation.

T   red, dry yellow coat

P   rapid, thin, or empty

✗   Do not use during pregnancy.

❂ **Major Formula**

MA ZI REN WAN

Hemp Seed Pill

Extract Formula Name: Apricot Seed and Linum Formula

Huo Ma Ren	Cannabis	6 - 12 g
Da Huang	Rheum	6 - 9 g
Xing Ren	Prunus	6 - 9 g
Zhi Shi	Citrus	3 - 6 g
Bai Shao Yao	Paeonia	6 - 9 g
Hou Po	Magnolia	6 - 12 g

Constipation due to yin/blood deficiency. This is commonly seen in the elderly, or after giving birth.

T   red or pale, dry

P   thin

RUN CHANG WAN I

Moisten the Intestines Pill from Master Shen's Book

Huo Ma Ren	Cannabis	9 - 15 g
Dang Gui	Angelica	9 - 12 g
Sheng Di Huang	Rehmannia	6 - 9 g
Tao Ren	Prunus	6 - 9 g
Zhi Ke	Citrus	6 - 9 g

Large Intestine damp heat with qi and blood stagnation causing hot dysentery with pain and abdominal spasms. This is often associated with food poisoning.

T   sticky yellow coat

P   rapid

❂ **Major Formula**

SHAO YAO TANG

Peony Decoction

Extract Formula Name: Peony Combination

Bai Shao Yao	Paeonia	9 - 25 g
Bing Lang	Areca	3 - 6 g
Da Huang	Rheum	6 - 9 g
Huang Qin	Scutellaria	6 - 15 g
Huang Lian	Coptis	3 - 9 g
Dang Gui	Angelica	6 - 9 g
Mu Xiang	Saussurea	3 - 6 g
Rou Gui	Cinnamomum	1 - 3 g
Gan Cao	Glycyrrhiza	3 - 6 g

Large
Intestine

Water accumulation with heat, damp and qi stagnation; or Stomach deficiency with food stagnation and water. Symptoms include diarrhea, borborygmus, or epigastric distention.

T   red, sticky yellow coat

P   slippery, rapid

SHENG JIANG XIE XIN TANG

Fresh Ginger Decoction to Drain the Epigastrium

Extract Formula Name: Pinellia and Ginger Combination

Sheng Jiang	Zingiber	9 - 12 g
Ban Xia	Pinellia	6 - 9 g
Ren Shen	Panax	6 - 12 g
Gan Jiang	Zingiber	3 - 6 g
Huang Qin	Scutellaria	6 - 9 g
Huang Lian	Coptis	3 - 6 g
Da Zao	Ziziphus	6 - 10 pc
Gan Cao	Glycyrrhiza	3 - 6 g

Blood stagnation with fire in the lower jiao causing constipation, sudden abdominal pain, dysmenorrhea, intestinal obstruction, or melena. In severe cases this may lead to restlessness, or even delirium.

T   purple

P   choppy or forceful

☞ Da Huang - Rheum should be added during the last 3 - 5 minutes of the decoction process. Mang Xiao - Mirabilitum should be added to the strained tea.

✘ Do not use during pregnancy.

TAO HE CHENG QI TANG

Peach Pit Decoction to Order the Qi

Extract Formula Name: Prunus and Rhubarb Combination

Tao Ren	Prunus	9 - 15 g
Gui Zhi	Cinnamomum	6 - 9 g
Mang Xiao	Mirabilitum	3 - 6 g
Da Huang	Rheum	9 - 12 g
Gan Cao	Glycyrrhiza	3 - 6 g

Kidney and Spleen yang deficiency which developed after a chronic damp heat dysentery causing damp cold. This obstructs the Large Intestines, manifesting as dark blood in the stools with pus.

T pale

P minute

☞ Ingredients should be ground into a powder.

TAO HUA TANG

Peach Blossom Decoction

Extract Formula Name: Kaolin and Oryza Combination

Chi Shi Zhi	Halloysitum Rubrum	20 - 30 g
Jing Mi	Oryza	20 - 30 g
Gan Jiang	Zingiber	6 - 9 g

---

1. Roundworms have migrated upward due to cold in the Large Intestines to the warmth of the epigastrium/chest. 2. Large Intestine cold and Stomach heat: mixed syndrome - jueyin syndrome.

T pale

P weak

☞ Wu Mei - Prunus should be soaked in vinegar for 12 hours.

WU MEI WAN

Mume Pill

Extract Formula Name: Mume Formula

Wu Mei	Prunus	20 - 25 g
Xi Xin	Asarum	1 - 3 g
Chuan Jiao	Zanthoxylum	1 - 3 g
Gan Jiang	Zingiber	12 - 15 g
Fu Zi	Aconitum	6 - 9 g
Huang Lian	Coptis	9 - 12 g
Huang Bai	Phellodendron	6 - 9 g
Gui Zhi	Cinnamomum	3 - 9 g
Dang Gui	Angelica	6 - 9 g
Ren Shen	Panax	6 - 9 g

Large Intestine

Blood deficiency causing constipation.

T pale

P weak, thin

WU REN WAN

Five-Seed Pill

Xing Ren	Prunus	9 - 20 g
Bai Zi Ren	Biota	3 - 6 g
Tao Ren	Prunus	9 - 15 g
Yu Li Ren	Prunus	3 - 6 g
Sha Ren	Amomum	3 - 6 g

Diarrhea due to Spleen qi deficiency with damp and Stomach heat causing dysentery with mucous and possible bleeding.

T   sticky yellow coat

P   slippery, rapid

XIANG LIAN WAN

Aucklandia and Coptis Pill

Extract Formula Name: Saussurea and Coptis Formula

Mu Xiang	Saussurea	6 - 9 g
Huang Lian	Coptis	3 - 6 g
Wu Zhu Yu	Evodia	3 - 12 g

Damp and blood stagnation causing intestinal abscess, colicky pain in the abdomen with urinary disturbances, or severe pain after menstruation or childbirth.

T   purple, sticky coat

P   wiry or choppy

YI YI REN TANG

Coix Decoction from the Standards

Yi Yi Ren	Coix	9 - 15 g
Mu Dan Pi	Paeonia	6 - 9 g
Gua Lou Ren	Trichosanthes	9 - 12 g
Tao Ren	Prunus	6 - 9 g

Chronic diarrhea has depleted Spleen and Kidney yang causing prolapse of the rectum or bowel incontinence.

T   pale, white coat

P   deep, slow

ZHEN REN YANG ZANG TANG

True Man's Decoction to Nourish the Organs

Ren Shen	Panax	6 - 9 g
Rou Gui	Cinnamomum	3 g
Bai Zhu	Atractylodes	6 - 12 g
He Zi	Terminalia	6 - 9 g
Rou Dou Kou	Myristica	9 - 12 g
Ying Su Ke	Papaver	6 - 15 g
Mu Xiang	Saussurea	3 - 9 g
Dang Gui	Angelica	6 - 15 g
Bai Shao Yao	Paeonia	9 - 12 g
Zhi Gan Cao	Glycyrrhiza	3- 6 g

Food stagnation in the middle jiao with damp and heat accumulation: cold and heat in the middle jiao with Spleen deficiency. Symptoms include fullness with pain, odorous diarrhea, mucus, tenesmus, gas, or constipation.

T red, red sides, rough, thick sticky yellow coat

P slippery, rapid, forceful

✗ Caution during pregnancy.

ZHI SHI DAO ZHI WAN

Immature Bitter Orange Pill to Guide Out Stagnation

Extract Formula Name: Chih-shih and Rhubarb Formula

Zhi Shi	Citrus	9 - 15 g
Shen Qu	Massa Fermentata	9 - 15 g
Da Huang	Rheum	15 - 25 g
Huang Qin	Scutellaria	6 - 9 g
Huang Lian	Coptis	6 - 9 g
Fu Ling	Poria	6 - 9 g
Ze Xie	Alisma	6 - 9 g
Bai Zhu	Atractylodes	6 - 9 g

Large Intestine

JIN YE (BODY FLUID) DISHARMONIES

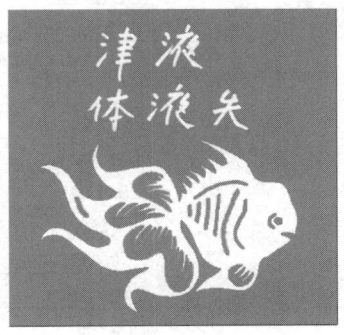

ACCUMULATION OF TAN YIN (DAMP AND PHLEGM)

- fullness in epigastrium or abdomen
- dizziness
- edema
- masses, lumps, or nodules

T thin or thick sticky white or yellowish coat

P slippery

Spleen/Stomach deficiency with damp causing vomiting or diarrhea.

T pale, sticky white coat

P weak, slippery

BAI ZHU SAN

Atractylodes Powder

Extract Formula Name: Atractylodes and Pueraria Formula

Ren Shen	Panax	6 - 9 g
Bai Zhu	Atractylodes	9 - 15 g
Ge Gen	Pueraria	9 - 15 g
Huo Xiang	Agastache	9 - 15 g
Fu Ling	Poria	9 - 15 g
Mu Xiang	Saussurea	3 - 6 g
Gan Cao	Glycyrrhiza	3 - 6 g

Jin Ye
(Body Fluid)

Liver wind and phlegm rises to the head leading to hypertension, dizziness, nausea, vomiting, or deviation of the eye or mouth.

T sticky white coat

P slippery

BAN XIA BAI ZHU TIAN MA TANG

Pinellia, Atractylodes, and Gastrodia Decoction

Extract Formula Name: Pinellia and Gastrodia Combination

Ban Xia	Pinellia	6 - 9 g
Bai Zhu	Atractylodes	6 - 15 g
Tian Ma	Gastrodia	6 - 9 g
Fu Ling	Poria	6 - 9 g
Chen Pi	Citrus	3 - 6 g
Sheng Jiang	Zingiber	3 - 6 g
Da Zao	Ziziphus	1 - 3 pc
Gan Cao	Glycyrrhiza	3 g

Phlegm and Liver qi stagnation causing hysteria, plumpit qi, or depression.

T light purple, sticky white or yellowish coat

P slippery or wiry

BAN XIA HOU PO TANG

Pinellia and Magnolia Bark Decoction

Extract Formula Name: Pinellia and Magnolia Combination

Ban Xia	Pinellia	6 - 9 g
Hou Po	Magnolia	6 - 15 g
Zi Su Ye	Perilla	3 - 6 g
Fu Ling	Poria	6 - 9 g
Sheng Jiang	Zingiber	9 - 12 g

Taiyang disease with high fever enters and damages the Stomach. It then fails to descend qi which leads to food, damp, or water accumulation (or heat and cold accumulation in the Stomach). This is known as firmness and fullness (pi man). Symptoms include epigastric fullness, gurgling, or loose stools.

T   yellow sticky coat

P   wiry, rapid

BAN XIA XIE XIN TANG

Pinellia Decoction to Drain the Epigastrium

Extract Formula Name: Pinellia Combination

Ban Xia	Pinellia	6 - 12 g
Huang Qin	Scutellaria	6 - 9 g
Huang Lian	Coptis	3 - 6 g
Gan Jiang	Zingiber	3 - 6 g
Ren Shen	Panax	6 - 9 g
Da Zao	Ziziphus	3 - 5 pc
Gan Cao	Glycyrrhiza	3 - 6 g

External wind cold entering the Stomach causing severe damp accumulation which then leads to fever and chills, diarrhea, vomiting, fullness, or abdominal bloating.

T   sticky white coat

P   slippery, superficial

BU HUAN JING ZHENG QI SAN

Rectify the Qi Powder Worth More Than Gold

Extract Formula Name: Pinellia, Atractylodes, and Agastache Formula

Hou Po	Magnolia	9 - 12 g
Cang Zhu	Atractylodes	3 - 9 g
Huo Xiang	Agastache	6 - 9 g
Ban Xia	Pinellia	6 - 9 g
Chen Pi	Citrus	3 - 6 g
Gan Cao	Glycyrrhiza	3 - 6 g
[Sheng Jiang	Zingiber	3 - 6 g]
[Da Zao	Ziziphus	3 - 5 pc]

Jin Ye
(Body Fluid)

Severe phlegm damp accumulation causing dizziness, headache, sticky phlegm expectoration, or amenorrhea due to phlegm obstruction.

T thick sticky white or slightly yellowish

P slippery

CANG FU DAO TAN TANG

Atractylodes, Cyperus, and Guide Out Phlegm Decoction

Ban Xia	Pinellia	6 - 9 g
Chen Pi	Citrus	3 - 6 g
Fu Ling	Poria	6 - 9 g
Tian Nan Xing	Arisaema	1 - 3 g
Zhi Shi	Citrus	3 - 9 g
Gan Cao	Glycyrrhiza	3 - 6 g
Cang Zhu	Atractylodes	3 - 9 g
Xiang Fu	Cyperus	3 - 9 g
Sheng Jiang	Zingiber	6 - 9 g

Spleen qi deficiency causing tan yin: damp or water accumulation. Symptoms include borborygmus, and loose, watery stools.

T pale, swollen, teethmarks, wet

P slippery

DA BAN XIA TANG

Major Pinellia Decoction

Ban Xia	Pinellia	6 - 9 g
Fu Ling	Poria	6 - 9 g
Bai Feng Mi	Mel	9 - 15 g

(Lung) phlegm damp with cough or coma causing wind phlegm, dizziness, or hypertension.

T thick sticky coat

P slippery

✗ Tian Nan Xing - Arisaema is slightly toxic.

DAO TAN TANG

Guide Out Phlegm Decoction

Ban Xia	Pinellia	6 - 9 g
Chen Pi	Citrus	3 - 6 g
Fu Ling	Poria	6 - 9 g
Gan Cao	Glycyrrhiza	3 - 6 g
Zhi Shi	Citrus	3 - 6 g
Tian Nan Xing	Arisaema	1 - 3 g
Sheng Jiang	Zingiber	3 g

Wind and phlegm accumulation causing hypertension, vertigo, and aphasia.

T rigid, sticky white or yellowish coat

P slippery

DI TAN TANG

Scour Phlegm Decoction

Extract Formula Name: Arisaema and Acorus Combination

Ban Xia	Pinellia	6 - 9 g
Fu Ling	Poria	6 - 9 g
Zhi Shi	Citrus	3 - 6 g
Chen Pi	Citrus	3 - 6 g
Zhu Ru	Bambusa	1 - 3 g
Dan Nan Xing	Arisaema	1 - 3 g
Ren Shen	Panax	3 - 6 g
Shi Chang Pu	Acorus	6 g
Gan Cao	Glycyrrhiza	3 - 6 g
[Sheng Jiang	Zingiber	3 - 6 g]
[Da Zao	Ziziphus	1 - 3 pc]

Basic formula for phlegm amd damp accumulation from Stomach and Spleen qi deficiency. Symptoms include nausea and vomiting, or epigastric distention.

T sticky coat

P slippery

✪ **Major Formula**

ER CHEN TANG

Two-Cured Decoction

Extract Formula Name: Citrus and Pinellia Combination

Ban Xia	Pinellia	6 - 9 g
Chen Pi	Citrus	3 - 6 g
Fu Ling	Poria	6 - 9 g
Gan Cao	Glycyrrhiza	3 - 6 g
[Sheng Jiang	Zingiber	3 - 6 g]
[Da Zao	Ziziphus	3 pc]

Jin Ye
(Body Fluid)

Damp heat in the lower jiao causing low back pain, hot, swollen knees or feet, or odorous leukorrhea.

T sticky yellow coat

P slippery, rapid

ER MIAO SAN

Two-Marvel Powder

Cang Zhu	Atractylodes	15 g
Huang Bai	Phellodendron	15 g

Wind heat with internal middle jiao heat and Large Intestine heat and damp causing dysentery: taiyang and yangming disease. Symptoms include fever, thirst, or burning anus.

T red, yellow coat

P rapid, slippery

GE GEN HUANG LIAN HUANG QIN TANG

Kudzu, Coptis, and Scutellaria Decoction

Extract Formula Name: Pueraria, Coptis and Scute Combination

Ge Gen	Pueraria	12 - 15 g
Huang Lian	Coptis	9 g
Huang Qin	Scutellaria	6 - 9 g
Gan Cao	Glycyrrhiza	3 - 6 g

Blood and phlegm stagnation in the uterus leading to masses or lumps, amenorrhea, dysmenorrhea, or restless fetus.

T purple, sticky coat

P wiry, slippery, choppy

GUI ZHI FU LING WAN

Cinnamon Twig and Poria Pill

Extract Formula Name: Cinnamon and Hoelen Formula

Gui Zhi	Cinnamomum	6 - 12 g
Fu Ling	Poria	6 - 12 g
Mu Dan Pi	Paeonia	6 - 12 g
Tao Ren	Prunus	6 - 12 g
Chi Shao Yao	Paeonia	9 - 12 g

Phlegm accumulation causing hardenings; or Liver qi stagnation leading to goiter or cancer.

T sticky coat

P slippery, wiry

HAI ZAO YU HU TANG

Sargassum Decoction for the Jade Flask

Hai Zao	Sargassum	3 - 6 g
Kun Bu	Laminaria	3 - 6 g
Hai Dai	Laminaria	1.5 g
Du Huo	Angelica	3 - 6 g
Lian Qiao	Forsythia	3 - 6 g
Zhe Bei Mu	Fritillaria	3 - 6 g
Chuan Xiong	Ligusticum	3 - 6 g
Ban Xia	Pinellia	3 - 6 g
Dang Gui	Angelica	3 - 6 g
Chen Pi	Citrus	3 - 6 g
Qing Pi	Citrus	3 - 6 g
Gan Cao	Glycyrrhiza	3 - 6 g

Cold in the Spleen/Stomach after ingestion of cold food with damp and qi stagnation in the center. Symptoms include lack of appetite, loose stools, or nausea and vomiting.

T pale, sticky white coat

P weak, deep, or tight

HOU PO WEN ZHONG TANG

Magnolia Bark Decoction for Warming the Middle

Extract Formula Name: Magnolia and Saussurea Combination

Hou Po	Magnolia	30 g
Gan Jiang	Zingiber	2 g
Mu Xiang	Saussurea	15 g
Chen Pi	Citrus	30 g
Fu Ling	Poria	15 g
Cao Dou Kou	Alpinia	15 g
Zhi Gan Cao	Glycyrrhiza	15 g
[Sheng Jiang	Zingiber	3 g]

Jin Ye (Body Fluid)

Wind damp heat invasion with internal pre-existing damp accumulation and qi/yang deficiency.

T   thin sticky white coat

P   slippery, soggy, slightly slow

HUO PO XIA LING TANG

Agastache, Magnolia Bark, Pinellia, and Poria Decoction

Huo Xiang	Agastache	6 g
Hou Po	Magnolia	3 g
Ban Xia	Pinellia	4.5 g
Chi Fu Ling	Poria	9 g
Zhu Ling	Polyporus	4.5 g
Dan Dou Chi	Glycine	9 g
Ze Xie	Alisma	4.5 g
Bai Dou Kou	Amomum	2 g
Yi Yi Ren	Coix	12 g
Xing Ren	Prunus	9 g

Wind damp heat invasion affecting the middle jiao causing recurring fevers and slight thirst.

T   sticky yellowish coat, moist

P   moderate

HUANG QIN HUA SHI TANG

Scutellaria and Talcum Decoction

Huang Qin	Scutellaria	6 - 9g
Hua Shi	Talcum	6 - 12 g
Bai Dou Kou	Amomum	1 - 3 g
Da Fu Pi	Areca	3 - 6 g
Fu Ling Pi	Poria	6 - 9 g
Zhu Ling	Polyporus	6 - 9 g
Tong Cao	Tetrapanax	3 - 6 g

Wind cold and damp accumulation, with qi stagnation in the middle jiao causing diarrhea, nausea, vomiting, headache, or fever and chills.

T white sticky coat

P soggy or slippery

☞ All ingredients should be ground into a powder. Take 6 g two to three times a day.

HUO XIANG ZHENG QI SAN

Agastache Powder to Rectify the Qi

Extract Formula Name: Agastache Formula

Huo Xiang	Agastache	9 g
Hou Po	Magnolia	6 - 9 g
Bai Zhi	Angelica	3 - 6 g
Zi Su Ye	Perilla	3 - 6 g
Chen Pi	Citrus	6 g
Bai Zhu	Atractylodes	6 g
Fu Ling	Poria	3 - 6 g
Ban Xia	Pinellia	6 g
Da Fu Pi	Areca	3 - 6 g
Jie Geng	Platycodon	6 g
Gan Cao	Glycyrrhiza	6 - 9 g
[Da Zao	Ziziphus	1 - 3 g]
[Sheng Jiang	Zingiber	3 - 6 g]

Heated water/phlegm in the Stomach and Large Intestines with qi stagnation causing edema with dyspnea, or a dry mouth.

T red, sticky yellow coat

P rapid, slippery

✘ Do not use during pregnancy.

JI JIAO LI HUANG WAN

Stephania, Zanthoxylum, Lepidium, and Rhubarb Pill

Extract Formula Name: Stephania and Lepidium Formula

Han Fang Ji	Stephania	3 g
Chuan Jiao	Zanthoxylum	3 g
Da Huang	Rheum	3 g
Ting Li Zi	Lepidium	3 g

Jin Ye
(Body Fluid)

Watery fluids in the Lungs and Spleen yang deficiency causing cough, wheezing, and a stuffy sensation in the chest.

T   pale, sticky or slippery white coat

P   slippery, wiry

LING GAN WU WEI JIANG XIN TANG

Poria, Licorice, Schisandra, Ginger, and Asarum Decoction

Fu Ling	Poria	6 - 12 g
Gan Cao	Glycyrrhiza	3 - 9 g
Wu Wei Zi	Schisandra	6 - 9 g
Gan Jiang	Zingiber	3 - 9 g
Xi Xin	Asarum	6 - 9 g

Spleen/Stomach yang deficiency causing phlegm accumulation which affects the Lungs; or taiyang disease was mistreated and guided into the Spleen leading to water accumulation. Symptoms include dyspnea, clear phlegm expectoration, and fullness in the chest and flanks.

T   pale, slippery white coat

P   slippery, weak, deep

LING GUI ZHU GAN TANG

Poria, Cinnamon Twig, Atractylodes, and Licorice Decoction

Extract Formula Name: Hoelen and Atractylodes Combination

Fu Ling	Poria	6 - 12 g
Gui Zhi	Cinnamomum	3 - 9 g
Bai Zhu	Atractylodes	6 - 9 g
Gan Cao	Glycyrrhiza	3 - 6 g

Spleen/Stomach qi deficiency with mild damp symptoms including decreased appetite, middle jiao distention, or nausea and vomiting.

T   pale, thin sticky coat

P   weak, slightly slippery

LIU JUN ZI TANG

Six-Gentlemen Decoction

Extract Formula Name: Six Major Herbs Combination

Ren Shen	Panax	6 - 9 g
Bai Zhu	Atractylodes	6 - 9 g
Fu Ling	Poria	6 - 9 g
Chen Pi	Citrus	3 - 6 g
Ban Xia	Pinellia	6 - 9 g
Gan Cao	Glycyrrhiza	3 - 6 g

Spleen deficiency with damp which is turning to heat in the middle jiao; or Stomach/Spleen deficiency causing a lack of fluids which leads to deficiency type heat.

T   pale or red, sticky coat

P   slippery, weak, thin

LIU SHEN SAN

Six-Miracle Powder from Standards of Patterns and Treatments

Ren Shen	Panax	6 - 9 g
Bai Zhu	Atractylodes	3 - 9 g
Fu Ling	Poria	6 - 9 g
Bian Dou	Dolichos	6 - 9 g
Huang Qi	Astragalus	6 - 12 g
Gan Cao	Glycyrrhiza	3 - 6 g
[Sheng Jiang	Zingiber	1 - 2 pc]
[Da Zao	Ziziphus	1 - 2 pc]

Damp heat in the lower jiao, or Liver fire. Symptoms include red and itchy eyes, temple headaches, odorous leukorrhea, or pruritus.

T   red, sticky yellow coating

P   wiry, rapid, slippery

LONG DAN XIE GAN TANG

Gentiana Decoction to Drain the Liver

Extract Formula Name: Gentiana Combination

Long Dan Cao	Gentiana	6 - 9 g
Zhi Zi	Gardenia	3 - 9 g
Mu Tong	Akebia	6 - 9 g
Huang Qin	Scutellaria	6 - 9 g
Ze Xie	Alisma	6 - 9 g
Che Qian Zi	Plantago	6 - 9 g
Dang Gui	Angelica	6 - 9 g
Sheng Di Huang	Rehmannia	6 - 12 g
Chai Hu	Bupleurum	6 - 9 g
Gan Cao	Glycyrrhiza	3 - 6 g

Jin Ye
(Body Fluid)

Stomach/Spleen deficiency with cold damp and middle jiao qi stagnation causing fullness and distention.

T thick sticky white coat

P slippery

PING WEI SAN

Calm the Stomach Powder

Extract Formula Name: Magnolia and Ginger Formula

Hou Po	Magnolia	6 - 12 g
Cang Zhu	Atractylodes	9 - 15 g
Chen Pi	Citrus	6 - 12 g
Gan Cao	Glycyrrhiza	3 - 6 g
[Da Zao	Ziziphus	3 - 6 pc]
[Sheng Jiang	Zingiber	3 - 6 g]

Phlegm damp leading to infertility or leukorrhea.

T thick sticky white coat

P slippery or soggy

QI GONG WAN

Open Uterus Pill

Ban Xia	Pinellia	6 - 9 g
Fu Ling	Poria	6 - 9 g
Cang Zhu	Atractylodes	6 - 9 g
Shen Qu	Massa Fermentata	6 - 12 g
Chen Pi	Citrus	3 - 6 g
Xiang Fu	Cyperus	6 - 9 g
Chuan Xiong	Ligusticum	3 - 6 g

Wind phlegm attacking the channels, especially the head and face with pre-existing qi and yang deficiency. This leads to paralysis, facial twitches, stiff muscles, spasms, or loose stools.

T pale, swollen, teethmarks, thick sticky coat

P slippery, deep, frail

✗ The formula is toxic and should not be taken over a long period of time. Do not use during pregnancy.

QIAN ZHENG SAN

Lead to Symmetry Powder

Jiang Can	Bombyx	6 g
Bai Fu Zi	Typhonium	6 g
Quan Xie	Buthus	6 g

Spleen qi deficiency with damp leading to diarrhea and irregular periods. Other symptoms include weight loss, fatigue, poor appetite, or pale face.

T pale, white coat

P weak or thin

SHEN LING BAI ZHU SAN

Ginseng, Poria, and Atractylodes Powder

Extract Formula Name: Ginseng and Atractylodes Formula

Ren Shen	Panax	9 - 15 g
Fu Ling	Poria	9 - 12 g
Bai Zhu	Atractylodes	3 - 9 g
Gan Cao	Glycyrrhiza	6 - 9 g
Lian Zi	Nelumbo	3 - 9 g
Yi Yi Ren	Coix	6 - 15 g
Shan Yao	Dioscorea	9 - 15 g
Bian Dou	Dolichos	6 - 9 g
Jie Geng	Platycodon	3 - 6 g
Sha Ren	Amomum	3 g

Damp heat in the lower jiao. Odorous leukorrhea, cloudy urine, and painful swollen feet.

T red, sticky yellow coat

P slippery, rapid

SI MIAO SAN

Four-Marvel Powder

Cang Zhu	Atractylodes	6 - 9 g
Huang Bai	Phellodendron	6 - 9 g
Yi Yi Ren	Coix	6 - 12 g
Huai Niu Xi	Achyranthes	6 - 12 g

Jin Ye
(Body Fluid)

Spleen qi deficiency with damp and watery leukorrhea, edema, or cramping pain. Other symptoms include loose stools, and urinary retention.

T   sticky white coat

P   weak, slippery

WEI LING TANG

Calm the Stomach and Poria Decoction

Extract Formula Name: Magnolia and Hoelen Combination

Ze Xie	Alisma	6 - 12 g
Zhu Ling	Polyporus	6 - 9 g
Fu Ling	Poria	6 - 9 g
Bai Zhu	Atractylodes	3 - 9 g
Gui Zhi	Cinnamomum	3 - 9 g
Hou Po	Magnolia	6 - 12 g
Cang Zhu	Atractylodes	3 - 9 g
Chen Pi	Citrus	3 - 6 g
Sheng Jiang	Zingiber	3 - 6 g
Da Zao	Ziziphus	3 - 6 pc
Gan Cao	Glycyrrhiza	3 - 6 g

Wind cold with internal damp causing a common cold without sweating. Stomach flu, heaviness in the head, cold intolerance, or nausea and vomiting may also be present.

T   white sticky coat

P   superficial

XIANG RU SAN

Elsholtzia Powder

Extract Formula Name: Elsholtzia Combination

Xiang Ru	Elsholtzia	9 - 12 g
Hou Po	Magnolia	9 - 12 g
Bian Dou	Dolichos	6 - 9 g

Spleen/Stomach qi deficiency with qi stagnation and cold damp in the middle jiao causing abdominal fullness or morning sickness.

T   pale, light purple, swollen, sticky white coat

P   slippery, weak

XIANG SHA LIU JUN ZI TANG

Six-Gentlemen Decoction with Aucklandia and Amomum

Extract Formula Name: Saussurea and Cardamon Combination

Ren Shen	Panax	6 - 9 g
Fu Ling	Poria	6 - 9 g
Bai Zhu	Atractylodes	3 - 9 g
Chen Pi	Citrus	3 - 6 g
Ban Xia	Pinellia	6 - 9 g
Sha Ren	Amomum	3 g
Mu Xiang	Saussurea	3 - 6 g
Zhi Gan Cao	Glycyrrhiza	3 - 6 g

Spleen and Stomach qi deficiency with damp accumulation. Symptoms include fullness, nausea and vomiting, loose stools, poor appetite, or morning sickness.

T   pale, thin sticky white coat

P   slippery, weak

XIANG SHA YANG WEI TANG

Nourish the Stomach Decoction with Aucklandia and Amomum

Extract Formula Name: Cyperus and Cluster Combination

Xiang Fu	Cyperus	6 - 9 g
Bai Dou Kou	Amomum	3 - 6 g
Sha Ren	Amomum	3 - 6 g
Mu Xiang	Saussurea	3 - 6 g
Bai Zhu	Atractylodes	6 - 9 g
Fu Ling	Poria	6 - 9 g
Chen Pi	Citrus	3 - 6 g
Dang Shen	Codonopsis	9 - 12 g
Hou Po	Magnolia	6 - 12 g
Cang Zhu	Atractylodes	3 - 9 g
Sheng Jiang	Zingiber	3 - 6 g
Da Zao	Ziziphus	3 - 6 pc
Zhi Gan Cao	Glycyrrhiza	3 - 6 g

Jin Ye
(Body Fluid)

Spleen qi and yang deficiency with damp and water accumulation causing loose stools with undigested food.

T   pale, swollen, teethmarks, white sticky coat

P   weak, deep, or frail

XIAO BAN XIA TANG

Minor Pinellia Decoction

Ban Xia	Pinellia	6 - 9 g
Sheng Jiang	Zingiber	3 - 6 g

Goiter, scrofula, and lumps due to yin deficieny with false heat. The false heat dries the fluids and causes phlegm accumulation.

T   red, coat

P   rapid, slippery, or wiry

XIAO LUO WAN

Reduce Scrofula Pill

Chuan Bei Mu	Fritiallaria	6 - 12 g
Mu Li	Ostrea	6 - 12 g
Xuan Shen	Scrophularia	6 - 12 g

Phlegm heat in the chest (Heart), or epigastrium (Stomach) leading to bronchitis, constipation, distending pain or pressure in the chest, numbness, or bitter taste.

T   red, sticky yellow coat

P   rapid, slippery

XIAO XIAN XIONG TANG

Minor Sinking Into the Chest Decoction

Extract Formula Name: Minor Trichosanthes Combination

Gua Lou	Trichosanthes	20 g
Huang Lian	Coptis	3 g
Ban Xia	Pinellia	6 - 9 g

Phlegm accumulation with Stomach qi deficiency causing hiccups, fullness, or nausea and vomiting.

T   pale, white sticky coat

P   frail, slippery, or wiry

☞ Xuan Fu Hua - Inula should be wrapped in a cheese cloth for decoction.

XUAN FU DAI ZHE TANG

Inula and Hematite Decoction

Extract Formula Name: Inula and Hematite Combination

Xuan Fu Hua	Inula	6 - 9 g
Dai Zhe Shi	Haematitum	6 - 12 g
Ren Shen	Panax	6 - 9 g
Ban Xia	Pinellia	6 - 9 g
Da Zao	Ziziphus	3 - 6 pc
Sheng Jiang	Zingiber	6 - 9 g
Zhi Gan Cao	Glycyrrhiza	3 - 6 g

Qi/blood/yang deficient patient gets a cold which leads to damp and phlegm accumulation in the channels, muscles, organs, or under the skin, causing swollen joints with atrophy, scrofula, or multiple abscesses.

T pale, thick sticky white coat

P weak, thin, deep

YANG HE TANG

Yang-Heartening Decoction

Shu Di Huang	Rehmannia	20 - 30 g
Rou Gui	Cinnamomum	6 - 9 g
Bai Jie Zi	Brassica	3 - 6 g
Lu Jiao Jiao	Cervus	9 - 12 g
Pao Jiang	Zingiber	1 - 3 g
Ma Huang	Ephedra	1 - 3 g
Gan Cao	Glycyrrhiza	3 - 6 g

Damp accumulation draining downward leading to clear white leukorrhea.

T swollen, thick white coat

P slippery

YI ZHI TANG

Boosting Wisdom Decoction

Bai Zhu	Atractylodes	9 g
Fu Ling	Poria	9 g
Chen Pi	Citrus	6 g
Cang Zhu	Atractylodes	6 g
Yi Yi Ren	Coix	6 g
Chai Hu	Bupleurum	6 g
Sheng Ma	Cimicifuga	2 g
Zhi Gan Cao	Glycyrrhiza	3 g

Damp heat accumulation in the middle jiao (Liver/Gallbladder) causing yang jaundice, dysurea, or hepatitis with mild fever.

T slightly red, thick sticky coat

P slippery, slightly rapid

YIN CHEN WU LING SAN

Artemisia Yinchenhao and Five-Ingredient Powder with Poria

Extract Formula Name: Capillaris and Hoelen Five Formula

Yin Chen Hao	Artemisia	10 - 20 g
Fu Ling	Poria	6 - 12 g
Zhu Ling	Polyporus	6 - 9 g
Bai Zhu	Atractylodes	3 - 9 g
Ze Xie	Alisma	6 - 9 g
Gui Zhi	Cinnamomum	3 - 9 g

Jin Ye
(Body Fluid)

Cold damp has entered the Spleen leading to water accumulation and Spleen yang deficiency. This causes damp in the middle jiao which bothers the Gallbladder so the bile cannot circulate properly. This manifests as yin-type jaundice.

T pale, white coat

P weak, deep

YIN CHEN ZHU FU TANG

Artemisia Yinchenhao, Atractylodes and Prepared Aconite Decoction

Extract Formula Name: Capillaris, Atractylodes and Aconite Combination

Yin Chen Hao	Artemisia	3 - 6 g
Gan Jiang	Zingiber	3 - 6 g
Bai Zhu	Atractylodes	6 - 9 g
Rou Gui	Cinnamomum	1 - 3 g
Fu Zi	Aconitum	1 - 3 g
Zhi Gan Cao	Glycyrrhiza	3 - 6 g

Stagnations of all kinds (qi, blood, food, damp, etc.). Symptoms include epigastric or chest fullness, nausea and vomiting, or poor appetite.

T depends on particular syndrome involved

P depends on particular syndrome involved

YUE JU WAN

Escape Restraint Pill

Chuan Xiong	Ligusticum	3 - 9 g
Cang Zhu	Atractylodes	3 - 9 g
Zhi Zi	Gardenia	3 - 9 g
Xiang Fu	Cyperus	3 - 9 g
Shen Qu	Massa Fermentata	3 - 9 g

Phlegm accumulation in the middle jiao restricts the Spleen. This leads to more damp and water accumulation which then overflows under the skin leading to edema.

T thick white sticky coat

P deep, slippery

ZHI MI FU LING TANG

Small Finger Poria Decoction

Ban Xia	Pinellia	6 - 15 g
Fu Ling	Poria	6 - 15 g
Zhi Ke	Citrus	3 - 9 g
Mang Xiao	Mirabilitum	1 - 3 g
[Sheng Jiang	Zingiber	3 - 6 g]

Food stagnation in the middle jiao with damp and heat accumulation: cold and heat in the middle jiao with Spleen deficiency. Symptoms include fullness with pain, odorous diarrhea, mucus, tenesmus, gas, or constipation.

T   red, red sides, rough, thick sticky yellow coat

P   slippery, rapid, forceful

✗   Caution during pregnancy.

ZHI SHI DAO ZHI WAN

Immature Bitter Orange Pill to Guide Out Stagnation

Extract Formula Name: Chih-shih and Rhubarb Formula

Zhi Shi	Citrus	9 - 15 g
Shen Qu	Massa Fermentata	9 - 15 g
Da Huang	Rheum	15 - 25 g
Huang Qin	Scutellaria	6 - 9 g
Huang Lian	Coptis	6 - 9 g
Fu Ling	Poria	6 - 9 g
Ze Xie	Alisma	6 - 9 g
Bai Zhu	Atractylodes	6 - 9 g

Damp heat accumulation in the middle jiao. There is more damp than heat causing fullness in the abdomen, thirst without desire to drink, or immediate fullness upon eating or drinking. This formula is also useful for yang jaundice.

T   red, thick sticky coat

P   slippery, rapid

ZHONG JIAO XIAN BI TANG

Middle Jiao and Clear Damp Decoction

Xing Ren	Prunus	3 - 6 g
Yi Yi Ren	Coix	9 - 12 g
Hua Shi	Talcum	6 g
Dou Juan	Glycine	9 g
Zhi Zi	Gardenia	6 - 9 g
Lian Qiao	Forsythia	6 g
Ban Xia	Pinellia	6 - 9 g
Han Fang Ji	Stephania	6 - 9 g
Can Sha	Bombyx	3 - 6 g
Shan Zha	Crataegus	3 - 9 g
Bian Dou	Dolichos	6 - 9 g

Jin Ye
(Body Fluid)

ACCUMULATION OF YING (WATER)

- borborygmus
- fullness sensation in the epigastrium or abdomen
- edema

T   wet, or white sticky coat

P   slippery

Taiyang disease with high fever enters and damages the Stomach. It then fails to descend qi which leads to food, damp, or water accumulation (or heat and cold accumulation in the Stomach). This is known as firmness and fullness (pi man). Symptoms include epigastric fullness, gurgling, or loose stools.

T   yellow sticky coat

P   wiry, rapid

BAN XIA XIE XIN TANG

Pinellia Decoction to Drain the Epigastrium

Extract Formula Name: Pinellia Combination

Ban Xia	Pinellia	6 - 12 g
Huang Qin	Scutellaria	6 - 9 g
Huang Lian	Coptis	3 - 6 g
Gan Jiang	Zingiber	3 - 6 g
Ren Shen	Panax	6 - 9 g
Da Zao	Ziziphus	3 - 5 pc
Gan Cao	Glycyrrhiza	3 - 6 g

Shaoyang disease with water and damp accumulation causing fullness in the hypochondriac area, malaria symptoms, and more chills than fever.

T   thin white coat

P   wiry

CHAI HU GUI ZHI GAN JIANG TANG

Bupleurum, Cinnamon Twig, and Ginger Decoction

Extract Formula Name: Bupleurum, Cinnamon and Ginger Combination

Chai Hu	Bupleurum	6 - 12 g
Gui Zhi	Cinnamomum	6 - 9 g
Gan Jiang	Zingiber	6 - 9 g
Huang Qin	Scutellaria	6 - 9 g
Mu Li	Ostrea	6 - 9 g
Tian Hua Fen	Trichosanthes	9 - 12 g
Gan Cao	Glycyrrhiza	3 - 6 g

Wind cold invasion which has turned to heat and entered the shaoyang level leading to water accumulation in the hypochondriac region.

T   red tip, thin yellow coat

P   superficial or wiry

CHAI ZHI BAN XIA TANG

Bupleurum, Bitter Orange and Pinellia Decoction

Chai Hu	Bupleurum	9 - 15 g
Zhi Ke	Citrus	3 - 9 g
Ban Xia	Pinellia	6 - 12 g
Huang Qin	Scutellaria	6 - 15 g
Jie Geng	Platycodon	3 - 6 g
Xing Ren	Prunus	6 - 9 g
Qing Pi	Citrus	3 - 9 g
Gan Cao	Glycyrrhiza	3 - 6 g

Kidney qi and yang deficiency causing edema which manifests mostly in the superficial and muscle layers.

T   pale, swollen, sticky white coat

P   weak, deep, slippery

FANG JI FU LING TANG

Stephania and Poria Decoction

Extract Formula Name: Stephania and Hoelen Combination

Han Fang Ji	Stephania	9 - 12 g
Fu Ling	Poria	9 - 18 g
Gui Zhi	Cinnamomum	9 - 12 g
Huang Qi	Astragalus	9 - 12 g
Gan Cao	Glycyrrhiza	3 - 6 g

Wind edema or wind damp with Spleen and wei qi deficiency causing sweating, urinary difficulty, or edema in the superficial layer.

T   pale, thin white coat

P   superficial

FANG JI HUANG QI TANG

Stephania and Astragalus Decoction

Extract Formula Name: Stephania and Astragalus Combination

Han Fang Ji	Stephania	9 - 12 g
Huang Qi	Astragalus	9 - 15 g
Bai Zhu	Atractylodes	6 - 9 g
Sheng Jiang	Zingiber	3 - 6 g
Da Zao	Ziziphus	3 - 4 pc
Gan Cao	Glycyrrhiza	3 - 6 g

Jin Ye
(Body Fluid)

Damp/water accumulation in the middle jiao causing abdominal fullness, ascites, or scanty urination.

T sticky white coat

P slippery

FEN XIAO TANG

Separate and Reduce Decoction

Extract Formula Name: Hoelen and Alisma Combination

Cang Zhu	Atractylodes	3 - 6 g
Bai Zhu	Atractylodes	3 - 6 g
Hou Po	Magnolia	6 - 9 g
Fu Ling	Poria	6 - 9 g
Chen Pi	Citrus	3 - 6 g
Zhu Ling	Polyporus	3 - 6 g
Deng Xin Cao	Juncus	1 pc
Ze Xie	Alisma	3 - 6 g
Xiang Fu	Cyperus	3 - 6 g
Mu Xiang	Saussurea	3 - 6 g
Zhi Shi	Citrus	3 - 6 g
Sha Ren	Amomum	1 - 3 g
Da Fu Pi	Areca	3 - 6 g
Sheng Jiang	Zingiber	3 - 6 g

Water accumulation in the middle jiao which restricts the Spleen function causing abdominal or epigastric fullness, borborygmus, fatigue, loose stools, or decreased appetite.

T pink or pale, wet

P slippery

FU LING GAN CAO TANG

Poria and Licorice Decoction

Extract Formula Name: Licorice and Hoelen Combination

Fu Ling	Poria	6 g
Gui Zhi	Cinnamomum	6 g
Sheng Jiang	Zingiber	9 g
Gan Cao	Glycyrrhiza	3 g

Heated water/phlegm in the Stomach and Large Intestines with qi stagnation causing edema with dyspnea, or a dry mouth.

T red, sticky yellow coat

P rapid, slippery

✗ Do not use during pregnancy.

JI JIAO LI HUANG WAN

Stephania, Zanthoxylum, Lepidium, and Rhubarb Pill

Extract Formula Name: Stephania and Lepidium Formula

Han Fang Ji	Stephania	3 g
Chuan Jiao	Zanthoxylum	3 g
Da Huang	Rheum	3 g
Ting Li Zi	Lepidium	3 g

Kidney yang deficiency causing edema, scanty urination, or benign prostate hypertrophy.

T pale, swollen, teethmarks, white sticky coat

P deep, wiry, slippery, thin

JI SHENG SHEN QI WAN

Kidney Qi Pill from Formulas to Aid the Living

Shu Di Huang	Rehmannia	6 - 12 g
Shan Yao	Dioscorea	6 - 12 g
Shan Zhu Yu	Cornus	6 - 9 g
Mu Dan Pi	Paeonia	6 - 12 g
Ze Xie	Alisma	6 - 9 g
Fu Ling	Poria	6 - 9 g
Fu Zi	Aconitum	6 - 9 g
Rou Gui	Cinnamomum	3 - 9 g
Che Qian Zi	Plantago	6 - 9 g
Chuan Niu Xi	Cyathula	6 - 9 g

Watery fluids in the Lungs and Spleen yang deficiency causing cough, wheezing, and a stuffy sensation in the chest.

T pale, sticky or slippery white coat

P slippery, wiry

LING GAN WU WEI JIANG XIN TANG

Poria, Licorice, Schisandra, Ginger, and Asarum Decoction

Fu Ling	Poria	6 - 12 g
Gan Cao	Glycyrrhiza	3 - 9 g
Wu Wei Zi	Schisandra	6 - 9 g
Gan Jiang	Zingiber	3 - 9 g
Xi Xin	Asarum	6 - 9 g

Jin Ye
(Body Fluid)

Heart yang is not warmed by the Kidneys leading to water accumulation which rises upwards causing abdominal pain, angina, Stomach cramping, tingling sensation in the abdomen, (ben ten qi - running piglet sensation), or scanty urine.

T   pale, wet, sticky white coat

P   deep, weak, slightly slow

LING GUI ZAO GAN TANG

Poria, Cinnamon Twig, Jujube, and Licorice Decoction

Fu Ling	Poria	9 - 12 g
Gui Zhi	Cinnamomum	3 - 9 g
Da Zao	Ziziphus	3 - 4 pc
Gan Cao	Glycyrrhiza	3 - 6 g

Spleen/Stomach yang deficiency causing phlegm accumulation which affects the Lungs; or taiyang disease was mistreated and guided into the Spleen leading to water accumulation. Symptoms include dyspnea, clear phlegm expectoration, and fullness in the chest and flanks.

T   pale, slippery white coat

P   slippery, weak, deep

✪ Major Formula

LING GUI ZHU GAN TANG

Poria, Cinnamon Twig, Atractylodes, and Licorice Decoction

Extract Formula Name: Hoelen and Atractylodes Combination

Fu Ling	Poria	6 - 12 g
Gui Zhi	Cinnamomum	3 - 9 g
Bai Zhu	Atractylodes	6 - 9 g
Gan Cao	Glycyrrhiza	3 - 6 g

Wind cold with pre-existing damp causing wind cold edema, and a headache which feels as if there is a belt around the head.

T   white coat

P   superficial, maybe slippery

MA HUANG JIA ZHU TANG

Ephedra Decoction plus Atractylodes

Ma Huang	Ephedra	6 - 9 g
Xing Ren	Prunus	6 - 9 g
Gui Zhi	Cinnamomum	3 - 6 g
Gan Cao	Glycyrrhiza	3 - 6 g
Bai Zhu	Atractylodes	6 - 9 g

Wind cold causes facial edema and scanty urination. This formula is also useful for jaundice accompanied by taiyang symptoms.

T   thin white coat

P   superficial, tight

MA HUANG LIAN QIAO CHI XIAO DOU TANG

Ephedra, Forsythia, and Aduki Bean Decoction

Ma Huang	Ephedra	3 - 9 g
Lian Qiao	Forsythia	6 - 9 g
Chi Xiao Dou	Phaseolus	6 - 9 g
Sang Bai Pi	Morus	6 - 9 g
Xing Ren	Prunus	6 - 9 g
Sheng Jiang	Zingiber	3 - 6 g
Da Zao	Ziziphus	3 - 4 pc
Gan Cao	Glycyrrhiza	3 - 6 g

Skin edema due to Spleen deficiency with abdominal fullness.

T   pale, swollen, teethmarks, white coat

P   weak

QI PI YIN

Seven-Peel Decoction

Fu Ling Pi	Poria	9 g
Chen Pi	Citrus	3 - 9 g
Da Fu Pi	Areca	3 - 9 g
Di Gu Pi	Lycium	9 g
Sheng Jiang Pi	Zingiber	3 - 9 g
Qing Pi	Citrus	3 - 9 g
Gan Cao Pi	Glycyrrhiza	3 - 6 g

Jin Ye
(Body Fluid)

Cold packs were used on a patient who had a common cold but also an underlying Spleen yang deficiency. Now the cold has moved into deeper layers and caused severe cold stagnation with water accumulation under the Heart. Symptoms include shortness of breath, watery sputum, angina, or stuffiness in the chest.

T pale, wet

P slow, slightly slippery

✗ Ba Dou - Croton is extremely toxic and should be used with extreme caution. Do not use during pregnancy.

SAN WU BAI SAN

Three-White Herbs Powder

Jie Geng	Platycodon	3 - 6 g
Bei Mu	Fritillaria	6 - 12 g
Ba Dou	Croton	1 - 3 g

Water accumulation with heat, damp and qi stagnation; or Stomach deficiency with food stagnation and water. Symptoms include diarrhea, borborygmus, or epigastric distention.

T red, sticky yellow coat

P slippery, rapid

SHENG JIANG XIE XIN TANG

Fresh Ginger Decoction to Drain the Epigastrium

Extract Formula Name: Pinellia and Ginger Combination

Sheng Jiang	Zingiber	9 - 12 g
Ban Xia	Pinellia	6 - 9 g
Ren Shen	Panax	6 - 12 g
Gan Jiang	Zingiber	3 - 6 g
Huang Qin	Scutellaria	6 - 9 g
Huang Lian	Coptis	3 - 6 g
Da Zao	Ziziphus	6 - 10 pc
Gan Cao	Glycyrrhiza	3 - 6 g

Spleen/Kidney qi and yang deficiency causing edema which manifests mostly in the lower body. Other symptoms include cold limbs, poor appetite, decreased urination, or heaviness.

T pale, sticky coat

P deep, slow, maybe thin

SHI PI YIN

Bolster the Spleen Decoction

Extract Brion Name: Magnolia and Atractylodes Combination

Fu Zi	Aconitum	6 - 9 g
Bai Zhu	Atractylodes	6 - 9 g
Mu Gua	Chaenomeles	6 - 9 g
Hou Po	Magnolia	6 - 12 g
Gan Jiang	Zingiber	6 - 9 g
Mu Xiang	Saussurea	6 - 9 g
Fu Ling	Poria	6 - 9 g
Da Fu Pi	Areca	3 - 6 g
Cao Guo	Amomum	3 - 6 g
Zhi Gan Cao	Glycyrrhiza	3 - 6 g
[Da Zao	Ziziphus	1 - 3 pc]
[Sheng Jiang	Zingiber	3 - 6 g]

Heart/Gallbladder qi deficiency with edema in the extremities, tight chest, palpitations, anxiety, or timidity.

T pale

P weak

SHI WEI WEN DAN TANG

Ten-Ingredient Decoction to Warm the Gallbladder

Ban Xia	Pinellia	6 - 9 g
Chen Pi	Citrus	3 - 6 g
Zhi Shi	Citrus	6 g
Fu Ling	Poria	6 g
Ren Shen	Panax	3 - 6 g
Suan Zao Ren	Ziziphus	3 - 6 g
Shu Di Huang	Rehmannia	3 - 9 g
Wu Wei Zi	Schisandra	3 - 6 g
Yuan Zhi	Polygala	3 - 6 g
Zhi Gan Cao	Glycyrrhiza	3 g
Da Zao	Ziziphus	2 pc
Sheng Jiang	Zingiber	5 pc

Jin Ye (Body Fluid)

Chronic water accumulation in the chest and hypochondrium causing cough and shortness of breath.

T white sticky coat

P deep, wiry

☞ Grind ingredients into a powder and take in 0.7 g doses in the morning with a warm tea made from ten pieces of Da Zao - Ziziphus. Between five and six bowel movements are expected after each dose.

✗ Do not use during pregnancy or in weak patients. Gan Sui - Euphorbia is toxic.

SHI ZAO TANG

Ten-Jujube Decoction

Extract Formula Name: Jujube Combination

Gan Sui	Euphorbia	6 g
Yuan Hua	Daphne	6 g
Jing Da Ji	Euphorbia	6 g

Damp heat accumulation causing edema.

T Swollen, white or sticky coat

P rapid, slippery

✗ This formula is slightly toxic due to the ingredient Shang Lu - Phytolacca. This prescription should not be taken during pregnancy.

SHU ZUO YIN ZI

Decoction for Diuresis

Extract Formula Name: Alisma and Areca Combination

Qiang Huo	Notopterygium	6 - 9 g
Qin Jiao	Gentiana	9 - 12 g
Da Fu Pi	Areca	6 - 9 g
Fu Ling Pi	Poria	20 - 40 g
Shang Lu	Phytolacca	3 - 6 g
Mu Tong	Akebia	9 - 12 g
Ze Xie	Alisma	9 - 15 g
Chi Xiao Dou	Phaseolus	15 - 30 g
Chuan Jiao	Zanthoxylum	6 - 9 g
Sheng Jiang	Zingiber	3 - 6 g

Spleen/Stomach deficiency with mild damp causing loose stools or urinary retention.

T pale, sticky white coat

P slippery, weak

SI LING SAN

Four-Ingredient Powder with Poria

Zhu Ling	Polyporus	6 - 9 g
Fu Ling	Poria	6 - 9 g
Ze Xie	Alisma	6 - 9 g
Bai Zhu	Atractylodes	3 - 9 g

Lung phlegm fluid causing eye/facial edema, cough or asthma, or Lung abscess with phlegm.

T sticky white coat

P slippery

TING LI DA ZAO XIE FEI TANG

Lepidium and Jujube Decoction to Drain the Lungs

Extract Formula Name: Lepidium and Jujube Combination

Ting Li Zi	Lepidium	6 - 9 g
Da Zao	Ziziphus	6 - 12 pc

Spleen qi deficiency with damp and watery leukorrhea, edema, or cramping pain. Other symptoms include loose stools, and urinary retention.

T sticky white coat

P weak, slippery

WEI LING TANG

Calm the Stomach and Poria Decoction

Extract Formula Name: Magnolia and Hoelen Combination

Ze Xie	Alisma	6 - 12 g
Zhu Ling	Polyporus	6 - 9 g
Fu Ling	Poria	6 - 9 g
Bai Zhu	Atractylodes	3 - 9 g
Gui Zhi	Cinnamomum	3 - 9 g
Hou Po	Magnolia	6 - 12 g
Cang Zhu	Atractylodes	3 - 9 g
Chen Pi	Citrus	3 - 6 g
Sheng Jiang	Zingiber	3 - 6 g
Da Zao	Ziziphus	3 - 6 pc
Gan Cao	Glycyrrhiza	3 - 6 g

Jin Ye
(Body Fluid)

Heat and water accumulation in the lower jiao (Bladder) with slight taiyang symptoms (wind cold); or Spleen qi deficiency with damp and water causing edema in the skin or muscle layer.

T   sticky white or yellow coat

P   slippery or superficial

WU LING SAN

Five-Ingredient Powder with Poria

Extract Formula Name: Hoelen Five Herbs Formula

Fu Ling	Poria	6 - 9 g
Zhu Ling	Polyporus	6 - 9 g
Ze Xie	Alisma	6 - 9 g
Gui Zhi	Cinnamomum	3 - 9 g
Bai Zhu	Atractylodes	6 - 9 g

Spleen qi deficiency with water/damp and qi stagnation causing edema, dyspnea, or urinary retention.

T   pale, swollen, teethmarks, sticky white coat

P   slippery

WU PI SAN

Five-Peel Powder

Extract Formula Name: Hoelen and Areca Combination

Sang Bai Pi	Morus	6 - 15 g
Sheng Jiang Pi	Zingiber	6 - 9 g
Chen Pi	Citrus	3 - 9 g
Da Fu Pi	Areca	6 - 12 g
Fu Ling Pi	Poria	6 - 15 g

Qi and blood stagnation causing chest pain with water/damp accumulation: Liver affects the Lungs. Symptoms include hypochondriac pain, possible coughing, or raspy voice.

T   purple, thick sticky coat

P   wiry

☞ Xuan Fu Hua - Inula should be wrapped in a cheesecloth.

XIANG FU XUAN FU TANG

Cyperus and Inula Decoction

Xiang Fu	Cyperus	6 - 9 g
Xuan Fu Hua	Inula	6 - 9 g
Yi Yi Ren	Coix	9 - 15 g
Chen Pi	Citrus	3 - 6 g
Zi Su Zi	Perilla	6 - 9 g
Ban Xia	Pinellia	6 - 9 g
Fu Ling	Poria	6 - 9 g

Wind cold with internal water accumulation causing profuse phlegm expectoration, body-aches, or superficial edema.

T   moist white coat

P   superficial, tight

XIAO QING LONG TANG

Minor Blue Dragon Decoction

Extract Formula Name: Minor Blue Dragon Combination

Ma Huang	Ephedra	6 - 9 g
Gui Zhi	Cinnamomum	6 - 9 g
Xi Xin	Asarum	3 g
Wu Wei Zi	Schisandra	6 - 9 g
Gan Jiang	Zingiber	3 g
Bai Shao Yao	Paeonia	6 - 9 g
Ban Xia	Pinellia	6 - 9 g
Gan Cao	Glycyrrhiza	3 - 6 g

Cold damp has entered the Spleen leading to water accumulation and Spleen yang deficiency. This causes damp in the middle jiao which bothers the Gallbladder so the bile cannot circulate properly. This manifests as yin-type jaundice.

T   pale, white coat

P   weak, deep

YIN CHEN ZHU FU TANG

Artemisia Yinchenhao, Atractylodes and Prepared Aconite Decoction

Extract Formula Name: Capillaris, Atractylodes and Aconite Combination

Yin Chen Hao	Artemisia	3 - 6 g
Gan Jiang	Zingiber	3 - 6 g
Bai Zhu	Atractylodes	6 - 9 g
Rou Gui	Cinnamomum	1 - 3 g
Fu Zi	Aconitum	1 - 3 g
Zhi Gan Cao	Glycyrrhiza	3 - 6 g

Jin Ye (Body Fluid)

Wind edema with fever and chills, or decreased urination.

T thin white coat

P superficial, slippery, or deep

YUE BI JIA ZHU TANG

Maidservant from Yue Decoction plus Atractylodes

Extract Formula Name: Atractylodes Combination

Ma Huang	Ephedra	6 - 9 g
Shi Gao	Gypsum	9 - 20 g
Bai Zhu	Atractylodes	6 - 9 g
Sheng Jiang	Zingiber	3 - 9 g
Da Zao	Ziziphus	3 - 7 pc
Gan Cao	Glycyrrhiza	3 - 6 g

Whole body edema due to wind causing wind intolerance, scanty urination, possible sweating, possible fever, or thirst.

T thin white coat

P superficial

YUE BI TANG

Maidservant from Yue Decoction

Extract Formula Name: Ma-Huang and Gypsum Combination

Ma Huang	Ephedra	6 - 15 g
Sheng Jiang	Zingiber	3 - 9 g
Shi Gao	Gypsum	15 - 30 g
Da Zao	Ziziphus	6 - 12 pc
Gan Cao	Glycyrrhiza	3 - 6 g

Spleen/Kidney qi and yang deficient patient suffers easily from wind cold with internal water accumulation, or experiences urinary difficulty, diarrhea, or edema.

T pale, swollen, teethmarks, moist, thin white coat

P frail or minute

ZHEN WU TANG

True Warrior Decoction

Extract Formula Name: Vitality Combination

Fu Zi	Aconitum	6 - 9 g
Bai Zhu	Atractylodes	6 - 9 g
Bai Shao Yao	Paeonia	6 - 9 g
Fu Ling	Poria	6 - 9 g
Sheng Jiang	Zingiber	6 - 9 g

Phlegm accumulation in the middle jiao restricts the Spleen. This leads to more damp and water accumulation which then overflows under the skin leading to edema.

T   thick white sticky coat

P   deep, slippery

ZHI MI FU LING TANG

Small Finger Poria Decoction

Ban Xia	Pinellia	6 - 15 g
Fu Ling	Poria	6 - 15 g
Zhi Ke	Citrus	3 - 9 g
Mang Xiao	Mirabilitum	1 - 3 g
[Sheng Jiang	Zingiber	3 - 6 g]

Severe edema (ascites), water and heat stagnation. This formula is a strong water purgative.

T   red, sticky coat

P   rapid, deep, forceful

☞ Grind herbs into a powder and take as a 3 - 6 g dose of pills in the morning. Only strong patients may take this dosage more than once.

✗ Do not use during pregnancy or in very weak patients. The formula is highly toxic, and should only be used for a limited time. Do not use with Gan Cao - Glycyrrhiza.

ZHOU CHE WAN

Vessel and Vehicle Pill

Gan Sui	Euphorbia	15 g
Yuan Hua	Daphne	15 g
Qian Niu Zi	Pharbitis	60 g
Jing Da Ji	Euphorbia	15 g
Qing Pi	Citrus	7.5 g
Chen Pi	Citrus	7.5 g
Da Huang	Rheum	30 g
Mu Xiang	Saussurea	7.5 g
Bing Lang	Areca	7.5 g
Qing Fen	Calomelas	1.5 g

Jin Ye
(Body Fluid)

SIX DIVISIONS

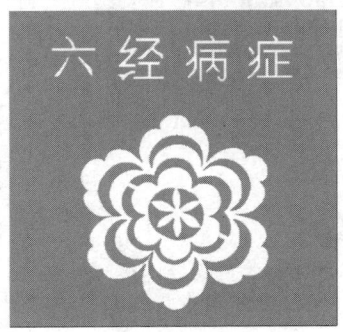

DISEASES IN THE TAIYANG STAGE

Please see WIND INVASIONS

DISEASES IN THE SHAOYANG STAGE

- bitter taste
- alternating chills and fever
- costal pain
- irritability

T white coat

P wiry

Shaoyang and yangming channel disease causing mild chills with severe fever, and thirst.

T red, thin yellow coat

P rapid, maybe flooding

CHAI HU BAI HU TANG

Bupleurum White Tiger Decoction

Chai Hu	Bupleurum	3 - 6 g
Huang Qin	Scutellaria	3 - 6 g
Shi Gao	Gypsum	12 - 20 g
Zhi Mu	Anemarrhena	6 - 12 g
Tian Hua Fen	Trichosanthes	6 - 9 g
Jing Mi	Oryza	6 - 9 g
Gan Cao	Glycyrrhiza	3 - 6 g

Six
Divisions

Phlegm damp obstruction in
the chest and epigastrium with
a complication of shaoyang disease. Symptoms include alternating fever and chills, bitter
taste, or cough with sticky
phlegm.

T   thick sticky white or yellow
     coat

P   slippery, wiry

CHAI HU DA YUAN YIN

Bupleurum Decoction to Reach the
Membrane Source

Zhi Ke	Citrus	5 g
Chai Hu	Bupleurum	6 - 9 g
Qing Pi	Citrus	3 - 6 g
Hou Po	Magnolia	6 - 12 g
Huang Qin	Scutellaria	6 - 9 g
Cao Guo	Amomum	3 - 6 g
He Ye	Nelumbo	6 - 15 g
Bing Lang	Areca	6 - 9 g
Jie Geng	Platycodon	3 - 6 g
Gan Cao	Glycyrrhiza	3 - 6 g

Shaoyang disease with water
and damp accumulation causing fullness in the hypochondriac area, malaria symptoms,
and more chills than fever.

T   thin white coat

P   wiry

CHAI HU GUI ZHI GAN JIANG TANG

Bupleurum, Cinnamon Twig, and Ginger Decoction

Extract Formula Name: Bupleurum,
Cinnamon and Ginger Combination

Chai Hu	Bupleurum	6 - 12 g
Gui Zhi	Cinnamomum	6 - 9 g
Gan Jiang	Zingiber	6 - 9 g
Huang Qin	Scutellaria	6 - 9 g
Mu Li	Ostrea	6 - 9 g
Tian Hua Fen	Trichosanthes	9 - 12 g
Gan Cao	Glycyrrhiza	3 - 6 g

Taiyang and shaoyang disease with joint congestion and intolerance to wind, or alternating fever and chills. Also useful for Liver overacting on Spleen.

T thin white coat

P possibly superficial

CHAI HU GUI ZHI TANG

Bupleurum and Cinnamon Twig Decoction

Extract Formula Name: Bupleurum and Cinnamon Combination

Gui Zhi	Cinnamomum	3 - 6 g
Chai Hu	Bupleurum	6 - 12 g
Ren Shen	Panax	3 - 6 g
Ban Xia	Pinellia	3 - 6 g
Huang Qin	Scutellaria	3 - 9 g
Bai Shao Yao	Paeonia	3 - 6 g
Sheng Jiang	Zingiber	3 - 6 g
Da Zao	Ziziphus	4 - 6 pc
Gan Cao	Glycyrrhiza	3 - 6 g

Qi deficient patient gets evil qi invading taiyang, shaoyang, and yangming channels. This causes irritability, constipation, full chest, or heaviness.

T red, sticky coat

P rapid, wiry

☞ Da Huang - Rheum should be added during the last 3 minutes of the decoction process.

✗ Qian Dan - Minium is toxic and should be substituted with Dai Zhe Shi - Haematitum or Sheng Tie Luo - Frusta Ferri. Caution during pregnancy.

CHAI HU JIA LONG GU MU LI TANG

Bupleurum plus Dragon Bone and Oyster Shell Decoction

Extract Formula Name: Bupleurum and D.B. Combination

Chai Hu	Bupleurum	9 - 12 g
Huang Qin	Scutellaria	6 g
Ren Shen	Panax	6 g
Gui Zhi	Cinnamomum	3 - 6 g
Ban Xia	Pinellia	6 g
Fu Ling	Poria	6 g
Da Huang	Rheum	6 g
Long Gu	Os Draconis	3 - 6 g
Mu Li	Ostrea	3 - 6 g
Sheng Jiang	Zingiber	3 - 6 g
Da Zao	Ziziphus	3 - 6 pc
Qian Dan	Minium	1 - 4 g

Six
Divisions

Shaoyang disorder with constipation, discomfort in the chest or flanks, or vomiting.

T thin yellow coat

P wiry

CHAI HU JIA MANG XIAO TANG

Bupleurum Decoction plus Mirabilite

Chai Hu	Bupleurum	6 - 9 g
Ren Shen	Panax	3 - 6 g
Ban Xia	Pinellia	3 - 6 g
Mang Xiao	Mirabilitum	3 - 6 g
Huang Qin	Scutellaria	3 - 9 g
Da Zao	Ziziphus	3 - 5 pc
Sheng Jiang	Zingiber	3 - 6 g
Gan Cao	Glycyrrhiza	3 - 6 g

Shaoyang disease with residual heat and injury to the yin. Symptoms include alternating fever and chills, malarflush, or night heat.

T red, scanty yellow coat, dry

P wiry, rapid, thin

CHAI HU QING ZAO TANG

Bupleurum Decoction to Clear Dryness

Chai Hu	Bupleurum	9 - 12 g
Huang Qin	Scutellaria	3 - 9 g
Tian Hua Fen	Trichosanthes	6 - 12 g
Zhi Mu	Anemarrhena	6 - 12 g
Chen Pi	Citrus	3 - 9 g
Sheng Jiang	Zingiber	3 - 6 g
Da Zao	Ziziphus	3 - 5 pc
Gan Cao	Glycyrrhiza	3 - 6 g

External invasion which has entered the jueyin level but shaoyang symptoms are present as well as blood deficiency and blood stagnation complaints. The main symptoms are alternating fever and chills with chest and back pain.

T   pale, purple, or purple spots

P   thin, wiry

CHAI HU SI WU TANG

Bupleurum and Four-Substance Decoction

Chai Hu	Bupleurum	6 - 12 g
Huang Qin	Scutellaria	6 - 9 g
Ren Shen	Panax	3 - 6 g
Ban Xia	Pinellia	6 g
Chuan Xiong	Ligusticum	6 - 15 g
Bai Shao Yao	Paeonia	6 - 15 g
Shu Di Huang	Rehmannia	6 - 15 g
Dang Gui	Angelica	6 - 15 g
Gan Cao	Glycyrrhiza	3 - 6 g

Shaoyang disease with accumulation of phlegm causing fullness and distention in the chest and diaphragm.

T   thick sticky yellow coat

P   wiry, rapid

CHAI HU XIAN XIONG TANG

Bupleurum Decoction for Sinking into the Chest

Chai Hu	Bupleurum	6 - 9 g
Huang Qin	Scutellaria	3 - 9 g
Huang Lian	Coptis	3 g
Ban Xia	Pinellia	6 - 12 g
Gua Lou Ren	Trichosanthes	9 - 18 g
Jie Geng	Platycodon	3 g
Zhi Ke	Citrus	3 - 6 g
Sheng Jiang	Zingiber	3 - 6 g

Six
Divisions

Shaoyang disorder with qi stagnation in the chest and diaphragm. Symptoms include fullness in the chest, dizziness, lack of hearing, headache, and alternating fever and chills.

T sticky white coat

P slippery, wiry

CHAI HU ZHI JIE TANG

Bupleurum, Bitter Orange, and Platycodon Decoction

Chai Hu	Bupleurum	6 - 9 g
Ban Xia	Pinellia	6 - 9 g
Huang Qin	Scutellaria	3 - 6 g
Zhi Ke	Citrus	3 - 6 g
Jie Geng	Platycodon	3 - 6 g
Chen Pi	Citrus	3 - 6 g
Sheng Jiang	Zingiber	3 - 6 g

Shaoyang disease with damp accumulation causing malaria with severe chills and mild fever.

T sticky white coat

P soggy

CHAI PING TANG

Bupleurum and Calm the Stomach Decoction

Chai Hu	Bupleurum	6 - 9 g
Huang Qin	Scutellaria	3 - 6 g
Ren Shen	Panax	3 - 6 g
Cang Zhu	Atractylodes	3 - 6 g
Chen Pi	Citrus	3 - 6 g
Hou Po	Magnolia	3 - 9 g
Ban Xia	Pinellia	3 - 6 g
Gan Cao	Glycyrrhiza	3 - 6 g

Wind cold invasion which has turned to heat and entered the shaoyang level leading to water accumulation in the hypochondriac region.

T red tip, thin yellow coat

P superficial or wiry

CHAI ZHI BAN XIA TANG

Bupleurum, Bitter Orange and Pinellia Decoction

Chai Hu	Bupleurum	9 - 15 g
Zhi Ke	Citrus	3 - 9 g
Ban Xia	Pinellia	6 - 12 g
Huang Qin	Scutellaria	6 - 15 g
Jie Geng	Platycodon	3 - 6 g
Xing Ren	Prunus	6 - 9 g
Qing Pi	Citrus	3 - 9 g
Gan Cao	Glycyrrhiza	3 - 6 g

Shaoyang disease with internal yangming channel heat. The formula purges internal heat stagnation. Symptoms include constipation, severe fever alternating with mild chills, bitter taste, thirst, or hypochondriac discomfort.

T red, yellow coat

P rapid, wiry, forceful

✗ Caution during pregnancy.

DA CHAI HU TANG

Major Bupleurum Decoction

Extract Formula Name: Major Bupleurum Combination

Chai Hu	Bupleurum	9 - 15 g
Da Huang	Rheum	6 - 9 g
Ban Xia	Pinellia	6 - 9 g
Huang Qin	Scutellaria	6 - 9 g
Bai Shao Yao	Paeonia	6 - 9 g
Zhi Shi	Citrus	6 - 9 g
Sheng Jiang	Zingiber	3 - 9 g
Da Zao	Ziziphus	3 - 6 pc

Shaoyang disease and damp accumulation leading to malaria, fullness in the chest, or nausea and vomiting.

T thick, sticky coat

P wiry, slippery

DA YUAN YIN

Reach the Membrane Source Decoction

Hou Po	Magnolia	6 - 9 g
Bing Lang	Areca	6 - 12 g
Zhi Mu	Anemarrhena	6 - 9 g
Bai Shao Yao	Paeonia	6 - 9 g
Cao Guo	Amomum	3 g
Huang Qin	Scutellaria	6 - 9 g
Gan Cao	Glycyrrhiza	3 - 6 g

Six Divisions

Yang jaundice from damp heat lodged in the shaoyang level; or damp heat in the Gallbladder causing alternating fever and chills, bitter taste, or malaria.

T red, thick sticky yellow coat

P slippery, wiry, rapid

☞ Bi Yu San - Green Jade Powder consists of: Hua Shi - Talcum, 3 - 6 g; Gan Cao - Glycyrrhiza, 3 - 6 g; and Qing Dai - Indigo, 9 - 12 g. All three ingredients should be cooked separately in a cheesecloth, then decocted with the rest of the herbs.

HAO QIN QING DAN TANG

Artemisia Annua and Scutellaria Decoction to Clear the Gallbladder

Qing Hao	Artemisia	6 g
Zhu Ru	Bambusa	9 g
Huang Qin	Scutellaria	6 g
Zhi Ke	Citrus	5 g
Chi Fu Ling	Poria	9 g
Ban Xia	Pinellia	5 g
Chen Pi	Citrus	5 g
Bi Yu San	Green Jade Powder	9 g

Chronic malaria has depleted Liver blood and Spleen qi and blood. The patient experiences alternating fever and chills which are aggravated with only mild stress.

T pale

P empty

HE REN YIN

Polygonum Multiflorum Root and Ginseng Decoction

He Shou Wu	Polygonum	9 - 20 g
Ren Shen	Panax	9 - 12 g
Chen Pi	Citrus	3 - 9 g
Dang Gui	Angelica	3 - 9 g
Wei Jiang	Zingiber	3 - 12 g

Pre-existing phlegm or damp accumulation with shaoyang disease leading to malaria. There is a slight possibility that this formula can cause vomiting.

T thick sticky white coat

P superficial, slippery, wiry

✘ Note that Chang Shan - Dichroa is an emetic. The formula may cause vomiting.

JIE NUE QI BAO YIN

Seven-Treasure Decoction to Check Malarial Conditions

Chang Shan	Dichroa	3 - 5 g
Bing Lang	Areca	3 g
Chen Pi	Citrus	3 g
Hou Po	Magnolia	3 g
Cao Guo	Amomum	3 g
Qing Pi	Citrus	3 g
Gan Cao	Glycyrrhiza	3 g

Excess fire cholecystitis with Liver qi and damp stagnation causing alternating fever and chills or severe hypochondriac pain.

T deep red, sticky yellow coat

P wiry, slippery, rapid, or flooding

☞ Mang Xiao - Mirabilitum should be dissolved into the strained tea. Da Huang - Rheum should be added within the last 3 - 5 minutes of the decoction process.

✗ Do not use during pregnancy

QING DAN XIE HUO TANG

Clear the Gallbladder and Drain Fire Decoction

Chai Hu	Bupleurum	9 - 15 g
Ban Xia	Pinellia	6 - 9 g
Yin Chen Hao	Artemisia	15 - 25 g
Long Dan Cao	Gentiana	6 - 9 g
Yu Jin	Curcuma	6 - 9 g
Da Huang	Rheum	6 - 9 g
Huang Qin	Scutellaria	6 - 15 g
Zhi Zi	Gardenia	6 - 9 g
Mang Xiao	Mirabilitum	6 - 9 g
Mu Xiang	Saussurea	3 - 6 g

Shaoyang disorder with severe fever and mild chills.

T red, dry

P wiry, rapid

QING PI TANG

Clear the Spleen Decoction

Qing Pi	Citrus	3 - 6 g
Chai Hu	Bupleurum	6 - 12 g
Ban Xia	Pinellia	6 - 12 g
Hou Po	Magnolia	6 - 12 g
Cao Guo	Amomum	3 - 9 g
Fu Ling	Poria	6 - 12 g
Huang Qin	Scutellaria	6 - 12 g
Bai Zhu	Atractylodes	6 - 12 g
Gan Cao	Glycyrrhiza	3 - 6 g
[Sheng Jiang	Zingiber	3 - 6 g]

Six
Divisions

Shaoyang level disease: symptoms include bitter taste, fullness in the abdomen and hypochondrium, intermittent fever and chills, dizziness, or belching.

T   red, dry, yellow or white coat

P   wiry, rapid

✪ Major Formula

XIAO CHAI HU TANG

Minor Bupleurum Decoction

Extract Formula Name: Minor Bupleurum Combination

Chai Hu	Bupleurum	9 - 15 g
Huang Qin	Scutellaria	6 - 9 g
Ban Xia	Pinellia	6 - 12 g
Ren Shen	Panax	9 - 12 g
Sheng Jiang	Zingiber	3 - 6 g
Da Zao	Ziziphus	3 - 4 pc
Gan Cao	Glycyrrhiza	3 - 6 g

DISEASES IN THE YANGMING STAGE

DISEASES IN THE YANGMING FU (ORGAN) STAGE

- severe constipation (pi man zhao shi - fullness, firmness, dryness, excess)
- abdominal bloating and pain
- profuse sweating, high fever
- severe thirst
- delirium

T red, yellow or dry black coat

P rapid, forceful

---

1. Yangming organ disease (pi man zhao shi - fullness, firmness, dryness, excess) causing masses in the abdomen; or yang jaundice with gallstones where the heat is greater than damp. 2. Fire and toxin are severe, so the water parts extravasate causing watery dysentery with odorous stools, bowel incontinence while in a coma, mania, or convulsions with high fever.

T bright red, dry yellow or black coat

P rapid, forceful

☞ Da Huang - Rheum should be added during the last 3 - 5 minutes of the decoction process, and Mang Xiao - Mirabilitum should be added into the strained tea.

✘ Do not use during pregnancy. The formula is very cold and can cause diarrhea and vomiting.

✪ **Major Formula**

DA CHENG QI TANG

Major Order the Qi Decoction

Extract Formula Name: Major Rhubarb Combination

Da Huang	Rheum	6 - 12 g
Mang Xiao	Mirabilitum	6 - 12 g
Zhi Shi	Citrus	6 - 9 g
Hou Po	Magnolia	6 - 15 g

Six
Divisions

Intestinal abscess or acute appendicitis due to heat and blood stagnation causing mass formation in the lower right quadrant with pain.

T yellow sticky

P rapid, slippery

☞ Da Huang - Rheum should be added during the last 3 - 5 minutes of the decoction process. Mang Xiao - Mirabilitum should be added to the strained tea..

✗ Do not use with appendicitis during pregnancy.

DA HUANG MU DAN TANG

Rhubarb and Moutan Decoction

Extract Formula Name: Rhubarb and Moutan Combination

Da Huang	Rheum	6 - 12 g
Mang Xiao	Mirabilitum	6 - 12 g
Dong Gua Ren	Benincasa	12 - 20 g
Tao Ren	Prunus	9 - 12 g
Mu Dan Pi	Paeonia	6 - 9 g

Heat in the middle and upper jiao with fullness as the main symptom (pi-syndrome from pi man zhao shi - firmness, fullness, dryness, excess). Symptoms include nausea and vomiting, possible hematemesis, red face, palpitations, diarrhea, or bleeding in the upper body.

T red, yellow coat

P rapid

✗ Do not use during pregnancy.

DA HUANG XIE XIN TANG

Rhubarb to Drain the Epigastrium Decoction

Da Huang	Rheum	6 - 12 g
Huang Lian	Coptis	3 - 9 g

Water/heat accumulation in the chest and abdomen causing qi obstruction which leads to pancreatitis with edema, intestinal obstruction, or lumps.

T red, dry coat

P rapid, slippery

☞ Soak and cook Gan Sui - Euphorbia, add Da Huang - Rheum during the last 3 - 5 minutes, then dissolve Mang Xiao - Mirabilitum into the strained tea.

✗ Gan Sui - Euphorbia is toxic, and should only be taken in small amounts. Do not use during pregnancy.

DA XIAN XIONG TANG

Major Sinking Into the Chest Decoction

Extract Formula Name: Rhubarb and Kansui Combination

Da Huang	Rheum	9 - 15 g
Mang Xiao	Mirabilitum	9 - 12 g
Gan Sui	Euphorbia	0.6 - 1 g

Wind heat with internal heat: taiyang and yangming organ disease. The heat is severe. Symptoms include dark yellow urine, constipation, severe fever and chills, heat sensations in the body, sores and carbuncles, skin disorders, and a bitter taste.

T bright or dark red, dry, yellow coat

P flooding, rapid, wiry

☞ Ingredients should be ground into powder, then made into a pill with water. Take 6 g each time, twice a day.

✗ Do not use during pregnancy.

FANG FENG TONG SHENG SAN

Ledebouriella Powder that Sagely Unblocks

Extract Formula Name: Siler and Platycodon Formula

Fang Feng	Ledebouriella	9 - 15 g
Ma Huang	Ephedra	9 - 15 g
Da Huang	Rheum	9 - 15 g
Mang Xiao	Mirabilitum	9 - 15 g
Jing Jie	Schizonepeta	9 - 15 g
Bo He	Mentha	9 - 15 g
Zhi Zi	Gardenia	9 - 15 g
Hua Shi	Talcum	60 - 90 g
Shi Gao	Gypsum	15 - 30 g
Huang Qin	Scutellaria	15 - 30 g
Lian Qiao	Forsythia	9 - 15 g
Jie Geng	Platycodon	15 - 30 g
Dang Gui	Angelica	9 - 15 g
Bai Shao Yao	Paeonia	9 - 15 g
Chuan Xiong	Ligusticum	9 - 15 g
Bai Zhu	Atractylodes	9 - 15 g
Gan Cao	Glycyrrhiza	30 - 60 g

Six Divisions

Blockage in the intestines with yangming organ disease and qi stagnation. Symptoms include no bowel movements or severe abdominal pain.

T   red, yellow coat

P   rapid, wiry, forceful

☞ Give one dose via nasogastric tube, and the next dose by enema a couple of hours later. Da Huang - Rheum is added during the last 3 minutes of the decoction process. Mang Xiao - Mirabilitum is added to the strained tea.

✘ Do not use during pregnancy.

FU FANG DA CHENG QI TANG

Revised Major Order the Qi Decoction

Lai Fu Zi	Raphanus	12 - 20 g
Hou Po	Magnolia	12 - 20 g
Da Huang	Rheum	9 - 12 g
Tao Ren	Prunus	6 g
Mang Xiao	Mirabilitum	9 - 12 g
Zhi Shi	Citrus	9 - 12 g
Chi Shao Yao	Paeonia	9 - 12 g

Yangming organ heat with qi/blood deficiency causing odorous urgent dysentery with abdominal pain which is worse with pressure, fatigue, or possible hallucinations.

T   dry yellow coat

P   weak

✘ Do not use during pregnancy.

HUANG LONG TANG

Yellow Dragon Decoction

Da Huang	Rheum	12 g
Mang Xiao	Mirabilitum	9 g
Hou Po	Magnolia	12 g
Zhi Shi	Citrus	9 g
Dang Gui	Angelica	9 g
Ren Shen	Panax	6 g
Jie Geng	Platycodon	3 - 6 g
Sheng Jiang	Zingiber	3 - 6 g
Da Zao	Ziziphus	1 - 3 pc
Gan Cao	Glycyrrhiza	3 g

Yangming organ syndrome in the abdomen (pi man zhao shi - firmness, fullness, dryness, excess) with blood stagnation causing acute yang jaundice, Gallbladder infection, intestinal obstruction, possible palpable mass, or nausea and vomiting.

T very red, maybe purplish, dry, rough surface, yellow/brown coat

P flooding, rapid

☞ Da Huang - Rheum should be added during the last 3 - 5 minutes of the decoction process. Mang Xiao - Mirabilitum should be dissolved into the strained tea.

✘ Do not use during pregnancy.

JIA JIAN CHENG QI TANG

Modified Order the Qi Decoction

Da Huang	Rheum	9 - 12 g
Mang Xiao	Mirabilitum	6 - 9 g
Hou Po	Magnolia	9 - 12 g
Zhi Shi	Citrus	6 g
Tao Ren	Prunus	9 - 15 g
Bai Shao Yao	Paeonia	9 - 15 g
Lai Fu Zi	Raphanus	6 - 12 g

Fire in the upper/middle jiao (chest/diaphragm) causing thirst, red lips, epistaxis, redness in the face, dark yellow urine, constipation, or delirium.

T red, dry yellow coat

P rapid

✘ Do not use during pregnancy.

LIANG GE SAN

Cool the Diaphragm Powder

Extract Formula Name: Forsythia and Rhubarb Formula

Da Huang	Rheum	6 - 9 g
Mang Xiao	Mirabilitum	6 - 9 g
Zhi Zi	Gardenia	3 - 6 g
Huang Qin	Scutellaria	6 - 9 g
Bo He	Mentha	3 - 6 g
Lian Qiao	Forsythia	9 - 12 g
Gan Cao	Glycyrrhiza	3 - 6 g
[Dan Zhu Ye	Lophatherum	3 - 6 g]

Six
Divisions

Yin/blood deficiency causing constipation with dry stools; or excess heat causing constipation.

T   red, dry yellow coat

P   rapid, thin, or empty

✘ Do not use during pregnancy.

MA ZI REN WAN

Hemp Seed Pill

Extract Formula Name: Apricot Seed and Linum Formula

Huo Ma Ren	Cannabis	6 - 12 g
Da Huang	Rheum	6 - 9 g
Xing Ren	Prunus	6 - 9 g
Zhi Shi	Citrus	3 - 6 g
Bai Shao Yao	Paeonia	6 - 9 g
Hou Po	Magnolia	6 - 12 g

Yangming heat with irritability and Spleen qi deficiency causing constipation with very dry feces, yellow urine, possible fever, or bleeding disorders.

T   red, yellow coat

P   deep, forceful, rapid

☞ Mang Xiao - Mirabilitum should be added to the strained tea.

✘ Do not use during pregnancy.

TIAO WEI CHENG QI TANG

Regulate the Stomach and Order the Qi Decoction

Extract Formula Name: Rhubarb and Mirabilitum Combination

Da Huang	Rheum	9 - 15 g
Mang Xiao	Mirabilitum	9 - 12 g
Zhi Gan Cao	Glycyrrhiza	3 - 9 g

Excess fire with qi stagnation causing fullness, possible palpable mass, or constipation. This is a mild yangming organ disease.

T   red, thin sticky yellow coat

P   rapid, slightly forceful

✘ Do not use during pregnancy.

XIAO CHENG QI TANG

Minor Order the Qi Decoction

Extract Formula Name: Minor Rhubarb Combination

Da Huang	Rheum	9 - 12 g
Zhi Shi	Citrus	6 g
Hou Po	Magnolia	6 - 12 g

Fire in the yangming organ with yin deficiency causing constipation with very dry stools.

T red, dry yellow coat

P rapid, thin, wiry

☞ Da Huang - Rheum should be added during the last 3 minutes of the cooking process. Mang Xiao - Mirabilitum should be added to the strained tea.

✗ Do not use during pregnancy.

ZENG YE CHENG QI TANG

Increase the Fluids and Order the Qi Decoction

Xuan Shen	Scrophularia	15 - 25 g
Sheng Di Huang	Rehmannia	15 - 20 g
Mai Men Dong	Ophiopogon	15 - 20 g
Mang Xiao	Mirabilitum	3 - 6 g
Da Huang	Rheum	6 - 9 g

Yangming fire causing jaundice, restlessness, fever, or constipation.

T red, yellow coat

P rapid, forceful

✗ Do not use during pregnancy.

ZHI ZI DA HUANG TANG

Gardenia and Rhubarb Decoction

Zhi Zi	Gardenia	6 - 12 g
Da Huang	Rheum	3 - 6 g
Zhi Shi	Citrus	3 - 9 g
Dan Dou Chi	Glycine	6 - 12 g

Six Divisions

DISEASES IN THE YANGMING JING (CHANNEL) STAGE

- high fever
- thirst
- profuse sweating
- irritability due to heat

T red, yellow coat

P flooding

Heat in the yangming channel with slight external cold and damp causing obstruction in the channels which leads to joint pain.

T red, yellow coat

P rapid, wiry

☞ Decoct the first four herbs, then add the rice at the end. It will absorb the water to make a thick liquid.

BAI HU JIA GUI ZHI TANG

White Tiger plus Cinnamon Twig Decoction

Shi Gao	Gypsum	20 - 30 g
Zhi Mu	Anemarrhena	9 - 12 g
Gan Cao	Glycyrrhiza	3 - 9 g
Gui Zhi	Cinnamomum	3 - 9 g
Jing Mi	Oryza	15 - 30 g

Upper jiao diabetes with heat: yangming channel syndrome with qi and yin deficiency causing severe sweating, fever, and thirst.

T red, dry yellow coat

P rapid, flooding, weak

☞ Decoct the first four herbs, then add the rice at the end. It will absorb the water to make a thick liquid.

BAI HU JIA REN SHEN TANG

White Tiger plus Ginseng Decoction

Extract Formula Name: Ginseng and Gypsum Combination

Shi Gao	Gypsum	15 - 20 g
Zhi Mu	Anemarrhena	9 - 12 g
Gan Cao	Glycyrrhiza	3 - 6 g
Ren Shen	Panax	3 - 9 g
Jing Mi	Oryza	9 - 12 g

Heat in the qi level/yangming channel syndrome causing severe fever, epidemic febrile disease, acute inflammation, encephalitis, or meningitis.

T   red, dry yellow coat

P   flooding, rapid

☞ Decoct the first five herbs, then add the rice at the end. It will absorb the water to make a thick liquid.

BAI HU JIA YIN QIAO TANG

White Tiger plus Lonicera and Forsythia Decoction

Shi Gao	Gypsum	20 - 30 g
Zhi Mu	Anemarrhena	9 - 12 g
Gan Cao	Glycyrrhiza	3 - 6 g
Jin Yin Hua	Lonicera	6 - 9 g
Lian Qiao	Forsythia	6 - 9 g
Jing Mi	Oryza	15 - 30 g

Summerheat with damp and yangming channel heat/qi level heat. This causes severe sweating, nausea, vomiting, thirst, or fever.

T   red, sticky yellow coat

P   slippery, rapid

☞ Decoct the first four herbs, then add the rice at the end. It will absorb the water to make a thick liquid.

BAI HU JIA ZHU TANG

White Tiger with White Atractylodes Decoction

Shi Gao	Gypsum	20 - 30 g
Zhi Mu	Anemarrhena	9 - 12 g
Gan Cao	Glycyrrhiza	3 - 6 g
Bai Zhu	Atractylodes	3 - 9 g
Jing Mi	Oryza	15 - 30 g

Heat in the qi level/yangming channel disease causing high fever, sweating, flooding pulse, or thirst.

T   red, yellow coat

P   flooding, rapid

☞ Decoct the first three herbs, then add the rice at the end. It will absorb the water to make a thick liquid.

❂ **Major Formula**

BAI HU TANG

White Tiger Decoction

Extract Formula Name: Gypsum Combination

Shi Gao	Gypsum	20 - 30 g
Zhi Mu	Anemarrhena	9 - 12 g
Gan Cao	Glycyrrhiza	3 - 6 g
Jing Mi	Oryza	15 - 30 g

Six
Divisions

Toxic heat in the yangming channel causing dysentery, or pus or blood in the stools.

T   red, yellow coat

P   wiry, rapid, rolling

BAI TOU WENG TANG

Pulsatilla Decoction

Extract Formula Name: Anemone Combination

Bai Tou Weng	Pulsatilla	20 - 40 g
Huang Bai	Phellodendron	9 - 12 g
Qin Pi	Fraxinus	9 - 15 g
Huang Lian	Coptis	6 - 9 g

Exterior wind cold or heat with internal heat which starts to go from the wei to the qi level into the yangming channel. Only mild exterior symptoms are present. Thirst, constipation, full and painful eye orbits, severe bodyaches, or restlessness are the main symptoms.

T   red, dry, thin yellow coat

P   superficial, slightly flooding, rapid

CHAI GE JIE JI TANG

Bupleurum and Kudzu Decoction to Release the Muscle Layer

Extract Formula Name: Bupleurum and Pueraria Combination

Chai Hu	Bupleurum	3 - 9 g
Ge Gen	Pueraria	9 - 12 g
Bai Zhi	Angelica	3 - 9 g
Shi Gao	Gypsum	6 - 15 g
Bai Shao Yao	Paeonia	6 - 9 g
Qiang Huo	Notopterygium	3 - 6 g
Huang Qin	Scutellaria	6 - 9 g
Jie Geng	Platycodon	3 - 6 g
Da Zao	Ziziphus	3 - 4 pc
Sheng Jiang	Zingiber	3 - 6 g
Gan Cao	Glycyrrhiza	3 - 6 g

Shaoyang and yangming channel disease causing mild chills with severe fever, and thirst.

T red, thin yellow coat

P rapid, maybe flooding

CHAI HU BAI HU TANG

Bupleurum White Tiger Decoction

Chai Hu	Bupleurum	3 - 6 g
Huang Qin	Scutellaria	3 - 6 g
Shi Gao	Gypsum	12 - 20 g
Zhi Mu	Anemarrhena	6 - 12 g
Tian Hua Fen	Trichosanthes	6 - 9 g
Jing Mi	Oryza	6 - 9 g
Gan Cao	Glycyrrhiza	3 - 6 g

Qi deficient patient gets evil qi invading taiyang, shaoyang, and yangming channels. This causes irritability, constipation, full chest, or heaviness.

T red, sticky coat

P rapid, wiry

☞ Da Huang - Rheum should be added during the last 3 minutes of the decoction process.

✗ Qian Dan - Minium is toxic and should be substituted with Dai Zhe Shi - Haematitum or Sheng Tie Luo - Frusta Ferri. Caution during pregnancy.

CHAI HU JIA LONG GU MU LI TANG

Bupleurum plus Dragon Bone and Oyster Shell Decoction

Extract Formula Name: Bupleurum and D.B. Combination

Chai Hu	Bupleurum	9 - 12 g
Huang Qin	Scutellaria	6 g
Ren Shen	Panax	6 g
Gui Zhi	Cinnamomum	3 - 6 g
Ban Xia	Pinellia	6 g
Fu Ling	Poria	6 g
Da Huang	Rheum	6 g
Long Gu	Os Draconis	3 - 6 g
Mu Li	Ostrea	3 - 6 g
Sheng Jiang	Zingiber	3 - 6 g
Da Zao	Ziziphus	3 - 6 pc
Qian Dan	Minium	1 - 4 g

Six
Divisions

Shaoyang disease with internal yangming channel heat. The formula purges internal heat stagnation. Symptoms include constipation, severe fever alternating with mild chills, bitter taste, thirst, or hypochondriac discomfort.

T red, yellow coat

P rapid, wiry, forceful

✗ Caution during pregnancy.

DA CHAI HU TANG

Major Bupleurum Decoction

Extract Formula Name: Major Bupleurum Combination

Chai Hu	Bupleurum	9 - 15 g
Da Huang	Rheum	6 - 9 g
Ban Xia	Pinellia	6 - 9 g
Huang Qin	Scutellaria	6 - 9 g
Bai Shao Yao	Paeonia	6 - 9 g
Zhi Shi	Citrus	6 - 9 g
Sheng Jiang	Zingiber	3 - 9 g
Da Zao	Ziziphus	3 - 6 pc

Heat in the yangming channel with pre-existing severe blood stagnation in the lower jiao which affects the uterus and the intestines. Symptoms include jaundice, mania, fever, melena with dry stools which are relatively easy to discharge, dysmenorrhea, amenorrhea, abdominal fullness, or bleeding in the stomach. This formula is stronger than 'Di Dang Wan - Resistance Pill.'

T red, dark purple

P wiry, rapid

✗ Do not use during pregnancy. Use only for a short duration.

DI DANG TANG

Resistance Decoction

Da Huang	Rheum	6 - 12 g
Tao Ren	Prunus	6 - 9 g
Shui Zhi	Hirudo	1 - 3 g
Meng Chong	Tabanus	1 - 3 g

Heat in the yangming channel with pre-existing severe blood stagnation in the lower jiao which affects the uterus and the intestines. Symptoms include jaundice, mania, fever, melena with dry stools which are relatively easy to discharge, dysmenorrhea, amenorrhea, abdominal fullness, or bleeding in the stomach. This formula is somewhat milder than 'Di Dang Tang - Resistance Decoction.'

T red, purple

P wiry, rapid

☞ Ingredients should all be ground up, then formed into pills.

✘ Caution during pregnancy.

DI DANG WAN

Resistance Pill

Da Huang	Rheum	12 g
Shui Zhi	Hirudo	20 - 30 g
Meng Chong	Tabanus	20 - 30 g
Tao Ren	Prunus	9 - 12 g

Yangming channel disease, damp stagnation and yin deficiency leading to mouth sores, swollen, red gums with pus, bad breath, sore throat, or eye disorders.

T thick sticky yellow coat

P rapid, slippery, thin

GAN LU YIN

Sweet Dew Decoction

Extract Formula Name: Sweet Combination

Shu Di Huang	Rehmannia	6 - 9 g
Sheng Di Huang	Rehmannia	6 - 9 g
Huang Qin	Scutellaria	6 - 9 g
Zhi Ke	Citrus	3 - 6 g
Mai Men Dong	Ophiopogon	6 - 9 g
Tian Men Dong	Asparagus	6 - 9 g
Pi Pa Ye	Eriobotrya	12 - 18 g
Yin Chen Hao	Artemisia	6 - 9 g
Shi Hu	Dendrobium	6 - 9 g
Gan Cao	Glycyrrhiza	3 - 6 g

Six
Divisions

Wind cold (deficiency type) with internal fire: taiyang and yangming disorder. This causes sweating, chills, nasal congestion, and constipation with abdominal fullness.

T   red, thin white or yellow coat

P   superficial, rapid

✗   Caution during pregnancy.

HOU PO QI WU TANG

Seven-Substance Decoction with Magnolia Bark

Extract Formula Name: Magnolia 7 Combination

Hou Po	Magnolia	15 g
Da Huang	Rheum	9 g
Gui Zhi	Cinnamomum	6 g
Zhi Shi	Citrus	9 g
Sheng Jiang	Zingiber	12 g
Da Zao	Ziziphus	12 pc
Gan Cao	Glycyrrhiza	6 g

Yangming channel disease/Stomach fire causing bleeding gums, toothache, soreness in the tongue, headaches, or red eyes.

T   red, dry

P   rapid, flooding

QING WEI SAN

Clear the Stomach Powder

Extract Formula Name: Coptis and Rehmannia Formula

Huang Lian	Coptis	3 - 6 g
Sheng Di Huang	Rehmannia	9 - 12 g
Mu Dan Pi	Paeonia	9 - 12 g
Dang Gui Shen	Angelica	9 - 12 g
Sheng Ma	Cimicifuga	9 - 15 g

Heat in the chest and Lungs due to taiyang disease; or lingering qi level heat manifesting in the yangming channel layer. In some patients this formula will induce vomiting, after which the symptoms will disappear.

T   red, especially the tip, yellow coat

P   rapid, forceful, superficial

✗   This prescription can cause vomiting.

ZHI ZI DOU CHI TANG

Gardenia and Prepared Soybean Decoction

Zhi Zi	Gardenia	6 - 9 g
Dan Dou Chi	Glycine	6 - 9 g

Yangming channel syndrome affecting the lower jiao; or wind cold causing heat in the Spleen/Stomach which burns the yin. This leads to water dysfunction and stagnation which heats up leading to Lin-syndrome: Heat Lin or damp heat edema.

T   red, sticky yellow coat

P   rapid

☞   E Jiao - Equus should be added to the strained tea.

ZHU LING TANG I

Polyporus Decoction

Extract Formula Name: Polyporus Combination

Zhu Ling	Polyporus	6 - 9 g
Fu Ling	Poria	6 - 9 g
Hua Shi	Talcum	6 - 9 g
Ze Xie	Alisma	6 - 9 g
E Jiao	Equus	6 - 9 g

DISEASES IN THE TAIYIN STAGE

- no appetite, no thirst
- vomiting
- abdominal fullness
- diarrhea

T   pale

P   deep, slow

Severe taiyin/taiyang disease with abdominal cramps as the main symptom.

T   thin white coat

P   superficial

GUI ZHI JIA SHAO YAO TANG

Cinnamon Twig Decoction plus Peony

Extract Formula Name: Cinnamon and Peony Combination

Gui Zhi	Cinnamomum	6 - 9 g
Bai Shao Yao	Paeonia	15 - 18 g
Sheng Jiang	Zingiber	3 - 6 g
Da Zao	Ziziphus	3 - 4 pc
Gan Cao	Glycyrrhiza	3 - 6 g

Six Divisions

Mild taiyin with taiyang syndrome: wind cold with mild Spleen qi deficiency. The chills are predominant, and the patient experiences diarrhea with epigastric fullness.

T pale, thin white coat

P weak, maybe superficial

GUI ZHI REN SHEN TANG

Cinnamon Twig and Ginseng Decoction

Extract Formula Name: Cinnamon and Ginseng Combination

Gui Zhi	Cinnamomum	9 - 12 g
Ren Shen	Panax	9 - 12 g
Gan Jiang	Zingiber	9 g
Bai Zhu	Atractylodes	9 g
Zhi Gan Cao	Glycyrrhiza	9 - 12 g

Kidney and Spleen yang deficiency with cold which has invaded all three yin channels (taiyin, shaoyin, and jueyin). Symptoms include shivering from cold, icy limbs and face, watery diarrhea, or cough with profuse saliva production.

T pale, wet, thin white moist coat

P minute or frail

☞ Remove She Xiang - Moschus, decoct the rest of the formula as usual, then add powdered Moschus to each dosage.

HUI YANG JIU JI TANG

Restore and Revive the Yang Decoction

Fu Zi	Aconitum	9 g
Rou Gui	Cinnamomum	3 - 6 g
Ren Shen	Panax	6 - 9 g
Gan Jiang	Zingiber	3 - 6 g
Fu Ling	Poria	6 - 9 g
Chen Pi	Citrus	3 - 6 g
Bai Zhu	Atractylodes	6 - 9 g
Wu Wei Zi	Schisandra	3 - 6 g
Ban Xia	Pinellia	6 - 9 g
Gan Cao	Glycyrrhiza	3 - 6 g
She Xiang	Moschus	0.3 g
[Sheng Jiang	Zingiber	1 - 3 g]

Blood level heat and taiyin level disease with lingering summerheat causing thirst and severe sweating.

T red or dark red

P rapid

JIA JIAN SHENG MAI SAN

Modified Generate the Pulse Powder

Mai Men Dong	Ophiopogon	6 - 12 g
Wu Wei Zi	Schisandra	6 - 12 g
Bei Sha Shen	Glehnia	6 - 12 g
Mu Dan Pi	Paeonia	6 - 12 g
Sheng Di Huang	Rehmannia	6 - 12 g

Middle jiao qi/yang deficiency resulting in loss of appetite, absence of thirst, watery diarrhea with undigested food, or cold or painful limbs.

T   pale, swollen, teethmarks, white coat

P   deep, weak

✪   Major Formula

LI ZHONG WAN

Regulate the Middle Pill

Extract Formula Name: Ginseng and Ginger Combination

Ren Shen	Panax	6 - 9 g
Gan Jiang	Zingiber	6 - 9 g
Bai Zhu	Atractylodes	6 - 9 g
Gan Cao	Glycyrrhiza	3 - 6 g

Exterior cold has gone internally. qi and yang are very weak and Kidney/Spleen yang have been damaged. Symptoms include low blood pressure, cold limbs, shock, or sweating.

T   pale, or purple, moist white coat

P   minute

☞ The raw type of Aconite is used here since it is much warmer than the prepared kind. 6 - 12 g of honey are often added for detoxification. Fu Zi - Aconitum is soaked in 8 - 10 cups of boiling water for 30 minutes to one hour. The remaining herbs should be added during the last 25 minutes and decocted as usual.

✗ Fu Zi - Aconitum in its raw form is toxic and is intended for short-term use only.

SI NI TANG

Frigid Extremities Decoction

Extract Formula Name: Aconite, Ginger and Licorice Combination

Fu Zi	Aconitum	9 - 15 g
Gan Jiang	Zingiber	6 - 12 g
Zhi Gan Cao	Glycyrrhiza	3 - 6 g

Six
Divisions

Cold damp has entered the Spleen leading to water accumulation and Spleen yang deficiency. This causes damp in the middle jiao which bothers the Gallbladder so the bile cannot circulate properly. This manifests as yin-type jaundice.

T   pale, white coat

P   weak, deep

YIN CHEN ZHU FU TANG

Artemisia Yinchenhao, Atractylodes and Prepared Aconite Decoction

Extract Formula Name: Capillaris, Atractylodes and Aconite Combination

Yin Chen Hao	Artemisia	3 - 6 g
Gan Jiang	Zingiber	3 - 6 g
Bai Zhu	Atractylodes	6 - 9 g
Rou Gui	Cinnamomum	1 - 3 g
Fu Zi	Aconitum	1 - 3 g
Zhi Gan Cao	Glycyrrhiza	3 - 6 g

DISEASES IN THE SHAOYIN STAGE

- 1. **Cold type**: cold limps with an aversion to cold and chills
- no appetite, diarrhea
- 2. **Heat type**: fever, irritability
- dry mouth

T   pale, or red

P   minute, or rapid

Severe yang deficiency and cold causes the yang to be pushed superficially leading to superficial false yang symptoms. The patient gives the appearance that he/she will get better but in reality may die soon. Symptoms include diarrhea, low fever, or red face. Internal cold with superficial false heat: shaoyin syndrome.

T   pale, red tip

P   deep, faint

BAI TONG TANG

White Penetrating Decoction

Gan Jiang	Zingiber	3 - 6 g
Fu Zi	Aconitum	3 - 9 g
Cong Bai	Allium	3 - 6 g

Stomach/Spleen yang defi-ciency causing watery diarrhea and epigastric pain. Severe cold symptoms such as cold limbs and vomiting of clear fluids.

T   pale, swollen, teethmarks, white coat

P   minute

✪ **Major Formula**

FU ZI LI ZHONG WAN

Prepared Aconite Pill to Regulate the Middle

Extract Formula Name: Aconite, Gin-seng, and Ginger Combination

Fu Zi	Aconitum	6 - 9 g
Ren Shen	Panax	3 - 9 g
Bai Zhu	Atractylodes	3 - 9 g
Gan Jiang	Zingiber	3 - 9 g
Zhi Gan Cao	Glycyrrhiza	3 - 6 g

Severe Kidney yang deficiency where the yang is unable to nourish the limbs leading to edema, and severe body aches with cold and damp symptoms: cold bi-syndrome.

T   pale, moist white coat

P   deep, minute, or choppy

FU ZI TANG

Prepared Aconite Decoction

Extract Formula Name: Aconite Com-bination

Fu Zi	Aconitum	9 - 15 g
Ren Shen	Panax	3 - 6 g
Fu Ling	Poria	9 - 12 g
Bai Zhu	Atractylodes	3 - 12 g
Bai Shao Yao	Paeonia	6 - 9 g

Heart/Kidney yin deficiency with fire after febrile disease leading to insomnia, palpita-tions, or tongue sores: shaoyin deficient heat syndrome.

T   red, scanty coat

P   rapid, thin

☞ E Jiao - Equus and egg yolks should be dissolved into the strained tea.

✪ **Major Formula**

HUANG LIAN E JIAO TANG

Coptis and Ass-Hide Gelatin Decoction

Extract Formula Name: Coptis and Gelatin Combination

Huang Lian	Coptis	9 - 12 g
E Jiao	Equus	6 - 9 g
Huang Qin	Scutellaria	6 - 9 g
Bai Shao Yao	Paeonia	6 - 9 g
Ji Zi Huang	Egg yolks	2

Six Divisions

Kidney and Spleen yang deficiency with cold which has invaded all three yin channels (taiyin, shaoyin, and jueyin). Symptoms include shivering from cold, icy limbs and face, watery diarrhea, or cough with profuse saliva production.

T pale, wet, thin white moist coat

P minute or frail

☞ Remove She Xiang - Moschus, decoct the rest of the formula as usual, then add powdered Moschus to each dosage.

HUI YANG JIU JI TANG

Restore and Revive the Yang Decoction

Fu Zi	Aconitum	9 g
Rou Gui	Cinnamomum	3 - 6 g
Ren Shen	Panax	6 - 9 g
Gan Jiang	Zingiber	3 - 6 g
Fu Ling	Poria	6 - 9 g
Chen Pi	Citrus	3 - 6 g
Bai Zhu	Atractylodes	6 - 9 g
Wu Wei Zi	Schisandra	3 - 6 g
Ban Xia	Pinellia	6 - 9 g
Gan Cao	Glycyrrhiza	3 - 6 g
She Xiang	Moschus	0.3 g
[Sheng Jiang	Zingiber	1 - 3 g]

Mild yang deficiency with external wind cold without sweating. (shaoyin and taiyang disease). Symptoms include extreme chilliness with mild fever and severe fatigue.

T pale, white coat

P minute

MA HUANG FU ZI XI XIN TANG

Ephedra, Prepared Aconite, and Asarum Decoction

Extract Formula Name: Ma-Huang and Asarum Combination

Ma Huang	Ephedra	6 - 9 g
Fu Zi	Aconitum	3 - 6 g
Xi Xin	Asarum	3 - 6 g

Shaoyin disease: severe yang deficiency with cold accumulation which causes false yang to be pushed to the exterior. The yang cannot stay in the interior causing icy limbs upon touch but no cold intolerance, flushed face, thirst without desire to drink, or a dry throat.

T pale, light purple, teethmarks, thin white coat

P slow, minute

TONG MAI SI NI TANG

Unblock the Pulse Decoction for Frigid Extremities

Extract Formula Name: Licorice, Aconite and Ginger Pulse Combination

Fu Zi	Aconitum	12 - 15 g
Gan Jiang	Zingiber	9 - 12 g
Gan Cao	Glycyrrhiza	3 - 6 g

Spleen/Kidney qi and yang deficient patient suffers easily from wind cold with internal water accumulation, or experiences urinary difficulty, diarrhea, or edema.

T pale, swollen, teethmarks, moist, thin white coat

P frail or minute

ZHEN WU TANG

True Warrior Decoction

Extract Formula Name: Vitality Combination

Fu Zi	Aconitum	6 - 9 g
Bai Zhu	Atractylodes	6 - 9 g
Bai Shao Yao	Paeonia	6 - 9 g
Fu Ling	Poria	6 - 9 g
Sheng Jiang	Zingiber	6 - 9 g

DISEASES IN THE JUEYIN STAGE

- heat sensation and pain in the chest
- hunger without desire to eat
- diarrhea, vomiting
- thirst

T red

P rapid, weak

Kidney and Spleen yang deficiency with cold which has invaded all three yin channels (taiyin, shaoyin, and jueyin). Symptoms include shivering from cold, icy limbs and face, watery diarrhea, or cough with profuse saliva production.

T pale, wet, thin white moist coat

P minute or frail

☞ Remove She Xiang - Moschus, decoct the rest of the formula as usual, then add powdered Moschus to each dosage.

HUI YANG JIU JI TANG

Restore and Revive the Yang Decoction

Fu Zi	Aconitum	9 g
Rou Gui	Cinnamomum	3 - 6 g
Ren Shen	Panax	6 - 9 g
Gan Jiang	Zingiber	3 - 6 g
Fu Ling	Poria	6 - 9 g
Chen Pi	Citrus	3 - 6 g
Bai Zhu	Atractylodes	6 - 9 g
Wu Wei Zi	Schisandra	3 - 6 g
Ban Xia	Pinellia	6 - 9 g
Gan Cao	Glycyrrhiza	3 - 6 g
She Xiang	Moschus	0.3 g
[Sheng Jiang	Zingiber	1 - 3 g]

Six Divisions

1. **Roundworms have migrated upward due to cold in the Large Intestines to the warmth of the epigastrium/chest. 2. Large Intestine cold and Stomach heat: mixed syndrome - jueyin syndrome.**

T   pale

P   weak

☞ Wu Mei - Prunus should be soaked in vinegar for 12 hours.

✪ **Major Formula**

WU MEI WAN

Mume Pill

Extract Formula Name: Mume Formula

Wu Mei	Prunus	20 - 25 g
Xi Xin	Asarum	1 - 3 g
Chuan Jiao	Zanthoxylum	1 - 3 g
Gan Jiang	Zingiber	12 - 15 g
Fu Zi	Aconitum	6 - 9 g
Huang Lian	Coptis	9 - 12 g
Huang Bai	Phellodendron	6 - 9 g
Gui Zhi	Cinnamomum	3 - 9 g
Dang Gui	Angelica	6 - 9 g
Ren Shen	Panax	6 - 9 g

FOUR STAGES

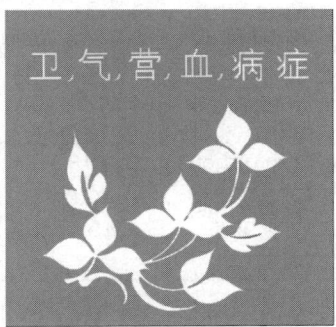

HEAT IN THE WEI (DEFENSIVE) LEVEL

Please see WIND INVASIONS

HEAT IN THE QI LEVEL

- high fever
- thirst
- profuse sweating
- cough or asthma with yellow expectoration

T red, dry, thick yellow coat

P flooding, rapid

Damp heat febrile disease or damp bi-syndrome with heat causing severe sweating and joint pain with swelling and redness. Joints feel hot to the touch.

T red, sticky yellow coat

P slippery, rapid, or flooding

☞ Decoct the first four herbs, then add the rice at the end. It will absorb the water to make a thick liquid.

BAI HU JIA CANG ZHU TANG

White Tiger plus Atractylodes Decoction

Shi Gao	Gypsum	20 - 30 g
Zhi Mu	Anemarrhena	9 - 12 g
Gan Cao	Glycyrrhiza	3 - 6 g
Cang Zhu	Atractylodes	3 - 9 g
Jing Mi	Oryza	15 - 30 g

Four Stages

Heat in the qi level/yangming channel syndrome causing severe fever, epidemic febrile disease, acute inflammation, encephalitis, or meningitis.

T red, dry yellow coat

P flooding, rapid

☞ Decoct the first five herbs, then add the rice at the end. It will absorb the water to make a thick liquid.

BAI HU JIA YIN QIAO TANG

White Tiger plus Lonicera and Forsythia Decoction

Shi Gao	Gypsum	20 - 30 g
Zhi Mu	Anemarrhena	9 - 12 g
Gan Cao	Glycyrrhiza	3 - 6 g
Jin Yin Hua	Lonicera	6 - 9 g
Lian Qiao	Forsythia	6 - 9 g
Jing Mi	Oryza	15 - 30 g

Summerheat with damp and yangming channel heat/qi level heat. This causes severe sweating, nausea, vomiting, thirst, or fever.

T red, sticky yellow coat

P slippery, rapid

☞ Decoct the first four herbs, then add the rice at the end. It will absorb the water to make a thick liquid.

BAI HU JIA ZHU TANG

White Tiger with White Atractylodes Decoction

Shi Gao	Gypsum	20 - 30 g
Zhi Mu	Anemarrhena	9 - 12 g
Gan Cao	Glycyrrhiza	3 - 6 g
Bai Zhu	Atractylodes	3 - 9 g
Jing Mi	Oryza	15 - 30 g

Heat in the qi level/yangming channel disease causing high fever, sweating, flooding pulse, or thirst.

T red, yellow coat

P flooding, rapid

☞ Decoct the first three herbs, then add the rice at the end. It will absorb the water to make a thick liquid.

✪ **Major Formula**

BAI HU TANG

White Tiger Decoction

Extract Formula Name: Gypsum Combination

Shi Gao	Gypsum	20 - 30 g
Zhi Mu	Anemarrhena	9 - 12 g
Gan Cao	Glycyrrhiza	3 - 6 g
Jing Mi	Oryza	15 - 30 g

Shaoyang and yangming channel disease causing mild chills with severe fever, and thirst.

T red, thin yellow coat

P rapid, maybe flooding

CHAI HU BAI HU TANG

Bupleurum White Tiger Decoction

Chai Hu	Bupleurum	3 - 6 g
Huang Qin	Scutellaria	3 - 6 g
Shi Gao	Gypsum	12 - 20 g
Zhi Mu	Anemarrhena	6 - 12 g
Tian Hua Fen	Trichosanthes	6 - 9 g
Jing Mi	Oryza	6 - 9 g
Gan Cao	Glycyrrhiza	3 - 6 g

Shaoyang disease with internal yangming channel heat. The formula purges internal heat stagnation. Symptoms include constipation, severe fever alternating with mild chills, bitter taste, thirst, or hypochondriac discomfort.

T red, yellow coat

P rapid, wiry, forceful

✗ Caution during pregnancy.

DA CHAI HU TANG

Major Bupleurum Decoction

Extract Formula Name: Major Bupleurum Combination

Chai Hu	Bupleurum	9 - 15 g
Da Huang	Rheum	6 - 9 g
Ban Xia	Pinellia	6 - 9 g
Huang Qin	Scutellaria	6 - 9 g
Bai Shao Yao	Paeonia	6 - 9 g
Zhi Shi	Citrus	6 - 9 g
Sheng Jiang	Zingiber	3 - 9 g
Da Zao	Ziziphus	3 - 6 pc

Damp accumulation with heat toxin in the qi level causing gastritis, hepatitis, fever, bodyaches, diarrhea, or vomiting.

T sticky yellow coat

P rapid, soggy

☞ All ingredients should be dried in sunlight and ground into powder. Take 9 g each time, twice a day.

GAN LU XIAO DU DAN

Sweet Dew Special Pill to Eliminate Toxin

Extract Formula Name: Talc and Scute Formula

She Gan	Belamcanda	120 g
Lian Qiao	Forsythia	120 g
Hua Shi	Talcum	450 g
Chuan Bei Mu	Fritillaria	150 g
Bo He	Mentha	120 g
Huang Qin	Scutellaria	300 g
Bai Dou Kou	Amomum	120 g
Yin Chen Hao	Artemisia	330 g
Shi Chang Pu	Acorus	180 g
Huo Xiang	Agastache	120 g
Mu Tong	Akebia	150 g

Heat in the qi and blood levels resulting in purpura.

T red, thin yellow coat

P flooding, rapid

☞ Shi Gao - Gypsum should be decocted first for 20 minutes. Xi Jiao - Rhinoceros is powdered and added to the strained decoction. Shui Niu Jiao - Bubalus should be substituted for Xi Jiao.

HUA BAN TANG

Transform Blotches Decoction

Shi Gao	Gypsum	30 g
Zhi Mu	Anemarrhena	12 g
Xuan Shen	Scrophularia	10 g
Xi Jiao	Rhinoceros	2 - 6 g
Jing Mi	Oryza	9 g
Gan Cao	Glycyrrhiza	10 g

Wind heat with fever, possible sweating, thirst, dyspnea, or asthma: heat in the qi level.

T red tip or border, yellow coat

P rapid, flooding

MA XING SHI GAN TANG

Ephedra, Apricot Kernel, Gypsum, and Licorice Decoction

Extract Formula Name: Ma-Huang and Apricot Seed Combination

Ma Huang	Ephedra	6 - 15 g
Xing Ren	Prunus	6 - 9 g
Shi Gao	Gypsum	6 - 20 g
Gan Cao	Glycyrrhiza	3 - 6 g

Mild summer heat invading the qi level with residual pathogens lingering causing mild superficial and damp symptoms. The patient feels thirst but can only sip fluids, and experiences diarrhea, gas, vomiting, or cold limbs.

T red, thin white coat

P rapid, maybe superficial

☞ The prepared form of Xi Gua - Citrullus is used.

☞ The outer skin of Si Gua Luo - Luffa is used.

QING LUO YIN

Clear the Collaterals Decoction

Bian Dou Hua	Dolichos	6 - 9 g
Xi Gua Shuang	Citrullus	6 - 9 g
Si Gua Pi	Luffa	6 - 9 g
Jin Yin Hua	Lonicera	6 - 9 g
He Ye	Nelumbo	6 g
Dan Zhu Ye	Lophatherum	6 - 9 g

Four Stages

Qi and blood level heat: qi level heat causing high fever, thirst, sweating; and blood level heat causing bleeding conditions, coma, or restlessness. This formula also treats toxic heat.

T   dark red, dry, yellow coat

P   flooding, rapid

☞ Shi Gao - Gypsum should be decocted first for 20 minutes. Xi Jiao - Rhinoceros should be powdered and added to the strained decoction. It should be substituted with 6 - 9 g of Shui Niu Jiao - Bubalus, or 30 g of Bai Mao Gen - Imperata.

QING WEN BAI DU YIN

Clear Epidemics and Overcome Toxin Decoction

Shi Gao	Gypsum	40 - 100 g
Zhi Mu	Anemarrhena	9 - 12 g
Xuan Shen	Scrophularia	6 - 9 g
Dan Zhu Ye	Lophatherum	3 - 6 g
Xi Jiao	Rhinoceros	1 - 3 g
Chi Shao Yao	Paeonia	6 - 9 g
Huang Qin	Scutellaria	6 - 9 g
Huang Lian	Coptis	3 - 6 g
Mu Dan Pi	Paeonia	6 - 9 g
Sheng Di Huang	Rehmannia	6 - 12 g
Zhi Zi	Gardenia	3 - 6 g
Jie Geng	Platycodon	3 - 6 g
Lian Qiao	Forsythia	6 - 9 g
Gan Cao	Glycyrrhiza	3 - 6 g

Qi level heat with toxin in the upper body causing throat swelling, fever, sweating, and thirst for cold fluids.

T   red, yellow coat

P   flooding, rapid

QING XIN LIANG GE SAN

Clear the Heart and Cool the Diaphragm Powder

Lian Qiao	Forsythia	6 - 15 g
Huang Qin	Scutellaria	6 - 9 g
Zhi Zi	Gardenia	3 - 6 g
Bo He	Mentha	3 - 6 g
Jie Geng	Platycodon	3 - 6 g
Shi Gao	Gypsum	12 - 15 g
Gan Cao	Glycyrrhiza	3 - 6 g

Heat or damp heat has entered the Stomach leading to fever, thirst, nausea and vomiting, and distention in the middle jiao.

T red

P rapid

ZHEN NI BAI HU TANG

White Tiger Decoction to Suppress Rebellion

Shi Gao	Gypsum	20 - 35 g
Zhi Mu	Anemarrhena	12 - 18 g
Zhu Ru	Bambusa	6 - 9 g
Ban Xia	Pinellia	6 - 12 g

Heat in the chest and Lungs due to taiyang disease; or lingering qi level heat manifesting in the yangming channel layer. In some patients this formula will induce vomiting, after which the symptoms will disappear.

T red, especially the tip, yellow coat

P rapid, forceful, superficial

✗ This prescription can cause vomiting.

ZHI ZI DOU CHI TANG

Gardenia and Prepared Soybean Decoction

Zhi Zi	Gardenia	6 - 9 g
Dan Dou Chi	Glycine	6 - 9 g

Qi level heat damaged the qi and yin. Now there is residual heat and a mild fever, dry mouth, and irritability.

T red

P rapid, weak, thin

ZHU YE SHI GAO TANG

Lophatherum and Gypsum Decoction

Extract Formula Name: Bamboo Leaves and Gypsum Combination

Dan Zhu Ye	Lophatherum	6 - 15 g
Shi Gao	Gypsum	20 - 30 g
Ban Xia	Pinellia	6 - 9 g
Ren Shen	Panax	3 - 6 g
Zhi Gan Cao	Glycyrrhiza	3 - 6 g
Jing Mi	Oryza	9 - 15 g
Mai Men Dong	Ophiopogon	12 - 15 g

Four Stages

HEAT IN THE YING (NUTRITIVE) LEVEL

- mental restlessness
- dry mouth without desire to drink
- night fevers
- skin eruptions

T   deep red, no coat

P   thin, rapid

Heat in the ying level with yin deficiency causing high fever which is worse at night, delirious speech, or mild purpura.

T   dark red and dry

P   rapid, thin

☞ Xi Jiao - Rhinoceros should be substituted with 9 g of Shui Niu Jiao - Bubalus or 30 g of Bai Mao Gen - Imperata.

QING YING TANG

Clear the Nutritive Level Decoction

Extract Formula Name: Rhinoceros and Scrophularia Combination

Xi Jiao	Rhinoceros	3 - 6 g
Sheng Di Huang	Rehmannia	9 - 12 g
Mai Men Dong	Ophiopogon	6 - 9 g
Huang Lian	Coptis	3 - 6 g
Xuan Shen	Scrophularia	6 - 9 g
Dan Zhu Ye	Lophatherum	6 g
Lian Qiao	Forsythia	6 g
Dan Shen	Salvia	6 - 9 g
Jin Yin Hua	Lonicera	6 - 9 g

HEAT IN THE XUE (BLOOD) LEVEL

- skin eruptions, purpura
- hematemesis, melena
- high fever
- mania

T dark red

P rapid, wiry

Heat in the qi and blood levels resulting in purpura.

T red, thin yellow coat

P flooding, rapid

☞ Shi Gao - Gypsum should be decocted first for 20 minutes. Xi Jiao - Rhinoceros is powdered and added to the strained decoction. Shui Niu Jiao - Bubalus should be substituted for Xi Jiao.

HUA BAN TANG

Transform Blotches Decoction

Shi Gao	Gypsum	30 g
Zhi Mu	Anemarrhena	12 g
Xuan Shen	Scrophularia	10 g
Xi Jiao	Rhinoceros	2 - 6 g
Jing Mi	Oryza	9 g
Gan Cao	Glycyrrhiza	10 g

Blood level heat and taiyin level disease with lingering summer-heat causing thirst and severe sweating.

T red or dark red

P rapid

JIA JIAN SHENG MAI SAN

Modified Generate the Pulse Powder

Mai Men Dong	Ophiopogon	6 - 12 g
Wu Wei Zi	Schisandra	6 - 12 g
Bei Sha Shen	Glehnia	6 - 12 g
Mu Dan Pi	Paeonia	6 - 12 g
Sheng Di Huang	Rehmannia	6 - 12 g

Four Stages

Heat in the blood level causing menorrhagia where the yin has already been damaged. Symptoms include thirst, dry mouth, and restlessness.

T red, yellow coat

P rapid, thin, forceful

☞ Ce Bai Ye Tan - Biota is charred to strenghten the stop bleeding effect.

QING RE ZHI BENG TANG

Clear Heat and Stop Excessive Uterine Bleeding Decoction

Huang Qin	Scutellaria	9 - 15 g
Huang Bai	Phellodendron	9 - 12 g
Zhi Zi	Gardenia	6 - 9 g
Mu Dan Pi	Paeonia	6 - 9 g
Chun Gen Bai Pi	Ailanthus	9 - 25 g
Sheng Di Huang	Rehmannia	9 - 18 g
Bai Shao Yao	Paeonia	9 - 25 g
Ce Bai Ye Tan	Biota	9 - 25 g
Gui Ban	Chinemys	9 - 15 g
Di Yu	Sanguisorba	9 - 18 g

Qi and blood level heat: qi level heat causing high fever, thirst, sweating; and blood level heat causing bleeding conditions, coma, or restlessness. This formula also treats toxic heat.

T dark red, dry, yellow coat

P flooding, rapid

☞ Shi Gao - Gypsum should be decocted first for 20 minutes. Xi Jiao - Rhinoceros should be powdered and added to the strained decoction. It should be substituted with 6 - 9 g of Shui Niu Jiao - Bubalus, or 30 g of Bai Mao Gen - Imperata.

QING WEN BAI DU YIN

Clear Epidemics and Overcome Toxin Decoction

Shi Gao	Gypsum	40 - 100 g
Zhi Mu	Anemarrhena	9 - 12 g
Xuan Shen	Scrophularia	6 - 9 g
Dan Zhu Ye	Lophatherum	3 - 6 g
Xi Jiao	Rhinoceros	1 - 3 g
Chi Shao Yao	Paeonia	6 - 9 g
Huang Qin	Scutellaria	6 - 9 g
Huang Lian	Coptis	3 - 6 g
Mu Dan Pi	Paeonia	6 - 9 g
Sheng Di Huang	Rehmannia	6 - 12 g
Zhi Zi	Gardenia	3 - 6 g
Jie Geng	Platycodon	3 - 6 g
Lian Qiao	Forsythia	6 - 9 g
Gan Cao	Glycyrrhiza	3 - 6 g

Severe toxin, epidemic summer heat, and blood heat causing delirious speech, purpura, or red eyes. This formula opens the orifice.

T   scarlet

P   rapid or flooding

☞ Herbs should be made into pills. Xi Jiao - Rhinoceros should be substituted with Shui Niu Jiao - Bubalus.

SHEN XI DAN

Magical Rhinoceros Special Pill

Xi Jiao	Rhinoceros	60 - 90 g
Jin Yin Hua	Lonicera	200 - 225 g
Ban Lan Gen	Isatis	100 - 135 g
Huang Qin	Scutellaria	60 - 90 g
Sheng Di Huang	Rehmannia	200 - 225 g
Lian Qiao	Forsythia	125 - 150 g
Xuan Shen	Scrophularia	90 - 105 g
Dan Dou Chi	Glycine	100 - 120 g
Shi Chang Pu	Acorus	60 - 90 g
Tian Hua Fen	Trichosanthes	40 - 60 g
Zi Cao	Lithospermum	40 - 60 g

Heat in the blood resulting in various types of upper jiao bleeding such as hemoptysis or epistaxis.

T   red or dark red

P   wiry, forceful, rapid

SI SHENG WAN

Four-Fresh Pill

Ce Bai Ye	Biota	9 - 12 g
Sheng Di Huang	Rehmannia	15 - 20 g
He Ye	Nelumbo	9 - 12 g
Ai Ye	Artemisia	6 - 9 g

Four
Stages

Blood level heat with blood stagnation causing various bleeding disorders such as melena, hematurea, hematemesis, purpura, or thirst but no desire to drink.

T dark red, or purple, dry, yellow coat

P rapid, thin

☞ Xi Jiao - Rhinoceros should be powdered and then added into the strained decoction. It should be substituted with 60 g Shui Niu Jiao - Bubalus. Powder and cook separately for 20 minutes before including the other herbs. Xi Jiao may also be substituted with 30 - 60 g of Bai Mao Gen - Imperata.

✪ **Major Formula**

XI JIAO DI HUANG TANG

Rhinoceros Horn and Rehmannia Decoction

Extract Formula Name: Rhinoceros and Rehmannia Combination

Xi Jiao	Rhinoceros	3 - 9 g
Sheng Di Huang	Rehmannia	15 - 30 g
Mu Dan Pi	Paeonia	9 - 15 g
Chi Shao Yao	Paeonia	9 - 15 g

INTERNAL MEDICINE DISHARMONIES AND MISCELLANEOUS SYNDROMES

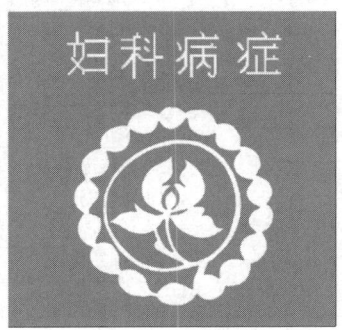

妇科病症

OB-GYN/MENSTRUAL DISORDERS

- irregular menstruation
- dysmenorrhea, amenorrhea
- uterine bleeding

T depends on involved syndrome

P depends on involved syndrome

Late periods due to yang deficiency or cold in the uterus. This formula is also useful during pregnancy to warm the uterus.

T pale, white coat

P frail

☞ Herbs should be ground into a powder and made into 6 g pills with rice vinegar.

AI FU NUAN GONG WAN

Mugwort and Aconite Pill for Warming the Womb

Ai Ye	Artemisia	60 - 90 g
Xiang Fu	Cyperus	150 - 180 g
Wu Zhu Yu	Evodia	40 - 60 g
Bai Shao Yao	Paeonia	40 - 60 g
Huang Qi	Astragalus	40 - 60 g
Dang Gui	Angelica	60 - 90 g
Xu Duan	Dipsacus	30 - 45 g
Shu Di Huang	Rehmannia	15 - 30 g
Chuan Xiong	Ligusticum	40 - 60 g
Rou Gui	Cinnamomum	9 - 15 g

Internal Medicine, Misc. Syndromes

Qi and blood deficiency with blood stagnation. This formula is for a restless fetus, infertility, irregular periods, poor appetite, weakness, or fatigue.

T   pale, thin white coat

P   weak, maybe wiry

BA ZHEN YI MU WAN

Eight-Treasure Pill to Benefit Mothers

Shu Di Huang	Rehmannia	6 - 15 g
Chuan Xiong	Ligusticum	3 - 9 g
Dang Gui	Angelica	6 - 9 g
Bai Shao Yao	Paeonia	6 - 12 g
Ren Shen	Panax	6 - 12 g
Bai Zhu	Atractylodes	3 - 9 g
Fu Ling	Poria	6 - 9 g
Yi Mu Cao	Leonurus	6 - 18 g
Gan Cao	Glycyrrhiza	3 - 6 g

Kidney qi/yin deficiency causing menorrhagia. Other symptoms may include low back pain, frequent urination, or weakness in the knees.

T   red or normal color, thin white coat

P   weak, especially in both chi (third) positions, slightly rapid

BAO YIN JIAN

Augment Yin Decoction

Huang Qin	Scutellaria	9 - 12 g
Huang Bai	Phellodendron	9 - 12 g
Sheng Di Huang	Rehmannia	9 - 15 g
Shu Di Huang	Rehmannia	9 - 15 g
Shan Yao	Dioscorea	6 - 9 g
Bai Shao Yao	Paeonia	6 - 12 g
Xu Duan	Dipsacus	6 - 9 g
Gan Cao	Glycyrrhiza	3 - 6 g

Spleen/Stomach qi deficiency where the Spleen qi is sinking, or the Spleen is not governing the blood. qi deficiency can lead to (morning) fever, early periods, weakness, diarrhea, or pallor.

T pale, swollen, teethmarks, thin white coat

P weak

BU ZHONG YI QI TANG

Tonify the Middle and Augment the Qi Decoction

Extract Formula Name: Ginseng and Astragalus Combination

Ren Shen	Panax	6 - 12 g
Huang Qi	Astragalus	9 - 15 g
Dang Gui	Angelica	6 - 9 g
Chen Pi	Citrus	3 - 6 g
Sheng Ma	Cimicifuga	3 - 6 g
Chai Hu	Bupleurum	3 - 9 g
Bai Zhu	Atractylodes	3 - 9 g
Zhi Gan Cao	Glycyrrhiza	3 - 6 g

Severe phlegm damp accumulation causing dizziness, headache, sticky phlegm expectoration, or amenorrhea due to phlegm obstruction.

T thick sticky white or slightly yellowish

P slippery

CANG FU DAO TAN TANG

Atractylodes, Cyperus, and Guide Out Phlegm Decoction

Ban Xia	Pinellia	6 - 9 g
Chen Pi	Citrus	3 - 6 g
Fu Ling	Poria	6 - 9 g
Tian Nan Xing	Arisaema	1 - 3 g
Zhi Shi	Citrus	3 - 9 g
Gan Cao	Glycyrrhiza	3 - 6 g
Cang Zhu	Atractylodes	3 - 9 g
Xiang Fu	Cyperus	3 - 9 g
Sheng Jiang	Zingiber	6 - 9 g

Yin and blood deficiency with blood stagnation causing emaciation, no appetite, amenorrhea, tidal fever, or abdominal distention.

T red, pale, purple or purple spots

P thin, choppy

✗ Do not use during pregnancy.

DA HUANG ZHE CHONG WAN

Rhubarb and Eupolyphaga Pill

Da Huang	Rheum	12 - 18 g
Tu Bie Chong	Eupolyphaga	3 g
Xing Ren	Prunus	3 - 6 g
Gan Qi	Sinica	3 g
Sheng Di Huang	Rehmannia	12 - 18 g
Bai Shao Yao	Paeonia	6 - 12 g
Meng Chong	Tabanus	3 - 6 g
Qi Cao	Holotrichia	3 - 6 g
Tao Ren	Prunus	6 - 9 g
Shui Zhi	Hirudo	3 - 6 g
Huang Qin	Scutellaria	6 g
Gan Cao	Glycyrrhiza	3 - 6 g

Liver/Spleen disharmony with heat. Symptoms include irregular menstruation, red or bloodshot eyes, or irritability.

T red sides, light purple, thin white coat

P wiry, rapid

DAN ZHI XIAO YAO SAN (JIA WEI XIAO YAO SAN)

Moutan, Gardenia, and Rambling Powder

Extract Formula Name: Bupleurum and Peony Formula

Mu Dan Pi	Paeonia	6 - 9 g
Zhi Zi	Gardenia	3 - 6 g
Chai Hu	Bupleurum	6 - 9 g
Bo He	Mentha	3 - 6 g
Dang Gui	Angelica	6 - 9 g
Bai Shao Yao	Paeonia	6 - 9 g
Bai Zhu	Atractylodes	3 - 9 g
Fu Ling	Poria	6 - 9 g
Gan Cao	Glycyrrhiza	3 - 6 g
[Sheng Jiang	Zingiber	3 - 6 g]

Qi/blood deficiency with bleeding, fever, heat feelings in the muscles, thirst with a desire for warm liquids, or irregular periods.

T pale, thin coat

P empty

DANG GUI BU XUE TANG

Dang Gui Decoction to Tonify the Blood

Extract Formula Name: Tang-Kuei and Astragalus Combination

Huang Qi	Astragalus	30 g
Dang Gui	Angelica	6 g

Kidney and Liver yin deficiency causing irregular menses a scanty menstrual flow, tinnitus, dizziness, or night sweating.

T red, scanty coat

P thin, rapid

DANG GUI DI HUANG YIN

Dang Gui and Rehmannia Decoction

Dang Gui	Angelica	6 - 9 g
Shu Di Huang	Rehmannia	6 - 12 g
Huai Niu Xi	Achyranthes	6 - 9 g
Shan Yao	Dioscorea	6 - 9 g
Du Zhong	Eucommia	6 - 9 g
Shan Zhu Yu	Cornus	6 - 9 g
Zhi Gan Cao	Glycyrrhiza	3 - 6 g

Heat in the yangming channel with pre-existing severe blood stagnation in the lower jiao which affects the uterus and the intestines. Symptoms include jaundice, mania, fever, melena with dry stools which are relatively easy to discharge, dysmenorrhea, amenorrhea, abdominal fullness, or bleeding in the stomach. This formula is stronger than 'Di Dang Wan - Resistance Pill.'

T red, dark purple

P wiry, rapid

✗ Do not use during pregnancy. Use only for a short duration.

DI DANG TANG

Resistance Decoction

Da Huang	Rheum	6 - 12 g
Tao Ren	Prunus	6 - 9 g
Shui Zhi	Hirudo	1 - 3 g
Meng Chong	Tabanus	1 - 3 g

Internal Medicine, Misc. Syndromes

Chronic uterine bleeding due to blood deficiency and cold. This formula is also useful for spotting or clear leukorrhea.

T   pale, white coat

P   weak, thin

☞ E Jiao - Equus should be dissolved into the strained tea.

DING XIANG JIAO AI TANG

Clove, Ass-Hide Gelatin, and Mugwort Decoction

Ding Xiang	Eugenia	3 - 6 g
E Jiao	Equus	3 - 9 g
Ai Ye	Artemisia	6 g
Shu Di Huang	Rehmannia	6 - 9 g
Dang Gui	Angelica	6 - 9 g
Bai Shao Yao	Paeonia	6 - 9 g
Chuan Xiong	Ligusticum	3 - 9 g

Kidney yin and yang deficiency with fire causing menopause, hot flashes, or urinary frequency.

T   red

P   rapid or normal rate, thin

ER XIAN TANG

Two-Immortal Decoction

Extract Formula Name: Curculigo and Epimedium Combination

Yin Yang Huo	Epimedium	9 - 15 g
Xian Mao	Curculigo	9 - 15 g
Dang Gui	Angelica	6 - 9 g
Huang Bai	Phellodendron	6 - 9 g
Zhi Mu	Anemarrhena	6 - 9 g
Ba Ji Tian	Morinda	6 - 9 g

Qi/blood stagnation under the diaphragm and epigastrium, or masses in the abdomen or epigastrium.

T purple

P wiry or choppy

✗ Do not use during pregnancy.

GE XIA ZHU YU TANG

Drive Out Blood Stasis Below the Diaphragm Decoction

Extract Formula Name: Persica and Carthamus Combination

Dang Gui	Angelica	6 - 9 g
Chuan Xiong	Ligusticum	6 - 9 g
Tao Ren	Prunus	6 - 9 g
Hong Hua	Carthamus	3 - 6 g
Mu Dan Pi	Paeonia	6 - 9 g
Chi Shao Yao	Paeonia	6 - 9 g
Yan Hu Suo	Corydalis	3 - 6 g
Xiang Fu	Cyperus	3 - 9 g
Zhi Ke	Citrus	3 - 6 g
Wu Ling Zhi	Trogopterus	6 - 9 g
Wu Yao	Lindera	3 - 6 g
Gan Cao	Glycyrrhiza	6 - 9 g

Spleen qi deficiency leading to uncontrolled menstrual bleeding which is pale and watery (ben lou syndrome).

T pale, swollen, teethmarks, thin coat

P hollow or thin, deep, weak

GU BEN ZHI BENG TANG

Stabilize the Root and Stop Excessive Uterine Bleeding Decoction

Shu Di Huang	Rehmannia	6 - 20 g
Bai Zhu	Atractylodes	6 - 15 g
Huang Qi	Astragalus	6 - 15 g
Dang Gui	Angelica	6 - 9 g
Ren Shen	Panax	6 - 9 g
Pao Jiang	Zingiber	3 - 6 g

Spleen qi deficiency causing ben lou syndrome - excessive uterine bleeding or spotting.

T pale, swollen, slight teeth-marks, thin white coat

P weak, thin

GU BEN ZHI LOU TANG

Stabilize the Root and Stop Spotting Decoction

Ren Shen	Panax	9 - 15 g
Bai Zhu	Atractylodes	6 - 12 g
Gan Jiang	Zingiber	3 - 6 g
Shu Di Huang	Rehmannia	9 - 12 g
Dang Gui	Angelica	9 - 12 g
Sheng Ma	Cimicifuga	6 - 9 g
Shan Yao	Dioscorea	6 - 12 g
Da Zao	Ziziphus	3 - 4 pc

Menorrhagia or spotting due to Kidney and Liver yin deficiency, false heat, blood stagnation, or Spleen qi deficiency.

T pale, thin coat

P weak, thin

☞ Zong Lu Pi Tan - Trachycarpus should be charred to maximize the stop bleeding function.

GU CHONG TANG

Stabilize Gushing Decoction

Bai Zhu	Atractylodes	9 - 30 g
Shan Zhu Yu	Cornus	9 - 24 g
Long Gu	Os Draconis	12 - 24 g
Mu Li	Ostrea	12 - 24 g
Zong Lu Pi Tan	Trachycarpus	3 - 6 g
Huang Qi	Astragalus	9 - 18 g
Bai Shao Yao	Paeonia	9 - 12 g
Qian Cao Gen	Rubia	6 - 9 g
Hai Piao Xiao	Sepia	9 - 12 g
Wu Bei Zi	Rhus/Melaphis	1 - 2 g

Liver qi stagnation with heat causing uterine bleeding which depletes yin (ben lou syndrome).

T rapid, no coat

P thin, rapid

GU JING WAN

Stabilize the Menses Pill

Extract Formula Name: Tortoise Shell and Scute Combination

Gui Ban	Chinemys	15 - 30 g
Chun Pi	Ailanthus	6 - 12 g
Bai Shao Yao	Paeonia	15 - 30 g
Huang Bai	Phellodendron	6 - 9 g
Huang Qin	Scutellaria	15 - 30 g
Xiang Fu	Cyperus	3 - 6 g

Kidney qi/yin deficiency causing irregular periods, leukorrhea, or a bearing-down sensation.

T red, thin white coat

P weak, especially the chi (third) positions

GU YIN JIAN

Stabilize the Yin Decoction

Shu Di Huang	Rehmannia	6 - 12 g
Shan Yao	Dioscorea	6 - 9 g
Wu Wei Zi	Schisandra	6 - 9 g
Shan Zhu Yu	Cornus	6 - 9 g
Tu Si Zi	Cuscuta	6 - 9 g
Ren Shen	Panax	6 - 9 g
Yuan Zhi	Polygala	3 g
Zhi Gan Cao	Glycyrrhiza	3 - 6 g

Blood deficiency with yang deficiency and cold causing coldness in the uterus with dysmenorrhea. The blood is scanty, pale, and watery. The patient experiences severe cramping upon menstrual onset.

T pale, light purple, some cracks, thin white coat

P slow, thin, weak

GUI FU SI WU TANG

Cinnamon Bark, Aconite, and Four-Substance Decoction

Sheng Di Huang	Rehmannia	6 - 12 g
Dang Gui	Angelica	6 - 9 g
Chuan Xiong	Ligusticum	3 - 9 g
Bai Shao Yao	Paeonia	6 - 9 g
Rou Gui	Cinnamomum	3 - 9 g
Fu Zi	Aconitum	1 - 6 g

Internal Medicine,
Misc. Syndromes

Kidney qi deficiency with Kidney/Liver yin deficiency causing amenorrhea, or back and knee pain.

T   pale or red, thin white or scanty coat

P   weak, maybe thin especially in the left chi (third) position

GUI SHEN TANG

Comeback Kidney Decoction

Shu Di Huang	Rehmannia	6 - 15 g
Shan Yao	Dioscorea	9 - 15 g
Shan Zhu Yu	Cornus	9 - 12 g
Gou Qi Zi	Lycium	9 - 15 g
Dang Gui	Angelica	9 - 12 g
Du Zhong	Eucommia	6 - 12 g
Fu Ling	Poria	6 - 12 g
Tu Si Zi	Cuscuta	9 - 12 g

Blood and phlegm stagnation in the uterus leading to masses or lumps, amenorrhea, dysmenorrhea, or restless fetus.

T   purple, sticky coat

P   wiry, slippery, choppy

GUI ZHI FU LING WAN

Cinnamon Twig and Poria Pill

Extract Formula Name: Cinnamon and Hoelen Formula

Gui Zhi	Cinnamomum	6 - 12 g
Fu Ling	Poria	6 - 12 g
Mu Dan Pi	Paeonia	6 - 12 g
Tao Ren	Prunus	6 - 12 g
Chi Shao Yao	Paeonia	9 - 12 g

Liver qi stagnation with blood deficiency causing delayed periods with clots.

T pale, purple

P choppy, wiry

GUO QI YIN

Delayed Menstruation Decoction

Shu Di Huang	Rehmannia	6 - 9 g
Dang Gui	Angelica	6 - 9 g
Bai Shao Yao	Paeonia	6 - 9 g
Chuan Xiong	Ligusticum	3 - 6 g
Hong Hua	Carthamus	3 - 6 g
Tao Ren	Prunus	3 - 6 g
Xiang Fu	Cyperus	3 - 6 g
Mu Tong	Akebia	3 - 6 g
E Zhu	Curcuma	3 - 6 g
Rou Gui	Cinnamomum	1 - 3 g
Gan Cao	Glycyrrhiza	3 - 6 g

Epistaxis or hematemesis during menses due to Stomach deficiency and rebellious qi.

T pale

P weak, thin

JIA WEI MAI MEN DONG TANG

Augmented Ophiopogon Decoction

Mai Men Dong	Ophiopogon	9 - 15 g
Shan Yao	Dioscorea	9 - 12 g
Ren Shen	Panax	9 - 12 g
Dan Shen	Salvia	9 - 12 g
Ban Xia	Pinellia	6 - 9 g
Bai Shao Yao	Paeonia	6 - 9 g
Tao Ren	Prunus	3 - 6 g
Da Zao	Ziziphus	3 - 5 pc
Gan Cao	Glycyrrhiza	3 - 6 g

Cold uterus with underlying blood deficiency causing excessive uterine bleed with pale, watery blood.

T   pale

P   slow, thin, weak

JIAO AI SI WU TANG

Gelatin and Artemisia and Four-Substance Decoction

Extract Formula Name: Gelatin and Artemisia Combination

Shu Di Huang	Rehmannia	6 - 12 g
Bai Shao Yao	Paeonia	6 - 9 g
Chuan Xiong	Ligusticum	3 - 6 g
Dang Gui	Angelica	6 - 9 g
E Jiao	Equus	3 - 9 g
Ai Ye	Artemisia	6 - 9 g
Gan Cao	Glycyrrhiza	3 - 6 g

Chong and Ren imbalance with blood deficiency causing restless fetus, pale post-partum bleeding, abdominal pain, a weak low back, or a cold uterus.

T   pale

P   frail, slow

☞ E Jiao - Equus should be dissolved at the end into the strained tea.

JIAO AI TANG

Ass-Hide Equus and Mugwort Decoction

Extract Formula Name: Tang-kuei and Equus Combination

E Jiao	Equus	6 - 9 g
Ai Ye	Artemisia	6 - 9 g
Dang Gui	Angelica	6 - 9 g
Sheng Di Huang	Rehmannia	18 g
Bai Shao Yao	Paeonia	12 g
Chuan Xiong	Ligusticum	6 g
Gan Cao	Glycyrrhiza	3 - 6 g

Spleen qi deficiency causing severe uterine bleeding which is pale in color, or early or irregular periods. The Spleen qi is sinking causing a restless fetus.

T   pale, swollen, teethmarks, thin white coat

P   weak

JU YUAN JIAN

Lift the Source Decoction

Ren Shen	Panax	6 - 9 g
Huang Qi	Astragalus	9 - 12 g
Sheng Ma	Cimicifuga	3 - 6 g
Bai Zhu	Atractylodes	3 - 6 g
Gan Cao	Glycyrrhiza	3 - 6 g

Liver qi stagnation with cold in the Stomach causing abdominal pain which is relieved by warmth. The Formula is also useful for dysmenorrhea.

T pale, white coat

P weak, slow, or wiry

LIANG FU WAN

Galanga and Cyperus Pill

Extract Formula Name: Galanga and Cyperus Formula

Gao Liang Jiang	Alpinia	6 - 9 g
Xiang Fu	Cyperus	6 - 9 g

Blood deficiency with deficient or excess heat causing purple menstrual blood, early periods, or thick leukorrhea with tidal fever.

T pale

P rapid, thin, weak

QIN LIAN SI WU TANG

Four-Substance Decoction with Scutellaria and Coptis

Huang Qin	Scutellaria	6 - 9 g
Huang Lian	Coptis	3 - 6 g
Chuan Xiong	Ligusticum	3 - 6 g
Bai Shao Yao	Paeonia	6 - 9 g
Dang Gui	Angelica	6 - 9 g
Mai Men Dong	Ophiopogon	6 - 9 g
Sheng Di Huang	Rehmannia	9 - 12 g

Yin deficiency with false heat causing early periods or constipation.

T red, scanty yellowish coat

P thin, rapid

QING JING SAN

Clear the Menses Powder

Shu Di Huang	Rehmannia	6 - 12 g
Mu Dan Pi	Paeonia	6 - 9 g
Di Gu Pi	Lycium	6 - 9 g
Qing Hao	Artemisia	3 - 6 g
Bai Shao Yao	Paeonia	6 - 9 g
Fu Ling	Poria	6 g
Huang Bai	Phellodendron	3 g

Internal Medicine,
Misc. Syndromes

Excess heat or heat in the blood leading to gushing uterine bleeding.

T   red, yellow coat

P   forceful, rapid, slippery

☞ Zong Lu Pi Tan - Trachycarpus is charred to maximize the stop bleeding function.

QING JING ZHI XUE TANG

Cool the Menses and Stop Bleeding Decoction

Sheng Di Huang	Rehmannia	6 - 25 g
Huang Bai	Phellodendron	6 - 12 g
Huang Qin	Scutellaria	9 - 15 g
Di Yu	Sanguisorba	9 - 25 g
Yi Mu Cao	Leonurus	9 - 15 g
Bai Mao Gen	Imperata	12 - 25 g
Mu Dan Pi	Paeonia	6 - 9 g
Pu Huang	Typha	9 - 15 g
Zong Lu Pi Tan	Trachycarpus	9 - 18 g

Blood heat causing severe uterine bleeding, heavy periods, and the blood is bright red and gushing (ben syndrome).

T   red

P   rapid, forceful

☞ Zong Lu Pi Tan - Trachycarpus and Di Yu Tan - Sanguisorba are charred to strengthen the stop bleeding effect. E Jiao - Equus should be dissolved into the strained tea.

QING RE GU JING TANG I

Clear Heat and Stabilize Menses Decoction I

Di Gu Pi	Lycium	6 - 9 g
Huang Qin	Scutellaria	6 - 9 g
Zhi Zi	Gardenia	6 - 9 g
Bai Mao Gen	Imperata	6 - 9 g
Mu Dan Pi	Paeonia	6 - 12 g
Sheng Di Huang	Rehmannia	6 - 12 g
Zong Lu Pi Tan	Trachycarpus	6 - 9 g
Di Yu Tan	Sanguisorba	6 - 9 g
Gan Cao	Glycyrrhiza	6 - 9 g
Ou Jie	Nelumbo	6 - 9 g
Gui Ban	Chinemys	12 g
Mu Li	Ostrea	12 g
E Jiao	Equus	12 g

Damp heat obstruction causing dysmenorrhea, pain prior to onset of the menstruation, cramps, or leukorrhea.

T light purple or red, thick sticky yellow coat

P slippery, slightly rapid, or wiry

QING RE GU JING TANG II

Clear Heat and Stabilize Menses Decoction II

Huang Bai	Phellodendron	6 - 9 g
Huang Lian	Coptis	3 - 9 g
Mu Dan Pi	Paeonia	6 - 12 g
Sheng Di Huang	Rehmannia	6 - 12 g
Dang Gui	Angelica	6 - 9 g
Chi Shao Yao	Paeonia	6 - 9 g
Chuan Xiong	Ligusticum	3 - 9 g
Yan Hu Suo	Corydalis	6 - 9 g

Heat in the blood level causing menorrhagia where the yin has already been damaged. Symptoms include thirst, dry mouth, and restlessness.

T red, yellow coat

P rapid, thin, forceful

☞ Ce Bai Ye Tan - Biota is charred to strenghten the stop bleeding effect.

QING RE ZHI BENG TANG

Clear Heat and Stop Excessive Uterine Bleeding Decoction

Huang Qin	Scutellaria	9 - 15 g
Huang Bai	Phellodendron	9 - 12 g
Zhi Zi	Gardenia	6 - 9 g
Mu Dan Pi	Paeonia	6 - 9 g
Chun Gen Bai Pi	Ailanthus	9 - 25 g
Sheng Di Huang	Rehmannia	9 - 18 g
Bai Shao Yao	Paeonia	9 - 25 g
Ce Bai Ye Tan	Biota	9 - 25 g
Gui Ban	Chinemys	9 - 15 g
Di Yu	Sanguisorba	9 - 18 g

Internal Medicine, Misc. Syndromes

Spleen/Lung qi and blood deficiency with Heart yang deficiency, or ying level deficiency. The patient is easily startled, experiences shortness of breath, lack of taste sensation, insomnia, or palpitations. This formula is also useful for irregular periods or uterine bleeding.

T pale, swollen

P weak

REN SHEN YANG RONG WAN

Ginseng Decoction to Nourish the Nutritive Qi

Extract Formula Name: Ginseng Combination

Bai Shao Yao	Paeonia	9 - 15 g
Chen Pi	Citrus	3 - 6 g
Dang Gui	Angelica	3 - 9 g
Ren Shen	Panax	6 - 9 g
Huang Qi	Astragalus	6 - 12 g
Bai Zhu	Atractylodes	6 - 9 g
Shu Di Huang	Rehmannia	3 - 6 g
Wu Wei Zi	Schisandra	3 - 6 g
Fu Ling	Poria	3 - 6 g
Yuan Zhi	Polygala	2 - 6 g
Rou Gui	Cinnamomum	6 - 9 g
Gan Cao	Glycyrrhiza	3 - 6 g
[Da Zao	Ziziphus	2 pc]
[Gan Jiang	Zingiber	3 pc]

Heart fire and excess heat leading to nose bleeding or premenstrual vomiting.

T red, yellow coat

P rapid, or empty

✗ Caution during pregnancy.

SAN HUANG SI WU TANG

Three-Yellow and Four-Substance Decoction

Shu Di Huang	Rehmannia	6 - 15 g
Bai Shao Yao	Paeonia	6 - 9 g
Chuan Xiong	Ligusticum	3 - 9 g
Dang Gui	Angelica	6 - 9 g
Huang Lian	Coptis	3 - 9 g
Da Huang	Rheum	6 - 12 g
Huang Qin	Scutellaria	6 - 9 g

Severe qi deficiency with yang and blood deficiency and cold symptoms. Irregular menstruation with a pale and watery flow, dizziness, pale or sallow face, cold limbs, or chills.

T pale, wet, thin white coat

P deep, weak, thready

SHAN HE YIN

Mountain and River Decoction

Shu Di Huang	Rehmannia	15 - 25 g
Dang Gui	Angelica	6 - 9 g
Bai Shao Yao	Paeonia	6 - 9 g
Chuan Xiong	Ligusticum	3 - 9 g
Rou Gui	Cinnamomum	3 - 9 g
Huang Qi	Astragalus	6 - 15 g

Blood and cold stagnation in the lower jiao with mass formation, blood clots, and dysmenorrhea. This formula is also useful for liver cirrhosis.

T pale, purple

P wiry or choppy

✗ Do not use during pregnancy.

SHAO FU ZHU YU TANG

Drive Out Blood Stasis in the Lower Abdomen Decoction

Extract Formula Name: Cnidium and Bulrush Combination

Yan Hu Suo	Corydalis	3 - 6 g
Dang Gui	Angelica	6 - 9 g
Mo Yao	Commiphora	3 - 6 g
Rou Gui	Cinnamomum	3 - 6 g
Xiao Hui Xiang	Foeniculum	1.5 - 3 g
Gan Jiang	Zingiber	3 - 6 g
Pu Huang	Typha	6 - 9 g
Chi Shao Yao	Paeonia	6 - 9 g
Wu Ling Zhi	Trogopterus	6 - 9 g
Chuan Xiong	Ligusticum	3 - 9 g

Internal Medicine, Misc. Syndromes

Spleen qi deficiency with damp leading to diarrhea and irregular periods. Other symptoms include weight loss, fatigue, poor appetite, or pale face.

T pale, white coat

P weak or thin, slow

SHEN LING BAI ZHU SAN

Ginseng, Poria, and Atractylodes Powder

Extract Formula Name: Ginseng and Atractylodes Formula

Ren Shen	Panax	9 - 15 g
Fu Ling	Poria	9 - 12 g
Bai Zhu	Atractylodes	3 - 9 g
Gan Cao	Glycyrrhiza	6 - 9 g
Lian Zi	Nelumbo	3 - 9 g
Yi Yi Ren	Coix	6 - 15 g
Shan Yao	Dioscorea	9 - 15 g
Bian Dou	Dolichos	6 - 9 g
Jie Geng	Platycodon	3 - 6 g
Sha Ren	Amomum	3 g

Post-partum retention of lochia due to blood and cold stagnation.

T pale, purple

P choppy

☞ Add yellow wine to the decoction.

SHENG HUA TANG

Generation and Transformation Decoction

Extract Formula Name: Tang-Kuei and Ginger Combination

Dang Gui	Angelica	15 - 28 g
Tao Ren	Prunus	6 - 9 g
Pao Jiang	Zingiber	3 - 6 g
Chuan Xiong	Ligusticum	6 - 9 g
Gan Cao	Glycyrrhiza	3 - 6 g

Spleen qi/blood deficiency causing slow blood circulation with deficiency type abdominal pain during menstruation, or bleeding sores.

T pale, light purple, thin white coat

P thin, weak

SHENG YU TANG

Sage-like Healing Decoction

Shu Di Huang	Rehmannia	15 - 25 g
Ren Shen	Panax	12 - 15 g
Dang Gui	Angelica	12 - 15 g
Huang Qi	Astragalus	15 - 20 g
Chuan Xiong	Ligusticum	6 - 9 g
Bai Shao Yao	Peonia	15 - 20 g

Qi/yang/blood deficiency. Symptoms include poor appetite, general malaise, mild cold symptoms, severe deficiency, rashes, dysmenorrhea, uterine bleeding, or post-partum deficiency.

T pale, thin white coat

P weak, thin, deep

SHI QUAN DA BU TANG

All-Inclusive Great Tonifying Decoction

Extract Formula Name: Ginseng and Tang-Kuei Ten Combination

Ren Shen	Panax	6 - 9 g
Fu Ling	Poria	9 - 12 g
Bai Zhu	Atractylodes	9 - 12 g
Gan Cao	Glycyrrhiza	3 - 6 g
Dang Gui	Angelica	12 - 15 g
Shu Di Huang	Rehmannia	15 - 20 g
Bai Shao Yao	Paeonia	12 - 15 g
Chuan Xiong	Ligusticum	3 - 9 g
Rou Gui	Cinnamomum	6 - 9 g
Huang Qi	Astragalus	15 - 20 g
[Da Zao	Ziziphus	1 - 3 g]
[Sheng Jiang	Zingiber	3 - 6 g]

Post-partum blood (lochia) retention with dark clots and severe abdominal pain. The stagnation is in the Chong and Ren channels.

T purple

P wiry

✗ Do not use during pregnancy.

SHI XIAO SAN

Sudden Smile Powder

Extract Formula Name: Pteropus and Bulrush Formula

Pu Huang	Typha	6 - 12 g
Wu Ling Zhi	Trogopterus	6 - 9 g

Internal Medicine, Misc. Syndromes

Spleen qi deficiency causing gushing uterine bleeding (ben syndrome).

T pale

P weak

SHOU PI JIAN

Consolidate Spleen Decoction

Cang Zhu	Atractylodes	3 - 6 g
Lian Zi	Nelumbo	3 - 9 g
Ren Shen	Panax	6 - 9 g
Suan Zao Ren	Ziziphus	6 - 12 g
Dang Gui	Angelica	3 - 9 g
Shan Yao	Dioscorea	6 - 9 g
Yuan Zhi	Polygala	3 - 6 g
Sheng Jiang	Zingiber	3 - 6 g
Zhi Gan Cao	Glycyrrhiza	3 - 6 g

Lung/Kidney yin deficiency with severe fire causing nosebleeds, or hemoptysis which occurs during or prior to the menses.

T red, cracks

P rapid, empty

SHUN JING TANG

Smooth the Menses Decoction

Shu Di Huang	Rehmannia	9 - 15 g
Mu Dan Pi	Paeonia	6 - 9 g
Dang Gui	Angelica	6 - 9 g
Bai Shao Yao	Paeonia	6 - 9 g
Bei Sha Shen	Glehnia	6 - 12 g
Jing Jie	Schizonepeta	6 - 9 g
Fu Ling	Poria	6 - 9 g

Blood stagnation with fire in the lower jiao causing constipation, sudden abdominal pain, dysmenorrhea, intestinal obstruction, or melena. In severe cases this may lead to restlessness, or even delirium.

T purple

P choppy or forceful

☞ Da Huang - Rheum should be added during the last 3 - 5 minutes of the decoction process. Mang Xiao - Mirabilitum should be added to the strained tea.

✘ Do not use during pregnancy.

TAO HE CHENG QI TANG

Peach Pit Decoction to Order the Qi

Extract Formula Name: Prunus and Rhubarb Combination

Tao Ren	Prunus	9 - 15 g
Gui Zhi	Cinnamomum	6 - 9 g
Mang Xiao	Mirabilitum	3 - 6 g
Da Huang	Rheum	9 - 12 g
Gan Cao	Glycyrrhiza	3 - 6 g

Mild blood deficiency with severe blood stagnation causing early periods or dysmenorrhea.

T pale or purple

P choppy or wiry

✘ Do not use during pregnancy.

TAO HONG SI WU TANG

Four-Substance Decoction with Safflower and Peach Pit

Shu Di Huang	Rehmannia	6 - 12 g
Bai Shao Yao	Paeonia	6 - 9 g
Chuan Xiong	Ligusticum	3 - 6 g
Dang Gui	Angelica	6 - 9 g
Tao Ren	Prunus	3 - 9 g
Hong Hua	Carthamus	3 - 6 g

Kidney and Liver yin deficiency causing amenorrhea, cold feeling in the abdomen, retarded growth in puberty, or clear leukorrhea.

T pale or slightly red

P weak, thin

☞ E Jiao - Equus should be added at the end to the strained tea.

TIAO GAN TANG

Regulating the Liver Decoction

Shan Yao	Dioscorea	9 - 12 g
E Jiao	Equus	6 - 12 g
Ba Ji Tian	Morinda	6 - 9 g
Dang Gui	Angelica	6 - 9 g
Ze Lan	Lycopus	6 - 12 g
Shan Zhu Yu	Cornus	6 - 9 g
Bai Shao Yao	Paeonia	6 - 9 g
Dan Shen	Salvia	6 - 9 g
Gan Cao	Glycyrrhiza	3 - 6 g

Internal Medicine, Misc. Syndromes

Deficient cold and blood stagnation causing menstrual irregularities, spotting between periods (lou syndrome), clots at the end of the period, coldness in the lower abdomen, or low-grade fever at night only.

T   pale, purple, dark purple spots

P   deep, slow, or tight

☞ E Jiao - Equus should be added at the end to the strained tea.

WEN JING TANG

Warm the Menses Decoction

Extract Formula Name: Tang-Kuei and Evodia Combination

Gui Zhi	Cinnamomum	6 - 9 g
Wu Zhu Yu	Evodia	6 - 9 g
Bai Shao Yao	Paeonia	6 - 9 g
Mai Men Dong	Ophiopogon	6 - 9 g
Mu Dan Pi	Paeonia	6 - 9 g
Ban Xia	Pinellia	6 - 9 g
Ren Shen	Panax	6 - 9 g
Dang Gui	Angelica	6 - 9 g
E Jiao	Equus	6 - 9 g
Chuan Xiong	Ligusticum	6 g
Sheng Jiang	Zingiber	3 - 6 g
Gan Cao	Glycyrrhiza	3 - 6 g

Liver qi stagnation causing late periods, irritability, premenstrual syndrome, or distention in the urinary tract.

T   light purple, thin coat

P   wiry

WU YAO TANG

Lindera Decoction

Wu Yao	Lindera	3 - 6 g
Dang Gui	Angelica	6 - 9 g
Xiang Fu	Cyperus	3 - 9 g
Mu Xiang	Saussurea	3 - 9 g
Gan Cao	Zingiber	3 - 6 g

Excess heat causing early periods, heavy periods with clots, flushed face, thirst, dry mouth, or irritability.

T red, cracks, rough, yellow coat

P rapid, forceful

☞ E Jiao - Equus should be dissolved into the strained tea.

XIANG QI TANG

Earlier-Time Decoction

Dang Gui	Angelica	6 - 9 g
Chuan Xiong	Ligusticum	3 - 9 g
Bai Shao Yao	Paeonia	6 - 9 g
Ai Ye	Artemisia	6 - 9 g
E Jiao	Equus	3 - 6 g
Huang Bai	Phellodendron	6 - 9 g
Huang Qin	Scutellaria	6 - 9 g
Huang Lian	Coptis	3 - 6 g
Zhi Mu	Anemarrhena	6 - 12g
Xiang Fu	Cyperus	6 - 9 g
Gan Cao	Glycyrrhiza	3 - 6 g

Liver qi stagnation manifesting mostly as irregular periods. Menstruation is sometimes early or sometimes late, and the patient experiences severe premenstrual syndrome, cramping prior to the onset of bleeding, or breast distention.

T light purple, thin coat

P wiry

XIANG WU SAN

Cyperus and Lindera Powder

Xiang Fu	Cyperus	6 - 12 g
Wu Yao	Lindera	3 - 9 g
Chai Hu	Bupleurum	6 - 9 g
Bai Zhu	Atractylodes	3 - 9 g
Bai Shao Yao	Paeonia	6 - 9 g
Dang Gui	Angelica	6 - 9 g
Fu Ling	Poria	6 - 9 g

Blood deficiency causing delayed periods, a pale watery flow, scanty period, dizziness, poor memory, blurry vision.

T pale

P weak, thin

XIAO YIN JIAN

Minor Yin Decoction

Dang Gui	Angelica	6 - 9 g
Sheng Di Huang	Rehmannia	12 - 25 g
Bai Shao Yao	Paeonia	6 - 12 g
Gou Qi Zi	Lycium	6 - 12 g
Shan Yao	Dioscorea	6 - 9 g
Gan Cao	Glycyrrhiza	3 - 6 g

Internal Medicine,
Misc. Syndromes

Blood stagnation in head, chest, and diaphragm causing angina, palpitations, insomnia, nightmares, or dysmenorrhea.

T purple or purple spots

P wiry

✗ Do not use during pregnancy.

XUE FU ZHU YU TANG

Drive out Stasis in the Mansion of Blood Decoction

Extract Formula Name: Persica and Achyranthes Combination

Dang Gui	Angelica	6 - 9 g
Chuan Xiong	Ligusticum	3 - 9 g
Sheng Di Huang	Rehmannia	6 - 9 g
Chi Shao Yao	Paeonia	6 - 9 g
Tao Ren	Prunus	6 - 12 g
Hong Hua	Carthamus	6 - 9 g
Chuan Niu Xi	Cyathula	9 - 12 g
Jie Geng	Platycodon	3 - 6 g
Zhi Ke	Citrus	3 - 6 g
Chai Hu	Bupleurum	3 - 9 g
Gan Cao	Glycyrrhiza	3 - 6 g

Blood stagnation with abdominal pain, severe spasms, and irregular periods.

T purple, or purple spots

P choppy, wiry

✗ Do not use during pregnancy.

YAN HU SUO TANG

Corydalis Decoction

Yan Hu Suo	Corydalis	30 - 45 g
Chi Shao Yao	Paeonia	9 - 15 g
Rou Gui	Cinnamomum	9 - 15 g
Ru Xiang	Boswellia	60 - 90 g
Mo Yao	Commiphora	60 - 90 g
Jiang Huang	Curcuma	60 - 90 g
Dang Gui	Angelica	9 - 15 g
Mu Xiang	Saussurea	60 - 90 g
Pu Huang	Typha	9 - 15 g
Gan Cao	Glycyrrhiza	6 - 9 g
[Sheng Jiang	Zingiber	3 - 6 g]

Spleen qi deficiency causing damp which heats up. This leads to heat type leukorrhea with a fishy smell or delayed periods from qi and blood deficiency.

T   pale, thin sticky yellow or white coat

P   slippery, weak

YI HUANG TANG

Change Yellow (Discharge) Decoction

Shan Yao	Dioscorea	9 - 30 g
Huang Bai	Phellodendron	6 - 9 g
Qian Shi	Euryale	9 - 30 g
Bai Guo	Gingko	6 - 10 pc
Che Qian Zi	Plantago	3 - 6 g

Kidney yang and essence deficiency causing amenorrhea, infertility, cold back or knees, pedal edema, or impotence.

T   pale, swollen, teethmarks, thin white coat

P   minute

YOU GUI WAN

Restore the Right Pill

Extract Formula Name: Eucommia and Rehmannia Formula

Rou Gui	Cinnamomum	6 - 9 g
Fu Zi	Aconitum	3 - 6 g
Gou Qi Zi	Lycium	6 - 9 g
Shan Yao	Dioscorea	6 - 9 g
Shu Di Huang	Rehmannia	12 - 20 g
Shan Zhu Yu	Cornus	6 - 9 g
Du Zhong	Eucommia	6 - 9 g
Dang Gui	Angelica	6 - 9 g
Tu Si Zi	Cuscuta	6 - 9 g
Lu Jiao Jiao	Cervus	6 - 9 g

Blood deficiency with interior excess heat causing constipation; or blood stagnation with excess heat resulting in amenorrhea.

T   red or purple, yellow coat

P   rapid

✗   Do not use during pregnancy.

YU ZHU SAN

Jade Candle Powder

Chuan Xiong	Ligusticum	3 - 9 g
Shu Di Huang	Rehmannia	6 - 12 g
Dang Gui	Angelica	6 - 9 g
Bai Shao Yao	Paeonia	6 - 9 g
Da Huang	Rheum	6 - 9 g
Mang Xiao	Mirabilitum	3 - 6 g
Gan Cao	Glycyrrhiza	3 - 6 g

Internal Medicine, Misc. Syndromes

Deficient cold with blood stagnation causing uterine bleeding with pain which is better with the passage of clots.

T pale, dark purple

P choppy or wiry

☞ The first seven ingredients (which may be calcined) should be ground and made into 9 - 12 g pills with glutinous rice and water. The pills should be coated with Zhu Sha - Cinnabaris. One pill per day with wine is the recommeded dosage.

✗ Do not use during pregnancy. Zhu Sha - Cinnabaris is toxic and should therefore not be taken long-term.

ZHEN LING DAN

Rouse the Spirits Special Pill

Zi Shi Ying	Fluoritum	60 g
Yu Liang Shi	Limonite	60 g
Dai Zhe Shi	Haematitum	60 g
Wu Ling Zhi	Trogopterus	30 g
Ru Xiang	Boswellia	30 g
Chi Shi Zhi	Halloysitum Rubrum	60 g
Mo Yao	Commiphora	30 g
Zhu Sha	Cinnabaris	15 g

Liver/Kidney yin and jing (essence) deficiency causing slow development in children; or premature aging in adults, in addition to common yin deficiency signs and symptoms. The formula is also for early menopause, spermatorrhea, low sex drive, infertility, or low sperm count.

T red, scanty coat

P thin, rapid

ZUO GUI YIN

Restore the Left [Kidney] Decoction

Shu Di Huang	Rehmannia	6 - 15 g
Shan Zhu Yu	Cornus	6 - 9 g
Shan Yao	Dioscorea	6 - 9 g
Gou Qi Zi	Lycium	6 - 9 g
Fu Ling	Poria	6 - 9 g
Zhi Gan Cao	Glycyrrhiza	3 - 6 g

OB-GYN/LEUKORRHEA

- vaginal discharge

T usually sticky coat

P usually slippery

Chronic uterine bleeding due to blood deficiency and cold. This formula is also useful for spotting or clear leukorrhea.

T pale, white coat

P weak, thin

☞ E Jiao - Equus should be dissolved into the strained tea.

DING XIANG JIAO AI TANG

Clove, Ass-Hide Gelatin, and Mugwort Decoction

Ding Xiang	Eugenia	3 - 6 g
E Jiao	Equus	3 - 9 g
Ai Ye	Artemisia	6 g
Shu Di Huang	Rehmannia	6 - 9 g
Dang Gui	Angelica	6 - 9 g
Bai Shao Yao	Paeonia	6 - 9 g
Chuan Xiong	Ligusticum	3 - 9 g

Damp heat in the lower jiao causing low back pain, hot, swollen knees or feet, or odorous leukorrhea.

T sticky yellow coat

P slippery, rapid

ER MIAO SAN

Two-Marvel Powder

Cang Zhu	Atractylodes	15 g
Huang Bai	Phellodendron	15 g

Turbid leukorrhea due to Kidney qi/yang deficiency. The Kidneys are unable to astringe.

T pale, swollen, slight teethmarks, wet, thin white coat

P minute or frail

FEN QING YIN

Separate Pure from Impure Powder

Bei Xie	Dioscorea	6 - 9 g
Yi Yi Ren	Coix	12 - 15 g
Wu Yao	Lindera	6 - 9 g
Shi Chang Pu	Acorus	6 - 9 g
Fu Ling	Poria	6 - 9 g
Chen Pi	Citrus	3 - 6 g
Gan Cao	Glycyrrhiza	3 - 6 g

Kidney qi/yin deficiency causing irregular periods, leukorrhea, or a bearing-down sensation.

T   red, thin white coat

P   weak, especially the chi (third) positions

GU YIN JIAN

Stabilize the Yin Decoction

Shu Di Huang	Rehmannia	6 - 12 g
Shan Yao	Dioscorea	6 - 9 g
Wu Wei Zi	Schisandra	6 - 9 g
Shan Zhu Yu	Cornus	6 - 9 g
Tu Si Zi	Cuscuta	6 - 9 g
Ren Shen	Panax	6 - 9 g
Yuan Zhi	Polygala	3 g
Zhi Gan Cao	Glycyrrhiza	3 - 6 g

Damp heat leukorrhea with low back pain, heat sensation along the leg, or eczema.

T   red, sticky yellow coat

P   wiry, rapid, slippery

JIA WEI ER MIAO SAN

Augmented Two-Marvel Powder

Huang Bai	Phellodendron	6 - 12 g
Cang Zhu	Atractylodes	9 - 15 g
Dang Gui Wei	Angelica	6 - 9 g
Bei Xie	Dioscorea	6 - 9 g
Han Fang Ji	Stephania	6 - 9 g
Chuan Niu Xi	Cyathula	6 - 9 g
Gui Ban	Chinemys	6 - 9 g

White turbid leukorrhea due to cold and deficiency in the lower jiao. This formula is also useful for spermatorrhea.

T pale

P weak

☞ This formula should be decocted twice. Stew tea into a thick paste. It should be taken on an empty stomach with three tablespoons of boiling water.

JIN YING GAO

Rosa Paste

Jin Ying Zi	Rosa	60 g
Ren Shen	Panax	60 g
Sang Piao Xiao	Paratenodera	60 g
Shan Yao	Dioscorea	60 g
Du Zhong	Eucommia	60 g
Yi Zhi Ren	Alpinia	30 g
Yi Yi Ren	Coix	30 g
Wu Zhu Yu	Evodia	30 g
Qian Shi	Euryale	30 g
Gou Qi Zi	Lycium	120 g
no pinyin name	Sodium Chloride	9 g

Black colored leukorrhea due to severe heat with abdominal pain, dysurea, genital swelling, thirst, increased appetite; purgative.

T very red, dry, sticky yellow coat

P rapid

✗ Caution during pregnancy

LI HUO TANG

Move Fire Decoction

Da Huang	Rheum	9 g
Bai Zhu	Atractylodes	15 g
Fu Ling	Poria	9 g
Che Qian Zi	Plantago	9 g
Huang Lian	Coptis	3 g
Zhi Zi	Gardenia	9 g
Bei Mu	Fritillaria	6 g
Wang Bu Liu Xing	Vaccaria	9 g

Damp heat in the lower jiao, or Liver fire. Symptoms include red and itchy eyes, temple headaches, odorous leukorrhea, or pruritus.

T red, sticky yellow coating

P wiry, rapid, slippery

LONG DAN XIE GAN TANG

Gentiana Decoction to Drain the Liver

Extract Formula Name: Gentiana Combination

Long Dan Cao	Gentiana	6 - 9 g
Zhi Zi	Gardenia	3 - 9 g
Mu Tong	Akebia	6 - 9 g
Huang Qin	Scutellaria	6 - 9 g
Ze Xie	Alisma	6 - 9 g
Che Qian Zi	Plantago	6 - 9 g
Dang Gui	Angelica	6 - 9 g
Sheng Di Huang	Rehmannia	6 - 12 g
Chai Hu	Bupleurum	6 - 9 g
Gan Cao	Glycyrrhiza	3 - 6 g

Kidney qi deficiency causing white leukorrhea.

T thin white coat

P weak

NEI BU WAN

Internal Tonification Pill

Lu Rong	Cervus	1 - 3 g
Rou Cong Rong	Cistanche	6 - 9 g
Tu Si Zi	Cuscuta	6 - 9 g
Huang Qi	Astralagus	6 -15 g
Rou Gui	Cinnamomum	6 - 9 g
Fu Zi	Aconitum	3 - 6 g
Sha Yuan Ji Li	Astragalus	6 - 9 g
Zi Wan	Aster	6 - 9 g
Sang Piao Xiao	Paratenodera	6 - 9 g

Phlegm damp leading to infertility or leukorrhea.

T   thick sticky white coat

P   slippery or soggy

QI GONG WAN

Open Uterus Pill

Ban Xia	Pinellia	6 - 9 g
Fu Ling	Poria	6 - 9 g
Cang Zhu	Atractylodes	6 - 9 g
Shen Qu	Massa Fermentata	6 - 12 g
Chen Pi	Citrus	3 - 6 g
Xiang Fu	Cyperus	6 - 9 g
Chuan Xiong	Ligusticum	3 - 6 g

Blood deficiency with deficient or excess heat causing purple menstrual blood, early periods, or thick leukorrhea with tidal fever.

T   pale

P   rapid, thin, weak

QIN LIAN SI WU TANG

Four-Substance Decoction with Scutellaria and Coptis

Huang Qin	Scutellaria	6 - 9 g
Huang Lian	Coptis	3 - 6 g
Chuan Xiong	Ligusticum	3 - 6 g
Bai Shao Yao	Paeonia	6 - 9 g
Dang Gui	Angelica	6 - 9 g
Mai Men Dong	Ophiopogon	6 - 9 g
Sheng Di Huang	Rehmannia	9 - 12 g

Spleen qi deficiency causing thin, clear or reddish leukorrhea, with low back pain.

T   pale, thin white coat

P   deep, thin, slippery

QING DAI TANG

Clear Discharge Decoction

Shan Yao	Dioscorea	9 - 30 g
Mu Li	Ostrea	9 - 15 g
Long Gu	Os Draconis	9 - 15 g
Qian Cao Gen	Rubia	6 - 9 g
Hai Piao Xiao	Sepia	9 - 12 g

Liver qi stagnation overacting on Spleen. This leads to damp which in turn heats up and then causes red leukorrhea. Or, the Liver fails to store the blood which also manifests as red leukorrhea.

T purple or pale

P wiry, or weak, thin

☞ E Jiao - Equus should be dissolved into the strained tea.

QING GAN ZHI LIN TANG

Clear Liver and Stop Leukorrhea Decoction

Bai Shao Yao	Paeonia	30 g
Dang Gui	Angelica	30 g
Shu Di Huang	Rehmannia	15 g
E Jiao	Equus	9 g
Mu Dan Pi	Paeonia	9 g
Huang Bai	Phellodendron	6 g
Huai Niu Xi	Achyranthes	6 g
Xiang Fu	Cyperus	3 g
Da Zao	Ziziphus	7 - 10 pc
no pinyin name	Small Black beans	30 g

Damp heat obstruction causing dysmenorrhea, pain prior to onset of the menstruation, cramps, or leukorrhea.

T light purple or red, thick sticky yellow coat

P slippery, slightly rapid, or wiry

QING RE GU JING TANG II

Clear Heat and Stabilize Menses Decoction II

Huang Bai	Phellodendron	6 - 9 g
Huang Lian	Coptis	3 - 9 g
Mu Dan Pi	Paeonia	6 - 12 g
Sheng Di Huang	Rehmannia	6 - 12 g
Dang Gui	Angelica	6 - 9 g
Chi Shao Yao	Paeonia	6 - 9 g
Chuan Xiong	Ligusticum	3 - 9 g
Yan Hu Suo	Corydalis	6 - 9 g

Yellow leukorrhea with dark yellow urination from heat and damp in the lower jiao.

T red, sticky yellowish coat

P slippery, rapid

QING XIN LIAN ZI YIN

Clear the Heart with Lotus Seed Decoction

Extract Formula Name: Lotus Seed Combination

Huang Qin	Scutellaria	6 - 9 g
Mai Men Dong	Ophiopogon	6 - 9 g
Ren Shen	Panax	6 - 9 g
Huang Qi	Astragalus	6 - 15g
Di Gu Pi	Lycium	6 - 9 g
Che Qian Zi	Plantago	6 - 9 g
Lian Zi	Nelumbo	3 - 9 g
Chai Hu	Bupleurum	6 - 9 g
Fu Ling	Poria	6 - 9 g

Trichomonas due to damp. External wash only!

T not important

P not important

☞ Herbs should be ground into a powder, then prepared as a draft.

✗ For external use only.

SHE CHUANG ZI SAN

Cnidium Powder

She Chuang Zi	Cnidium	9 - 15 g
Bai Bu	Stemona	9 - 15 g
Chuan Jiao	Zanthoxylum	9 - 15 g
Ming Fan	Alumen	9 - 15 g
Ku Shen	Sophora	9 - 15 g

Leukorrhea or cloudy spermatorrhea due to Kidney yang deficiency.

T pale

P frail

SHUI LU ER XIAN DAN

Water and Earth Immortals Special Pill

Qian Shi	Euryale	10 g
Jin Ying Zi	Rosa	10 g

External cold causing stagnation in the Liver channel. This leads to testicle pain and swelling in men, or to clear leukorrhea in women.

T   pale, purple, thin white coat

P   slow, wiry, or tight

☞ Ba Dou - Croton and Chuan Lian Zi - Melia should be dry fried for 5 - 10 minutes. Discard Ba Dou, then decoct as usual. This way the effect of Chuan Lian Zi is to actually warm the Liver channel.

TIAN TAI WU YAO SAN

Top-Quality Lindera Powder

Wu Yao	Lindera	6 - 9 g
Xiao Hui Xiang	Foeniculum	3 - 6 g
Gao Liang Jiang	Alpinia	3 - 6 g
Mu Xiang	Saussurea	3 - 6 g
Qing Pi	Citrus	3 - 6 g
Chuan Lian Zi	Melia	6 - 9 g
Bing Lang	Areca	6 - 9 g
Ba Dou	Croton	6 - 15 g

Spleen qi deficiency with Liver qi stagnation causing leukorrhea. The discharge is thin, watery, or white. Other symptoms include loose stools, poor appetite, and possible irritability.

T   pale, light purple, swollen, sticky white coat

P   slippery, slow

WAN DAI TANG

End Discharge Decoction

Bai Zhu	Atractylodes	20 - 30 g
Cang Zhu	Atractylodes	3 - 6 g
Shan Yao	Dioscorea	20 - 30 g
Chen Pi	Citrus	3 - 6 g
Bai Shao Yao	Paeonia	6 - 12 g
Chai Hu	Bupleurum	3 - 6 g
Jing Jie	Schizonepeta	6 - 9 g
Che Qian Zi	Plantago	6 - 9 g
Ren Shen	Panax	6 - 9 g
Gan Cao	Glycyrrhiza	3 - 6 g

Spleen qi deficiency with damp and watery leukorrhea, edema, or cramping pain. Other symptoms include loose stools, and urinary retention.

T   sticky white coat

P   weak, slippery

WEI LING TANG

Calm the Stomach and Poria Decoction

Extract Formula Name: Magnolia and Hoelen Combination

Ze Xie	Alisma	6 - 12 g
Zhu Ling	Polyporus	6 - 9 g
Fu Ling	Poria	6 - 9 g
Bai Zhu	Atractylodes	3 - 9 g
Gui Zhi	Cinnamomum	3 - 9 g
Hou Po	Magnolia	6 - 12 g
Cang Zhu	Atractylodes	3 - 9 g
Chen Pi	Citrus	3 - 6 g
Sheng Jiang	Zingiber	3 - 6 g
Da Zao	Ziziphus	3 - 6 pc
Gan Cao	Glycyrrhiza	3 - 6 g

Trichomonas infection: damp heat causing yellow, odorous leukorrhea, and severe itching.

T   red, sticky yellow coat

P   rapid, slippery

WU MEI YIN CHEN TANG

Mume and Artemisia Yinchenhao Decoction

Wu Mei	Prunus	20 - 30 g
Yin Chen Hao	Artemisia	9 - 15 g
Chuan Jiao	Zanthoxylum	6 - 9 g
Jin Yin Hua	Lonicera	6 - 12 g
Bian Xu	Polygonum	6 - 9 g
Bai Zhu	Atractylodes	6 - 9 g
Fu Ling	Poria	6 - 15 g
Long Dan Cao	Gentiana	6 - 9 g
Huang Bai	Phellodendron	6 - 9 g

Spleen qi deficiency causing damp which heats up. This leads to heat type leukorrhea with a fishy smell, or delayed periods from qi and blood deficiency.

T   pale, thin sticky yellow or white coat

P   slippery, weak

YI HUANG TANG

Change Yellow (Discharge) Decoction

Shan Yao	Dioscorea	9 - 30 g
Huang Bai	Phellodendron	6 - 9 g
Qian Shi	Euryale	9 - 30 g
Bai Guo	Gingko	6 - 10 pc
Che Qian Zi	Plantago	3 - 6 g

Kidney qi deficiency leading to spermatorrhea, or white leukorrhea in women.

T   pale or normal color, thin white coat

P   weak

YI YUAN JIAN

Benefit the Source Decoction

Yuan Zhi	Polygala	3 g
Shan Yao	Dioscorea	6 g
Qian Shi	Euryale	6 g
Suan Zao Ren	Ziziphus	6 g
Bai Zhu	Atractylodes	4.5 g
Fu Ling	Poria	4.5 g
Ren Shen	Panax	3 - 6 g
Wu Wei Zi	Schisandra	14 pc
Jin Ying Zi	Rosa	6 g
Gan Cao	Glycyrrhiza	3 g

Damp accumulation draining downward leading to clear white leukorrhea.

T   swollen, thick white coat

P   slippery

YI ZHI TANG

Boosting Wisdom Decoction

Bai Zhu	Atractylodes	9 g
Fu Ling	Poria	9 g
Chen Pi	Citrus	6 g
Cang Zhu	Atractylodes	6 g
Yi Yi Ren	Coix	6 g
Chai Hu	Bupleurum	6 g
Sheng Ma	Cimicifuga	2 g
Zhi Gan Cao	Glycyrrhiza	3 g

Damp heat accumulation causing leukorrhea which smells fishy and is thick, yellow, or reddish.

T   red, sticky yellow coat

P   rapid, slippery

☞ Herbs should be ground and made into pills of 3 g with glutenous rice. Take 2 - 3 pills once or twice daily. Huang Bai - Phellodendron and Gao Liang Jiang - Alpinia should both be charred.

YU DAI WAN

Cure Discharge Pill

Bai Shao Yao	Paeonia	20 - 30 g
Chun Pi	Ailanthus	60 - 90 g
Huang Bai	Phellodendron	9 - 12 g
Gao Liang Jiang	Alpinia	9 - 18 g

Damp heat accumulation leading to leukorrhea. The discharge is very odorous, yellow, thick, and may be profuse.

T   red, thick yellow sticky coat

P   slippery, rapid

ZHI DAI TANG

Stop Leukorrhea Decoction

Fu Ling	Poria	6 - 9 g
Zhu Ling	Polyporus	6 - 9 g
Ze Xie	Alisma	6 - 9 g
Che Qian Zi	Plantago	3 - 9 g
Yin Chen Hao	Artemisia	15 g
Zhi Zi	Gardenia	3 - 6 g
Huang Bai	Phellodendron	3 - 9 g
Mu Dan Pi	Paeonia	6 - 12 g
Chi Shao Yao	Paeonia	6 - 9 g
Huai Niu Xi	Achyranthes	3 - 6 g

OB-GYN/PREGNANCY DISORDERS AND INFERTILITY

- spotting during pregnancy
- threatened miscarriage
- infertility

T depends on involved syndrome

P depends on involved syndrome

Late periods due to yang deficiency or cold in the uterus. This formula is also useful during pregnancy to warm the uterus.

T pale, white coat

P frail

☞ Herbs should be ground into a powder and made into 6 g pills with rice vinegar.

AI FU NUAN GONG WAN

Mugwort and Aconite Pill for Warming the Womb

Ai Ye	Artemisia	60 - 90 g
Xiang Fu	Cyperus	150 - 180 g
Wu Zhu Yu	Evodia	40 - 60 g
Bai Shao Yao	Paeonia	40 - 60 g
Huang Qi	Astragalus	40 - 60 g
Dang Gui	Angelica	60 - 90 g
Xu Duan	Dipsacus	30 - 45 g
Shu Di Huang	Rehmannia	15 - 30 g
Chuan Xiong	Ligusticum	40 - 60 g
Rou Gui	Cinnamomum	9 - 15 g

Kidney/Liver yin deficiency with blood deficiency causing post-partum sweating, or night sweats.

T red, thin yellow coat

P thin, rapid

BA WEI DI HUANG WAN

Eight-Ingredient Pill with Rehmannia

Sheng Di Huang	Rehmannia	6 - 12 g
Shan Zhu Yu	Cornus	6 - 9 g
Shan Yao	Dioscorea	6 - 9 g
Fu Ling	Poria	6 - 9 g
Ze Xie	Alisma	6 - 9 g
Mu Dan Pi	Paeonia	6 - 9 g
Wu Wei Zi	Schisandra	6 - 9 g
Huang Qi	Astragalus	9 - 15 g

Qi and blood deficiency with blood stagnation. This formula is for a restless fetus, infertility, irregular periods, poor appetite, weakness, or fatigue.

T pale, thin white coat

P weak, maybe wiry

BA ZHEN YI MU WAN

Eight-Treasure Pill to Benefit Mothers

Shu Di Huang	Rehmannia	6 - 15 g
Chuan Xiong	Ligusticum	3 - 9 g
Dang Gui	Angelica	6 - 9 g
Bai Shao Yao	Paeonia	6 - 12 g
Ren Shen	Panax	6 - 12 g
Bai Zhu	Atractylodes	3 - 9 g
Fu Ling	Poria	6 - 9 g
Yi Mu Cao	Leonurus	6 - 18 g
Gan Cao	Glycyrrhiza	3 - 6 g

Spleen qi deficiency causing morning sickness, a restless fetus, loose stools, or poor appetite.

T pale, swollen, white coat

P weak

BAO TAI ZI SHENG WAN

Protect the Fetus and Aid Life Pill

Ren Shen	Panax	6 - 9 g
Fu Ling	Poria	6 - 9 g
Bai Zhu	Atractylodes	6 - 9 g
Gan Cao	Glycyrrhiza	3 - 6 g
Lian Zi	Nelumbo	6 - 9 g
Bian Dou	Dolichos	6 - 9 g
Huo Xiang	Agastache	6 - 9 g
Bai Dou Kou	Amomum	3 - 6 g
Chen Pi	Citrus	3 - 6 g
Jie Geng	Platycodon	3 - 6 g
Shan Yao	Dioscorea	6 - 9 g
Yi Yi Ren	Coix	6 - 12 g
Ze Xie	Alisma	6 - 9 g
Mai Ya	Hordeum	12 - 20 g
Qian Shi	Euryale	6 - 9 g
Shan Zha	Crataegus	6 - 12 g
Huang Lian	Coptis	3 g

Post-partum abdominal pain of the deficiency type after qi and blood loss from giving birth.

T pale

P frail

☞ E Jiao - Equus should be added to the strained tea.

CHANG NING TANG

Intestinal Serenity Decoction

Shu Di Huang	Rehmannia	6 - 12 g
Dang Gui	Angelica	6 - 12 g
Mai Men Dong	Ophiopogon	6 - 9 g
Ren Shen	Panax	6 - 9 g
Xu Duan	Dipsacus	6 - 9 g
Rou Gui	Cinnamomum	3 g
E Jiao	Equus	6 - 9 g
Shan Yao	Dioscorea	6 - 9 g
Gan Cao	Glycyrrhiza	3 - 6 g

Kidney yin and Spleen qi/blood deficiency causing uterine prolapse with low back pain, night urination, or hearing loss and tinnitus.

T red or pale

P frail

DA BU YUAN JIAN

Great Tonify the Basal Decoction

Ren Shen	Panax	6 - 12 g
Shu Di Huang	Rehmannia	9 - 25 g
Shan Yao	Dioscorea	6 - 9 g
Shan Zhu Yu	Cornus	3 - 6 g
Gou Qi Zi	Lycium	6 - 9 g
Dang Gui	Angelica	6 - 9 g
Du Zhong	Eucommia	6 - 9 g
Gan Cao	Glycyrrhiza	3 - 6 g

Spleen qi and blood deficiency with slight cold leading to spasm pain or post-partum emaciation.

T   pale, white coat

P   weak

☞ Yi Tang - Saccharum Granorum is added to the strained tea.

DANG GUI JIAN ZHONG TANG

Dang Gui Decoction to Construct the Middle

Extract Formula Name: Tang-Kuei, Cinnamon and Peony Combination

Yi Tang	Saccharum Granorum	6 - 20 g
Gui Zhi	Cinnamomum	3 - 9 g
Bai Shao Yao	Paeonia	6 - 9 g
Sheng Jiang	Zingiber	3 - 6 g
Da Zao	Ziziphus	3 - 6 pc
Gan Cao	Glycyrrhiza	3 - 6 g
Dang Gui	Angelica	6 - 9 g

Spleen qi and blood deficiency with yin deficiency and restless fetus. This prescription can be taken as a preventative during pregnancy.

T   pale or red

P   thin, weak

DANG GUI SAN

Dang Gui Powder

Extract Formula Name: Tang-Kuei Formula

Dang Gui	Angelica	6 - 12 g
Huang Qin	Scutellaria	6 - 12 g
Chuan Xiong	Ligusticum	3 g
Bai Zhu	Atractylodes	3 - 9 g
Bai Shao Yao	Paeonia	6 - 9 g

Liver overacting on Spleen causing mild cramping in the abdomen with Liver blood deficiency and some damp accumulation. Symptoms include urinary retention and lower body edema. This is often seen during pregnancy.

T   pale, orange color on the sides

P   weak, thin, or slightly wiry

DANG GUI SHAO YAO SAN

Dang Gui and Peony Powder

Extract Formula Name: Tang-Kuei and Peony Formula

Dang Gui	Angelica	6 - 9 g
Bai Shao Yao	Paeonia	3 - 9 g
Bai Zhu	Atractylodes	3 - 9 g
Fu Ling	Poria	6 - 9 g
Chuan Xiong	Ligusticum	3 - 6 g
Ze Xie	Alisma	6 - 9 g

Internal Medicine, Misc. Syndromes

Blood deficiency with external cold after childbirth. This leads to spasms or hernia pain which are both relieved by pressure.

T pale

P deep, wiry, weak

☞ This formula should be prepared as a stew with eight cups of water. Simmer until it is reduced to three to four cups.

DANG GUI SHENG JIANG YANG ROU TANG

Mutton Stew with Dang Gui and Fresh Ginger Decoction

Dang Gui	Angelica	9 - 12 g
Sheng Jiang	Zingiber	9 - 15 g
Yang Rou	Mutton	40 - 50 g

Spleen/Stomach qi deficiency and cold causing vomiting during pregnancy.

T pale, thin white coat

P weak

GAN JIANG REN SHEN BAN XIA WAN

Ginger, Ginseng, and Pinellia Pill

Extract Formula Name: G.P. and Ginseng Formula

Gan Jiang	Zingiber	3 g
Ren Shen	Panax	3 g
Ban Xia	Pinellia	6 g
[Sheng Jiang	Zingiber	1 - 3 g]

Spleen qi deficiency during pregnancy with lethargy, spotting, or low back pain.

T pale, swollen, teethmarks, thin white coat

P weak, thin

☞ E Jiao - Equus should be added at the end to the strained tea.

JIA JIAN BU ZHONG YI QI TANG

Modified Tonify the Middle and Augment the Qi Decoction

Ren Shen	Panax	6 - 9 g
Huang Qi	Astragalus	6 - 12 g
Chen Pi	Citrus	3 - 6 g
Bai Zhu	Atractylodes	3 - 9 g
Sheng Ma	Cimicifuga	3 - 6 g
Chai Hu	Bupleurum	3 - 9 g
E Jiao	Equus	3 - 9 g
Ai Ye	Artemisia	3 - 9 g
Gan Cao	Glycyrrhiza	3 - 6 g

Chong and Ren imbalance with blood deficiency causing restless fetus, pale post-partum bleeding, abdominal pain, a weak low back, or a cold uterus.

T pale

P frail, slow

☞ E Jiao - Equus should be dissolved at the end into the strained tea.

JIAO AI TANG

Ass-Hide Equus and Mugwort Decoction

Extract Formula Name: Tang-kuei and Equus Combination

E Jiao	Equus	6 - 9 g
Ai Ye	Artemisia	6 - 9 g
Dang Gui	Angelica	6 - 9 g
Sheng Di Huang	Rehmannia	18 g
Bai Shao Yao	Paeonia	12 g
Chuan Xiong	Ligusticum	6 g
Gan Cao	Glycyrrhiza	3 - 6 g

Spleen qi deficiency causing severe uterine bleeding which is pale in color, or early or irregular periods. The Spleen qi is sinking causing a restless fetus.

T pale, swollen, teethmarks, thin white coat

P weak

JU YUAN JIAN

Lift the Source Decoction

Ren Shen	Panax	6 - 9 g
Huang Qi	Astragalus	9 - 12 g
Sheng Ma	Cimicifuga	3 - 6 g
Bai Zhu	Atractylodes	3 - 6 g
Gan Cao	Glycyrrhiza	3 - 6 g

Phlegm damp leading to infertility or leukorrhea.

T thick sticky white coat

P slippery or soggy

QI GONG WAN

Open Uterus Pill

Ban Xia	Pinellia	6 - 9 g
Fu Ling	Poria	6 - 9 g
Cang Zhu	Atractylodes	6 - 9 g
Shen Qu	Massa Fermentata	6 - 12 g
Chen Pi	Citrus	3 - 6 g
Xiang Fu	Cyperus	6 - 9 g
Chuan Xiong	Ligusticum	3 - 6 g

Internal Medicine, Misc. Syndromes

Post-partum retention of lochia due to blood and cold stagnation.

T pale, purple

P choppy

☞ Add yellow wine to the decoction.

SHENG HUA TANG

Generation and Transformation Decoction

Extract Formula Name: Tang-Kuei and Ginger Combination

Dang Gui	Angelica	15 - 28 g
Tao Ren	Prunus	6 - 9 g
Pao Jiang	Zingiber	3 - 6 g
Chuan Xiong	Ligusticum	6 - 9 g
Gan Cao	Glycyrrhiza	3 - 6 g

Kidney qi deficiency causing a restless fetus with spotting, threatened miscarriage, or frequent urination.

T pale

P frail

☞ E Jiao - Equus should be dissolved in water and used to form the other herbs into 6 g pills .

SHOU TAI WAN

Fetus Longevity Pill

Loranthus and Cuscuta Combination

E Jiao	Equus	30
Sang Ji Sheng	Loranthus	30 g
Tu Si Zi	Cuscuta	60 g
Xu Duan	Dipsacus	30 g

Spleen qi/blood deficiency during pregnancy causing restless fetus, or use formula if the woman has a history of miscarriage or infertility.

T pale, thin white coat

P weak, thin, slippery

TAI SHAN PAN SHI WAN

Powder that Gives the Stability of Mount Tai

Ren Shen	Panax	6 - 9 g
Huang Qi	Astragalus	12 - 15 g
Shu Di Huang	Rehmannia	9 - 12 g
Chuan Xiong	Ligusticum	3 - 6 g
Bai Zhu	Atractylodes	9 - 12 g
Sha Ren	Amomum	1 - 3 g
Huang Qin	Scutellaria	6 - 9 g
Xu Duan	Dipsacus	3 - 6 g
Bai Shao Yao	Paeonia	6 - 9 g
Zhi Gan Cao	Glycyrrhiza	3 - 6 g
Nuo Mi	Glutinous Oryza	3 - 6 g

Kidney qi deficiency causing infertility, urinary frequency, or incontinence.

T pale or normal color, thin white coat

P weak

☞ For infertility and a stronger qi and blood tonifying effect add 'Dang Gui Bu Xue Tang - Dang Gui Decoction to Tonify the Blood' and 'Si Jun Zi Tang - Four-Gentlemen Decoction.'

WU ZI YAN ZONG WAN

Five-Seeds Normalizing Pill

Wu Wei Zi	Schisandra	6 - 12 g
Fu Pen Zi	Rubus	6 - 9 g
Tu Si Zi	Cuscuta	6 - 9 g
Che Qian Zi	Plantago	6 - 9 g
Gou Qi Zi	Lycium	6 - 12 g

Spleen/Stomach qi deficiency with qi stagnation and cold damp in the middle jiao causing abdominal fullness or morning sickness.

T pale, light purple, swollen, sticky white coat

P slippery, weak

XIANG SHA LIU JUN ZI TANG

Six-Gentlemen Decoction with Aucklandia and Amomum

Extract Formula Name: Saussurea and Cardamon Combination

Ren Shen	Panax	6 - 9 g
Fu Ling	Poria	6 - 9 g
Bai Zhu	Atractylodes	3 - 9 g
Chen Pi	Citrus	3 - 6 g
Ban Xia	Pinellia	6 - 9 g
Sha Ren	Amomum	3 g
Mu Xiang	Saussurea	3 - 6 g
Zhi Gan Cao	Glycyrrhiza	3 - 6 g

Pronounced wind cold with mild qi stagnation, or wind cold invasion during pregnancy.

T thin white coat

P superficial, tight

XIANG SU CONG CHI TANG

Cyperus, Perilla Leaf, Scallion, and Prepared Soybean Decoction

Zi Su Ye	Perilla	6 - 9 g
Xiang Fu	Cyperus	6 - 9 g
Cong Bai	Allium	2 - 4 pc
Dan Dou Chi	Glycine	9 - 12 g
Chen Pi	Citrus	3 - 6 g
Zhi Gan Cao	Glycyrrhiza	3 - 6 g

Internal Medicine, Misc. Syndromes

Kidney yang and essence deficiency causing amenorrhea, infertility, cold back or knees, pedal edema, or impotence.

T pale, swollen, teethmarks, thin white coat

P minute

YOU GUI WAN

Restore the Right Pill

Extract Formula Name: Eucommia and Rehmannia Formula

Rou Gui	Cinnamomum	6 - 9 g
Fu Zi	Aconitum	3 - 6 g
Gou Qi Zi	Lycium	6 - 9 g
Shan Yao	Dioscorea	6 - 9 g
Shu Di Huang	Rehmannia	12 - 20 g
Shan Zhu Yu	Cornus	6 - 9 g
Du Zhong	Eucommia	6 - 9 g
Dang Gui	Angelica	6 - 9 g
Tu Si Zi	Cuscuta	6 - 9 g
Lu Jiao Jiao	Cervus	6 - 9 g

Infertility due to Kidney qi deficiency.

T normal color or pale, thin white coat

P weak, especially in both chi (third) positions

YU LIN WAN

Nourish Cute Animal Pill

Lu Jiao Shuang	Cervus	6 - 9 g
Tu Si Zi	Cuscuta	6 - 9 g
Du Zhong	Eucommia	6 - 12 g
Chuan Jiao	Zanthoxylum	3 - 6 g
Zi He Che	Placenta Hominis	3 - 9 g
Xiang Fu	Cyperus	6 - 9 g

Impotence or infertility due to Kidney yang deficiency with simultaneous qi and blood deficiency. Symptoms include blurry vision, low back pain, and poor memory.

T   pale, thin white coat

P   frail

ZAN YU DAN

Special Pill to Aid Fertility

Rou Cong Rong	Cistanche	6 - 12 g
Fu Zi	Aconitum	6 g
Ba Ji Tian	Morinda	6 - 12 g
Rou Gui	Cinnamomum	6 g
She Chuang Zi	Cnidium	6 g
Xian Mao	Curculigo	6 - 12 g
Dang Gui	Angelica	9 - 15 g
Bai Zhu	Atractylodes	12 - 18 g
Gou Qi Zi	Lycium	9 - 15 g
Yin Yang Huo	Epimedium	6 - 12 g
Shan Zhu Yu	Cornus	6 - 12 g
Shu Di Huang	Rehmannia	6 - 12 g
Jiu Zi	Allium	6 - 12 g
Du Zhong	Eucommia	6 - 12 g

Liver/Kidney yin and jing (essence) deficiency causing slow development in children; or premature aging in adults, in addition to common yin deficiency signs and symptoms. The formula is also for early menopause, spermatorrhea, low sex drive, infertility, or low sperm count.

T   red, scanty coat

P   thin, rapid

ZUO GUI YIN

Restore the Left [Kidney] Decoction

Shu Di Huang	Rehmannia	6 - 15 g
Shan Zhu Yu	Cornus	6 - 9 g
Shan Yao	Dioscorea	6 - 9 g
Gou Qi Zi	Lycium	6 - 9 g
Fu Ling	Poria	6 - 9 g
Zhi Gan Cao	Glycyrrhiza	3 - 6 g

Internal Medicine, Misc. Syndromes

WIND DAMP BI - SYNDROME

- joint pain
- joint deformities
- heaviness
- numbness or paralysis in the extremities

T   sticky coat

P   slippery

Damp heat febrile disease or damp bi-syndrome with heat causing severe sweating and joint pain with swelling and redness. Joints feel hot to the touch.

T   red, sticky yellow coat

P   slippery, rapid, or flooding

☞ Decoct the first four herbs, then add the rice at the end. It will absorb the water to make a thick liquid.

BAI HU JIA CANG ZHU TANG

White Tiger plus Atractylodes Decoction

Shi Gao	Gypsum	20 - 30 g
Zhi Mu	Anemarrhena	9 - 12 g
Gan Cao	Glycyrrhiza	3 - 6 g
Cang Zhu	Atractylodes	3 - 9 g
Jing Mi	Oryza	15 - 30 g

Heat in the yangming channel with slight external cold and damp causing obstruction in the channels which leads to joint pain.

T   red, yellow coat

P   rapid, wiry

☞ Decoct the first four herbs, then add the rice at the end. It will absorb the water to make a thick liquid.

BAI HU JIA GUI ZHI TANG

White Tiger plus Cinnamon Twig Decoction

Shi Gao	Gypsum	20 - 30 g
Zhi Mu	Anemarrhena	9 - 12 g
Gan Cao	Glycyrrhiza	3 - 9 g
Gui Zhi	Cinnamomum	3 - 9 g
Jing Mi	Oryza	15 - 30 g

Dysentery weakens the legs severely causing difficulty walking; or wind invades the knees causing atrophy in the legs with severe swelling and pain in one or both knees.

T pale, sticky coat

P slippery

DA FANG FENG TANG

Major Ledebouriella Decoction

Extract Formula Name: Major Siler Combination

Fu Zi	Aconitum	6 - 9 g
Chuan Xiong	Ligusticum	6 - 9 g
Fang Feng	Ledebouriella	6 - 12 g
Shu Di Huang	Rehmannia	6 - 12 g
Qiang Huo	Notopterygium	6 - 12 g
Bai Shao Yao	Paeonia	6 - 12 g
Dang Gui	Angelica	6 - 12 g
Bai Zhu	Atractylodes	3 - 9 g
Huang Qi	Astragalus	6 - 12 g
Ren Shen	Panax	3 - 9 g
Du Zhong	Eucommia	6 - 12 g
Huai Niu Xi	Achyranthes	3 - 9 g
Gan Jiang	Zingiber	3 g
Da Zao	Ziziphus	1 - 3 pc
Zhi Gan Cao	Glycyrrhiza	3 - 6 g

External wind attacks the channels where there is an underlying qi and blood deficiency. Wind cold changes to heat causing chronic hemiplegia, spasms, numbness and pain, or slurred speech.

T red, yellow coat, deviated

P wiry, rapid

DA QIN JIAO TANG

Major Gentiana Qinjiao Decoction

Qin Jiao	Gentiana	9 - 12 g
Chuan Xiong	Ligusticum	6 - 9 g
Dang Gui	Angelica	6 - 9 g
Bai Shao Yao	Paeonia	6 - 9 g
Shu Di Huang	Rehmannia	9 - 15 g
Sheng Di Huang	Rehmannia	9 - 15 g
Fu Ling	Poria	6 - 9 g
Bai Zhu	Atractylodes	6 - 9 g
Qiang Huo	Notopterygium	6 - 9 g
Du Huo	Angelica	6 - 9 g
Fang Feng	Ledebouriella	6 - 9 g
Bai Zhi	Angelica	3 - 6 g
Xi Xin	Asarum	3 - 6 g
Huang Qin	Scutellaria	6 - 12 g
Shi Gao	Gypsum	6 - 9 g
Gan Cao	Glycyrrhiza	3 - 6 g

Heat bi-syndrome: wind damp heat causing redness and heat in the joints, stabbing or severe fullness pain, or restlessness. The symptoms are better with cold weather. This formula is also useful for damp heat skin disorders.

T normal color or red, dry, rough texture, yellow coat

P rapid, superficial, slightly slippery

DANG GUI LIAN TONG TANG

Dang Gui and Anemarrhena Decoction

Extract Formula Name: Tang-Kuei and Anemarrhena Combination

Ren Shen	Panax	6 - 9 g
Huang Qin	Scutellaria	9 - 12 g
Bai Zhu	Atractylodes	6 - 9 g
Cang Zhu	Atractylodes	3 - 9 g
Dang Gui	Angelica	6 - 9 g
Ze Xie	Alisma	6 - 9 g
Zhu Ling	Polyporus	6 - 9 g
Yin Chen Hao	Artemisia	6 - 12 g
Ge Gen	Pueraria	6 - 12 g
Zhi Mu	Anemarrhena	9 - 12 g
Sheng Ma	Cimicifuga	6 - 9 g
Qiang Huo	Notopterygium	6 - 12 g
Fang Feng	Ledebouriella	6 - 12 g
Ku Shen	Sophora	6 - 9 g
Gan Cao	Glycyrrhiza	3 - 6 g

Blood and yin deficient patient with cold evil qi which leads to obstruction of the channels which causes pain. The patient feels cold subjectively and may feel cold to the touch. Raynaud's disease.

T pale, white coat

P deep, thin, or minute

DANG GUI SI NI TANG

Dang Gui Decoction for Frigid Extremities

Extract Formula Name: Tang-Kuei and Jujube Combination

Dang Gui	Angelica	6 - 12 g
Gui Zhi	Cinnamomum	3 - 9 g
Bai Shao Yao	Paeonia	6 - 9 g
Mu Tong	Akebia	6 - 9 g
Xi Xin	Asarum	3 - 6 g
Da Zao	Ziziphus	3 - 5 pc
Gan Cao	Glycyrrhiza	3 - 6 g

Internal Medicine, Misc. Syndromes

Bone bi-syndrome: wind cold damp with Kidney yang deficiency and yin and blood deficiency. Symptoms include chronic joint pain, cold knees, joint deformities, or stiffness or weakness in the joints.

T   pale, thin white coat

P   frail

✪ Major Formula

DU HUO JI SHENG TANG

Angelica Pubescens and Sangjisheng Decoction

Extract Formula Name: Tuhuo and Loranthus Combination

Du Huo	Angelica	6 - 9 g
Sang Ji Sheng	Loranthus	6 - 12 g
Qin Jiao	Gentiana	6 - 9 g
Fang Feng	Ledebouriella	6 - 9 g
Dang Gui	Angelica	6 - 9 g
Rou Gui	Cinnamomum	6 g
Ren Shen	Panax	6 - 9 g
Huai Niu Xi	Achyranthes	6 - 9 g
Du Zhong	Eucommia	6 - 9 g
Sheng Di Huang	Rehmannia	6 - 9 g
Fu Ling	Poria	6 - 9 g
Chuan Xiong	Ligusticum	3 - 6 g
Bai Shao Yao	Paeonia	6 - 9 g
Xi Xin	Asarum	3 - 6 g
Gan Cao	Glycyrrhiza	3 - 6 g

Wind bi-syndrome: wind cold damp causing migrating joint pain.

T pale, sticky white coat, wet

P maybe superficial, slow, slippery

FANG FENG TANG

Ledebouriella Decoction

Fang Feng	Ledebouriella	12 g
Qin Jiao	Gentiana	9 -12 g
Dang Gui	Angelica	6 - 9 g
Fu Ling	Poria	6 - 9 g
Xing Ren	Prunus	6 - 9 g
Qiang Huo	Notopterygium	3 - 6 g
Gui Zhi	Cinnamoum	3 - 6 g
Ge Gen	Pueraria	9 - 12 g
Sheng Jiang	Zingiber	3 - 6 g
Da Zao	Ziziphus	3 - 4 pc
Gan Cao	Glycyrrhiza	3 - 6 g
For the lower limbs add:		
Du Huo	Angelica	6 - 9 g
Huai Niu Xi	Achyranthes	6 - 12 g
Bei Xie	Dioscorea	6 - 9 g
For the upper limbs:		
Bai Zhi	Angelica	6 - 9 g
Wei Ling Xian	Clematis	6 - 9 g
Chuan Xiong	Ligusticum	3 - 9 g
Jiang Huang	Curcuma	6 - 9 g
For the low back add:		
Du Zhong	Eucommia	6 - 12 g
Sang Ji Sheng	Loranthus	6 - 12 g
Xu Duan	Dipsacus	6 - 9 g
Ba Ji Tian	Morinda	6 - 9 g

Severe Kidney yang deficiency where the yang is unable to nourish the limbs leading to edema, and severe body aches with cold and damp symptoms: cold bi-syndrome.

T   pale, moist white coat

P   deep, minute, or choppy

FU ZI TANG

Prepared Aconite Decoction

Extract Formula Name: Aconite Combination

Fu Zi	Aconitum	9 - 15 g
Ren Shen	Panax	3 - 6 g
Fu Ling	Poria	9 - 12 g
Bai Zhu	Atractylodes	3 - 12 g
Bai Shao Yao	Paeonia	6 - 9 g

Chronic wind cold damp causing heat which is worse at night, or joints which are swollen, hot, and painful.

T   sticky white coat

P   slippery, wiry

GUI ZHI SHAO YAO ZHI MU TANG

Cinnamon Twig, Peony, and Anemarrhena Decoction

Extract Formula Name: Cinnamon and Anemarrhena Combination

Gui Zhi	Cinnamomum	9 - 12 g
Bai Shao Yao	Paeonia	9 - 12 g
Zhi Mu	Anemarrhena	9 - 12 g
Ma Huang	Ephedra	3 - 6 g
Bai Zhu	Atractylodes	12 - 15 g
Fu Zi	Aconitum	3 - 6 g
Fang Feng	Ledebouriella	9 - 12 g
Sheng Jiang	Zingiber	12 - 15 g
Gan Cao	Glycyrrhiza	3 - 6 g

Kidney and Liver yin deficiency causing bone bi-syndrome or wei syndrome. Deficient yin cannot nourish tendons and false heat burns tendons and muscles. This leads to atrophy, joint swelling, or deformities. The pain tends to be more fixed.

T   red, scanty coat

P   thin, rapid, weak

☞ All ingredients should be ground up as powder. Take 10 g each time, twice a day.

✪ Major Formula

HU QIAN WAN

Hidden Tiger Pill

Extract Formula Name: Tiger Bone and Tortoise Shell Formula

Gui Ban	Chinemys	120 g
Huang Bai	Phellodendron	150 g
Shu Di Huang	Rehmannia	60 g
Zhi Mu	Anemarrhena	60 g
Bai Shao Yao	Paeonia	60 g
Suo Yang	Cynomorium	45 g
Hu Gu	Panthera	30 g
Chen Pi	Citrus	60 g
Gan Jiang	Zingiber	15 g

Blood stagnation in the channels with a mild wind invasion. This leads to a superficial numbness sensation without pain.

T   purple or pale

P   choppy or tight

HUANG QI GUI ZHI WU WU TANG

Astragalus and Cinnamon Twig Five-Substance Decoction

Extract Formula Name: Astragalus and Cinnamon Five Herb Combination

Huang Qi	Astragalus	9 g
Gui Zhi	Cinnamomum	9 g
Bai Shao Yao	Paeonia	9 g
Sheng Jiang	Zingiber	18 g
Da Zao	Ziziphus	9 - 12 pc

Cold damp stagnation in the channels of the legs causing weakness in the legs, difficulty walking, spasms, numbness, polio, or cold intolerance.

T sticky white coat

P rolling, slow

JI MING SAN

Powder to Take at Cock's Crow

Extract Formula Name: Areca Seed and Chaenomeles Formula

Bing Lang	Areca	15 g
Wu Zhu Yu	Evodia	1 - 3 g
Mu Gua	Chaenomeles	9 g
Chen Pi	Citrus	9 g
Zi Su Ye	Perilla	3 g
Jie Geng	Platycodon	5 g
Sheng Jiang	Zingiber	5 g

Weakness in the extremities with difficulty walking and muscle atrophy due to blood deficiency and damp stagnation.

T pale, sticky coat

P thin, slippery

JIA WEI SI WU TANG

Augmented Four-Substance Decoction

Dang Gui	Angelica	6 - 9 g
Huang Bai	Phellodendron	6 - 9 g
Mai Men Dong	Ophiopogon	6 - 9 g
Shu Di Huang	Rehmannia	9 - 12 g
Cang Zhu	Atractylodes	3 - 9 g
Du Zhong	Eucommia	3 - 6 g
Bai Shao Yao	Paeonia	3 - 9 g
Ren Shen	Panax	3 g
Wu Wei Zi	Schisandra	3 - 6 g
Zhi Mu	Anemarrhena	6 - 9 g
Huai Niu Xi	Achyranthes	3 - 9 g
Huang Lian	Coptis	3 g
Chuan Xiong	Ligusticum	3 - 6 g

Wind damp cold bi-syndrome with qi deficiency leading to numbness, heavy sensation, cold and wind intolerance, slight joint swelling, or acute rheumatic fever.

T pale, thin white coat

P superficial, slightly slow

JUAN BI TANG I

Remove Painful Obstruction Decoction from Selected Formulas

Extract Formula Name: Chianghuo and Turmeric Combination

Qiang Huo	Notopterygium	6 - 15 g
Huang Qi	Astragalus	6 - 15
Dang Gui	Angelica	6 - 12 g
Chi Shao Yao	Paeonia	6 - 12 g
Fang Feng	Ledebouriella	6 - 9 g
Jiang Huang	Curcuma	6 - 9 g
Sheng Jiang	Zingiber	3 - 6 g
Da Zao	Ziziphus	3 - 6 pc
Gan Cao	Glycyrrhiza	3 - 6 g

Wind damp cold bi-syndrome with numbness, heavy sensation, migrating joint pain, or cold and wind intolerance.

T sticky white coat

P slippery, slow

JUAN BI TANG II

Remove Painful Obstruction from Medical Revelations

Qiang Huo	Notopterygium	6 - 12 g
Du Huo	Angelica	6 - 12 g
Sang Zhi	Morus	9 - 18 g
Dang Gui	Angelica	6 - 12 g
Mu Xiang	Saussurea	3 - 9 g
Hai Feng Teng	Piper	9 - 18 g
Gui Zhi	Cinnamomum	6 - 9 g
Qin Jiao	Gentiana	6 - 12 g
Chuan Xiong	Ligusticum	3 - 9 g
Ru Xiang	Boswellia	3 - 6 g
Gan Cao	Glycyrrhiza	3 - 6 g

Wind cold damp with pre-existing internal damp causing muscle aches; or external wind damp cold and internal heat causing intolerance to wind and cold, joint- or bodyaches, lack of sweating, or thirst.

T normal color, or red, thin yellowish coat

P superficial, rapid, maybe slippery

JIU WEI QIANG HUO TANG

Nine-Ingredient Decoction with Notopterygium

Extract Formula Name: Chianghuo Combination

Qiang Huo	Notopterygium	3 - 6 g
Cang Zhu	Atractylodes	3 - 6 g
Xi Xin	Asarum	1 - 3 g
Fang Feng	Ledebouriella	3 - 6 g
Chuan Xiong	Ligusticum	3 - 6 g
Huang Qin	Scutellaria	3 - 9 g
Bai Zhi	Angelica	3 - 6 g
Sheng Di Huang	Rehmannia	3 - 9 g
Gan Cao	Glycyrrhiza	3 - 6 g

Acute wind damp cold lodged in the channels causing acute bi-syndrome. Symptoms include heaviness and pain in the body, belt-type headache, or lack of sweating.

T normal color, thin white coat

P superficial

✪ Major Formula

QIANG HUO SHENG SHI TANG

Notopterygium Decoction to Overcome Dampness

Extract Formula Name: Chianghuo and Vitex Combination

Qiang Huo	Notopterygium	3 - 6 g
Gao Ben	Ligusticum	3 - 6 g
Fang Feng	Ledebouriella	6 - 9 g
Du Huo	Angelica	6 - 9 g
Chuan Xiong	Ligusticum	3 - 9 g
Man Jing Zi	Vitex	3 - 9 g
Gan Cao	Glycyrrhiza	3 - 6 g

Qi and blood stasis with underlying Kidney and Liver yin deficiency and qi/blood deficiency manifesting as wind damp bi-syndrome. Symptoms include tremors and weakness in the extremities.

T pale

P wiry, weak, thin

SAN BI TANG

Three-Painful Obstruction Decoction

Xu Duan	Dipsacus	6 - 9 g
Fang Feng	Ledebouriella	6 - 9 g
Rou Gui	Cinnamomum	6 - 9 g
Dang Gui	Angelica	6 - 9 g
Xi Xin	Asarum	3 g
Fu Ling	Poria	6 - 9 g
Qin Jiao	Gentiana	6 - 9 g
Du Zhong	Eucommia	6 - 9 g
Ren Shen	Panax	3 - 6 g
Huai Niu Xi	Achyranthes	6 - 9 g
Bai Shao Yao	Paeonia	6 - 9 g
Huang Qi	Astragalus	6 - 9 g
Du Huo	Angelica	6 - 9 g
Chuan Xiong	Ligusticum	3 - 9 g
Sheng Di Huang	Rehmannia	6 - 9 g
Gan Cao	Glycyrrhiza	3 - 6 g
Gan Jiang	Zingiber	3 - 6 g

Kidney and Liver yin deficiency with blood deficiency and wind damp. This leads to blurry vision, cough, constipation, or bi-syndrome.

T red, scanty yellow coat

P thin

☞ Herbs should be formed into 9 g pills. Adults take one pill two times a day.

SANG MA WAN

Mulberry Leaf and Sesame Seed Pill

Sang Ye	Morus	250 - 300 g
Hei Zhi Ma	Sesamum	100 - 120 g
Feng Mi	Mel	250 - 300 g

Qi and blood stagnation in the channels causing pain in the extremities or muscles.

T purple

P wiry

SHEN TONG ZHU YU TANG

Drive Out Blood Stasis from a Painful Body Decoction

Chuan Xiong	Ligusticum	3 - 9 g
Tao Ren	Prunus	6 - 9 g
Hong Hua	Carthamus	6 - 9 g
Qin Jiao	Gentiana	6 - 9 g
Qiang Huo	Notopterygium	3 - 6 g
Dang Gui	Angelica	6 - 9 g
Chuan Niu Xi	Cyathula	6 - 12 g
Mo Yao	Commiphora	6 - 9 g
Wu Ling Zhi	Trogopterus	6 - 9 g
Di Long	Pheretima	6 - 9 g
Xiang Fu	Cyperus	3 - 6 g
Gan Cao	Glycyrrhiza	3 - 6 g

Wind damp bi-syndrome with phlegm and blood stagnation causing sharp piercing pain in all joints.

T purple, sticky coat

P wiry, slippery

SHU FENG HUO XUE TANG

Disperse Wind and Invigorate the Blood Decoction

Extract Formula Name: Stephania and Carthamus Combination

Dang Gui	Angelica	6 - 9 g
Han Fang Ji	Stephania	6 - 9 g
Chuan Xiong	Ligusticum	3 - 9 g
Bai Zhi	Angelica	6 - 9 g
Wei Ling Xian	Clematis	3 - 9 g
Cang Zhu	Atractylodes	3 - 9 g
Hong Hua	Carthamus	3 - 9 g
Dan Nan Xing	Arisaema	3 g
Huang Bai	Phellodendron	6 - 9 g
Gui Zhi	Cinnamomum	3 - 9 g
Qiang Huo	Notopterygium	6 - 9 g
Gan Jiang	Zingiber	3 - 6 g

Lower body wind cold damp bi-syndrome with blood stagnation causing low back pain, muscle aches, sciatica, or hemiplegia.

T purple

P wiry, slippery

✗ Do not use during pregnancy.

SHU JING HUO XUE TANG

Relax the Channels and Invigorate the Blood Decoction

Extract Formula Name: Clematis and Stephania Combination

Bai Shao Yao	Paeonia	6 - 9 g
Chuan Xiong	Ligusticum	3 - 9 g
Sheng Di Huang	Rehmannia	6 - 9 g
Dang Gui	Angelica	6 - 9 g
Cang Zhu	Atractylodes	3 - 6 g
Fu Ling	Poria	6 - 9 g
Long Dan Cao	Gentiana	6 - 9 g
Tao Ren	Prunus	3 - 6 g
Wei Ling Xian	Clematis	3 - 6 g
Huai Niu Xi	Achyranthes	6 - 9 g
Qiang Huo	Notopterygium	3 - 6 g
Chen Pi	Citrus	3 - 6 g
Fang Feng	Ledebouriella	6 - 9 g
Han Fang Ji	Stephania	6 - 9 g
Bai Zhi	Angelica	3 - 6 g
Sheng Jiang	Zingiber	3 - 6 g
Gan Cao	Glycyrrhiza	3 - 6 g

Blood stagnation in the head, face, and neck area leading to migraines or cyanotic lips.

T   purple or purple spots

P   wiry or choppy

☞ Decoct all herbs except She Xiang - Moschus for 15 minutes. Add 230 cc of rice wine and let cook for another 5 - 10 minutes, then add powdered She Xiang - Moschus and dissolve into the tea.

✘ Do not use during pregnancy.

TONG QIAO HUO XUE TANG

Unblock the Orifices and Invigorate the Blood Decoction

Extract Formula Name: Persica and Cnidium Combination

Hong Hua	Carthamus	6 - 9 g
Tao Ren	Prunus	6 - 9 g
Chuan Xiong	Ligusticum	3 - 9 g
Chi Shao Yao	Paeonia	6 - 9 g
Cong Bai	Allium	3 - 6 g
She Xiang	Moschus	0.1 - 0.3 g
Da Zao	Ziziphus	3 - 6 pc
Sheng Jiang	Zingiber	3 - 6 g

Severe joint pain due to wind damp cold bi-syndrome with significant pain in the hands and feet.

T   moist, white

P   slow, slippery

☞ Decoct Chuan Wu - Aconitum one hour prior to adding the other herbs. The prepared type of Aconite should be used.

✘ This formula can be somewhat toxic. Caution during pregnancy.

WU TOU TANG

Aconite Decoction

Zhi Chuan Wu	Aconitum	6 - 15 g
Huang Qi	Astragalus	9 - 12 g
Ma Huang	Ephedra	6 - 9 g
Bai Shao Yao	Paeonia	6 - 9 g
Gan Cao	Glycyrrhiza	3 - 6 g

Wind stroke leading to paralysis and numbness; or wind cold damp in the channels resulting in wandering or fixed pain in the joints and muscles. The patient has difficulty controlling the muscles due to weakness and spasms.

T moist, white coat

P slow, slippery

☞ The formula should be taken as a powder. The prepared types of Aconite are used here.

✘ Do not use during pregnancy. It is a very strong prescription. Use only for a short period of time.

XIAO HUO LUO DAN

Minor Invigorate the Collaterals Special Pill

Cao Wu	Aconitum	60 g
Chuan Wu	Aconitum	60 g
Tian Nan Xing	Arisaema	60 g
Di Long	Pheretima	60 g
Ru Xiang	Boswellia	30 g
Mo Yao	Commiphora	30 g

Damp heat obstruction in the channels causing joint pain with fever and shivering.

T red, sticky coat

P slippery, rapid

XUAN BI TANG

Disband Painful Obstruction Decoction

Guang Fang Ji	Aristolochia	9 - 15 g
Lian Qiao	Forsythia	6 - 9 g
Xing Ren	Prunus	9 - 15 g
Yi Yi Ren	Coix	9 - 15 g
Zhi Zi	Gardenia	6 - 9 g
Hua Shi	Talcum	9 - 15 g
Ban Xia	Pinellia	6 - 9 g
Can Sha	Bombyx	6 - 9 g
Chi Xiao Dou	Phaseolus	6 - 9 g

Wind damp heat causing joint pain with swelling and pain in hands and feet, and fever.

T red, sticky coat

P rapid, slippery

YI YI REN TANG II

Coix Decoction from the Enlightened Physicians

Extract Formula Name: Coix Combination

Yi Yi Ren	Coix	9 - 20 g
Dang Gui	Angelica	6 - 9 g
Ma Huang	Ephedra	6 - 9 g
Cang Zhu	Atractylodes	6 - 9 g
Bai Shao Yao	Paeonia	6 - 9 g
Gui Zhi	Cinnamomum	6 - 9 g
Zhi Gan Cao	Glycyrrhiza	3 - 6 g

BLOOD STAGNATION DUE TO TRAUMA

- pain caused by a traumatic injury
- swelling and/or hematoma

T purple or unremarkable

P tends to be wiry

Trauma causing qi and blood stagnation which leads to bruising and swelling.

T purple

P wiry

☞ Herbs should be made into 3 g pills with honey. Adults take one or two pills two times a day.

✘ Do not use during pregnancy.

✪ **Major Formula**

DIE DA WAN

Trauma Pill

Chuan Xiong	Ligusticum	20 - 30 g
Dang Gui	Angelica	20 - 30 g
Mo Yao	Commiphora	20 - 30 g
Tu Bie Chong	Eupolyphaga	20 - 30 g
Ma Huang	Ephedra	50 - 60 g
Ru Xiang	Boswellia	20 - 30 g
Xue Jie	Dracaena	20 - 30 g
Zi Ran Tong	Pyritum	20 - 30 g

Blood stagnation due to trauma. The pain is mostly in the chest and flanks. Symptoms include large bruises or stabbing pain.

T purple

P wiry, slippery

☞ A few drops of wine should be added at the end.

✘ Do not use during pregnancy.

FU YUAN HUO XUE TANG

Revive Health by Invigorating the Blood Decoction

Extract Formula Name: Tang-Kuei and Persica Combination

Tao Ren	Prunus	6 - 9 g
Hong Hua	Carthamus	6 - 9 g
Da Huang	Rheum	9 - 30 g
Chai Hu	Bupleurum	6 - 15 g
Tian Hua Fen	Trichosanthes	9 - 12 g
Dang Gui	Angelica	6 - 9 g
Chuan Shan Jia	Manis	6 - 9 g
Gan Cao	Glycyrrhiza	3 - 6 g

Qi and blood stagnation in the channels causing pain, ulcerations, or swellings.

T purple

P wiry, choppy

✘ Do not use during pregnancy.

HUO LUO XIAO LING DAN

Fantastically Effective Pill to Invigorate the Collaterals

Dan Shen	Salvia	15 g
Dang Gui	Angelica	15 g
Mo Yao	Commiphora	15 g
Ru Xiang	Boswellia	15 g

Qi/blood stagnation from external or internal injury of all kinds causing pain and bleeding.

T purple

P wiry or choppy

☞ Powder herbs and take in a 0.2 - 1.5 g dosage internally. For external use mix herbs with wine.

✘ Do not use during pregnancy. Zhu Sha - Cinnabaris is toxic, and should only be used short-term.

✪ Major Formula

QI LI SAN

Seven-Thousandths of a Tael Powder

Extract Formula Name: Musk and Catechu Formula

Xue Jie	Dracaena	30 g
Ru Xiang	Boswellia	3 - 6 g
Hong Hua	Carthamus	3 - 6 g
Mo Yao	Commiphora	3 - 6 g
Er Cha	Acacia	6 - 9 g
Zhu Sha	Cinnabaris	3 - 5 g
She Xiang	Moschus	0.5 g
Bing Pian	Dryobalanops	0.5 g

TOXIC HEAT

- fever
- bleeding disorders
- sore, swollen throat or diptheria
- boils, carbuncles

T red, yellow coat

P rapid, forceful

Heart/Pericardium fire with toxic heat and fever which congeals into phlegm. This leads to delirium, coma, aphasia, or convulsions in children.

T dark red, sticky yellow coat

P rapid, forceful, wiry

☞ Herbs should be ground and made into 3 g pills. The adult dosage is one pill two to three times a day. Xi Jiao - Rhinoceros should be substituted with Shui Niu Jiao - Bubalus.

✗ Do not use during pregnancy. Do not take over a prolonged period of time. Note that Zhu Sha - Cinnabaris is toxic.

AN GONG NIU HUANG WAN

Calm the Palace Pill with Cattle Gallstone

Extract Formula Name: Bos and Curcuma Formula

Niu Huang	Bos	25 - 30 g
Xi Jiao	Rhinoceros	25 - 30 g
She Xiang	Moschus	7.5 g
Huang Lian	Coptis	25 - 30 g
Zhi Zi	Gardenia	25 - 30 g
Huang Qin	Scutellaria	25 - 30 g
Bing Pian	Dryobalanops	7.5 g
Zhen Zhu Mu	Pteria	12 - 15 g
Yu Jin	Curcuma	25 - 30 g
Xiong Huang	Realgar	25 - 30 g
Zhu Sha	Cinnabaris	25 - 30 g

Heat in the qi level/yangming channel syndrome causing severe fever, epidemic febrile disease, acute inflammation, encephalitis, or meningitis.

T red, dry yellow coat

P flooding, rapid

☞ Decoct the first five herbs, then add the rice at the end. It will absorb the water to make a thick liquid.

BAI HU JIA YIN QIAO TANG

White Tiger plus Lonicera and Forsythia Decoction

Shi Gao	Gypsum	20 - 30 g
Zhi Mu	Anemarrhena	9 - 12 g
Gan Cao	Glycyrrhiza	3 - 6 g
Jin Yin Hua	Lonicera	6 - 9 g
Lian Qiao	Forsythia	6 - 9 g
Jing Mi	Oryza	15 - 30 g

Toxic heat in the yangming channel causing dysentery, or pus or blood in the stools.

T red, yellow coat

P wiry, rapid, rolling

BAI TOU WENG TANG

Pulsatilla Decoction

Extract Formula Name: Anemone Combination

Bai Tou Weng	Pulsatilla	20 - 40 g
Huang Bai	Phellodendron	9 - 12 g
Qin Pi	Fraxinus	9 - 15 g
Huang Lian	Coptis	6 - 9 g

Damp accumulation with heat toxin in the qi level causing gastritis, hepatitis, fever, body-aches, diarrhea, or vomiting.

T sticky yellow coat

P rapid, soggy

☞ All ingredients should be dried in sunlight and ground into powder. Take 9 g each time, twice a day.

GAN LU XIAO DU DAN

Sweet Dew Special Pill to Eliminate Toxin

Extract Formula Name: Talc and Scute Formula

She Gan	Belamcanda	120 g
Lian Qiao	Forsythia	120 g
Hua Shi	Talcum	450 g
Chuan Bei Mu	Fritillaria	150 g
Bo He	Mentha	120 g
Huang Qin	Scutellaria	300 g
Bai Dou Kou	Amomum	120 g
Yin Chen Hao	Artemisia	330 g
Shi Chang Pu	Acorus	180 g
Huo Xiang	Agastache	120 g
Mu Tong	Akebia	150 g

Heat is creating fire, then toxin which affects the three jiaos. The heat may be internal or external. Symptoms include high fever, mania, delirium, or bleeding in the upper parts.

T red, dry, rough

P rapid, forceful

✪ **Major Formula**

HUANG LIAN JIE DU TANG

Coptis Decoction to Relieve Toxicity

Extract Formula Name: Coptis and Scute Combination

Huang Lian	Coptis	3 - 9 g
Huang Bai	Phellodendron	6 g
Huang Qin	Scutellaria	6 g
Zhi Zi	Gardenia	9 g

Internal Medicine, Misc. Syndromes

Toxic heat with underlying Kidney and Lung yin deficiency causing diptheria, laryngitis, or tonsillitis. The patient experiences sore, swollen throat, dry nose and lips, cough, or wheezing.

T red, scanty yellow coat

P rapid

KANG BAI HOU HE JI

Treat Diptheria Decoction

Sheng Di Huang	Rehmannia	12 - 30 g
Huang Qin	Scutellaria	6 - 18 g
Lian Qiao	Forsythia	6 - 18 g
Mai Men Dong	Ophiopogon	6 - 9 g
Xuan Shen	Scrophularia	6 - 9 g

Toxic heat and phlegm from chronic heat in the middle jiao complicated by wind heat affects the throat leading to tonsillitis with pus and difficulty swallowing.

T red, sticky yellow coat

P rapid, forceful

☞ Herbs should be powdered and mixed with wine. Adults should take 3 - 8 small pills each time.

✘ Do not use during pregnancy.

LIU SHEN WAN

Six-Miracle Pill

Niu Huang	Bos	3 - 6 g
Xiong Huang	Realgar	2 - 3 g
Chan Su	Bufo	2 - 3 g
Bing Pian	Dryobalanops	2 - 3 g
She Xiang	Moschus	3 - 6 g
Zhen Zhu	Pteria	3 - 6 g

Toxic heat causing swelling and abscess, fever, thirst, or scanty urination.

T red or dark red, yellow coat

P rapid, forceful

✘ Formula is very cold. Use caution during pregnancy.

NEI SHU HUANG LIANG TANG

Internal Dispersing Decoction with Coptis

Huang Lian	Coptis	3 - 9 g
Zhi Zi	Gardenia	3 - 9 g
Huang Qin	Scutellaria	6 - 9 g
Da Huang	Rheum	3 - 6 g
Lian Qiao	Forsythia	3 - 9 g
Dang Gui	Angelica	6 - 9 g
Bing Lang	Areca	3 - 6 g
Bo He	Mentha	6 - 9 g
Bai Shao Yao	Paeonia	3 - 9 g
Mu Xiang	Saussurea	3 - 6 g
Jie Geng	Platycodon	3 - 6 g
Gan Cao	Glycyrrhiza	3 - 6 g

Wind heat with toxic fire causing throat and gum swelling or oral ulcers.

T red or dark red, cracked

P rapid, forceful

✗ Do not use during pregnancy.

NIU HUANG SHANG QING WAN

Cattle Gallstone Pill to Ascend and Clear

Huang Lian	Coptis	3 - 9 g
Huang Bai	Phellodendron	6 - 9 g
Zhi Zi	Gardenia	3 - 6 g
Huang Qin	Scutellaria	6 - 9 g
Da Huang	Rheum	9 - 20 g
Fang Feng	Ledebouriella	6 - 9 g
Jing Jie	Schizonepeta	6 - 9 g
Chuan Xiong	Ligusticum	3 - 6 g
Niu Huang	Bos	2 - 3 g
Shi Gao	Gypsum	9 - 20 g
Bing Pian	Dryobalanops	3 - 9 g
Bai Zhi	Angelica	3 - 6 g
Bo He	Mentha	3 - 6 g
Dang Gui	Angelica	6 - 9 g
Chi Shao Yao	Paeonia	6 - 12 g
Lian Xin	Nelumbo	9 - 15 g
Lian Qiao	Forsythia	6 - 9 g
Xiong Huang	Realgar	3 - 6 g
Ju Hua	Chrysanthemum	6 - 9 g
Jie Geng	Platycodon	3 g
Gan Cao	Glycyrrhiza	3 g

Toxic heat with wind heat, sore, swollen throat, and facial swelling.

T   red, dry yellow coat

P   forceful, rapid

PU JI XIAO DU YIN

Universal Benefit Decoction to Eliminate Toxin

Extract Formula Name: Scute and Cimicifuga Combination

Huang Qin	Scutellaria	6 - 18 g
Huang Lian	Coptis	6 - 18 g
Ban Lan Gen	Isatis	3 - 6 g
Lian Qiao	Forsythia	3 - 6 g
Niu Bang Zi	Arctium	3 - 6 g
Chen Pi	Citrus	3 - 6 g
Sheng Ma	Cimicifuga	1 - 3 g
Jiang Can	Bombyx	1 - 3 g
Bo He	Mentha	3 - 6 g
Ma Bo	Lasiosphaera	3 - 6 g
Chai Hu	Bupleurum	3 - 6 g
Xuan Shen	Scrophularia	3 - 6 g
Jie Geng	Platycodon	3 - 6 g
Gan Cao	Glycyrrhiza	3 - 6 g

Wind heat with toxin affecting the neck and head with swollen sore throat or glands, tonsillitis, or pharyngitis.

T   red

P   rapid

QIANG LAN TANG

Notopterygium and Isatis Root Decoction

Qiang Huo	Notopterygium	9 - 12 g
Ban Lan Gen	Isatis	12 - 20 g

Qi and blood level heat: qi level heat causing high fever, thirst, sweating; and blood level heat causing bleeding conditions, coma, or restlessness. This formula also treats toxic heat.

T dark red, dry, yellow coat

P flooding, rapid

☞ Shi Gao - Gypsum should be decocted first for 20 minutes. Xi Jiao - Rhinoceros should be powdered and added to the strained decoction. It should be substituted with 6 - 9 g of Shui Niu Jiao - Bubalus, or 30 g of Bai Mao Gen - Imperata.

QING WEN BAI DU YIN

Clear Epidemics and Overcome Toxin Decoction

Shi Gao	Gypsum	40 - 100 g
Zhi Mu	Anemarrhena	9 - 12 g
Xuan Shen	Scrophularia	6 - 9 g
Dan Zhu Ye	Lophatherum	3 - 6 g
Xi Jiao	Rhinoceros	1 - 3 g
Chi Shao Yao	Paeonia	6 - 9 g
Huang Qin	Scutellaria	6 - 9 g
Huang Lian	Coptis	3 - 6 g
Mu Dan Pi	Paeonia	6 - 9 g
Sheng Di Huang	Rehmannia	6 - 12 g
Zhi Zi	Gardenia	3 - 6 g
Jie Geng	Platycodon	3 - 6 g
Lian Qiao	Forsythia	6 - 9 g
Gan Cao	Glycyrrhiza	3 - 6 g

Qi level heat with toxin in the upper body causing throat swelling, fever, sweating, and thirst for cold fluids.

T red, yellow coat

P flooding, rapid

QING XIN LIANG GE SAN

Clear the Heart and Cool the Diaphragm Powder

Lian Qiao	Forsythia	6 - 15 g
Huang Qin	Scutellaria	6 - 9 g
Zhi Zi	Gardenia	3 - 6 g
Bo He	Mentha	3 - 6 g
Jie Geng	Platycodon	3 - 6 g
Shi Gao	Gypsum	12 - 15 g
Gan Cao	Glycyrrhiza	3 - 6 g

Qi and blood deficiency with toxic abscess causing mastitis, intestinal abscess, or fever and chills.

T pale or red, yellow coat

P rapid

SHEN XIAO TUO LI SAN

Miraculous Powder for Supporting the Interior

Ren Dong Cao	Lonicera	15 g
Dang Gui	Angelica	9 g
Huang Qi	Astragalus	15 g
Gan Cao	Glycyrrhiza	15 - 20 g

Toxic heat with blood stagnation causing gangrene or ulcers in the extremities.

T red or purple spots

P rapid, wiry

☞ To ensure effectiveness, one package a day is administered for at least one week.

SI MIAO YONG AN TANG

Four-Valiant Decoction for Well-Being

Jin Yin Hua	Lonicera	60 - 90 g
Dang Gui	Angelica	35 g
Xuan Shen	Scrophularia	60 - 90 g
Gan Cao	Glycyrrhiza	20 g

Phlegm heat toxin and blood stagnation with pus causing Lung abscess, measles, whooping cough, cough with blood-streaked sputum, chest congestion, or low-grade fever.

T red, sticky yellow coat

P rapid, slippery

WEI JING TANG

Reed Decoction

Phragmites Combination

Lu Gen	Phragmitis	40 - 60 g
Dong Gua Ren	Benincasa	15 - 25 g
Yi Yi Ren	Coix	15 - 20 g
Tao Ren	Prunus	6 - 9 g

Damp heat with toxin causing abscess, skin rash in the lower limbs, or erysipelas.

T red, sticky coat

P rapid, slippery

WU SHEN TANG

Five-Miracle Decoction

Jin Yin Hua	Lonicera	30 - 60 g
Zi Hua Di Ding	Viola	15 - 20 g
Fu Ling	Poria	9 - 12 g
Huai Niu Xi	Achyranthes	3 - 6 g
Che Qian Zi	Plantago	6 - 9 g

Any organ heat or toxin causing boils or sores. They are painful, hot, swollen, and may be hard to the touch.

T red or dark red, yellow dry coat

P rapid

WU WEI XIAO DU YIN

Five-Ingredient Decoction to Eliminate Toxin

Jin Yin Hua	Lonicera	12 - 15 g
Zi Hua Di Ding	Viola	9 - 15 g
Pu Gong Ying	Taraxacum	9 - 15 g
Zi Bei Tian Kuei	Begonia	9 - 15 g
Ye Ju Hua	Chrysanthemum	9 - 15 g

Phlegm fire or toxic fire causing qi and blood stagnation. This manifests as carbuncles and boils with redness, mild chills, and severe fever.

T red, thin yellow coat

P rapid, forceful

☞ The formula should be decocted with 50 % wine and 50 % water. It may also be applied topically.

✗ Zao Jiao Ci - Gleditsia is slightly toxic and should not be used during pregnancy.

XIAN FANG HUO MING YIN

Sublime Formula for Sustaining Life

Extract Formula Name: Angelica and Mastic Combination

Jin Yin Hua	Lonicera	6 - 9 g
Zhe Bei Mu	Fritillaria	3 - 6 g
Dang Gui Wei	Angelica	9 - 12 g
Tian Hua Fen	Trichosanthes	3 - 6 g
Ru Xiang	Boswellia	2 - 3 g
Zao Jiao Ci	Gleditsia	2 - 3 g
Fang Feng	Ledebouriella	3 - 6 g
Chi Shao Yao	Paeonia	6 g
Mo Yao	Commiphora	3 - 6 g
Bai Zhi	Angelica	3 g
Chuan Shan Jia	Manis	3 - 6 g
Chen Pi	Citrus	3 - 6 g
Gan Cao	Glycyrrhiza	3 - 6 g

External invasion with toxic heat causing carbuncles, mastitis, or red rashes.

T red, thin yellow coat

P superficial, rapid

XIAO YAN JIE DU WAN

Reduce Inflammation and Relieve Toxicity Pill

Jin Yin Hua	Lonicera	9 - 20 g
Pu Gong Ying	Taraxacum	9 - 20 g
Fang Feng	Ledebouriella	6 - 9 g
Lian Qiao	Forsythia	9 - 15 g
Gan Cao	Glycyrrhiza	3 - 6 g

Wind heat and toxin causing measles, lack of sweating, cough, dark urine, or severe sore throat.

T red tip

P superficial, rapid

XUAN DU FA BIAO TANG

Dissipate Toxin and Release the Exterior Decoction

Sheng Ma	Cimicifuga	6 - 9 g
Ge Gen	Pueraria	6 - 9 g
Xing Ren	Prunus	6 - 9 g
Qian Hu	Peucedanum	6 - 9 g
Jie Geng	Platycodon	3 - 6 g
Bo He	Mentha	3 - 6 g
Fang Feng	Ledebouriella	3 - 6 g
Jing Jie	Schizonepeta	3 - 6 g
Lian Qiao	Forsythia	3 - 9 g
Niu Bang Zi	Arctium	3 - 6 g
Dan Zhu Ye	Lophatherum	3 - 6 g
Zhi Ke	Citrus	3 - 6 g
Mu Tong	Akebia	6 - 9 g
Gan Cao	Glycyrrhiza	3 - 6 g

Lung/Kidney yin deficiency with toxin causing diptheria, laryngitis, coarse breathing, or dry hacking cough.

T   red, dry, yellow coat

P   thin, rapid, or empty

YANG YIN QING FEI TANG

Nourish the Yin and Clear the Lungs Decoction

Sheng Di Huang	Rehmannia	6 - 12 g
Xuan Shen	Scrophularia	6 - 9 g
Bai Shao Yao	Paeonia	6 - 9 g
Mai Men Dong	Ophiopogon	6 - 12 g
Bo He	Mentha	3 - 6 g
Chuan Bei Mu	Fritillaria	3 - 6 g
Mu Dan Pi	Paeonia	6 - 9 g
Gan Cao	Glycyrrhiza	3 - 6 g

Fire toxin from wind damp heat causing skin lesions with pus and redness.

T   red

P   rapid, slippery

☞ Xi Jiao - Rhinoceros should be substituted with 6 - 9 g of Shui Niu Jiao - Bubalus or 30 g of Bai Mao Gen - Imperata.

YIN HUA JIE DU TANG

Honeysuckle Decoction to Relieve Toxicity

Jin Yin Hua	Lonicera	9 - 20 g
Zi Hua Di Ding	Viola	9 - 20 g
Lian Qiao	Forsythia	6 - 18 g
Huang Lian	Coptis	6 g
Xia Ku Cao	Prunella	6 - 18 g
Xi Jiao	Rhinoceros	2 - 3 g
Mu Dan Pi	Paeonia	6 - 9 g
Chi Fu Ling	Poria	6 - 9 g

Wind/toxic heat with damp and qi deficiency causing red, swollen sores or carbuncles.

T thin sticky white coat

P superficial

YIN QIAO BAI DU SAN

Honeysuckle and Forsythia Powder to Overcome Pathogenic Influences

Qiang Huo	Notopterygium	6 - 9 g
Chuan Xiong	Ligusticum	3 - 6 g
Du Huo	Angelica	3 - 6 g
Chai Hu	Bupleurum	6 - 9 g
Qian Hu	Peucedanum	6 - 9 g
Ren Shen	Panax	6 - 9 g
Jie Geng	Platycodon	3 - 6 g
Zhi Ke	Citrus	3 - 6 g
Fu Ling	Poria	3 - 6 g
Gan Cao	Glycyrrhiza	3 - 6 g
Jin Yin Hua	Lonicera	6 - 9 g
Lian Qiao	Forsythia	6 - 9 g

Damp heat in the Lungs causing toxin in the throat with obstruction and soreness.

T red, sticky yellow coat

P rapid, slippery

YIN QIAO MA BO SAN

Honeysuckle, Forsythia, and Puffball Powder

Lian Qiao	Forsythia	15 - 25 g
Jin Yin Hua	Lonicera	9 - 12 g
Niu Bang Zi	Arctium	12 - 15 g
Ma Bo	Lasiosphaera	6 - 9 g
She Gan	Belamcanda	6 - 9 g
[Lu Gen	Phragmites	12 - 20 g]

SUMMERHEAT INVASION

- fever and chills after exposure to the sun
- nausea and vomiting
- thirst
- sweating

T red tip, yellow coat

P superficial, rapid

Summerheat with damp and yangming channel heat/qi level heat. This causes severe sweating, nausea, vomiting, thirst, or fever.

T red, sticky yellow coat

P slippery, rapid

☞ Decoct the first four herbs, then add the rice at the end. It will absorb the water to make a thick liquid.

BAI HU JIA ZHU TANG

White Tiger with White Atractylodes Decoction

Shi Gao	Gypsum	20 - 30 g
Zhi Mu	Anemarrhena	9 - 12 g
Gan Cao	Glycyrrhiza	3 - 6 g
Bai Zhu	Atractylodes	3 - 9 g
Jing Mi	Oryza	15 - 30 g

Longstanding summer damp heat with urinary problems and fever.

T red, thin yellow coat

P rapid

CHUN ZE TANG

Spring Pond Decoction

Fu Ling	Poria	6 - 9 g
Zhu Ling	Polyporus	6 - 9 g
Ze Xie	Alisma	6 - 9 g
Gui Zhi	Cinnamomum	3 - 9 g
Bai Zhu	Atractylodes	6 - 9 g
Chai Hu	Bupleurum	6 - 9 g
Mai Men Dong	Ophiopogon	6 - 9 g
Ren Shen	Panax	6 - 9 g

Summerheat with internal water and damp accumulation leading to headaches and fever. This leads to depletion of qi and yin. Symptoms include nausea and vomiting, thirst and dry mouth, diarrhea, or restlessness.

T   red, sticky yellowish coat

P   rapid, superficial

GUI LING GAN LU YIN

Cinnamon and Poria Sweet Dew Decoction

Hua Shi	Talcum	15 - 30 g
Shi Gao	Gypsum	15 - 30 g
Han Shui Shi	Calcitum	12 - 30 g
Rou Gui	Cinnamomum	6 - 9 g
Fu Ling	Poria	12 - 30 g
Ze Xie	Alisma	9 - 15 g
Zhu Ling	Polyporus	9 - 15 g
Bai Zhu	Atractylodes	9 - 12 g
Gan Cao	Glycyrrhiza	6 - 9 g
Sheng Jiang	Zingiber	1 - 3 g

Summer damp heat, mostly manifesting in the upper jiao with fever, chills, sweating, or dizziness.

T   thin sticky coat

P   rapid, slippery

LEI SHI QING LIANG DI SHU TANG

Master Lei's Decoction to Clear, Cool and Remove Summerheat

Hua Shi	Talcum	12 - 15 g
Qing Hao	Artemisia	3 - 6 g
Bian Dou	Dolichos	6 - 9 g
Lian Qiao	Forsythia	6 - 9 g
Tong Cao	Tetrapanax	3 - 9 g
Fu Ling	Poria	6 - 9 g
Gan Cao	Glycyrrhiza	3 - 6 g
Xi Gua	Citrullus	1 pc

A patient with pre-existing qi deficiency gets a summerheat and damp invasion leading to dizziness, headache, diarrhea, heaviness, and fever and chills.

T   red or normal color

P   rapid, weak

LI SHI QING SHU YI QI TANG

Master Li's Decoction to Clear Summerheat and Augment the Qi

Ren Shen	Panax	6 - 9 g
Cang Zhu	Atractylodes	3 - 9 g
Bai Zhu	Atractylodes	6 - 9 g
Huang Qi	Astragalus	6 - 12 g
Ge Gen	Pueraria	6 - 9 g
Mai Men Dong	Ophiopogon	6 - 9 g
Wu Wei Zi	Schisandra	3 - 9 g
Qing Pi	Citrus	3 - 6 g
Chen Pi	Citrus	3 - 6 g
Sheng Ma	Cimicifuga	3 - 6 g
Dang Gui	Angelica	3 - 6 g
Shen Qu	Massa Fermentata	6 - 9 g
Ze Xie	Alisma	6 - 9 g
Huang Bai	Phellodendron	6 - 9 g
Gan Cao	Glycyrrhiza	3 - 6 g

Summer heat with damp causing nausea and vomiting, thirst, fullness in the chest, or diarrhea.

T   sticky coat

P   slippery, superficial

LIU HE TANG

Harmonize the Six Decoction

Extract Formula Name: Cardamon Combination

Huo Xiang	Agastache	6 - 9 g
Sha Ren	Amomum	3 - 9 g
Hou Po	Magnolia	6 - 9 g
Dang Shen	Codonopsis	6 - 9 g
Xing Ren	Prunus	3 - 6 g
Bian Dou	Dolichos	6 - 9 g
Ban Xia	Pinellia	6 - 9 g
Mu Gua	Chaenomeles	6 - 9 g
Bai Zhu	Atractylodes	6 - 9 g
Chi Fu Ling	Poria	6 - 9 g
Gan Cao	Glycyrrhiza	3 - 6 g

Internal Medicine, Misc. Syndromes

Summerheat with damp causing fever, nausea, vomiting, thirst, irritability, or sweating.

T sticky yellow coat

P rapid, slippery

⊗ Major Formula

LIU YI SAN

Six-to-One Powder

Hua Shi	Talcum	6 parts
Zhi Gan Cao	Glycyrrhiza	1 part

Mild summer heat invading the qi level with residual pathogens lingering causing mild superficial and damp symptoms. The patient feels thirst but can only sip fluids, and experiences diarrhea, gas, vomiting, or cold limbs.

T red, thin white coat

P rapid, maybe superficial

☞ The prepared form of Xi Gua - Citrullus is used. The outer skin of Si Gua Luo - Luffa is used.

QING LUO YIN

Clear the Collaterals Decoction

Bian Dou Hua	Dolichos	6 - 9 g
Xi Gua Shuang	Citrullus	6 - 9 g
Si Gua Pi	Luffa	6 - 9 g
Jin Yin Hua	Lonicera	6 - 9 g
He Ye	Nelumbo	6 g
Dan Zhu Ye	Lophatherum	6 - 9 g

Summerheat opens the pores so the patient sweats which leads to qi and yin deficiency; or yin deficient patient gets a summerheat invasion. Symptoms include thirst, high fever, or profuse sweating.

T red

P frail, rapid

☞ Lian Geng - Nelumbo is Lotus stem.

QING SHU YI QI TANG

Clear Summerheat and Augment the Qi Decoction

Extract Formula Name: Lotus Stem and Ginseng Combination

Xi Gua Pi	Citrullus	20 -30 g
Xi Yang Shen	Panax	6 - 9 g
Mai Men Dong	Ophiopogon	6 - 9 g
Lian Geng	Nelumbo	6 - 9 g
Shi Hu	Dendrobium	6 - 9 g
Dan Zhu Ye	Lophatherum	3 - 6 g
Fu Ling	Poria	6 - 9 g
Huang Lian	Coptis	3 - 6 g
Zhi Mu	Anemarrhena	6 - 9 g
Gan Cao	Glycyrrhiza	3 - 6 g
Jing Mi	Oryza	10 - 15 g

Pre-existing Spleen qi deficiency leading to damp and water in the middle jiao. This creates damp heat. The formula is also used for summer heat invasions. Symptoms include fever and chills, poor appetite, and headache.

T thin white coat

P soggy, wiry, thin

SAN REN TANG

Three-Nut Decoction

Extract Formula Name: Apricot, Coix, and Cluster Combination

Xing Ren	Prunus	6 - 12 g
Yi Yi Ren	Coix	12 - 15 g
Bai Dou Kou	Amomum	3 - 6 g
Hou Po	Magnolia	6 - 9 g
Ban Xia	Pinellia	6 - 9 g
Dan Zhu Ye	Lophatherum	6 - 9 g
Tong Cao	Tetrapanax	3 g
Hua Shi	Talcum	12 - 15 g

Severe toxin, epidemic summer heat, and blood heat causing delirious speech, purpura, or red eyes. This formula opens the orifice.

T scarlet

P rapid or flooding

☞ Herbs should be made into pills. Xi Jiao - Rhinoceros should be substituted with Shui Niu Jiao - Bubalus.

SHEN XI DAN

Magical Rhinoceros Special Pill

Xi Jiao	Rhinoceros	60 - 90 g
Jin Yin Hua	Lonicera	200 - 225 g
Ban Lan Gen	Isatis	100 - 135 g
Huang Qin	Scutellaria	60 - 90 g
Sheng Di Huang	Rehmannia	200 - 225 g
Lian Qiao	Forsythia	125 - 150 g
Xuan Shen	Scrophularia	90 - 105 g
Dan Dou Chi	Glycine	100 - 120 g
Shi Chang Pu	Acorus	60 - 90 g
Tian Hua Fen	Trichosanthes	40 - 60 g
Zi Cao	Lithospermum	40 - 60 g

Internal Medicine, Misc. Syndromes

Severe early-stage summer heat (excess type) causing lack of sweating, nausea and vomiting, or high fever.

T   thin sticky white coat

P   superficial, rapid

XIN JIA XIANG RU YIN

Newly-Augmented Elsholtzia Decoction

Bian Dou Hua	Dolichos	6 - 9 g
Xiang Ru	Elsholtzia	6 - 9 g
Jin Yin Hua	Lonicera	6 - 9 g
Lian Qiao	Forsythia	6 - 9 g
Hou Po	Magnolia	6 - 12 g

Summer damp heat in all three jiaos leading to sweating, diarrhea, nausea, scanty urination, or tidal fever.

T   red tip, sticky yellow coat

P   superficial, rapid, slippery

XING REN HUA SHI TANG

Apricot Kernel and Talcum Decoction

Xing Ren	Prunus	6 - 9 g
Hua Shi	Talcum	9 - 12 g
Huang Lian	Coptis	3 - 6 g
Huang Qin	Scutellaria	6 - 9 g
Hou Po	Magnolia	6 - 12 g
Chen Pi	Citrus	3 - 6 g
Ban Xia	Pinellia	6 - 9 g
Tong Cao	Tetrapanax	3 - 6 g
Yu Jin	Curcuma	6 - 9 g

OPEN THE ORIFICE, COMA

- paralysis
- coma or delirium
- aphasia

T depends on the involved syndrome

P depends on the involved syndrome

Heart/Pericardium fire with toxic heat and fever which congeals into phlegm. This leads to delirium, coma, aphasia, or convulsions in children.

T dark red, sticky yellow coat

P rapid, forceful, wiry

☞ Herbs should be ground and made into 3 g pills. The adult dosage is one pill two to three times a day. Xi Jiao - Rhinoceros should be substituted with Shui Niu Jiao - Bubalus.

✘ Do not use during pregnancy. Do not take over a prolonged period of time. Note that Zhu Sha - Cinnabaris is toxic.

✪ **Major Formula**

AN GONG NIU HUANG WAN

Calm the Palace Pill with Cattle Gallstone

Extract Formula Name: Bos and Curcuma Formula

Niu Huang	Bos	25 - 30 g
Xi Jiao	Rhinoceros	25 - 30 g
She Xiang	Moschus	7.5 g
Huang Lian	Coptis	25 - 30 g
Zhi Zi	Gardenia	25 - 30 g
Huang Qin	Scutellaria	25 - 30 g
Bing Pian	Dryobalanops	7.5 g
Zhen Zhu Mu	Pteria	12 - 15 g
Yu Jin	Curcuma	25 - 30 g
Xiong Huang	Realgar	25 - 30 g
Zhu Sha	Cinnabaris	25 - 30 g

Qi and blood stagnation with qi deficiency and blockage in the channels leading to wind stroke, hemiplegia, and atrophy in the lower limbs. The patient has difficulty walking.

T purple, thin white coat

P wiry, weak, slow

BU YANG HUAN WU TANG

Tonify the Yang to Restore Five-tenths Decoction

Extract Formula Name: Astragalus and Peony Combination

Huang Qi	Astragalus	60 - 120 g
Chuan Xiong	Ligusticum	3 - 6 g
Chi Shao Yao	Paeonia	3 - 6 g
Dang Gui Wei	Angelica	6 - 9 g
Hong Hua	Carthamus	3 - 6 g
Tao Ren	Prunus	3 - 6 g
Di Long	Pheretima	3 - 6 g

Internal Medicine,
Misc. Syndromes

Kidney yin/yang deficiency with false fire and phlegm leading to depletion of Heart qi. Symptoms include paraplegia, aphasia, and blockage of the orifice.

T red or normal color, sticky yellow coat

P slippery, slightly rapid, weak, or thin, deep

DI HUANG YIN ZI

Rehmannia Decoction

Shu Di Huang	Rehmannia	12 - 15 g
Shan Zhu Yu	Cornus	6 - 9 g
Ba Ji Tian	Morinda	6 - 9 g
Rou Cong Rong	Cistanche	6 - 9 g
Rou Gui	Cinnamomum	3 - 9 g
Shi Hu	Dendrobium	6 - 9 g
Shi Chang Pu	Acorus	6 - 9 g
Yuan Zhi	Polygala	3 - 6 g
Mai Men Dong	Ophiopogon	6 - 9 g
Fu Ling	Poria	6 - 9 g
Wu Wei Zi	Schisandra	6 - 9 g
Fu Zi	Aconitum	3 - 6 g
[Bo He	Mentha	1 - 3 g]
[Sheng Jiang	Zingiber	3 - 6 g]
[Da Zao	Ziziphus	1 g]

Wind and phlegm accumulation causing hypertension, vertigo, and aphasia.

T rigid, sticky white or yellowish coat

P slippery

DI TAN TANG

Scour Phlegm Decoction

Extract Formula Name: Arisaema and Acorus Combination

Ban Xia	Pinellia	6 - 9 g
Fu Ling	Poria	6 - 9 g
Zhi Shi	Citrus	3 - 6 g
Chen Pi	Citrus	3 - 6 g
Zhu Ru	Bambusa	1 - 3 g
Dan Nan Xing	Arisaema	1 - 3 g
Ren Shen	Panax	3 - 6 g
Shi Chang Pu	Acorus	6 g
Gan Cao	Glycyrrhiza	3 - 6 g
[Sheng Jiang	Zingiber	3 - 6 g]
[Da Zao	Ziziphus	1 - 3 pc]

Phlegm fire obstructing the orifice causing mania, severe palpitations, cough with profuse phlegm, dizziness, wheezing, anxiety, bad dreams, or lumps in the neck.

T red, thick yellow sticky coat

P wiry, rapid, forceful

☞ Herbs should be made into 6 - 9 g pills. Adults take one pill one or two times a day.

✗ Do not use during pregnancy or post-partum.

GUN TAN WAN

Vaporize Phlegm Pill

Extract Formula Name: Lapis and Scute Formula

Da Huang	Rheum	200 - 240 g
Huang Qin	Scutellaria	200 - 240 g
Meng Shi	Lapis Micae Seu Chloriti	20 - 30 g
Chen Xiang	Aquilaria	9 - 15 g

Phlegm heat invading the Pericardium giving rise to wind. Symptoms include spasms, convulsions, loss of consciousness, or nausea and vomiting from phlegm in the middle jiao. This is seen most commonly in small children and infants.

T red, sticky yellow coat

P rapid, wiry, slippery

☞ Herbs should be powdered and made into very tiny pills. For infants the dosage is one pill 2 - 3 times a day.

✗ Do not use during pregnancy. Zhu Sha - Cinnabaris is toxic. The formula should not be used over a long period of time.

HUI CHUN DAN (XIAO ER HUI CHUN DAN)

Return of the Spring Special Pill

Niu Huang	Bos	9 - 12 g
Dan Nan Xing	Arisaema	50 - 60 g
Tian Zhu Huang	Bambusa	35 - 40 g
Chuan Bei Mu	Fritillaria	35 - 40 g
Ban Xia	Pinellia	35 - 40 g
Chen Xiang	Aquilaria	35 - 40 g
Jiang Can	Bombyx	35 - 40 g
Quan Xie	Buthus	35 - 40 g
She Xiang	Moschus	9 - 12 g
Gou Teng	Uncaria	20 - 25 g
Tian Ma	Gastrodia	35 - 40 g
Zhu Sha	Cinnabaris	0.2 - 1.5 g
Bai Dou Kou	Amomum	35 - 40 g
Tan Xiang	Santalum	35 - 40 g
Da Huang	Rheum	50 - 60 g
Mu Xiang	Saussurea	35 - 40 g
Chen Pi	Citrus	35 - 40 g
Zhi Ke	Citrus	35 - 40 g
Gan Cao	Glycyrrhiza	25 - 27 g

Heat settles into the Pericardium causing irritability, delirious speech, or childhood convulsions.

T dark red

P rapid, wiry

☞ Herbs should be powdered and made into 3 g pills. Take one pill 2 - 3 times a day.

✘ Zhu Sha - Cinnabaris is toxic and should only be used short-term.

NIU HUANG QING XIN WAN

Cattle Gallstone Pill to Clear the Heart

Extract Formula Name: Bovis Bezoar and Coptis Formula

Niu Huang	Bos	0.5 - 0.75 g
Huang Lian	Coptis	9 - 15 g
Zhi Zi	Gardenia	6 - 9 g
Huang Qin	Scutellaria	6 - 9 g
Yu Jin	Curcuma	6 - 9 g
Zhu Sha	Cinnabaris	3 - 5 g

Wind phlegm attacking the channels, especially the head and face with pre-existing qi and yang deficiency. This leads to paralysis, facial twitches, stiff muscles, spasms, or loose stools.

T pale, swollen, teethmarks, thick sticky coat

P slippery, deep, frail

✘ The formula is toxic and should not be taken over a long period of time. Do not use during pregnancy.

QIAN ZHENG SAN

Lead to Symmetry Powder

Jiang Can	Bombyx	6 g
Bai Fu Zi	Typhonium	6 g
Quan Xie	Buthus	6 g

Wind heat with wind stroke causing paraplegia, or facial paralysis with severe heat symptoms.

T red, yellow coat

P rapid

✗ Caution during pregnancy.

QU FENG ZHI BAO DAN

Greatest Treasure Special Pill to Dispel Wind

Hua Shi	Talcum	12 - 15 g
Dang Gui	Angelica	9 - 12 g
Chuan Xiong	Ligusticum	9 g
Gan Cao	Glycyrrhiza	6 g
Fang Feng	Ledebouriella	6 - 9 g
Bai Shao Yao	Paeonia	6 - 9 g
Bai Zhu	Atractylodes	6 g
Du Huo	Angelica	6 g
Ren Shen	Panax	3 g
Qiang Huo	Notopterygium	3 - 6 g
Shu Di Huang	Rehmannia	6 g
Tian Ma	Gastrodia	6 g
Shi Gao	Gypsum	6 g
Huang Qin	Scutellaria	6 g
Jie Geng	Platycodon	3 g
Zhi Zi	Gardenia	1 - 3 g
Jing Jie	Schizonepeta	6 g
Bo He	Mentha	3 g
Da Huang	Rheum	6 g
Mang Xiao	Mirabilitum	6 g
Lian Qiao	Forsythia	3 - 6 g
Ma Huang	Ephedra	6 g
Huang Lian	Coptis	3 g
Huang Bai	Phellodendron	3 g
Xi Xin	Asarum	3 g
Quan Xie	Buthus	3 g

Wind stroke with phlegm accumulation causing hemiplegia, facial paralysis, aphasia, or seizures from wind phlegm.

T sticky coat

P slippery, forceful

☞ Herbs should be ground into a powder and then taken as a draft. The actual dosage of Li Lu - Veratrum depends on the constitution of the patient.

✗ This formula causes vomiting.

SAN SHENG SAN

Three-Sage Powder

Gua Di	Cucumis	100 - 150 g
Li Lu	Veratrum	6 - 25 g
Fang Feng	Ledebouriella	100 - 150 g

Damp cold and phlegm causing sudden collapse, clenched jaw, or coma; or qi stagnation or damp cold leading to coldness in the chest and abdomen or chest pain, coma, or qi stagnation from an epidemic manifesting in fullness in the chest. The patient feels the urge to vomit or defecate but is unable to do so, which then leads to sudden loss of consciousness.

T pale

P slow, slippery

☞ The prescription is made into pills. Xi Jiao - Rhinoceros should be substituted with Shui Niu Jiao - Bubalus.

✗ Do not use during pregnancy. Zhu Sha - Cinnabaris is toxic, and should only be used short-term.

✪ **Major Formula**

SU HE XIANG WAN

Liquid Styrax Pill

Extract Formula Name: Styrax Formula

Su He Xiang	Liquidambar	30 g
She Xiang	Moschus	60 g
Bing Pian	Dryobalanops	30 g
An Xi Xiang	Styrax	60 g
Ru Xiang	Boswellia	30 g
Tan Xiang	Santalum	60 g
Ding Xiang	Eugenia	60 g
Bi Ba	Piper	60 g
Xiang Fu	Cyperus	60 g
Xi Jiao	Rhinoceros	60 g
Bai Zhu	Atractylodes	60 g
He Zi	Terminalia	60 g
Zhu Sha	Cinnabaris	60 g
Mu Xiang	Saussarea	60 g
Chen Xiang	Aguilaria	60 g

Exposure to bad smells with phlegm obstruction causing clenched jaw, difficulty breathing, and loss of consciousness. This may be a life-threatening disorder.

T thick sticky coat

P slippery

☞ Equal amounts of the two herbs should be made into a powder. A very small amount of the powder should be blown into the nose, but inhalation into the lungs should be avoided.

✗ Do not use during pregnancy. Do not use for loss of consciousness from cerebral hemorrhage or traumatic head injuries.

TONG GUAN SAN

Open the Gate Powder

Zao Jiao	Gleditsia	10 g
Xi Xin	Asarum	10 g

Liver wind due to fire in the pericardium, or phlegm heat obstructing the orifice causing stroke, high fever, irritability, loss of consciousness, or a raspy voice.

T dark red, sticky yellow grey coat

P rapid, slippery

☞ Herbs should be ground separately, then sifted together. Make into 3 g pills. Adults take one pill 2 - 3 times a day. Xi Jiao - Rhinoceros should be substituted with Shui Niu Jiao - Bubalus or 50 - 60 g of Bai Mao Gen - Imperata.

✗ Do not use during pregnancy. Zhu Sha - Cinnabaris is toxic and should not be used over a prolonged period of time.

ZHI BAO DAN

Greatest Treasure Special Pill

Extract Formula Name: Rhinoceros and Succinum Formula

Xi Jiao	Rhinoceros	20 - 30 g
Niu Huang	Bos	12 - 15 g
She Xiang	Moschus	0.1 - 0.3 g
Dai Mao	Eretmochelydis	20 - 30 g
An Xi Xiang	Styrax	30 - 45 g
Hu Po	Succinum	20 - 30 g
Xiong Huang	Realgar	20 - 30 g
Zhu Sha	Cinnabaris	20 - 30 g
Bing Pian	Dryobalanops	0.1 - 0.3 g

Severe heat enters the Pericardium causing Liver wind which leads to delirious speech, fever, twitches, and convulsions.

T red, yellow coat

P wiry, rapid, forceful

☞ Available in prepared form.

✗ Do not use during pregnancy. Zhu Sha - Cinnabaris is toxic and should not be used over a long period of time.

ZI XUE DAN

Purple Snow Special Pill

Extract Formula Name: Rhinoceros and Antelope Horn Formula

Han Shui Shi	Calcitum	6 - 9 g
Hua Shi	Talcum	9 - 15 g
Ling Yang Jiao	Saiga	0.5 - 1 g
She Xiang	Moschus	0.3 g
Chen Xiang	Aquilaria	1 - 3 g
Qing Mu Xiang	Aristolochia	3 - 6 g
Xi Jiao	Rhinoceros	0.5 - 1 g
Shi Gao	Gypsum	6 - 9 g
Xuan Shen	Scrophularia	9 - 15 g
Sheng Ma	Cimicifuga	6 - 9 g
Zhu Sha	Cinnabaris	1 g
Ci Shi	Magnetitum	6 - 9 g
Ding Xiang	Eugenia	2 g
Xiao Shi	Niter	9 - 15 g
Mang Xiao	Mirabilitum	9 - 15 g
Huang Jin	Aurum	9 - 15 g
Zhi Gan Cao	Glycyrrhiza	3 - 6 g

TUMOR OR NODULE DISSOLVING

- masses or lumps anywhere in the body
- subcutaneous nodules

T depends on the involved syndrome

P depends on the involved syndrome

Blood and phlegm stagnation in the uterus leading to masses or lumps, amenorrhea, dysmenorrhea, or restless fetus.

T purple, sticky coat

P wiry, slippery, choppy

GUI ZHI FU LING WAN

Cinnamon Twig and Poria Pill

Extract Formula Name: Cinnamon and Hoelen Formula

Gui Zhi	Cinnamomum	6 - 12 g
Fu Ling	Poria	6 - 12 g
Mu Dan Pi	Paeonia	6 - 12 g
Tao Ren	Prunus	6 - 12 g
Chi Shao Yao	Paeonia	9 - 12 g

Phlegm accumulation causing hardenings; or Liver qi stagnation leading to goiter or cancer.

T sticky coat

P slippery, wiry

✪ **Major Formula**

HAI ZAO YU HU TANG

Sargassum Decoction for the Jade Flask

Hai Zao	Sargassum	3 - 6 g
Kun Bu	Laminaria	3 - 6 g
Hai Dai	Ecklonia	1.5 g
Du Huo	Angelica	3 - 6 g
Lian Qiao	Forsythia	3 - 6 g
Zhe Bei Mu	Fritillaria	3 - 6 g
Chuan Xiong	Ligusticum	3 - 6 g
Ban Xia	Pinellia	3 - 6 g
Dang Gui	Angelica	3 - 6 g
Chen Pi	Citrus	3 - 6 g
Qing Pi	Citrus	3 - 6 g
Gan Cao	Glycyrrhiza	3 - 6 g

Blood and phlegm accumulation leading to solid scrofula due to Liver yang excess with a mild heat aspect.

T red, sticky yellow coat

P wiry, rapid

☞ Xia Ku Cao - Prunella should be decocted until it is very thick. The other herbs should be added to the strained tea and decocted until they become like syrup.

XIA KU CAO GAO

Prunella Syrup

Xia Ku Cao	Prunella	500 - 700 g
Wu Yao	Lindera	9 - 15 g
Xuan Shen	Scrophularia	9 - 15 g
Dang Gui	Angelica	9 - 15 g
Zhe Bei Mu	Fritillaria	9 - 15 g
Kun Bu	Laminaria	9 - 15 g
Jie Geng	Platycodon	6 - 9 g
Bai Shao Yao	Paeonia	9 - 15 g
Jiang Can	Bombyx	9 - 15 g
Chuan Xiong	Ligusticum	6 - 9 g
Chen Pi	Citrus	6 - 9 g
Xiang Fu	Cyperus	20 - 25 g
Hong Hua	Carthamus	6 - 9 g
Da Zao	Ziziphus	200 - 230 g
Gan Cao	Glycyrrhiza	6 - 9 g

Qi and blood deficiency with qi/blood and phlegm stagnation causing masses on the neck, breasts, or axilla areas.

T pale or purple

P weak or choppy

XIANG BEI YANG YING TANG

Cyperus and Fritillaria Decoction to Nourish the Nutritive Qi

Ren Shen	Panax	6 - 9 g
Bai Zhu	Atractylodes	3 - 6 g
Fu Ling	Poria	6 - 9 g
Chuan Xiong	Ligusticum	3 - 6 g
Chen Pi	Citrus	3 - 6 g
Dang Gui	Angelica	6 - 9 g
Xiang Fu	Cyperus	6 - 9 g
Shu Di Huang	Rehmannia	6 - 12 g
Bei Mu	Fritillaria	3 - 6 g
Bai Shao Yao	Paeonia	6 - 9 g
Jie Geng	Platycodon	3 - 6 g
Da Zao	Ziziphus	3 - 6 pc
Sheng Jiang	Zingiber	3 - 6 g
Gan Cao	Glycyrrhiza	1 - 3 g

Goiter, scrofula, and lumps due to yin deficieny with false heat. The false heat dries the fluids and causes phlegm accumulation.

T red, coat

P rapid, slippery, or wiry

XIAO LUO WAN

Reduce Scrofula Pill

Chuan Bei Mu	Fritiallaria	6 - 12 g
Mu Li	Ostrea	6 - 12 g
Xuan Shen	Scrophularia	6 - 12 g

WIND ATTACKING THE CHANNELS OR SKIN

- skin rashes which move around
- itchy rashes
- muscle spasms
- various types of paralysis

T   unremarkable

P   superficial

Wind phlegm attacking the channels, especially the head and face with pre-existing qi and yang deficiency. This leads to paralysis, facial twitches, stiff muscles, spasms, or loose stools.

T   pale, swollen, teethmarks, thick sticky coat

P   slippery, deep, frail

✗   The formula is toxic and should not be taken over a long period of time. Do not use during pregnancy.

QIAN ZHENG SAN

Lead to Symmetry Powder

Jiang Can	Bombyx	6 g
Bai Fu Zi	Typhonium	6 g
Quan Xie	Buthus	6 g

Blood deficiency which gives rise to wind. This causes an itchy rash which is dry and pale red.

T   pale or purple

P   thin

SI WU XIAO FENG SAN

Eliminate Wind Decoction with the Four-Substances

Sheng Di Huang	Rehmannia	6 - 9 g
Dang Gui	Angelica	6 - 9 g
Chi Shao Yao	Paeonia	3 - 6 g
Chuan Xiong	Ligusticum	3 - 6 g
Jing Jie	Schizonepeta	3 - 6 g
Fang Feng	Ledebouriella	3 - 6 g
Bai Xian Pi	Dictamnus	3 - 6 g
Bo He	Mentha	3 - 6 g
Chai Hu	Bupleurum	2 g
Du Huo	Angelica	3 g
Chan Tui	Cryptotympana	3 - 6 g
Da Zao	Ziziphus	2 - 3 pc

Wind phlegm in the channels with severe spasms, stiffness in the jaw, or rigidity of the whole body. This formula is a strong anti-spasmodic.

T   deviated, sticky white coat

P   variable

☞ Zhu Sha - Cinnabaris and 60 ml of yellow wine should be added at the end to the strained tea.

✗ Do not use during pregnancy. Do not use over long periods of time. Tian Nan Xing - Arisaema is slightly toxic and Zhu Sha - Cinnabaris is very toxic.

WU HU ZHUI FENG SAN

Five-Tiger Powder to Pursue Wind

Chan Tui	Cryptotympana	30 g
Tian Ma	Gastrodia	6 g
Tian Nan Xing	Arisaema	3 - 6 g
Jiang Can	Bombyx	6 g
Quan Xie	Buthus	7 - 9 g
Zhu Sha	Cinnabaris	1 g

Liver wind or external wind with phlegm accumulation in the channels causing stroke, aphasia, cerebral hemorrhage, or numbness; or cold attacking the chest and axillae causing severe localized pain in the flanks.

T   sticky white coat

P   slippery or wiry

WU YAO SHUN QI SAN

Lindera Powder to Smooth the Flow of Qi

Extract Formula Name: Lindera Formula

Wu Yao	Lindera	9 - 15 g
Chen Pi	Citrus	9 - 15 g
Ma Huang	Ephedra	6 - 9 g
Bai Zhi	Angelica	3 - 9 g
Zhi Ke	Citrus	3 - 6 g
Jiang Can	Bombyx	3 g
Jie Geng	Platycodon	3 g
Chuan Xiong	Ligusticum	3 - 9 g
Pao Jiang	Zingiber	3 - 6 g
Gan Cao	Glycyrrhiza	3 - 6 g
[Da Zao	Ziziphus	3 - 8 pc]
[Sheng Jiang	Zingiber	3 - 6 g]

Internal Medicine, Misc. Syndromes

Wind heat and damp with preexisting damp heat lodged in the skin and muscles. This causes an itchy, weepy rash, or bleeding under the skin (purpura) with heat or wind intolerance.

T   red tip or border, white or yellow coat

P   superficial, rapid

⭐ Major Formula

XIAO FENG SAN I

Eliminate Wind Powder from True Lineage

Extract Formula Name: Tang-Kuei and Arctium Formula

Fang Feng	Ledebouriella	3- 6 g
Jing Jie	Schizonepeta	3 - 6 g
Chan Tui	Cryptotympana	3 g
Ku Shen	Sophora	3 g
Niu Bang Zi	Arctium	3 g
Hei Zhi Ma	Sesamum	3 g
Shi Gao	Gypsum	3 g
Zhi Mu	Anemarrhena	3 g
Cang Zhu	Atractylodes	3 g
Sheng Di Huang	Rehmannia	3 g
Dang Gui	Angelica	3 g
Mu Tong	Akebia	2 g
Gan Cao	Glycyrrhiza	2 g

Wind damp with qi stagnation causes a rash, dizziness, headache, and numbness of the skin.

T   sticky coat

P   slippery

XIAO FENG SAN II

Eliminate Wind Powder from Imperial Grace Formulary

Jing Jie	Schizonepeta	6 - 9 g
Bo He	Mentha	6 g
Chan Tui	Cryptotympana	6 g
Jiang Can	Bombyx	6 g
Hou Po	Magnolia	3 - 6 g
Qiang Huo	Notopterygium	6 g
Fang Feng	Ledebouriella	6 g
Ren Shen	Panax	6 g
Chuan Xiong	Ligusticum	6 g
Fu Ling	Poria	6 g
Chen Pi	Citrus	3 - 6 g

Wind heat with pre-existing heat and lumps leading to dizziness during pregnancy or swellings around the jaw and neck.

T   red tip and body, sticky coat

P   rapid

XIAO FENG SAN III

Eliminate Wind Powder from Effective Formulas

Shi Gao	Gypsum	20 g
Chuan Xiong	Ligusticum	3 - 9 g
Jing Jie	Schizonepeta	3 - 6 g
Ju Hua	Chrysanthemum	3 - 6 g
Fang Feng	Ledebouriella	6 - 9 g
Dang Gui	Angelica	6 - 9 g
Bai Zhi	Angelica	3 - 9 g
Qiang Huo	Notopterygium	6 - 9 g
Dou Juan	Glycine	3 - 6 g
Ling Yang Jiao	Saiga	6 g
Gan Cao	Glycyrrhiza	6 - 15 g

Wind stroke leading to paralysis and numbness; or wind cold damp in the channels resulting in wandering or fixed pain in the joints and muscles. The patient has difficulty controlling the muscles due to weakness and spasms.

T   moist, white coat

P   slow, slippery

☞ The formula should be taken as a powder. The prepared types of Aconite are used here.

✗ Do not use during pregnancy. It is a very strong prescription. Use only for a short period of time.

XIAO HUO LUO DAN

Minor Invigorate the Collaterals Special Pill

Cao Wu	Aconitum	60 g
Chuan Wu	Aconitum	60 g
Tian Nan Xing	Arisaema	60 g
Di Long	Pheretima	60 g
Ru Xiang	Boswellia	30 g
Mo Yao	Commiphora	30 g

Wind stroke with wind cold invasion and pre-existing qi deficiency causing fever and chills, hemiplegia, aphasia, or facial paralysis.

T pale, deviated, thin white coat

P superficial, or deep, frail

☞ Fu Zi - Aconitum should be cooked 30 - 60 minutes prior to adding the other herbs.

XIAO XU MING TANG

Minor Prolong Life Decoction

Extract Formula Name: Ma-Huang and Peony Combination

Chuan Xiong	Ligusticum	3 - 6 g
Ma Huang	Ephedra	3 - 6 g
Bai Shao Yao	Paeonia	6 - 12 g
Guang Fang Ji	Aristolochia	6 - 12 g
Fang Feng	Ledebouriella	9 - 12 g
Ren Shen	Panax	3 - 6 g
Fu Zi	Aconitum	3 - 6 g
Rou Gui	Cinnamomum	3 - 6 g
Huang Qin	Scutellaria	3 - 9 g
Xing Ren	Prunus	9 - 12 g
Sheng Jiang	Zingiber	9 - 12 pc
Gan Cao	Glycyrrhiza	3 - 6 g

External wind attacks the channels with pre-existing qi/Blood deficiency; or Liver wind with heat causing flaccid hemiplegia, aphasia, or mild fever. There may also be slight mental confusion.

T sticky yellow coat

P wiry, forceful, or rapid, slippery

XU MING TANG

Prolong Life Decoction

Extract Formula Name: Ma-Huang and Ginseng Combination

Gui Zhi	Cinnamomum	6 - 9 g
Ma Huang	Ephedra	6 - 9 g
Chuan Xiong	Ligusticum	3 - 6 g
Xing Ren	Prunus	6 - 9 g
Shi Gao	Gypsum	6 - 9 g
Ren Shen	Panax	6 - 9 g
Dang Gui	Angelica	6 - 9 g
Gan Jiang	Zingiber	6 - 9 g
Gan Cao	Glycyrrhiza	3 - 9 g

Wind with phlegm causing muscle spasms, lockjaw, tetanus, kyphotic arch, or spasms in the trachea.

T   deviated or stiff

P   tight or wiry

✗   Do not use during pregnancy. The formula is toxic and should not be taken over a long period of time.

YU ZHEN SAN

True Jade Powder

Tian Nan Xing	Arisaema	10 g
Bai Fu Zi	Typhonium	10 g
Qiang Huo	Notopterygium	10 g
Tian Ma	Gastrodia	10 g
Fang Feng	Ledebouriella	10 g
Bai Zhi	Angelica	10 g

Severe heat causing Liver wind. This causes muscle twitches, convulsions, or spasms.

T   red, deviated, yellow coat

P   forceful

✗   Do not use during pregnancy. The formula is toxic and should not be taken over a prolonged period of time.

ZHI JING SAN

Stop Spasms Powder

Wu Gong	Scolopendra	10 g
Quan Xie	Buthus	10 g

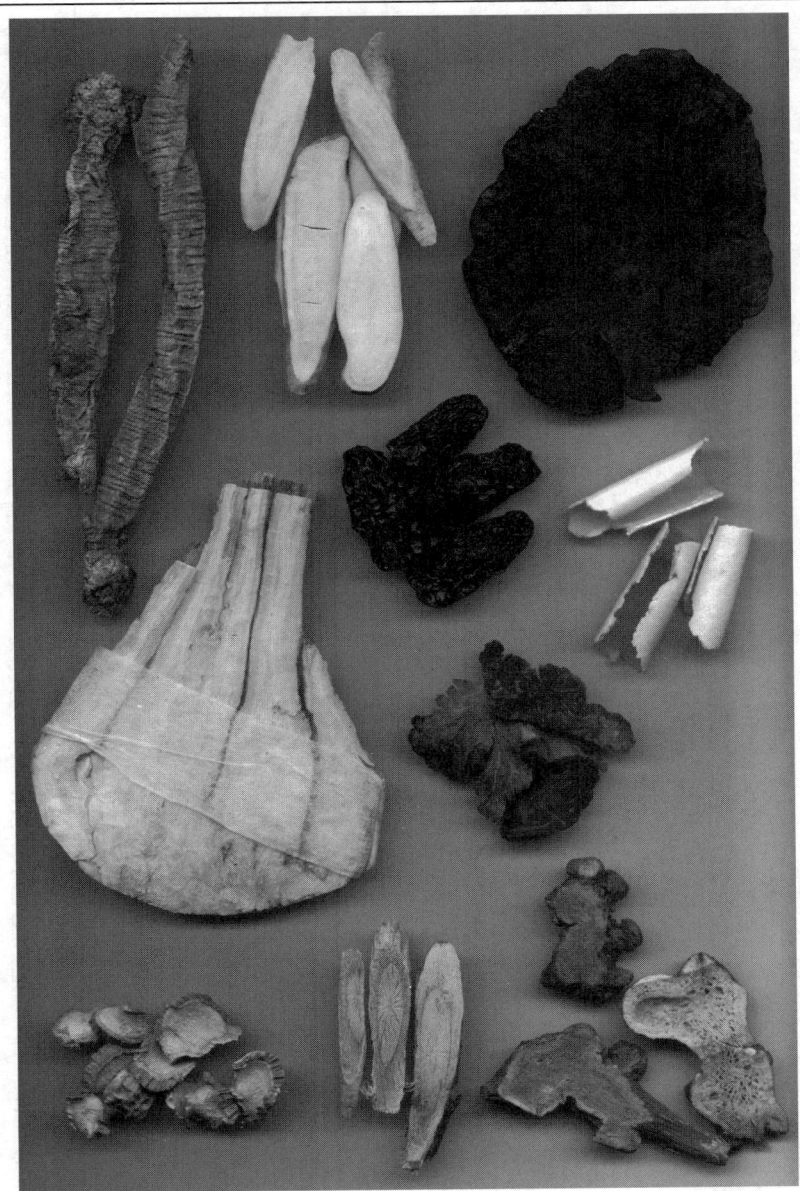

Ba Zhen Tang

Clockwise from top left: Dang Shen/Codonopsis, Bai Shao Yao/Paeonia, Shu Di Huang/Rehmannia, Da Zao/Ziziphus (center), Fu Ling/Poria (right), Chuan Xiong/Ligusticum, Bai Zhu/Atractylodes, Gan Cao/Glycyrrhiza, Sheng Jiang/Zingiber, Dang Gui/Angelica. Shown at one-half actual size.

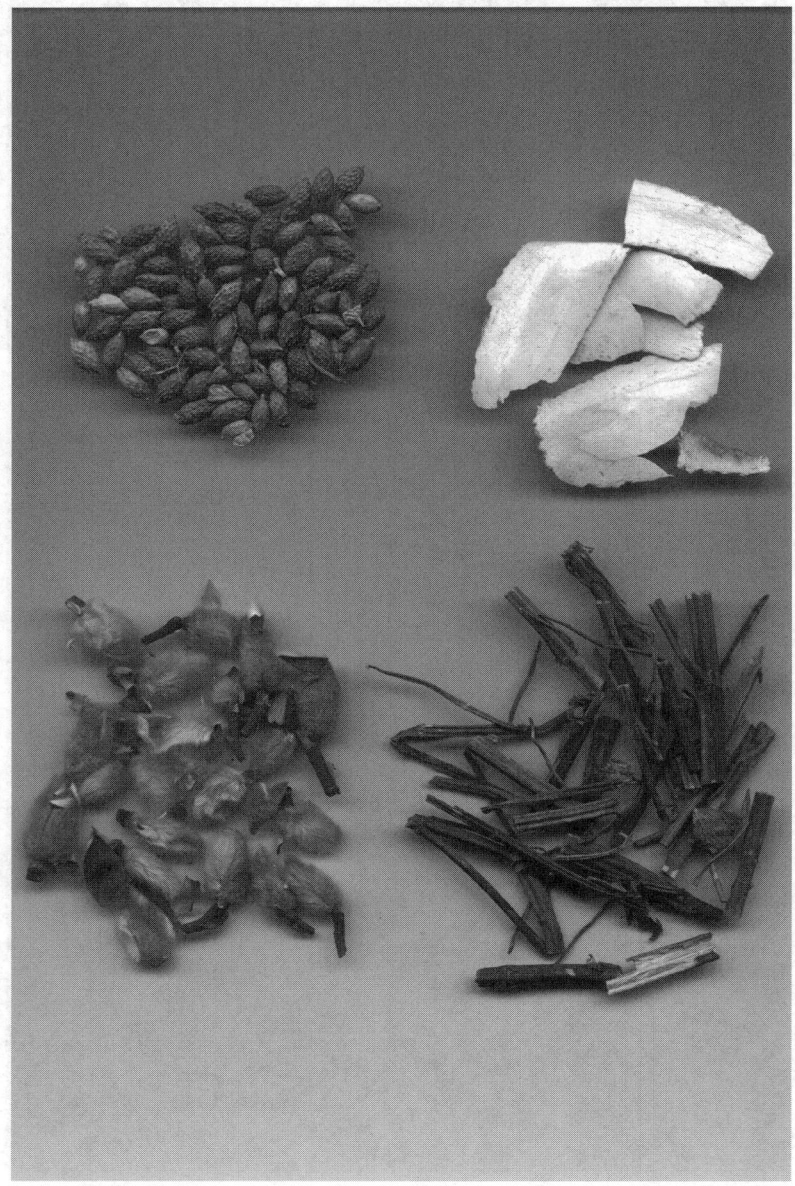

Cang Er Zi San

Clockwise from top left: Cang Er Zi/Xanthium, Bai Zhi/Angelica, Bo He/Mentha, Xin Yi Hua/Magnolia. Shown at one-half actual size.

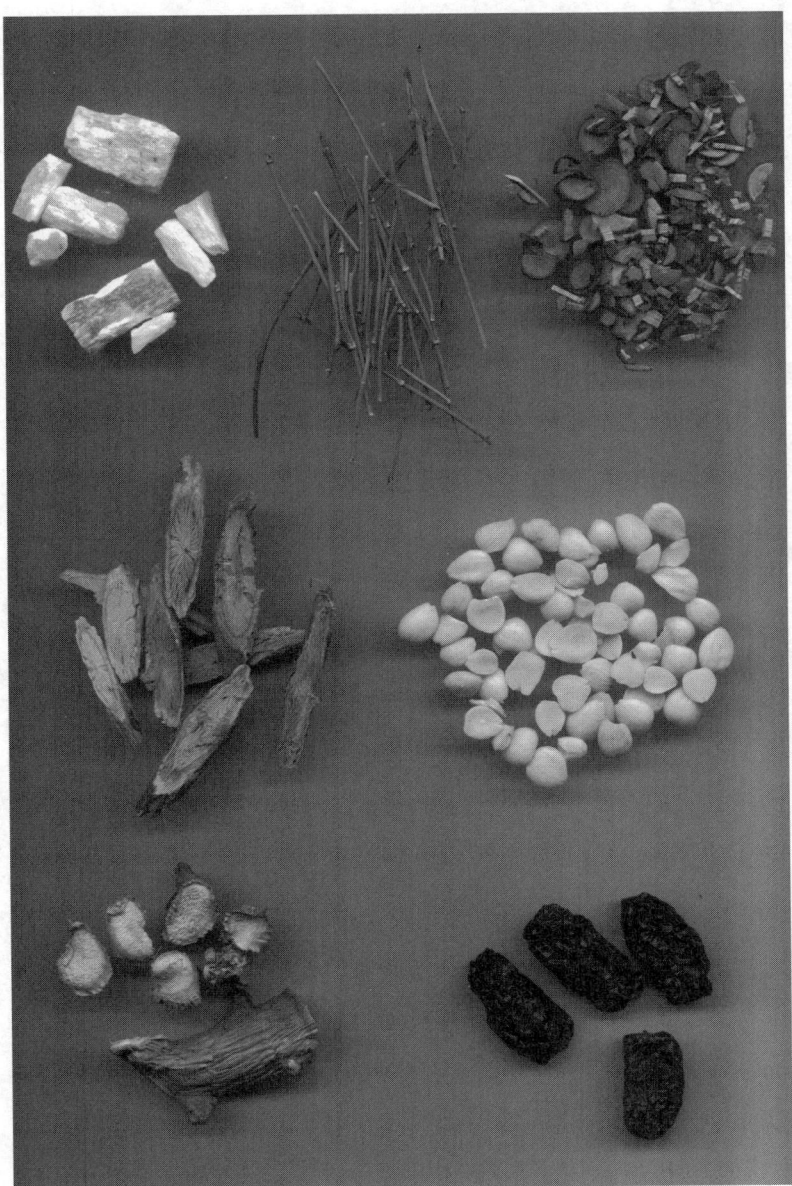

Da Qing Long Tang

Clockwise from top left: Shi Gao/Gypsum, Ma Huang/Ephedra, Gui Zhi/Cinnamomum, Xing Ren/Prunus, Da Zao/Ziziphus, Sheng Jiang/Zingiber, Gan Cao/Glycyrrhiza. Shown at one-half actual size.

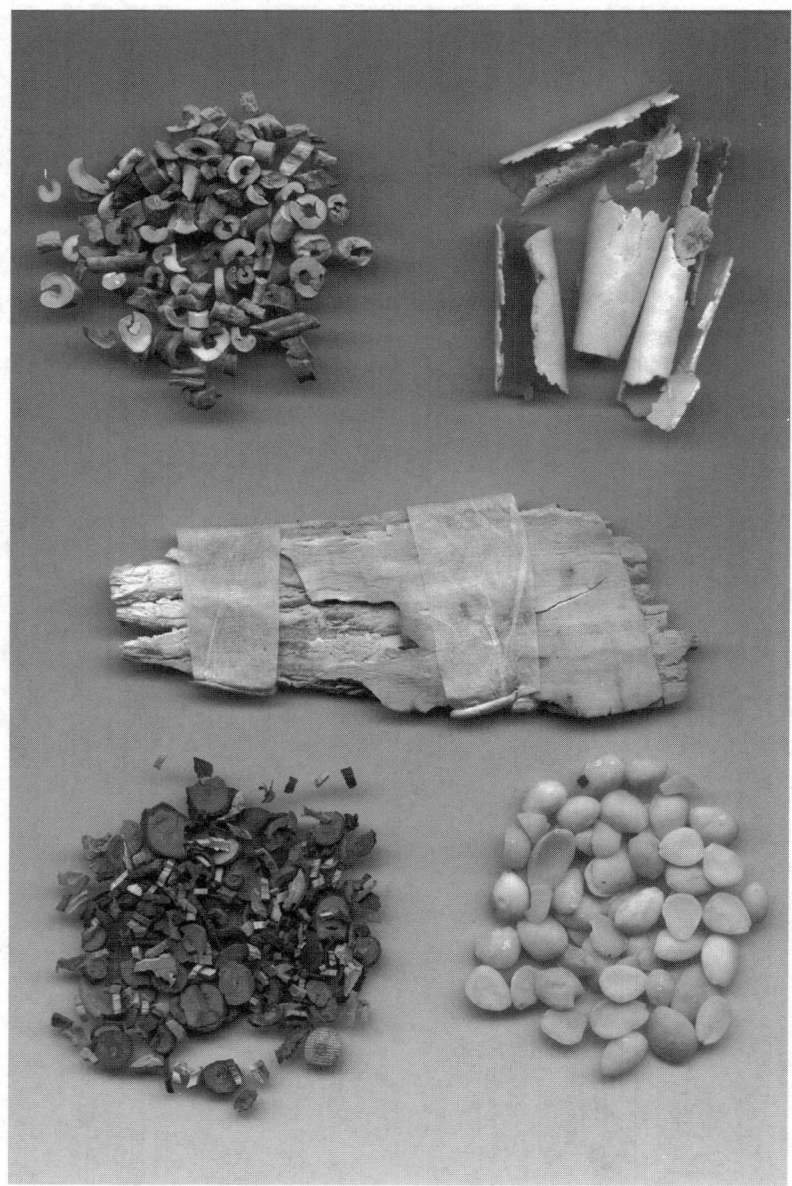

Gui Zhi Fu Ling Wan

Top row left to right: Mu Dan Pi/Paeonia, Fu Ling/Poria. Middle: Chi Shao Yao/Paeonia. Bottom row: Gui Zhi/Cinnamomum, Tao Ren/Prunus. Shown at one-half actual size.

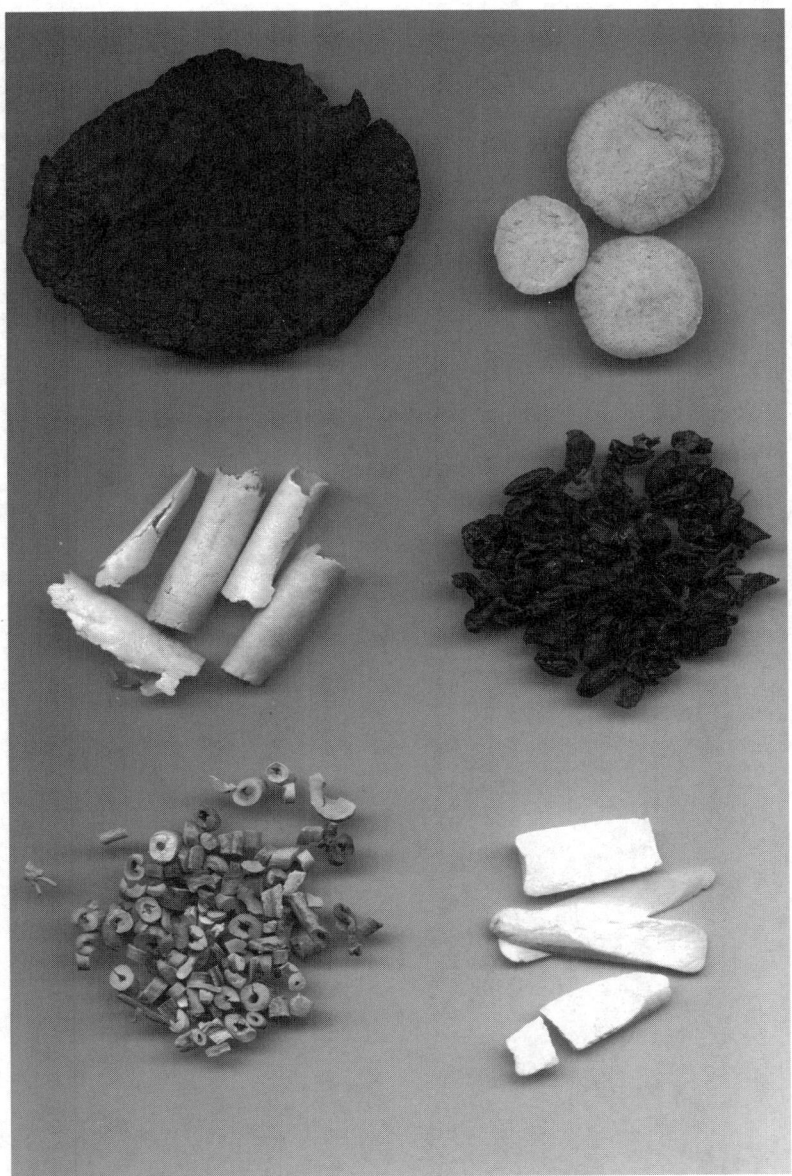

Liu Wei Di Huang Wan

Clockwise from top left: Shu Di Huang/Rehmannia, Ze Xie/Alisma, Shan Zhu Yu/Comus, Shan Yao/Dioscorea, Mu Dan Pi/Paeonia, Fu Ling/Poria. Shown at one-half actual size.

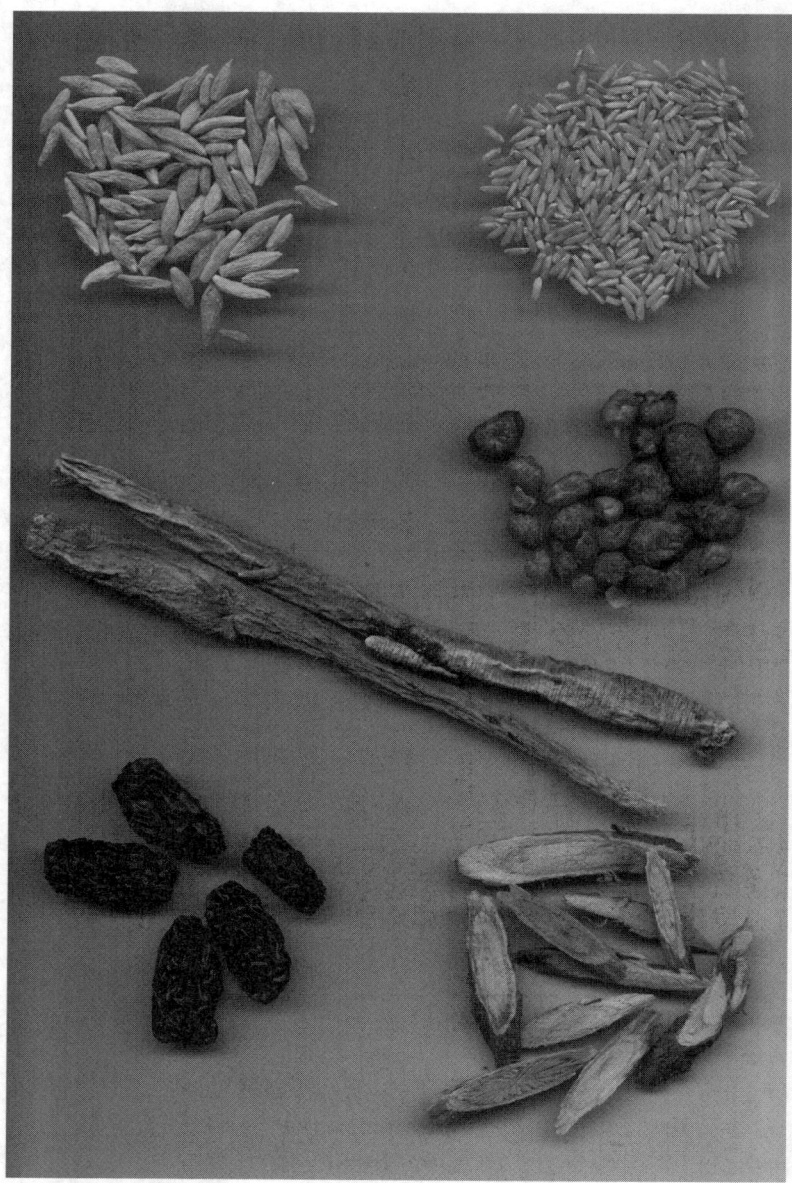

Mai Men Dong Tang

Clockwise from top left: Mai Men Dong/Ophiopogon, Jing Mi/Oryza, Ban Xia/Pinellia, Dang Shen/Codonopsis (long sticks), Gan Cao/Glycyrrhiza, Da Zao/Ziziphus. Shown at one-half actual size.

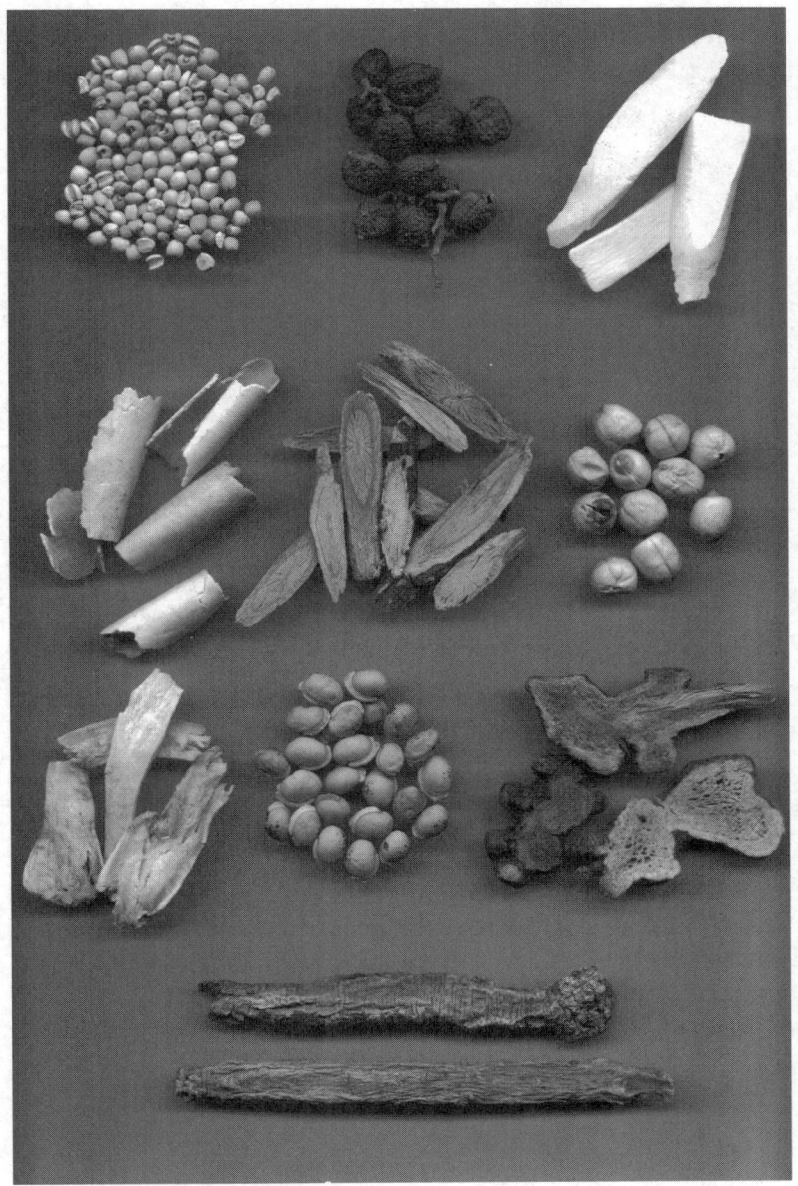

Shen Ling Bai Zhu San

Top row left to right: Yi Yi Ren/Coix, Sha Ren/Amomum, Shan Yao/Discorea. Second row: Fu Ling/Poria, Gan Cao/Glycyrrhiza, Lian Zi/Nelumbo. Third row: Jie Geng/Platycodon, Bian Dou/ Dolichos, Bai Zhu/Atractylodes. Bottom: Dang Shen/Codonopsis. Shown at one-half actual size.

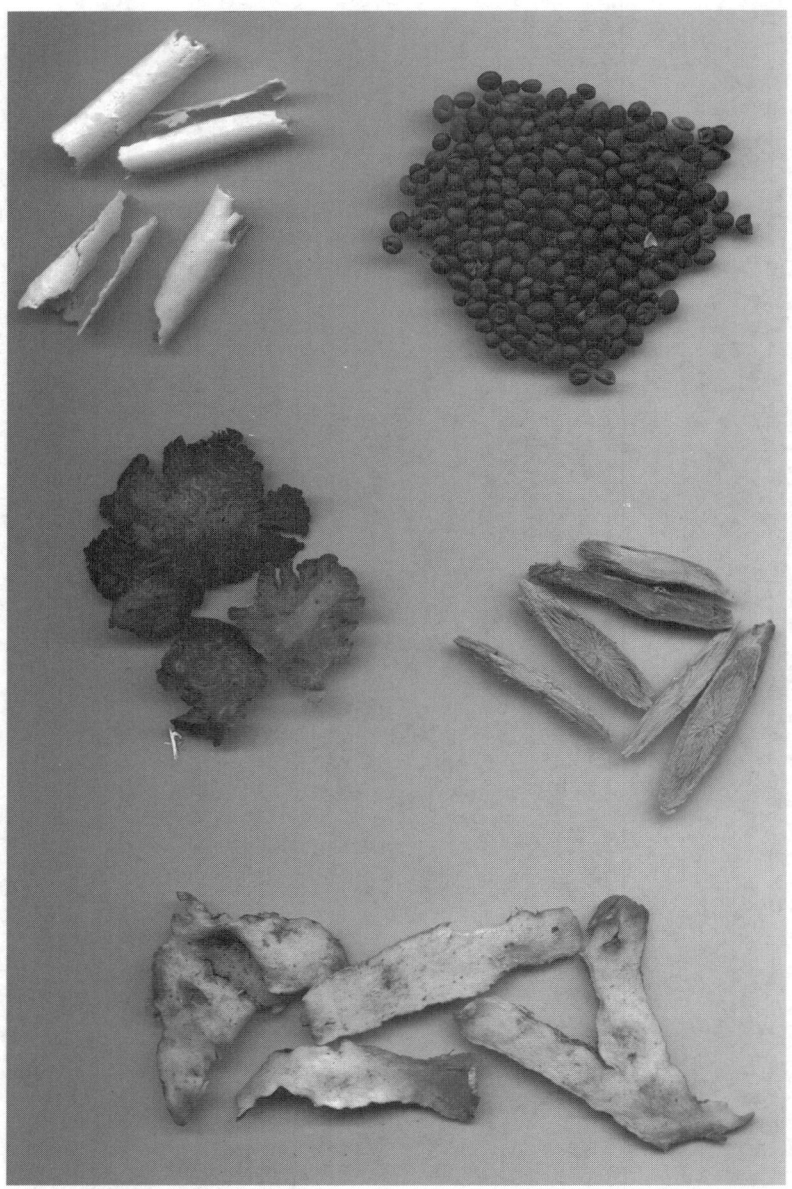

Suan Zao Ren Tang

Clockwise from top left: Fu Ling/Poria, Suan Zao Ren/Ziziphus, Gan Cao/Glycyrrhiza, Zhi Mu/Ane-marrhena, Chuan Xiong/Ligusticum. Shown at one-half actual size.

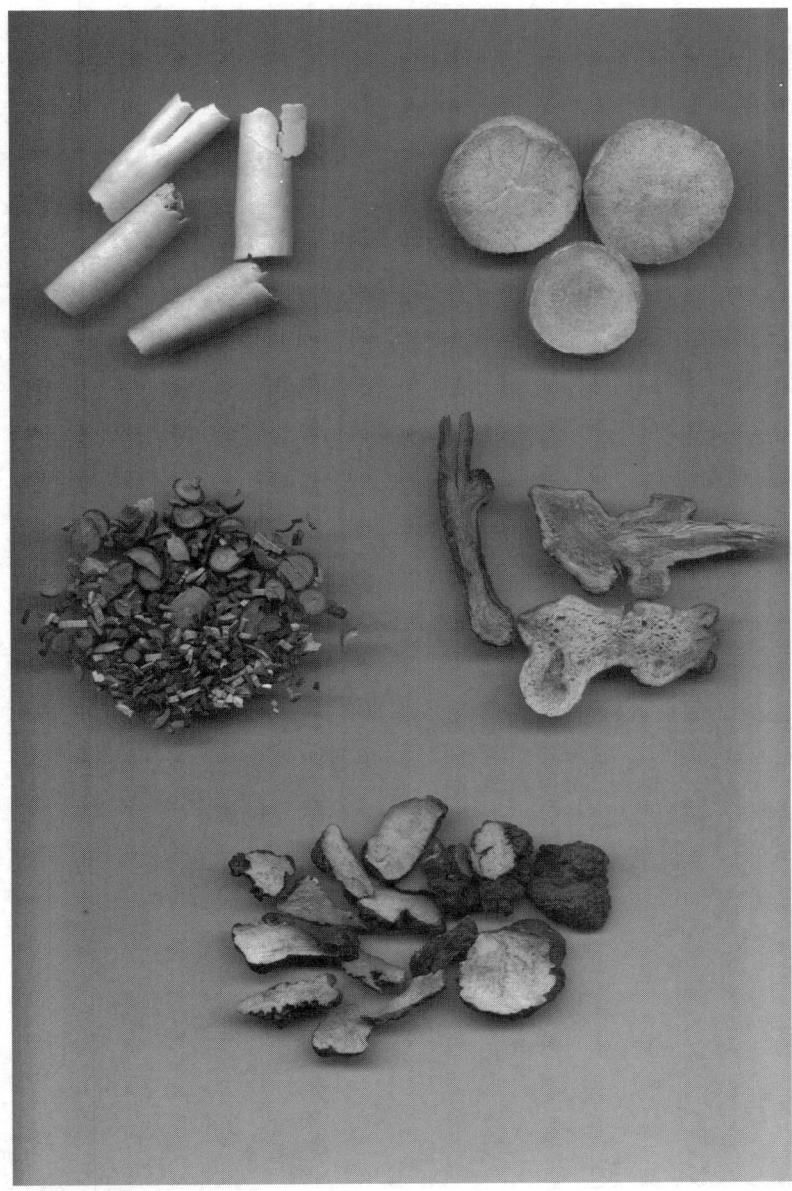

Wu Ling San

Clockwise from top left: Fu Ling/Poria, Ze Xie/Alisma, Bai Zhu/Atractylodes, Zhu Ling/Polyporus, Gui Zhi/Cinnamomum. Shown at one-half actual size.

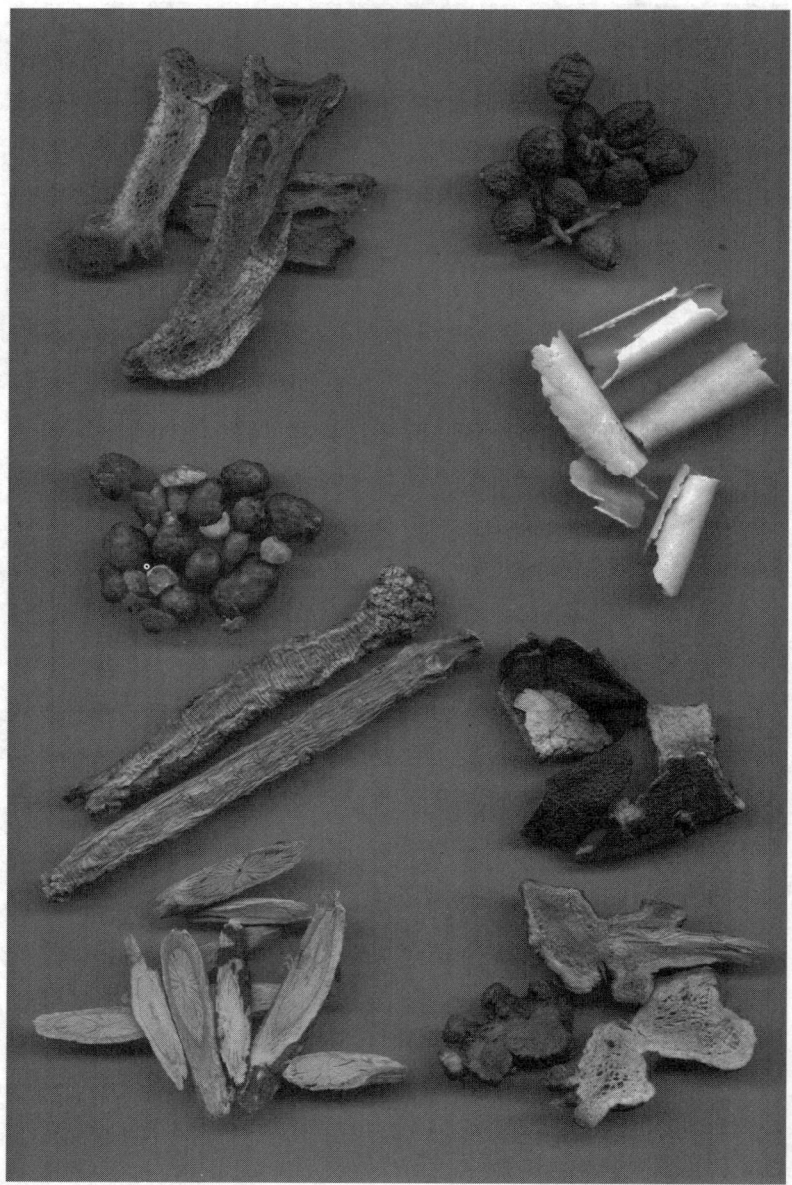

Xiang Sha Liu Jun Zi Tang

Clockwise from top left: Mu Xiang/Saussurea, Sha Ren/Amomum, Fu Ling/Poria, Chen Pi/Citrus, Bai Zhu/Atractylodes, Gan Cao/Glycyrrhiza, Dang Shen/Codonopsis, Ban Xia/Pinellia. Shown at one-half actual size.

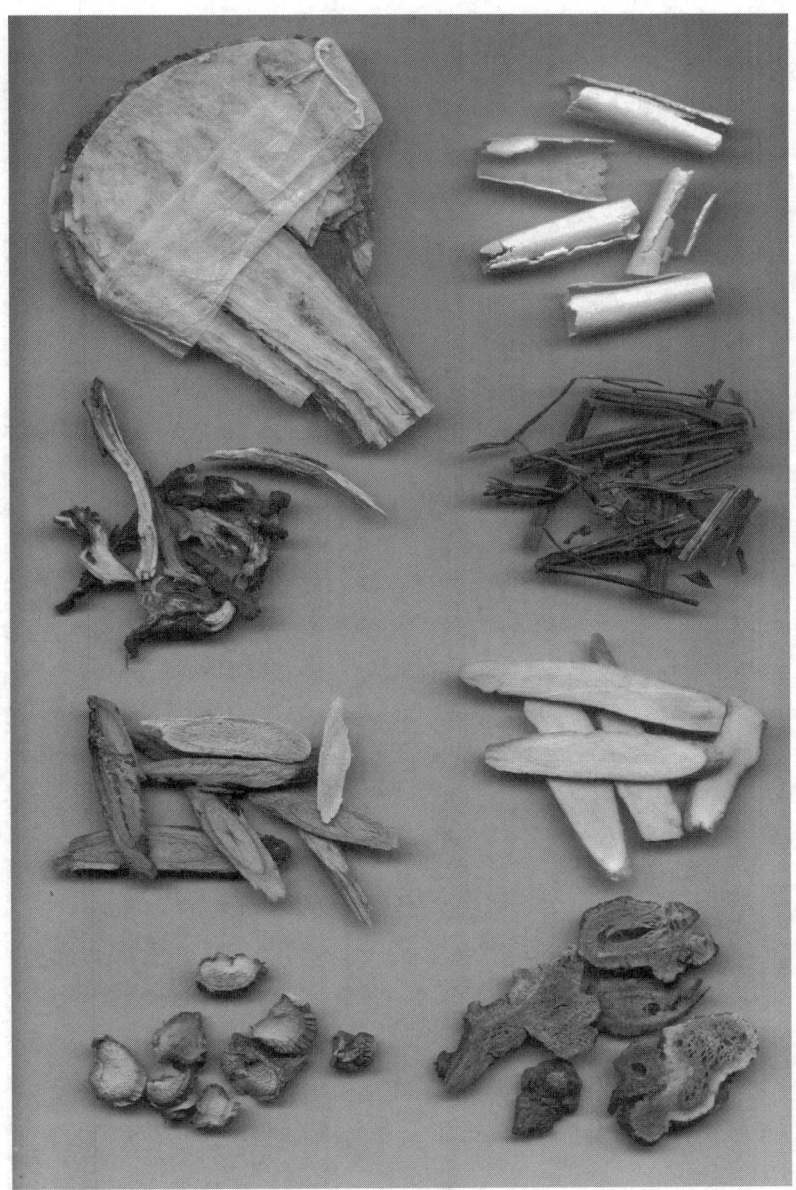

Xiao Yao San

Clockwise from top left: Dang Gui/Angelica, Fu Ling/Poria, Bo He/Mentha, Bai Shao Yao/Paeonia, Bai Zhu/Atractylodes, Sheng Jiang/Zingiber, Gan Cao/Glycyrrhiza, Chai Hu/Bupleurum. Shown at one-half actual size.

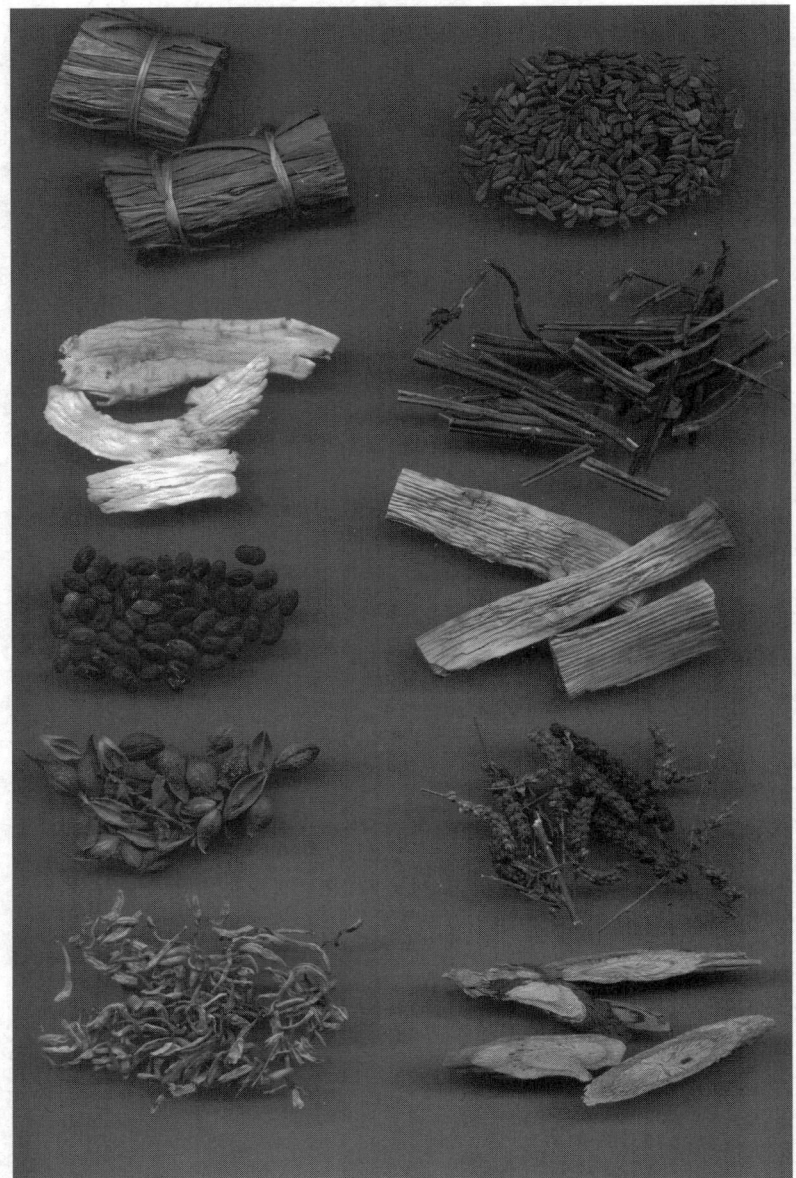

Yin Qiao San

Clockwise from top left: Dan Zhu Ye/Lophatherum, Niu Bang Zi/Arctium, Bo He/Mentha, Lu Gen/Phragmites, Jing Jie/Schizonepeta, Gan Cao/Glycyrrhiza, Jin Yin Hua/Lonicera, Lian Qiao/Forsythia, Dan Dou Chi/Glycine, Jie Geng/Platycodon. Shown at one-half actual size.

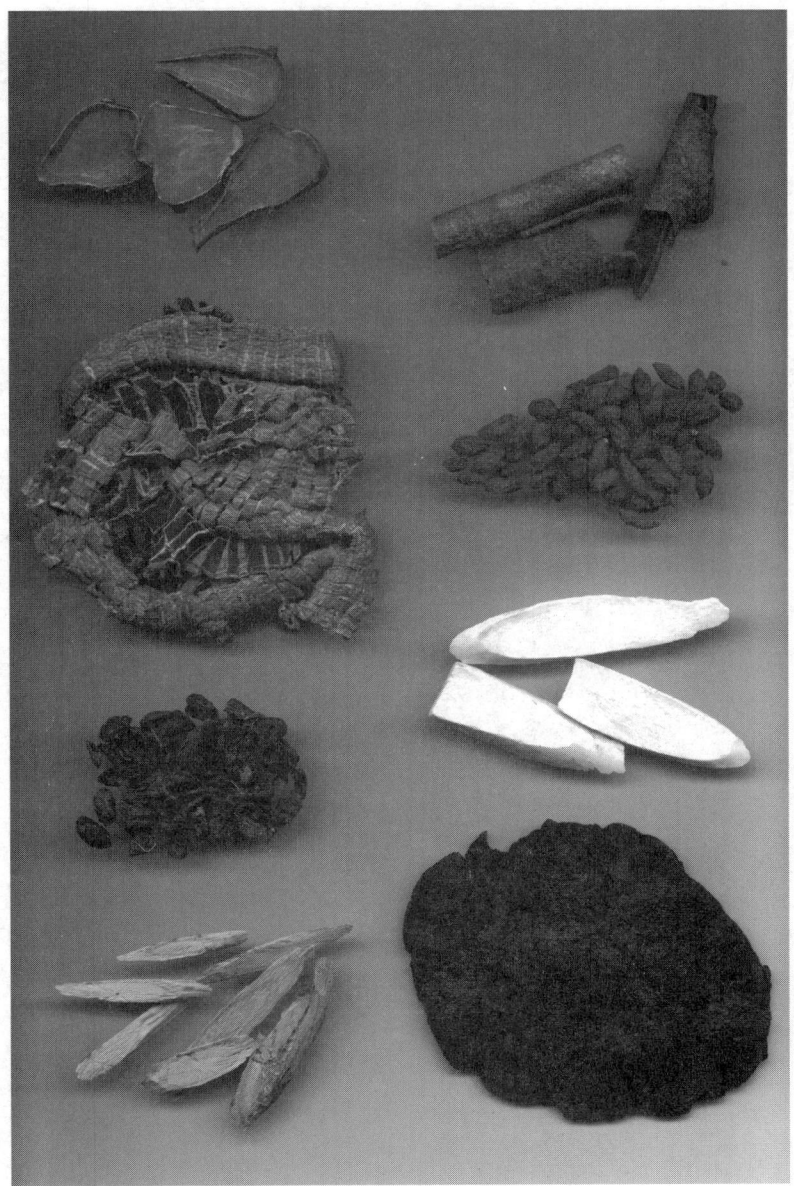

You Gui Yin

Clockwise from top left: Fu Zi/Aconitum, Rou Gui/Cinnamomum, Gou Qi Zi/Lycium, Shan Yao/Dioscorea, Shu Di Huang/Rehmannia, Gan Cao/Glycyrrhiza, Shan Zhu Yu/Comus, Du Zhong/ Eucommia. Shown at one-half actual size.

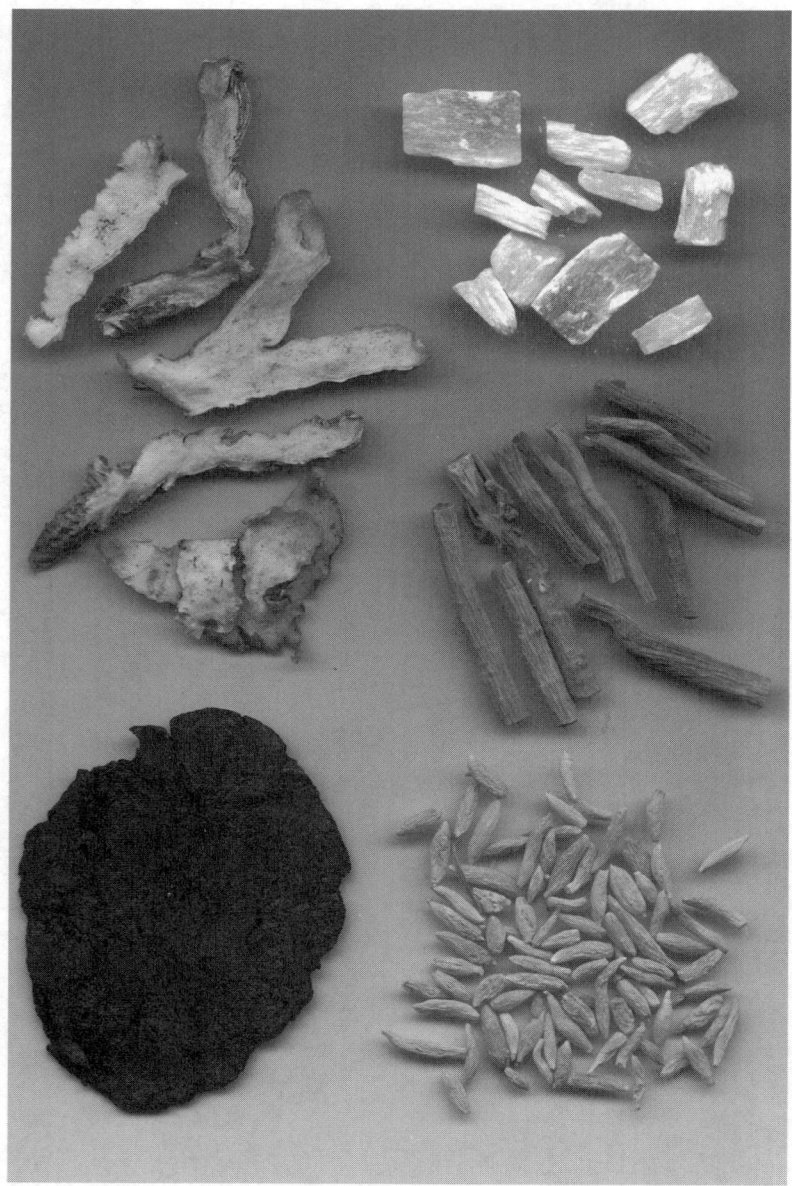

Yu Nu Jian

Clockwise from top left: Zhi Mu/Anemarrhena, Shi Gao/Gypsum, Huai Niu Xi/Achyranthes, Mai Men Dong/Ophlopogon, Sheng Di Huang/Rehmannia. Shown at one-half actual size.

Part 2

Clinical Quick Reference for Single Herbs

Many inexperienced practitioners of Chinese herbal medicine rely on standard formulas. This is both unfortunate and prudent. It takes solid knowledge of herbs and clinical experience to gain the confidence necessary to modify and individualize formulas. Yet customizing formulas can produce effectiveness far beyond that of standard formulas.

This chapter is a selected listing of single herbs organized by traditional categories. However, within the traditional categories, there are innovative subdivisions intended to help steer the practitioner toward choosing the most likely herbs to add or subtract from formulas.

The herb lists selected for this chapter are purposely limited in scope. The herbs within each subdivision are only the most important or commonly used herbs for a given energetic function. Furthermore, herbs are listed only in places where they have primary relevance. (Secondary uses for herbs are not covered here.) Herbs in a given category possess specific properties which particularly suggest their use for that function.

For the practitioner with limited experience using loose herbs, the authors suggest narrowing down the choices for herbs to modify a formula by consulting this chapter. Then it will be helpful to check a materia medica for a full understanding of the final few choices.

This section does not detail the many complex functions and applications of single herbs. It is designed as a learning tool for the most basic energetic functions of the herbs. A more in-depth discussion is beyond the scope of this work. An understanding of the complete range of possible functions and indications of any single herb can be found in a materia medica.

Please note that particular functions and applications of any herb may be changed by how that herb is used in a prescription. The total synergistic complex of other herbs in a formula may change the actions of an herb. For example, an herb that is energetically warm and dispels wind damp cold may be used in a prescription that treats wind damp heat if the formula contains other herbs which give it an overall cool or cold temperature.

Finally, it is important to remember that in Chinese medicine it is common to find many differing subjective interpretations on the uses of herbs. Over time, a practitioner develops an intuitive feel for specific herbs, the relationships between herbs, and which herbs are best for a given patient's needs.

Herbs that Clear Exterior Conditions (Diaphoretics)

Warm, Pungent Herbs that Clear Exterior Conditions

Treat Wind Cold Excess (Strong Wind Cold Dispersing Function)

Ma Huang / Ephedra
Xi Xin / Asarum
Zi Su Ye / Perilla
Gui Zhi / Cinnamomum

Treat Wind Cold Deficiency (Mild, Moderate Wind Cold Dispersing Function)

Jing Jie / Schizonepeta
Fang Feng / Ledebouriella
Gui Zhi / Cinnamomum

Dispel Wind Cold Damp and Alleviate Headaches

Qiang Huo / Notopterygium
Gao Ben / Ligusticum
Bai Zhi / Angelica
Xi Xin / Asarum

Dispel Wind Cold and Open the Nasal Passages

Xin Yi Hua / Magnolia
Cang Er Zi / Xanthium
Xi Xin/ Asarum

Warm Herbs with Multiple Functions and Wide Applications

Sheng Jiang / Zingiber
Cong Bai / Allium
Xiang Ru / Elsholtzia
E Bu Shi Cao / Centipeda
Sheng Liu / Tamarix

Cool, Pungent Herbs that Clear Exterior Conditions

Dispel Wind Heat and Promote the Surfacing of Rashes

Bo He / Mentha
Niu Bang Zi / Arctium
Chan Tui / Cryptotympana

Dispel Wind Heat and Clear Vision

Mu Zei / Equisetum
Gu Jing Cao / Eriocaulon

Dispel Wind Heat, Clear Vision, and Clear the Liver

Sang Ye / Morus
(Huang) Ju Hua / Chrysanthemum

Dispel Wind Heat and Raise Yang Qi

Chai Hu / Bupleurum
Sheng Ma / Cimicifuga

Dispel Wind Heat Trapped in the Muscles

Ge Gen / Pueraria

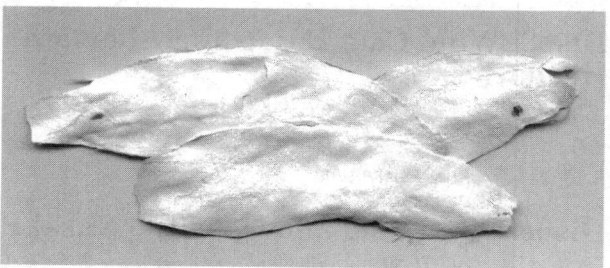

Ge Gen / Pueraria (Shown at one-half actual size)

Cool Herbs with Multiple Functions and Wide Applications

Fu Ping / Spirodela
Dan Dou Chi / Glycine
Man Jing Zi / Vitex
Chai Hu / Bupleurum
Ge Gen / Pueraria

Herbs that Clear Heat

Herbs that Extinguish Fire by Clearing Internal Heat

Clear Heat in the Qi (Yangming) Stage

Clear Lung and Stomach Heat
Shi Gao / Gypsum
Zhi Mu / Anemarrhena
Lu Gen / Phragmites
Ya Zhi Cao / Commelina

Clear Heart and Stomach Heat
Dan Zhu Ye / Lophatherum

Clear Heart Fire
Lian Xin / Nelumbo

Clear Heat (and Damp) from the Liver and Three Burners
Zhi Zi / Gardenia

Clear Fire and Summer Heat
Han Shui Shi / Calcitum

Clear Heat, Spasms, and Fire Poison
Xiong Dan / Ursus
Niu Dan / Bos

Clear Heat and Brighten the Eyes

Clear Both Excess Liver Heat and Wind Heat and Brighten Eyes
Jue Ming Zi / Cassia
Qing Xiang Zi / Celosia

Clear Both Excess and Deficient Liver Heat and Brighten the Eyes
Xia Ku Cao / Prunella
Mi Meng Hua / Buddleia
Chong Wei Zi / Leonurus
(Bai) Ju Hua / Chrysanthemum

Clear Excess Liver Heat Only
Ye Ming Sha / Vespertilio

Herbs that Clear Heat and Cool the Blood

Cool the Blood and Clear Heart Fire
Xi Jiao / Rhinoceros
Shui Niu Jiao / Bubalus

Cool the Blood and Clear Large Intestine and Liver Heat
Huai Jiao / Sophora

Cool the Blood and Detoxify Fire Poison
Zi Cao / Lithospermum
Mu Dan Pi / Paeonia

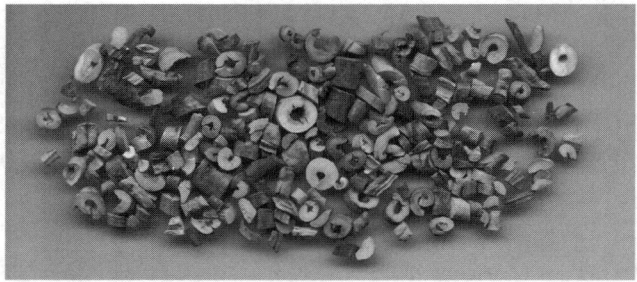

Mu Dan Pi / Paeonia (Shown at one-half actual size)

Cool the Blood and Clear Yin Deficient Heat
Di Gu Pi / Lycium
Yin Chai Hu / Stellaria
Bai Wei / Cynanchum

Cool the Blood, Nourish Yin, and Produce Fluids
Sheng Di Huang / Rehmannia
Xuan Shen / Scrophularia

Additional Herb with Multiple Functions and Wide Applications
Mu Dan Pi / Paeonia

Herbs that Clear Heat and Dry Damp

Target the Three Burners

Upper Burner
Huang Qin / Scutellaria
Tang Song Cao / Thalictrum

Middle Burner
Huang Lian / Coptis
Xiao Nie / Berberis
Shi Da Gong Lao / Mahonia

Lower Burner
Huang Bai / Phellodendron

Targets the Liver/Gallbladder
Long Dan Cao / Gentiana

Targets the Liver and Large Intestine
Qin Pi / Fraxinus

Targets the Large Intestine and Skin
Ku Shen / Sophora

Clears Heat, Dries Dampness, and Clears Yin Deficient Heat
Hu Huang Lian / Picrorhiza

Herbs that Clear Heat and Toxins

Treat Febrile Disease and Epidemic Poison

Particularly Throat and Lung Fire Poison
Da Qing Ye / Isatis
Ban Lan Gen / Isatis

Particularly Toxic Abscesses and Swellings
Jin Yin Hua / Lonicera
Lian Qiao / Forsythia

Treat a Wide Range of Heat Patterns Including Fire Poison, Toxic Abscesses and Swellings
Pu Gong Ying / Taraxacum
Chuan Xin Lian / Andrographis
Zao Xiu / Paris
Qing Mu Xiang / Aristolochia
Zi Bei Tian Kui / Begonia

Treat Toxic Swelling: Internal and External Abscesses, Nodules, Sores, Carbuncles, Boils, etc. (Including Some Tumors)

Primarily Administered Internally
Ban Zhi Lian / Scutellaria
Tu Fu Ling / Smilax

Breast Abscess
Lou Lu / Rhaponticum

Lung Abscess
Yu Xing Cao / Houttuynia

Intestinal Abscess
Bai Hua She She Cao / Oldenlandia
Hong Teng / Sargentodoxa

Administered Both Internally and Externally
Bai Xian Pi / Dictamnus
Bai Lian / Ampelopsis
Lu Jiao / Cervus
Si Ji Qing / Ilex
Zao Jiao Ci / Gleditsia

Lung Abscess
Hu Er Cao / Saxifraga

Intestinal Abscess
Bai Jiang Cao / Patrinia

Breast or Intestinal Abscess
Pu Gong Ying / Taraxacum

Benefit the Throat and Clear Throat Inflammation

Clear Heat and Fire Poison
Jin Sha Teng / Lygodium
Ma Bo / Lasiosphaera
Shan Dou Gen / Sophora
Qing Dai / Indigo
Dian Di Mei / Androsace
Zhu Sha Gen / Ardisia
Jin Guo Lan / Tinospora
Wan Nian Qing / Rhodea

Clear Heat, Fire Poison and Hot Poisonous Phlegm (such as Diptheria)
She Gan / Belamcanda
Suan Jiang / Physalis

Treat Throat Inflammation and Toxic Abscesses

Ye Ju Hua / Chrysanthemum
Zi Hua Di Ding / Viola
Tu Niu Xi / Achyranthes
Shi Shang Bai / Selaginella
Qian Li Guang / Senecio
Guan Ye Liao / Polygonum
Jin Qiao Mai / Fagopyrum

Treat Toxic Dysentery-Like Disorders

Treat Acute Disorders: Epidemic Damp Heat, Fire Poison and Bleeding

Bai Tou Weng / Pulsatilla
Ma Chi Xian / Portulaca
Tie Xian / Acalypha
Feng Wei Cao / Pteris
Fan Bai Cao / Potentilla

Treat Chronic, Recurring and Cold Stagnation Disorders

Ya Dan Zi / Brucea

Herbs that Clear and Alleviate Summerheat

Summerheat with Thirst

Lu Dou / Phaseolus
Ren Shen Ye / Panax

Summerheat with Thirst and Scanty Urine

Xi Gua / Citrullus
Dong Gua Pi / Benincasa

Summerheat with Chest Discomfort

Lian Geng / Nelumbo

Summerheat with Diarrhea

He Ye / Nelumbo

Summerheat with Diarrhea and Vomiting

Bian Dou / Dolichos

Summerheat with Multiple Signs and Symptoms of Damp Heat

Dou Juan / Glycine

Clear Summerheat, Cool the Blood and Clear
Deficient Blood or Yin Fevers
Qing Hao / Artemisia

Herbs that Treat Malaria

Chang Shan / Dichroa
Shu Qi / Dichroa
Qing Hao / Artemisia
Ma Bian Cao / Verbena
Ya Dan Zi / Brucea
Yan Fu Mu / Rhus
Tian Ming Jing / Carpesium
Ba Xian Hua / Hydrangea

Herbs that Drain Downward

Purgatives

Treat Acute Excess Heat Accumulation

Da Huang / Rheum
Mang Xiao / Mirabilitum
Fan Xie Ye / Cassia

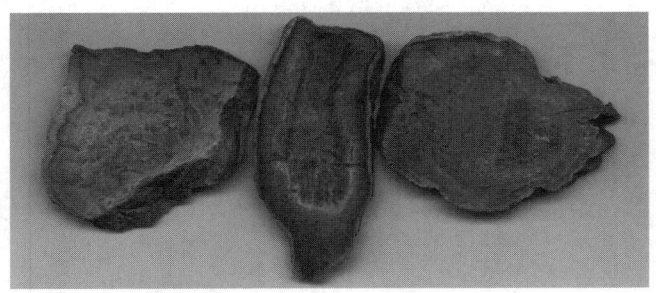

Da Huang / Rheum (Shown at one-half actual size)

Treat Chronic Accumulation of Heat

Lu Hui / Aloe

Moist Lubricants

Gentle, Nourishing Moist Laxatives for Deficient Conditions

Huo Ma Ren / Cannabis
Feng Mi / Mel

Strong Moist Laxative for Excess Conditions

Yu Li Ren / Prunus

Severe Expellants (Cathartics)

Moderate Expellant Herb that Can Be Used for a Longer Period of Time

Qian Nui Zi / Pharbitis

Severe Cathartic Herbs that Should Be Used for Short Periods of Time Only

Shang Lu / Phytolacca
Yuan Hua / Daphne
Gan Sui / Euphorbia
Jing Da Ji / Euphorbia
Xu Sui Zi / Euphorbia
Wu Jiu Gen Pi / Sapium

Severe Cathartic Herb for Cold Conditions that Should Be Used for Short Periods of Time Only

Ba Dou / Croton

Herbs that Drain Damp (Diuretics)

Anti-edemic Herbs that Regulate Water Metabolism

Promote Urination and Drain Damp

Fu Ling / Poria
Fu Ling Pi / Poria
Ze Xie / Alisma
Zhu Ling / Polyporus
Dong Gua Pi / Benincasa
Sheng Jiang Pi / Zingiber
Pu Hui / Typha

Promote Urination, Drain Damp and Fortify the Spleen

Fu Ling / Poria
Shu Yi Ren / Coix

Clear Heat and Drain Damp

Chi Fu Ling / Poria
Yi Yi Ren / Coix
Han Fang Ji / Stephania
Guang Fang Ji / Aristolochia
Dong Gua Ren / Benincasa
Chi Xiao Dou / Phaseolus
Ban Bian Lian / Lobelia
Lu Ying / Sambucus
San Bai Cao / Saururus

Urinary Soothing Herbs that Treat Painful Urinary Disorder

With Equal Heat and Damp

Mu Tong / Akebia
Tong Cao / Tetrapanax
Di Fu Zi / Kochia
Bian Xu / Polygonum

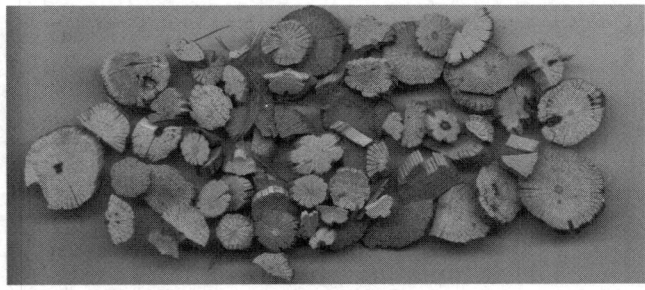

Mu Tong / Akebia (Shown at one-half actual size)

With Predominant Heat
Shi Wei / Pyrrosia
Deng Xin Cao / Juncus
Qu Mai / Dianthus
Che Qian Cao / Plantago
Hai Jin Sha / Lygodium

With Predominant Dampness
Bei Xie / Dioscorea

With Stones
Jin Qian Cao / Lysimachia
Yu Mi Xu / Zea
Hai Jin Sha / Lygodium
Lou Gu / Gryllotalpa

With Concomitant Diarrhea
Che Qian Zi / Plantago
Hua Shi / Talcum

With Concomitant Constipation
Dong Kui Zi / Abutilon

Herbs that Relieve Jaundice
Yin Chen Hao / Artemisia
Jin Qian Cao / Lysimachia
Yu Mi Xu / Zea
Hu Zhang / Polygonum
Chui Pen Cao / Sedum

Herbs that Resolve Phlegm and Stop Cough

Herbs that Resolve Phlegm

Cool Herbs that Resolve Hot Phlegm

Hot Phlegm Accumulation in the Lungs
Chuan Bei Mu / Fritillaria
Qian Hu / Peucedanum
Gua Luo / Trichosanthes
Gua Lua Ren / Trichosanthes
Tian Hua Fen / Trichosanthes
Tian Zhu Huang / Bambusa
Pang Da Hai / Sterculia
Bai Mao Xia Ku Cao / Ajuga
Gan Jie Geng / Adenophora

Hot Phlegm Accumulation in the Stomach
Zhu Ru / Bambusa

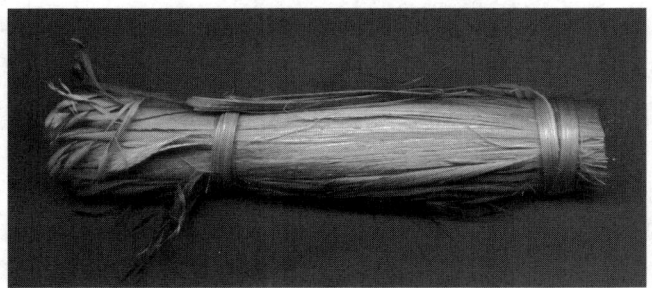

Zhu Ru / Bambusa (Shown at one-half actual size)

Turbid Phlegm Blocking the Channels
Kun Bu / Laminaria
Hai Dai / Laminaria
Hai Zao / Sargassum
Zhe Bei Mu / Fritillaria
Fu Hai Shi / Pumice
Ze Qi / Euphorbia
Huang Yao Zi / Dioscorea

Turbid Phlegm Obstructing the Orifices
Zhu Li / Bambusa
Hou Zao / Macaque

Warm Herbs that Resolve Cold Phlegm

Cold Phlegm Accumulation in the Lungs
Bai Qian / Cynanchum
Ju Hong / Citrus

Cold Damp Phlegm Accumulation in the Stomach/Spleen
(Fa) Ban Xia / Pinellia
Xuan Fu Hua / Inula
Jin Fei Cao / Inula

Turbid Phlegm Blocking the Channels
Bai Jie Zi / Brassica

Turbid Phlegm Obstructing the Orifices
Bai Fu Zi / Typhonium
Zao Jiao / Gleditsia
Zhi Nan Xing / Arisaema

Neutral Temperature Herbs that Resolve Both Hot and Cold Phlegm

Phlegm Accumulation in the Lungs
(Ku) Jie Geng / Platycodon
Han Cai / Rorippa

Turbid Phlegm Blocking the Channels
Hai Ge Ke / Cyclina
Wa Leng Zi / Arca
Mao Zhao Cao / Ranunculus

Turbid Phlegm Obstructing the Orifices
Meng Shi / Lapis Micae seu Chloriti

Herbs that Alleviate Cough and Wheezing

Cough from Many Different Etiologies
(Bei) Xing Ren / Prunus
Zi Wan / Aster
Kuan Dong Hua / Tussilago

Externally Contracted Cough
Kuan Dong Hua / Tussilago
(Bei) Xing Ren / Prunus
Gua Lou Pi / Trichosanthes

Cold Induced Cough

Zi Wan / Aster
Zi Su Zi / Perilla
Hu Tui Ye / Eleagnus
(Bei)Xing Ren / Prunus

Heat Induced Cough

Sang Bai Pi / Morus
Pi Pa Ye / Eriobotrya
Ma Dou Ling / Aristolochia
Bao Ma Zi / Syringa
(Bei) Xing Ren / Prunus
Da Juan Hua Ye / Rhododendron
Ji Ning / Salvia

Cough with Phlegm Accumulation in the Lungs

Kuan Dong Hua / Tussilago
Zi Su Zi / Perilla
Zi Wan / Aster
(Bei) Xing Ren / Prunus
Zi Jin Niu / Ardisia
Da Juan Hua Ye / Rhododendron
Ji Ning / Salvia
Bao Ma Zi / Syringa

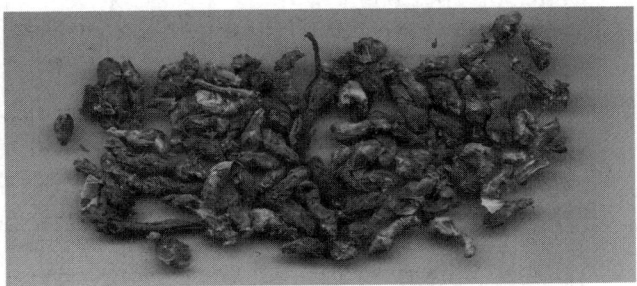

Kuan Dong Hua / Tussilago (Shown at one-half actual size)

Cough with Phlegm Accumulation in the Stomach and/or Lungs

Pi Pa Ye / Eriobotrya

Dry Cough

Kuan Dong Hua / Tussilago
Pi Pa Ye / Eriobotrya
(Nan) Xing Ren / Prunus
Gua Lou Pi / Trichosanthes

Nan Wu Wei Zi / Schisandra

Cough with Wheezing
Kuan Dong Hua / Tussilago
Zi Su Zi / Perilla
Sang Bai Pi / Morus
Ma Dou Ling / Aristolochia
(Bei) Xing Ren / Prunus
Sha Ren Hua / Amomum
Fo Shou Hua / Citrus
Ting Li Zi / Lepidium

Chronic, Deficient Cough Stemming from Internal Damage

Cold Deficient Cough
Zi Wan / Aster
Bai Bu / Stemona
Hu Tui Ye / Eleagnus

Lung Deficient Cough with Phlegm Heat
Ma Dou Ling / Aristolochia
Ba Mao Zi / Syringa

Deficient Yin Cough
Bai Bu / Stemona
Nan Sha Shen / Adenophora

Cough with Hoarseness
Mu Hu Die / Oroxylum
Ren Shen Ye / Panax

Cough with a Sensation of Chest Constriction
Zi Su Zi / Perilla
Zi Su Geng / Perilla

Cough accompanied by Edema
Sang Bai Pi / Morus
Zi Jin Niu / Ardisia
Jiao Mu / Zanthoxylum

Herbs that Expel Phlegm Through Vomiting (Emetics)
Li Lu / Veratrum
Gua Di / Cucumis
Chang Shan / Dichroa
Shu Qi / Dichroa
Ren Shen Lu / Panax

Herbs that Expel Wind Damp (Anti-rheumatics)

Pain Relieving Herbs that Target the Muscle Layer

Wind Damp Cold in the Upper Body
Qiang Huo / Notopterygium

Wind Damp Cold in the Lower Body
Du Huo / Angelica
Can Sha / Bombyx

Wind Damp Cold in Both the Upper and Lower Body
Fang Feng / Ledebouriella
Wei Ling Xian / Clematis
Cang Er Zi / Xanthium
Song Jie / Pinus
Cang Er Cao / Xanthium
Chuan Wu / Aconitum
Wu Tou / Aconitum
Cao Wu / Aconitum

Wind Damp Heat in Both the Upper and Lower Body
Guang Fang Ji / Aristolochia

Neutral Temperature Herbs that Dispel Wind Damp in Both the Upper and Lower Body
Qin Jiao / Gentiana
She Tui / Zaocys
Chuan Shan Long / Dioscorea
Xun Gu Feng / Aristolochia
Ba Qia / Smilax

Invigorating Herbs that Target the Channel Layer

Wind Damp Cold in the Lower Body
Mu Gua / Chaenomeles

Wind Damp Cold in Both the Upper and Lower Body
Hai Feng Teng / Piper
Wei Ling Xian / Clematis
Bai Hua She / Agkistrodon
Shen Jin Cao / Lycopodium

Wind Damp Heat in Both the Upper and Lower Body

Xi Xian Cao / Siegesbeckia
Luo Shi Teng / Trachelospermum
Kuan Jin Teng / Tinospora
Si Gua Luo / Luffa
Chou Wu Tong / Clerodendron
Ren Dong Teng / Lonicera

Neutral Temperature Herbs that Dispel Wind Damp in the Upper Body

Sang Zhi / Morus

Neutral Temperature Herbs that Dispel Wind Damp in the Lower Body

Lu Lu Tong / Liquidambar
Chuan Niu Xi / Cyathula
Hai Tong Pi / Erythrina

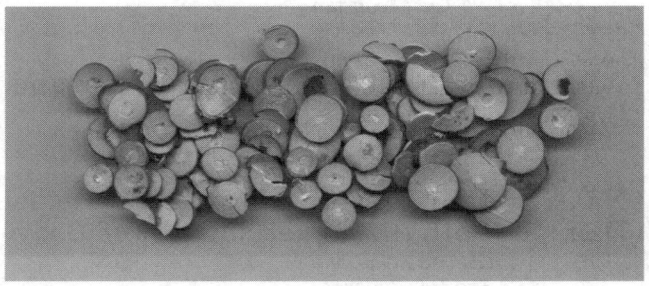

Sang Zhi / Morus (Shown at one-half actual size)

Neutral Temperature Herbs that Dispel Wind Damp in Both the Upper and Lower Body

Wu Shao She / Zaocys
Lao Guan Cao / Erodium

Strengthening Herbs that Target the Bone and Tendon Layer

Wind Damp Cold in the Lower Body

Xu Duan / Dipsacus
Lu Xian Cao / Pyrola
Gou Ji / Cibotium
Sang Ji Sheng / Loranthus
Du Huo / Angelica

Wind Damp Cold in Both the Upper and Lower Body

Wu Jia Pi / Acanthopanax
Hu Gu / Panthera
Bao Gu / Panthera
Gou Gu / Canis
Qian Nian Jian / Homalomena
Chang Chun Teng / Hedera

Aromatic Herbs that Resolve Middle Jiao Damp

Release Exterior Damp Summerheat Patterns with Digestive Symptoms

> Huo Xiang / Agastache
> Pei Lan / Eupatorium

Dispel Damp which Distresses the Middle Jiao

> Huo Xiang / Agastache
> Hou Po / Magnolia
> Hou Po Hua / Magnolia
> Cang Zhu / Atractylodes
> Bai Dou Kou / Amomum
> Sha Ren / Amomum
> Sha Ren Ke / Amomum

Dispel Cold and Dry Damp Due to Cold, Deficient Middle Jiao

> Cao Guo / Amomum
> Cao Dou Kou / Alpinia

Herbs that Alleviate Food Stagnation

Alleviate Food Stagnation and Accumulation Due to Meat

Shan Zha / Crataegus

Alleviate Food Stagnation and Accumulation Due to Grains

Hot Food Stagnation
Gu Ya / Oryza

Cold Food Stagnation and Deficient Middle Jiao
Mai Ya / Hordeum

Treat Cold Food Stagnation Due to Cold, Deficient Middle Jiao

Shen Qu / Massa Fermentata
Ji Nei Jin / Gallus
E Wei / Ferula
Ji Shi Teng / Paederia
Ge Shan Xiang / Cynanchum

Treat Food and Phlegm Stagnation

Lai Fu Zi / Raphanus

Herbs that Warm the Interior and Dispel Cold

Warm Endogenous Spleen Cold Deficiency

Fu Zi / Aconitum
Rou Gui / Cinnamomum
Gan Jiang / Zingiber

Warm Kidneys and Tonify Yang

Fu Zi / Aconitum
Rou Gui / Cinnamomum

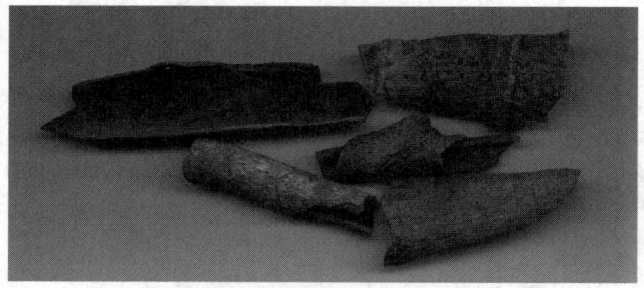

Rou Gui / Cinnamomum (Shown at one-half actual size)

Dispel Cold Pathogenic Influence in the Stomach

Bi Ba / Piper
Hu Jiao / Piper
Bi Cheng Qie / Piper

Dispel Cold Pathogenic Influence in the Middle Jiao

Chuan Jiao / Zanthoxylum
Ding Xiang / Caryophyllum
Gao Liang Jiang / Alpinia
Ba Jiao Hui Xiang / Illicium

Dispel Cold Pathogenic Influence in the Stomach/Liver and their Respective Channels

Wu Zhu Yu / Evodia
Xiao Hui Xiang / Foeniculum

Alleviate the Pain of Cold Pathogenic Influence in the Low Back and Lower Abdomen

Dou Chi Jiang / Litsea

Herbs that Regulate the Qi

Regulate Middle Jiao Qi Stagnation

Zhi Shi / Citrus
Zhi Ke / Citrus
Da Fu Pi / Areca
Bing Lang / Areca
Shi Di / Diospyros

Regulate Liver Qi Stagnation

Qing Pi / Citrus
Ju He / Citrus
Mei Gui Hua / Rosa
Xiang Fu / Cyperus
Chuan Lian Zi / Melia

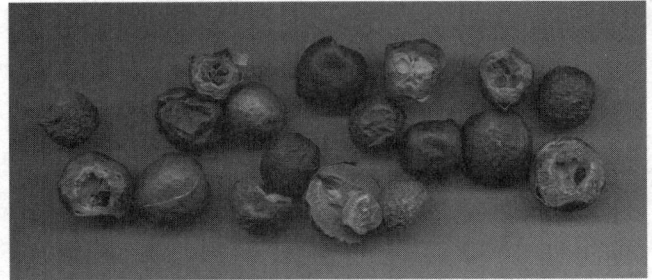

Chuan Lian Zi / Melia (Shown at one-half actual size)

Regulate Mixed Qi Stagnation

Lung, Spleen and Stomach Qi Stagnation
Chen Pi / Citrus
Chen Xiang / Aquilaria

Liver and Stomach Qi Stagnation
Li Zhi He / Litchi
Ba Yue Zha / Akebia

Liver and Spleen/Stomach Qi Stagnation
Mu Xiang / Saussurea
Fo Shou / Citrus

Multiple Mixed Qi Stagnation
Tan Xiang / Santalum
Xie Bai / Allium
Wu Yao / Lindera
Yan Hu Suo / Corydalis

Herbs that Regulate the Blood

Herbs that Arrest Bleeding (Hemostatics)

Hemostatic Herbs with Astringent Action

Stop Coughing and Vomiting of Blood
Bai Ji / Bletilla

Arrest Excessive Uterine Bleeding
Xue Yu Tan / Homo Sapiens

Arrest Urinary Bleeding
Zi Zhu / Callicarpa

Arrest the Bleeding Diarrhea of Chronic Dysentery-like Disorders
Shan Zha Tan / Crataegus
Shi Bing / Diospyros

Arrest Bleeding in Miscellaneous Locations
Xian He Cao / Agrimonia
Zong Lu Pi Tan / Trachycarpus
Hua Sheng Yi / Arachis
Ji Mu / Loropetalum

Hemostatic Herbs with Astringent and Invigorating Actions that Dispel Congealed Blood Stasis

Stop Coughing and Vomiting of Blood
Ou Jie / Nelumbo

Stop Excessive Menstrual or Uterine Bleeding
Chong Wei Zi / Leonurus

Stop Bleeding Due to Trauma
Jiang Xiang / Dalbergia

Arrest Bleeding in Miscellaneous Locations
Pu Huang Tan / Typha
Lian Fang / Nelumbo
Hua Rui Shi / Ophicalcitum
Jing Tian San Qi / Sedum
Mao Mei / Rubus

Hemostatic Herbs that are Unobstructing and Dispel Congealed Blood Stasis

San Qi / Panax
Ju Ye San Qi / Gynura

Blood Cooling Hemostatic Herbs

Arrest Nasal Bleeding

Bai Mao Gen / Imperata
Bai Mao Hua / Imperata

Stop Coughing and Vomiting of Blood

Qian Cao Gen / Rubia

Arrest Excessive Uterine Bleeding

Zhu Ma Gen / Boehmeria

Arrest Urinary Bleeding

Xiao Ji / Cephalanoplos

Stop Bloody Stool

Di Yu / Sanguisorba
Huai Hua Mi / Sophora
Ji Guan Hua / Celosia

Arrest Bleeding in Miscellaneous Locations

Ce Bai Ye / Biota
Da Ji / Cirsium
Ji Cai / Capsella

Warming Hemostatic Herbs that Arrest Cold Induced Bleeding

Cold Induced Stomach and Intestinal Bleeding

Pao Jiang / Zingiber
Fu Long Gan / Terra Flava Usta

Cold Deficient Uterine Bleeding

Lu Jiao Shuang / Cervus

Channel Warming Hemostatic for Cold Induced Uterine and Menstrual Bleeding

Ai Ye / Artemisia

Herbs that Invigorate the Blood

Harmonize the Blood and Promote Menses
Ji Xue Teng / Millettia

Move the Blood and Promote Menses
Chuan Xiong / Ligusticum
Yi Mu Cao / Leonurus
Wang Bu Liu Xing / Vaccaria
Yue Ji Hua / Rosa
(Sheng) Pu Huang / Typha

Dispel Congealed Blood and Promote Menses
Dan Shen / Salvia
Ze Lan / Lycopus
Chi Shao Yao / Paeonia
Tao Ren / Prunus
Hong Hua / Carthamus
Huai Niu Xi / Achyranthes

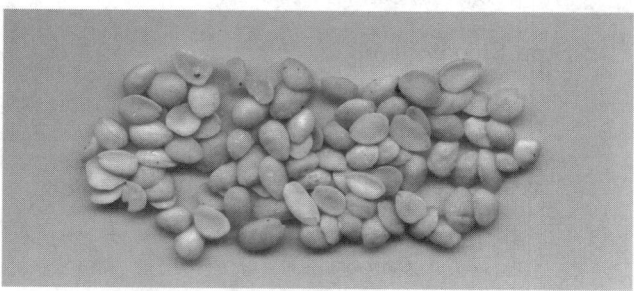

Tao Ren / Prunus (Shown at one-half actual size)

Resolve Congealed Blood and Masses and Move Qi
Yu Jin / Curcuma
Jiang Huang / Curcuma
San Leng / Sparganium
E Zhu / Curcuma
Gan Qi / Rhus

Strong Animal Substances that Break Up Congealed Blood Stasis and Masses
Shui Zhi / Hirudo
Tu Bie Chong / Eupolyphaga
Meng Chong / Tabanus

Alleviate Internal Pain

Yan Hu Suo / Corydalis
Wu Ling Zhi / Trogopterus
Lu Jiao / Cervus

Reduce Swelling and Pain due to Trauma

Ru Xiang / Boswellia
Mo Yao / Commiphora
Zi Ran Tong / Pyritum
Xue Jie / Dracaena
Su Mu / Caesalpinia
Liu Ji Nu / Artemisia

Blood Invigorating Herbs with Multiple Functions

Wa Leng Zi / Arca
Chuan Niu Xi / Cyathula
Lu Lu Tong / Liquidambar
Chuan Shan Jia / Manis
Mao Dong Qing / Ilex
Hu Zhang / Polygonum

Herbs that Tonify

Herbs that Tonify the Qi

Tonify Qi of the Middle Jiao (Spleen/Stomach)

Bai Zhu / Atractylodes
Da Zao / Ziziphus
Hong Zao / Ziziphus
Zhi Gan Cao / Glycyrrhiza
Jing Mi / Oryza

Tonify Qi of the Middle and Upper Jiaos (Spleen/Lungs)

Dang Shen / Codonopsis
Huang Qi / Astragalus
Gan Cao / Glycyrrhiza
Yi Tang / Saccharum Granorum
Feng Mi / Mel
Mian Hua Gen / Gossypium

Qi and Yang of the Middle and Upper Jiaos

(Hong) Ren Shen / Panax
Ye Shan Shen / Panax
Ji Lin Shen / Panax

Qi and Yin of the Middle and Upper Jiaos

Tai Zi Shen / Pseudostellaria
Huang Jing / Polygonatum
Bai Shen / Panax
Shen Xu / Panax

Tonify Qi of the Upper, Middle and Lower Jiaos (Lungs/Stomach/Spleen/Kidney)

Shan Yao / Dioscorea

Herbs that Tonify the Blood

Nourish Blood and Tonify the Heart and Spleen

Long Yan Rou / Euphoria

Nourish Liver Blood

He Shou Wu / Polygonum

Nourish Blood and Kidney Yin

Shu Di Huang / Rehmannia

Nourish Liver and Kidney Blood and Yin
Gou Qi Zi / Lycium
Sang Shen / Morus
Chu Shi Zi / Broussonetia

Tonify, Invigorate and Harmonize the Blood
Dang Gui / Angelica
Dang Gui Tou / Angelica
Dang Gui Wei / Angelica

Tonify Blood, Retain Yin and Soothe the Liver
Bai Shao Yao / Paeonia

Tonify Blood, Nourish Yin or Essence and Arrest Bleeding
E Jiao / Equus
Lu Jiao Jiao / Cervus

Herbs that Tonify the Yin

Tonify Lung Yin
Bai He / Lilium
Luo Han Guo / Momordica
Luo Han Ye / Momordica

Tonify Lung and Stomach Yin
Bei Sha Shen / Glehnia
Mai Men Dong / Ophiopogon
Yu Zhu / Polygonatum
Shi Hu / Dendrobium
Ming Dang Shen / Changium
Tian Hua Fen / Trichosanthes

Tonify Lung and Kidney Yin
Tian Men Dong / Asparagus

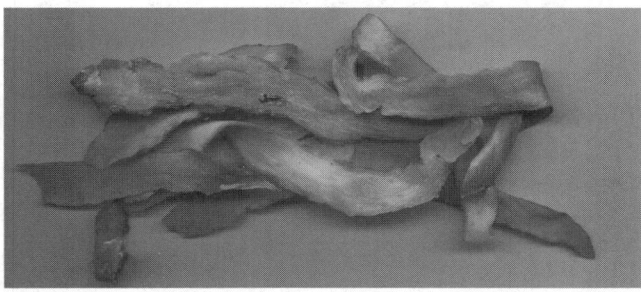

Yu Zhu / Polygonatum (Shown at one-half actual size)

Tonify Liver and Kidney Yin

Nu Zhen Zi / Ligustrum
Han Lian Cao / Eclipta
Sang Ji Sheng / Loranthus
Hei Zhi Ma / Sesamum
Gui Ban Jiao / Chinemys
Bie Jia Jiao / Amyda

Yin and Qi

Xi Yang Shen / Panax
Sheng Shai Shen / Panax
Nan Sha Shen / Adenophora

Yin Deficiency accompanied by Yang Rising

Gui Ban / Chinemys
Bie Jia / Amyda
Bai Mu Er / Tremella
Huai Niu Xi / Achyranthes

Herbs that Tonify the Yang

Tonify Kidney and Lung Deficiency

Dong Chong Xia Cao / Cordyceps
Hu Tao Ren / Juglans
Ge Jie / Gekko
E Guan Shi / Stalactitum
Zi He Che / Placenta Hominis

Tonify the Kidneys, Warm the Spleen Yang and Treat Urinary Incontinence and Diarrhea due to Cold Deficiency

Bu Gu Zhi / Psoralea
Yi Zhi Ren / Alpinia
Jiu Xiang Chong / Aspongopus

Warm Cold Deficient Kidneys

Hu Lu Ba / Trigonella
Jiu Zi / Allium
Yang Qi Shi / Actinolitum

Tonify Kidney Yang, Benefit the Essence and Moisten the Intestines

Rou Cong Rong / Cistanche
Suo Yang / Cynomorium

Tonify Kidney Yang, Strengthen the Sinews and Expel Wind Cold Damp
Ba Ji Tian / Morinda
Yin Yang Huo / Epimedium
Xian Mao / Curculigo

Tonify the Liver and Kidneys, Strengthen the Sinews and Bones and Treat Pain and Weakness in Low Back and Knees
Du Zhong / Eucommia
Xu Duan / Dipsacus
Gou Ji / Cibotium
Gu Sui Bu / Drynaria

Tonify/Nourish Liver and Kidney Essence and Brighten the Eyes
Tu Si Zi / Cuscuta
Sha Yuan Ji Li / Astragalus

Animal Substances that Tonify the Kidneys, Fortify the Yang and Essence, and Strengthen Sexual Functioning
Guang Gou Shen / Canis
Hai Gou Shen / Phoca
Hei Lu Shen / Equus
Hua Lu Shen / Cervus
Hai Ma / Hippocampus
Hai Long / Solenognathus
Hai Shen / Strichopus

Animal Substances that Strongly Tonify the Yang, Essence, Blood and Qi
Lu Rong / Cervus
Zi He Che / Homo Sapiens

Astringents

Primarily for the Upper Jiao

Prevent and Stop Abnormal Sweating

Fu Xiao Mai / Triticum
Ma Huang Gen / Ephedra
Nuo Dao Gen / Oryza

Restrain Lung Qi and Repress Coughing

Bai Guo / Ginkgo
Yin Guo Ye/ Ginkgo

Primarily for the Middle Jiao

Stop Chronic Diarrhea

Rou Dou Kou / Myristica
Chun Pi / Ailanthus
Shi Liu Pi / Punica

Stop Chronic Diarrhea, Restrain Lung Qi and Repress Cough

He Zi / Terminalia
Wu Mei / Prunus
Ying Su Ke / Papaver
Wu Bei Zi / Rhus/Melaphis

Stop Chronic Diarrhea, Stabilize the Menses and Arrest Abnormal Uterine Bleeding

Chi Shi Zhi / Halloysitum Rubrum
Yu Liang Shi / Limonite

Primarily for the Lower Jiao

Preserve the Essence, Stabilize the Menses and Arrest Abnormal Uterine Bleeding

Hai Piao Xiao / Sepia

Benefit and Stabilize the Kidney, Preserve the Essence and Stop Frequent Urination and Incontinence

Sang Piao Xiao / Paratenodera
Fu Pen Zi / Rubus
Lian Xu / Nelumbo

Preserve the Essence and Stop Chronic Diarrhea

Qian Shi / Euryale
Jin Ying Zi / Rosa
Lian Zi / Nelumbo

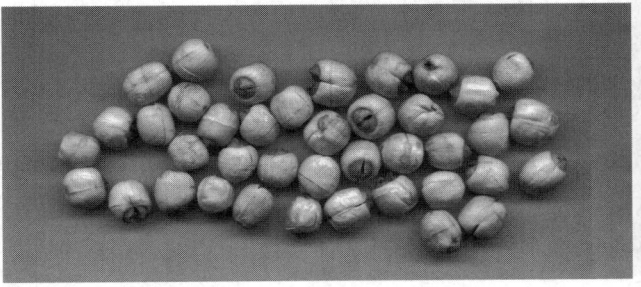

Lian Zi / Nelumbo (Shown at one-half actual size)

Astringents with Multiple Functions and Wide Applications

Shan Zhu Yu / Cornus
Wu Wei Zi / Schisandra

Substances that Calm the Shen (Tranquilizers)

Herbs that Nurture the Heart, Calm the Shen and:

Tonify Heart Blood
Bai Zi Ren / Biota

Tonify Liver Yin
Suan Zao Ren / Ziziphus

Tonify Blood and Yin and Balance Yin and Yang
Ye Jiao Teng / Polygonum

Tonify Qi and Blood
Ling Zhi / Ganoderma

Astringents

Substances the Calm the Shen
(Tranquilizers)

Drain Damp
Fu Shen / Poria

Release Constrained Emotions Due to Liver Qi Stagnation
He Huan Pi / Albizzia
He Huan Hua / Albizzia

Release Constrained Emotions and Expel Phlegm
Yuan Zhi / Polygala

Substances that Calm the Shen, Subdue Liver Yang and:

Subdue Rising Liver Yang
Dai Zhe Shi / Hematitum
Ci Shi / Magnetitum
Zhen Zhu Mu / Pteria
Sheng Tie Luo / Frusta Ferri

Subdue Rising Liver Yang and Possess Astringent Properties
Long Gu / Os Draconis
Mu Li / Ostrea
Long Chi / Dens Draconis
Duan Mu Li / Ostrea
Duan Long Gu / Os Draconis

Sedate the Heart and Treat Palpitations, Emotional Distress, Seizures and Convulsions
Zi Shi Ying / Fluoritum
Hu Po / Succinum
Zhen Zhu / Pteria
Zhu Sha / Cinnabaris

Herbs that Subdue Wind, Stop Tremors and Sedate Liver Yang

Strongly Calm and Suppress Convulsions, Seizures and Spasms

Treat Wind, Convulsions and Seizures due to Extreme Heat

Clear Blazing Heat, Soothe the Liver and Subdue Rising Liver Yang

Ling Yang Jiao / Saiga
Shan Yang Jiao / Naemorhedis
Gou Teng / Uncaria
Dai Mao / Eretmochelydis
Ren Gong Niu Huang / Bos

Clear Blazing Heat, Dispel Wind and Open the Channels in Windstroke Patterns

Di Long / Pheretima

Treat Wind and Spasms in Wind Phlegm Heat Patterns

Quan Xie / Buthus
Jiang Can / Bombyx
Meng Shi / Lapis Micae seu Chloriti
Dan Nan Xing / Arisaema

Treat Wind and Spasms in Wind Cold Patterns

Wu Gong / Scolopendra

Soothe the Liver and Subdue Rising Liver Yang and Fire

Bai Ji Li / Tribulus
Shi Jue Ming / Haliotis
San Qi Hua / Panax
Luo Bu Ma / Apocynum

Pacify the Liver and Subdue Wind in Patterns of Heat, Deficient Blood, Wind Phlegm and Windstroke

Tian Ma / Gastrodia

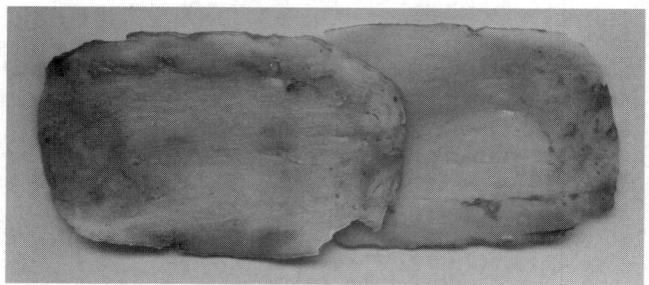

Tian Ma / Gastrodia (Shown at one-half actual size)

Aromatic Substances that Open the Orifices

Particularly Strong for Opening the Orifices

She Xiang / Moschus

Open Orifices and Clear Heat

Niu Huang / Bos
Bing Pian / Dryobalanops

Open Orifices and Penetrate Turbid Phlegm

Su He Xiang / Liquidambar
Shi Chang Pu / Acorus
Jiu Jie Chang Pu / Anemone

Open Orifices and Invigorate Qi and Blood

An Xi Xiang / Styrax

Herbs that Expel Parasites (Anti-helminthics)

Roundworms

Shi Jun Zi / Quisqualis
Ku Lian Gen Pi / Melia
Ku Lian Mu Pi / Melia
Wu Yi / Ulmus
Nan Gua Zi / Cucurbita
Shi Liu Gen Pi / Punica
Fei Zi / Torreya
He Shi / Carpesium

Tapeworms

Bing Lang / Areca
Lei Wan / Omphalia
Wu Yi / Ulmus
Nan Gua Zi / Cucurbita
Shi Liu Gen Pi / Punica
Fei Zi / Torreya
He Shi / Carpesium

Hookworms

Guan Zhong / Dryopteris
Da Suan / Allium
Fei Zi / Torreya
He Shi / Carpesium

Pinworms

Da Suan / Allium
Fei Zi / Torreya
He Shi / Carpesium

Substances For Topical Use

Kill Parasites and Treat Damp Skin Rash

Ming Fan / Alumen
Ku Fan / Alumen

Dry Damp, Kill Parasites and Strengthen the Yang

Liu Huang / Sulphur
She Chuang Zi / Cnidium

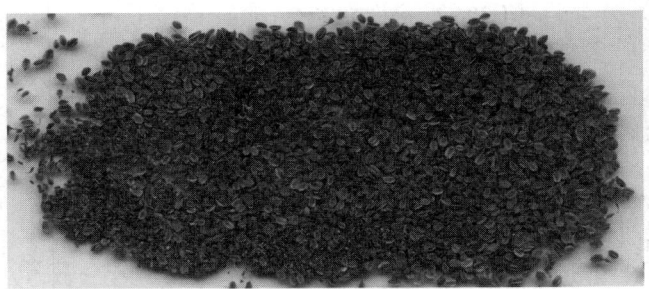

She Chuang Zi / Cnidium (image 3 x actual size)

Expel Wind Damp and Kill Parasites

Da Feng Zi / Hydnocarpus
Zhang Nao / Cinnamomum
Zao Jiao Ci / Gleditsia

Detoxify Poison and Kill Parasites

Qing Fen / Calomelas
Xiong Huang / Realgar
Shui Yin / Hydrargyrum

Detoxify Poison and Invigorate Blood

Mu Bie Zi / Momordica
Ban Mao / Mylabris

Detoxify Poison and Diminish Swelling

Peng Sha / Borax
Chan Su / Bufo
Xuan Ming Fan / Mirabilitum
(Sheng) Ban Xia / Pinellia
(Sheng) Tian Nan Xing / Arisaema

Detoxify Poison, Expel Wind and Damp, and Stop Pain

Lu Feng Fang / Polistes

Drain Poison and Regenerate Flesh

Lu Gan Shi / Smithsonitum
Qian Dan / Minium
Pi Shi / Arsenolite
Dan Fan / Chalcanthitum

Clear Heat, Detoxify Fire Toxin and Treat Nodules

Shan Ci Gu / Tulipa

Activate the Channels, Stop Pain, Move Blood and Diminish Swelling

Ma Qian Zi / Strychnos

Absorb Fluid Leakage and Alleviate Bleeding and Chronic Dysentery

Mi Tuo Seng / Lithargyrum
Er Cha / Acacia
Chen Shi Huei / Calcaria

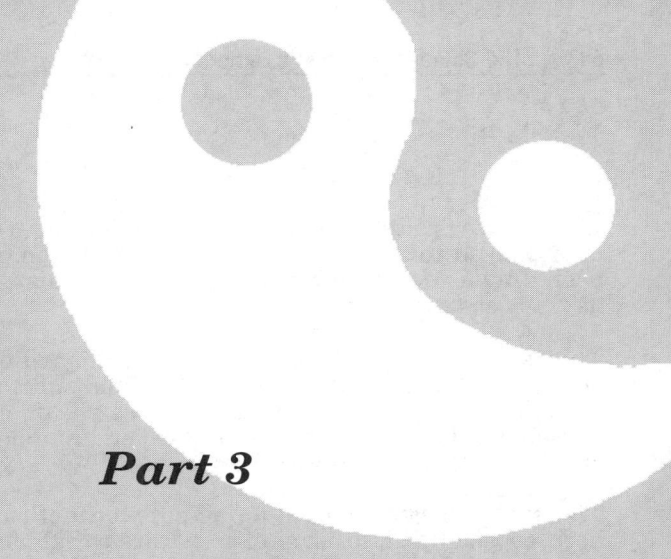

Part 3

Table of Herbal Preparation Procedures

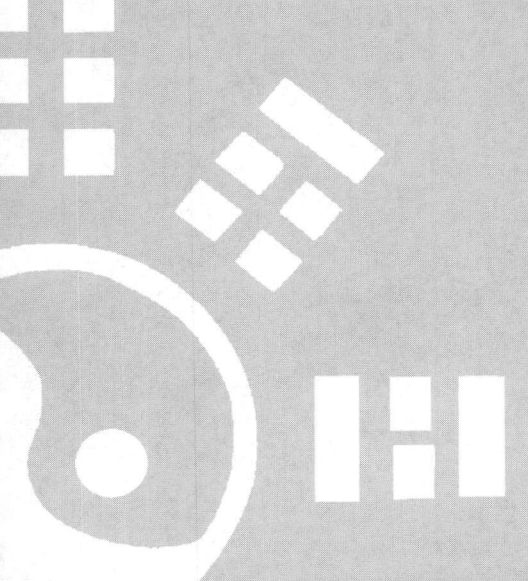

Part Three is a table of herbal preparations for a clinical setting. It is organized to aid in the preparation of herbs. Its contents have been drawn from traditional sources and the authors' experiences as Chinese herbal pharmacists.

This table is organized alphabetically by Pinyin herb name, with the botanical herb name following. For animal substances, the zoological name is used. For mineral substances, the pharmaceutical name is used. For botanical, pharmaceutical and common name cross-referencing, please consult Part Four.

This table does not account for all possible methods of preparing an herb, especially those forms of preparation that have been developed in modern Western countries. The forms of preparation listed here are either readily available from Chinese herbal sources or are easily prepared in a clinical setting. Unusual forms of preparation not readily available are beyond the scope of this book.

The last page of this chapter lists the combining cautions generally observed for certain herbs. These cautions are noted by number in the second to last column of the table.

The last column lists standard adult dosages. In cases where herbs have no dosage listed, the standard dosage is either unavailable or the herb is generally used externally.

Name of herb or substance	Decoction	Powder/Pills taken internally: O may be ☺ commonly ● always	Used with wine or extracted	Whole substance often eaten separately	External use: O possible ☺ mainly (internal caution) ● only	Do not cook substance ● Refrigerate	Add near end of cooking: O last 5 min ☺ 10 min ● 15 min	Cook 30 - 60 minutes before adding other herbs	Dissolve/steep in strained previously cooked decoction	Wrap in separate porous bag (cheesecloth)	Slice or Crush: ☺ small pieces ● powder	May be used: ☺ fresh or dried ● fresh only	May be available in prepared form - less toxic or stronger this way	Available in charred form	Toxic: ☺ slightly ● very toxic	Contraindicated in pregnancy: ☺ caution ● never use	Combining Cautions... See page 620	Standard Dosage Range in Grams
Ai Ye/ Artemisia	✓				O									✓				3-8
An Xi Xiang/ Styrax	✓	☺																0.3-1
Ba Dou/ Croton		●													●	☺	2	0.1-0.3
Ba Jiao Hui Xiang/ Illicium	✓	O																3-8
Ba Ji Tian/ Morinda	✓																	6-15
Ba Qia/ Smilax	✓				O													12-30
Ba Xian Hua/ Hydrangea	✓															☺		9-12
Bai Bu/ Stemona	✓				O													3-9
Bai Dou Kou/ Amomum	✓	☺					☺				☺							1.5-10
Bai Fu Zi/ Typhonium	✓				O										●	●		1.5-5
Bai Guo/ Ginkgo	✓														☺			4.5-9
Bai He/ Lilium	✓																	15-30
Bai Hua She/ Agkistrodon	✓	O	✓	✓											☺			1-10
Bai Hua She She Cao/ Oldenlandia	✓											☺				☺		15-60
Bai Ji/ Bletilla	✓				O												1	5-15
Bai Ji Li/ Tribulus	✓															☺		5-12
Bai Jiang Cao/ Patrinia	✓				O							☺						6-15

A, B

Legend for symbol columns:
- **Powder/Pills taken internally:** ○ may be ◐ commonly ● always
- **External use:** ○ possible ◐ mainly (internal caution) ● only
- **Do not cook substance** ● Refrigerate
- **Add near end of cooking:** ○ last 5 min ◐ 10 min ● 15 min
- **Slice or Crush:** ◐ small pieces ● powder
- **May be used:** ◐ fresh or dried ● fresh only
- **Toxic:** ◐ slightly ● very toxic
- **Contraindicated in pregnancy:** ◐ caution ● never use

Name of herb or substance	Decoction	Powder/Pills taken internally	Used with wine or extracted	Whole substance often eaten separately	External use	Do not cook substance / Refrigerate	Add near end of cooking	Cook 30-60 minutes before adding other herbs	Dissolve/steep in strained previously cooked decoction	Wrap in separate porous bag (cheesecloth)	Slice or Crush	May be used	May be available in prepared form - less toxic or stronger this way	Available in charred form	Toxic	Contraindicated in pregnancy	Combining Cautions... See page 620	Standard Dosage Range in Grams
Bai Jie Zi/ Brassica	✓																	3-9
Bai Lian/ Ampelopsis	✓				○												9	3-10
Bai Mao Gen/ Imperata	✓											◐						15-30
Bai Mao Hua/ Imperata	✓																	10-20
Bai Mao Xia Ku Cao/ Ajuga	✓																	15-30
Bai Mu Er/ Tremella	✓			✓														5-10
Bai Qian/ Cynanchum	✓																	3-9
Bai Shao Yao/ Paeonia	✓																28	9-18
Bai Tou Weng/ Pulsatilla	✓				○													6-15
Bai Wei/ Cynanchum	✓		✓														39	3-9
Bai Xian Pi/ Dictamnus	✓				○													4-10
Bai Zhi/ Angelica	✓	○			○												34	3-10
Bai Zhu/ Atractylodes	✓																	3-12
Bai Zi Ren/ Biota	✓				○	●												9-18
Ban Bian Lian/ Lobelia	✓				○							◐						9-30

Legend for symbols used in the table:
- Powder/Pills taken internally: ○ may be · ◉ commonly · ● always
- External use: ○ possible · ◉ mainly (internal caution) · ● only
- Do not cook substance: ● Refrigerate
- Add near end of cooking: ○ last 5 min · ○ 10 min · ● 15 min
- Slice or Crush: ◉ small pieces · ● powder
- May be used: ◉ fresh or dried · ● fresh only
- Toxic: ◉ slightly · ● very toxic
- Contraindicated in pregnancy: ◉ caution · ● never use
- Combining Cautions... See page 620

Name of herb or substance	Decoction	Powder/Pills taken internally	Used with wine or extracted	Whole substance often eaten separately	External use	Do not cook substance / Refrigerate	Add near end of cooking	Cook 30-60 minutes before adding other herbs	Dissolve/steep in strained previously cooked decoction	Wrap in separate porous bag (cheesecloth)	Slice or Crush	May be used	May be available in prepared form - less toxic or stronger this way	Available in charred form	Toxic	Contraindicated in pregnancy	Combining Cautions... See page 620	Standard Dosage Range in Grams
Ban Lan Gen/ Isatis	✓																	15-30
Ban Mao/ Mylabris	✓	◉			◉										●	●	8	0.03-0.06
(Fa) Ban Xia/ Pinellia	✓												✓		◉	●	9	5-9
(Sheng) Ban Xia/ Pinellia					●										●			
Ban Zhi Lian/ Scutellaria	✓				○						◉					◉		15-60
Bao Gu/ Panthera	✓	◉	✓	✓							◉							9-15
Bao Ma Zi/ Syringa	✓											◉						20-50
Bei Sha Shen/ Glehnia	✓																4	9-30
Bei Xie/ Dioscorea	✓																	9-15
Bi Ba/ Piper	✓	◉			○						◉							2-5
Bi Cheng Qie/ Litsea	✓																	2-5
Bian Dou/ Dolichos	✓											◉						9-18
Bian Xu/ Polygonum	✓				○													9-15
Bie Jia/ Amyda	✓							✓			◉					●	63	9-30
Bing Lang/ Areca	✓			✓											◉	◉		6-15
Bing Pian/ Dryobalanops		●			○											◉		0.3-0.9

B

Name of herb or substance	Decoction	Powder/Pills taken internally: ○ may be ⊛ commonly ● always	Used with wine or extracted	Whole substance often eaten separately	External use: ○ possible ⊛ mainly (internal caution) ● only	Do not cook substance; ● Refrigerate	Add near end of cooking: ○ last 5 min ⊛ 10 min ● 15 min	Cook 30 - 60 minutes before adding other herbs	Dissolve/steep in strained previously cooked decoction	Wrap in separate porous bag (cheesecloth)	Slice or Crush: ⊛ small pieces ● powder	May be used: ⊛ fresh or dried ● fresh only	May be available in prepared form - less toxic or stronger this way	Available in charred form	Toxic: ⊛ slightly ● very toxic	Contraindicated in pregnancy: ⊛ caution ● never use	Combining Cautions... See page 620	Standard Dosage Range in Grams
Bo He/ Mentha	✓						○											2-10
Bu Gu Zhi/ Psoralea	✓				○												8	3-10
Can Sha/ Bombyx	✓			✓	○					✓								3-10
Cang Er Zi/ Xanthium	✓				○										⊛			3-10
Cang Zhu/ Atractylodes	✓																	3-10
Cao Dou Kou/ Alpinia	✓						⊛				⊛							2-6
Cao Guo/ Amomum	✓						⊛				⊛				⊛			3-6
Ce Bai Ye/ Biota	✓				○									✓				10-15
Chai Hu/ Bupleurum	✓																	3-10
Chan Su/ Bufo		●			⊛										●	●		0.02-0.03
Chan Tui/ Cryptotympana	✓															⊛		3-10
Chang Chun Teng/ Hedera	✓				○													9-15
Chang Shan/ Dichroa	✓												✓		●	⊛		4-9
Che Qian Cao/ Plantago	✓			✓	○							⊛						9-20
Che Qian Zi/ Plantago	✓									✓						●		3-12
Chen Pi/ Citrus	✓						●											3-9

Name of herb or substance	Decoction	Powder/Pills taken internally: ○ may be ◐ commonly ● always	Used with wine or extracted	Whole substance often eaten separately	External use: ○ possible ◐ mainly (internal caution) ● only	Do not cook substance ● Refrigerate	Add near end of cooking: ○ last 5 min ◐ 10 min ● 15 min	Cook 30-60 minutes before adding other herbs	Dissolve/steep in strained previously cooked decoction	Wrap in separate porous bag (cheesecloth)	Slice or Crush: ◐ small pieces ● powder	May be used: ◐ fresh or dried ● fresh only	May be available in prepared form - less toxic or stronger this way	Available in charred form	Toxic: ◐ slightly ● very toxic	Contraindicated in pregnancy: ◐ caution ● never use	Combining Cautions... See page 620	Standard Dosage Range in Grams
Chen Shi Huei/ Calcaria		○			◐										●			
Chen Xiang/ Aquilaria		◐						✓			◐							1-3
Cheng Liu/ Tamarix	✓																	3-10
Chi Fu Ling/ Poria	✓																	6-18
Chi Shao Yao/ Paeonia	✓																4	6-9
Chi Shi Zhi/ Halloysitum Rubrum	✓				○			✓			◐		✓			◐	66	9-30
Chi Xiao Dou/ Phaseolus	✓		✓		○													9-30
Chong Wei Zi/ Leonurus	✓															●		3-9
Chou Wu Tong/ Clerodendron	✓						○											10-30
Chu Shi Zi/ Broussonetia	✓																	9-15
Chuan Bei Mu/ Fritillaria	✓	○						✓			◐						30	3-9
Chuan Jiao/ Zanthoxylum	✓				○										◐	◐	56	2-5
Chuan Lian Zi/ Melia	✓				○						◐				◐			3-9
Chuan Niu Xi/ Cyathula	✓															●		6-12

Legend for symbols used in the table:
- Powder/Pills taken internally: ○ may be, ❂ commonly, ● always
- External use: ○ possible, ❂ mainly (internal caution), ● only
- ❂ Do not cook substance, ● Refrigerate
- Add near end of cooking: ○ last 5 min, ❂ 10 min, ● 15 min
- Slice or Crush: ❂ small pieces, ● powder
- May be used: ❂ fresh or dried, ● fresh only
- Toxic: ❂ slightly, ● very toxic
- Contraindicated in pregnancy: ❂ caution, ● never use
- Combining Cautions... See page 620

Name of herb or substance	Decoction	Powder/Pills taken internally	Used with wine or extracted	Whole substance often eaten separately	External use	Do not cook / Refrigerate	Add near end of cooking	Cook 30-60 minutes before adding other herbs	Dissolve/steep in strained previously cooked decoction	Wrap in separate porous bag (cheesecloth)	Slice or Crush	May be used	May be available in prepared form - less toxic or stronger this way	Available in charred form	Toxic	Contraindicated in pregnancy	Combining Cautions... See page 620	Standard Dosage Range in Grams
Chuan Shan Jia/ Manis	✓	❂			○											●		1-9
Chuan Shan Long/ Dioscorea	✓																	9-20
Chuan Xin Lian/ Andrographis	✓	○			○							❂						1-15
Chuan Xiong/ Ligusticum	✓															●		3-9
Chui Pen Cao/ Sedum	✓				○							❂						15-30
Chun Pi/ Ailanthus	✓				○													3-15
Ci Shi/ Magnetitum	✓							✓			●			✓				9-30
Cong Bai/ Allium	✓				○	●	●					❂						3-10
Da Feng Zi/ Hydnocarpus	✓	○			❂										●			0.3-0.9
Da Fu Pi/ Areca	✓																	3-9
Da Huang/ Rheum	✓	○			○		○										❂	3-12
Da Ji/ Cirsium	✓				○							❂						4.5-15
Da Qing Ye/ Isatis	✓											❂						10-30
Da Suan/ Allium	✓				○							❂						5-15
Da Zao/ Ziziphus	✓																	10-30
Dai Mao/ Eretmochelys	✓							✓			❂							3-6

Name of herb or substance	Decoction	Powder/Pills taken internally: ○ may be ❋ commonly ● always	Used with wine or extracted	Whole substance often eaten separately	External use: ○ possible ❋ mainly (internal caution) ● only	❋ Do not cook substance ● Refrigerate	Add near end of cooking: ○ last 5 min ❋ 10 min ● 15 min	Cook 30 - 60 minutes before adding other herbs	Dissolve/steep in strained previously cooked decoction	Wrap in separate porous bag (cheesecloth)	Slice or Crush: ❋ small pieces ● powder	May be used: ❋ fresh or dried ● fresh only	May be available in prepared form - less toxic or stronger this way	Available in charred form	Toxic: ❋ slightly ● very toxic	Contraindicated in pregnancy: ❋ caution ● never use	Combining Cautions... See page 620	Standard Dosage Range in Grams
Dai Zhe Shi/ Haematitum	✓							✓			❋		✓				❋	10-30
Dan Dou Chi/ Glycine	✓												✓					10-15
Dan Fan/ Chalcanthitum					●										●			0.1-0.3
Dan Nan Xing/ Arisaema	✓												✓		❋	●		3-6
Dan Shen/ Salvia	✓																4	3-15
Dan Zhu Ye/ Lophatherum	✓															❋		10-15
Dang Gui/ Angelica	✓																	3-15
Dang Gui Tou/ Angelica	✓																	3-15
Dang Gui Wei/ Angelica	✓																	3-15
Dang Shen/ Codonopsis	✓																4	9-15
Deng Xin Cao/ Juncus	✓																	1.5-3
Di Er Cao/ Hypericum	✓				○							❋						20-50
Di Feng/ Illicium	✓																	
Di Fu Zi/ Kochia	✓				○												46	6-15
Di Gu Pi/ Lycium	✓				○													6-15
Di Long/ Pheretima	✓	○									●							5-15

Name of herb or substance	Decoction	Powder/Pills taken internally: ○ may be ✿ commonly ● always	Used with wine or extracted	Whole substance often eaten separately	External use: ○ possible ✿ mainly (internal caution) ● only	✿ Do not cook substance ● Refrigerate	Add near end of cooking: ○ last 5 min ✿ 10 min ● 15 min	Cook 30 - 60 minutes before adding other herbs	Dissolve/steep in strained previously cooked decoction	Wrap in separate porous bag (cheesecloth)	Slice or Crush: ✿ small pieces ● powder	May be used: ✿ fresh or dried ● fresh only	May be available in prepared form - less toxic or stronger this way	Available in charred form	Toxic: ✿ slightly ● very toxic	Contraindicated in pregnancy: ✿ caution ● never use	Combining Cautions... See page 620	Standard Dosage Range in Grams
Di Yu/ Sanguisorba	✓				○									✓				10-15
Dian Di Mai/ Androsace	✓																	3-9
Ding Xiang/ Eugenia	✓	○															3	0.5-4.5
Dong Bei Guan Zhong/ Dryopteris	✓														✿	●		6-15
Dong Chong Xia Cao/ Cordyceps	✓	○		✓														3-9
Dong Gua Pi/ Benincasa	✓																	15-30
Dong Gua Ren/ Benincasa	✓										✿							3-12
Dong Kui Zi/ Malva	✓															✿		9-15
Dou Chi Jiang/ Litsea	✓																	1.5-6
Dou Juan/ Glycine	✓																5	9-15
Du Huo/ Angelica	✓																	3-9
Du Zhong/ Eucommia	✓																	9-15
E Bu Shi Cao/ Centipeda	✓																	3-6
E Guan Shi/ Stalactitum	✓							✓			✿							9-30
E Jiao/ Equus		○	✓			✿			✓		●						57	6-15

Name of herb or substance	Decoction	Powder/Pills taken internally	Used with wine or extracted	Whole substance often eaten separately	External use	Do not cook substance / Refrigerate	Add near end of cooking	Cook 30-60 min before adding other herbs	Dissolve/steep in strained previously cooked decoction	Wrap in separate porous bag (cheesecloth)	Slice or Crush	May be used (fresh/dried)	May be available in prepared form	Available in charred form	Toxic	Contraindicated in pregnancy	Combining Cautions (See page 620)	Standard Dosage Range in Grams
E Wei/ Ferula	✓															●		1-2
E Zhu/ Curcuma	✓															●		3-9
Er Cha/ Acacia		●			◐							◐						0.1-0.9
Fan Bai Cao/ Potentilla	✓				○						◐							9-15
Fan Xie Ye/ Cassia	✓						●									●		3-9
Fang Feng/ Ledebouriella	✓																33	5-9
Fei Zi/ Torreya	✓	◐																9-15
Feng Mi/ Mel	✓		✓															15-50
Feng Wei Cao/ Pteris	✓				○						◐							9-18
Fo Shou/ Citrus	✓																	3-9
Fo Shou Hua/ Citrus	✓																	3-6
Fu Hai Shi/ Pumice	✓	○								✓								9-15
Fu Ling/ Poria	✓																44	9-15
Fu Ling Pi/ Poria	✓																	9-15
Fu Long Gan/ Terra Flava Usta	✓									✓								15-60
Fu Pen Zi/ Rubus	✓																	4.5-9
Fu Ping/ Spirodela	✓				○													3-6

E, F

Column key (legend):
- Powder/Pills taken internally: ○ may be ◉ commonly ● always
- External use: ○ possible ◉ mainly (internal caution) ● only
- Do not cook substance ● Refrigerate
- Add near end of cooking: ○ last 5 min ◉ 10 min ● 15 min
- Slice or Crush: ◉ small pieces ● powder
- May be used: ◉ fresh or dried ● fresh only
- Toxic: ◉ slightly ● very toxic
- Contraindicated in pregnancy: ◉ caution ● never use
- Combining Cautions... See page 620

Name of herb or substance	Decoction	Powder/Pills taken internally	Used with wine or extracted	Whole substance often eaten separately	External use	Do not cook substance ● Refrigerate	Add near end of cooking	Cook 30 - 60 minutes before adding other herbs	Dissolve/steep in strained previously cooked decoction	Wrap in separate porous bag (cheesecloth)	Slice or Crush	May be used	May be available in prepared form - less toxic or stronger this way	Available in charred form	Toxic	Contraindicated in pregnancy	Combining Cautions	Standard Dosage Range in Grams
Fu Shen/ Poria	✓																	9-15
Fu Xiao Mai/ Triticum	✓																	9-30
(Hei) Fu Zi/ Aconitum	✓							✓					✓		●	●	6	3-15
Gan Cao/ Glycyrrhiza	✓				○												7	3-9
Gan Jiang/ Zingiber	✓															◉		3-9
Gan Sui/ Euphorbia	✓	◉			○								✓		●	●	43	0.5-1
Gao Ben/ Ligusticum	✓																	2-10
Gao Liang Jiang/ Alpinia	✓																	1.5-9
Ge Gen/ Pueraria	✓																	5-20
Ge Hua/ Pueraria	✓																	5-9
Ge Jie/ Gekko	✓	◉																3-15
Ge Shan Xiang/ Cynanchum	✓																	
Gou Gu/ Canis	✓	◉	✓	✓				✓										9-15
Gou Ji/ Cibotium	✓																59	5-9
Gou Qi Zi/ Lycium	✓																	6-18
Gou Teng/ Uncaria	✓						◉											6-15

Name of herb or substance	Decoction	Powder/Pills taken internally: (○ may be / ✿ commonly / ● always)	Used with wine or extracted	Whole substance often eaten separately	External use: (○ possible / ✿ mainly (internal caution) / ● only)	✿ Do not cook substance / ● Refrigerate	Add near end of cooking: (○ last 5 min / ✿ 10 min / ● 15 min)	Cook 30-60 minutes before adding other herbs	Dissolve/steep in strained previously cooked decoction	Wrap in separate porous bag (cheesecloth)	Slice or Crush: (✿ small pieces / ● powder)	May be used: (✿ fresh or dried / ● fresh only)	May be available in prepared form - less toxic or stronger this way	Available in charred form	Toxic: (✿ slightly / ● very toxic)	Contraindicated in pregnancy: (✿ caution / ● never use)	Combining Cautions... See page 620	Standard Dosage Range in Grams
Gu Jing Cao/ Eriocaulon	✓																	6-15
Gu Sui Bu/ Drynaria	✓			○														9-15
Gu Ya/ Oryza					✿			✓				●						9-15
Gua Di/ Cucumis	✓	○			○										✿	●		0.3-1.0
Gua Lou/ Trichosanthes	✓										✿						10	9-30
Gua Lou Pi/ Trichosanthes	✓																10	6-12
Gua Lou Ren/ Trichosanthes	✓										✿						10	9-15
Guan Ye Liao/ Polygonum	✓																	
Guan Zhong/ Dryopteris	✓														✿	●		6-16
Guang Fang Ji/ Aristolochia	✓																	3-15
Guang Gou Shen/ Canis		●		✓								●						3-15
Gui Ban/ Chinemys	✓							✓			✿					●	62	9-30
Gui Zhi/ Cinnamomum	✓															✿		3-15
Hai Dai/ Laminaria	✓																	5-15
Hai Feng Teng/ Piper	✓															●		6-15
Hai Ge Ke/ Cyclina	✓	○								✓	●		✓					1-15

G, H

Legend for columns:

- Decoction
- Powder/Pills taken internally: ○ may be ⊕ commonly ● always
- Used with wine or extracted
- Whole substance often eaten separately
- External use: ○ possible ⊕ mainly (internal caution) ● only
- ⊕ Do not cook substance ● Refrigerate
- Add near end of cooking: ○ last 5 min ⊕ 10 min ● 15 min
- Cook 30 - 60 minutes before adding other herbs
- Dissolve/steep in strained previously cooked decoction
- Wrap in separate porous bag (cheesecloth)
- Slice or Crush: ⊕ small pieces ● powder
- May be used: ⊕ fresh or dried ● fresh only
- May be available in prepared form - less toxic or stronger this way
- Available in charred form
- Toxic: ⊕ slightly ● very toxic
- Contraindicated in pregnancy: ⊕ caution ● never use
- Combining Cautions... See page 620
- Standard Dosage Range in Grams

Name of herb or substance	Decoct	Powder	Wine	Whole	External	No cook/Refrig	Add end	Cook first	Dissolve	Wrap bag	Slice/Crush	Fresh	Prepared	Charred	Toxic	Pregnancy	Combining	Dosage (g)
Hai Gou Shen/ Phoca		●		✓							●							3-15
Hai Jin Sha/ Lygodium	✓									✓								6-15
Hai Long/ Solenognathus	✓	⊕		✓							⊕					●		1.5-2.4
Hai Ma/ Hippocampus	✓	⊕	✓	✓							⊕					●		3-9
Hai Piao Xiao/ Sepia	✓				○						⊕						11	5-9
Hai Tong Pi/ Erythrina	✓				○						⊕							6-12
Hai Zao/ Sargassum	✓																8	5-15
Han Cai/ Rorippa	✓			✓								⊕					27	20-50
Han Fang Ji/ Stephania	✓																	5-9
Han Lian Cao/ Eclipta	✓											⊕						9-30
Han Shui Shi/ Calcitum	✓				○		✓					●						9-30
He Huan Hua/ Albizzia	✓																	3-9
He Huan Pi/ Albizzia	✓																	9-15
He Shi/ Carpesium	✓	⊕													⊕			9-15
He Shou Wu/ Polygonum	✓																12	9-30

Name of herb or substance	Decoction	Powder/Pills taken internally: ○ may be ◐ commonly ● always	Used with wine or extracted	Whole substance often eaten separately	External use: ○ possible ◐ mainly (internal caution) ● only	◐ Do not cook substance ● Refrigerate	Add near end of cooking: ○ last 5 min ◐ 10 min ● 15 min	Cook 30 - 60 minutes before adding other herbs	Dissolve/steep in strained previously cooked decoction	Wrap in separate porous bag (cheesecloth)	Slice or Crush: ◐ small pieces ● powder	May be used: ◐ fresh or dried ● fresh only	May be available in prepared form - less toxic or stronger this way	Available in charred form	Toxic: ◐ slightly ● very toxic	Contraindicated in pregnancy: ◐ caution ● never use	Combining Cautions... See page 620	Standard Dosage Range in Grams
He Zi/ Terminalia	✓										◐							3-9
Hei Lu Shen/ Equus		●	✓									●						3-15
Hei Zhi Ma/ Sesamum	✓																	9-30
Hong Hua/ Carthamus	✓						●									●		3-9
Hong Teng/ Sargentodoxa	✓		✓													◐		15-30
Hou Po/ Magnolia	✓															◐	50	3-9
Hou Po Hua/ Magnolia	✓																	3-6
Hou Zao/ Macaca		●	✓									●						0.3-1
Hu Er Cao/ Saxifraga	✓				○							◐			◐			9-15
Hu Gu/ Panthera	✓	◐	✓	✓	○						◐							3-6
Hu Huang Lian/ Picrorhiza	✓																	3-9
Hu Jiao/ Piper	✓																	2-3
Hu Lu Ba/ Trigonella	✓															●		3-9
Hu Po/ Succinum		●			○						●							1.5-3
Hu Tao Ren/ Juglans	✓			✓														9-30
Hu Tui Ye/ Eleagnus	✓																	9-15

H

Name of herb or substance	Decoction	Powder/Pills taken internally: ○ may be ⊗ commonly ● always	Used with wine or extracted	Whole substance often eaten separately	External use: ○ possible ⊗ mainly (internal caution) ● only	Do not cook substance ● Refrigerate	Add near end of cooking: ○ last 5 min ⊗ 10 min ● 15 min	Cook 30 - 60 minutes before adding other herbs	Dissolve/steep in strained previously cooked decoction	Wrap in separate porous bag (cheesecloth)	Slice or Crush: ⊗ small pieces ● powder	May be used: ⊗ fresh or dried ● fresh only	May be available in prepared form - less toxic or stronger this way	Available in charred form	Toxic: ⊗ slightly ● very toxic	Contraindicated in pregnancy: ⊗ caution ● never use	Combining Cautions... See page 620	Standard Dosage Range in Grams
Hu Zhang/ Polygonum	✓				○						⊗					●		6-12
Hua Lu Shen/ Cervus		●		✓								●						6-15
Hua Rui Shi/ Ophicalcitum		⊗	✓		○	⊗						●				●		3-9
Hua Sheng Yi/ Arachis	✓																	6-10
Hua Shi/ Talcum	✓				○					✓	●					⊗		9-12
Huai Hua Mi/ Sophora	✓													✓				6-15
Huai Jiao/ Sophora	✓															●		6-15
Huai Niu Xi/ Achyranthes	✓	○	✓													●	54	9-15
Huang Bai/ Phellodendron	✓				○													3-12
Huang Jing/ Polygonatum	✓																	9-15
Huang Lian/ Coptis	✓	○			○												41	1.5-9
Huang Qi/ Astragalus	✓				○													9-25
Huang Qin/ Scutellaria	✓																40	6-15
Huang Yao Zi/ Dioscorea	✓	⊗	✓		○										⊗			4.5-9
Huo Ma Ren/ Cannabis	✓										⊗							9-15

Name of herb or substance	Decoction	Powder/Pills taken internally: ○ may be ✿ commonly ● always	Used with wine or extracted	Whole substance often eaten separately	External use: ○ possible ✿ mainly (internal caution) ● only	✿ Do not cook substance ● Refrigerate	Add near end of cooking: ○ last 5 min ✿ 10 min ● 15 min	Cook 30 - 60 minutes before adding other herbs	Dissolve/steep in strained previously cooked decoction	Wrap in separate porous bag (cheesecloth)	Slice or Crush: ✿ small pieces ● powder	May be used: ✿ fresh or dried ● fresh only	May be available in prepared form - less toxic or stronger this way	Available in charred form	Toxic: ✿ slightly ● very toxic	Contraindicated in pregnancy: ✿ caution ● never use	Combining Cautions... See page 620	Standard Dosage Range in Grams
Huo Xiang/ Agastache	✓						●											4.5-9
Ji Cai/ Capsella	✓											✿						9-15
Ji Gu Cao/ Abrus	✓											✿						9-15
Ji Guan Hua/ Celosia	✓																	10-15
Ji Mu/ Loropetalum	✓																	20-100
Ji Nei Jin/ Gallus	✓	✿																1.5-9
Ji Ning/ Salvia	✓																	9-15
Ji Shi Teng/ Paederia	✓				○													9-15
Ji Xue Teng/ Millettia	✓																	9-15
Jiang Can/ Bombyx	✓	✿									●							1-9
Jiang Huang/ Curcuma	✓				○											✿		3-9
Jiang Xiang/ Dalbergia	✓	○			○													1.5-9
(Ku) Jie Geng/ Platycodon	✓																5	3-6
Jin Guo Lan/ Tinospora	✓				○													3-9
Jin Qian Cao/ Lysimachia	✓			✓								✿						15-60
Jin Sha Teng/ Lygodium	✓				○													15-60

Legend:
- Powder/Pills taken internally: ○ may be ✿ commonly ● always
- External use: ○ possible ✿ mainly (internal caution) ● only
- Do not cook substance: ● Refrigerate
- Add near end of cooking: ○ last 5 min ✿ 10 min ● 15 min
- Slice or Crush: ✿ small pieces ● powder
- May be used: ✿ fresh or dried ● fresh only
- Toxic: ✿ slightly ● very toxic
- Contraindicated in pregnancy: ✿ caution ● never use

Name of herb or substance	Decoction	Powder/Pills taken internally	Used with wine or extracted	Whole substance often eaten separately	External use	Do not cook substance	Add near end of cooking	Cook 30-60 minutes before adding other herbs	Dissolve/steep in strained previously cooked decoction	Wrap in separate porous bag (cheesecloth)	Slice or Crush	May be used	May be available in prepared form - less toxic or stronger this way	Available in charred form	Toxic	Contraindicated in pregnancy	Combining Cautions... See page 620	Standard Dosage Range in Grams
Jin Yin Hua/ Lonicera	✓																	9-15
Jin Yin Teng/ Lonicera	✓																	15-30
Jin Ying Zi/ Rosa	✓																	5-9
Jing Da Ji/ Euphorbia	✓	✿													●	●	13	1-3
Jing Jie/ Schizonepeta	✓						✿											4.5-9
Jing Mi/ Oryza	✓			✓														50-100
Jing Tian San Qi/ Sedum	✓			○								✿						9-15
Jiu Jie Chang Pu/ Anemone	✓																	2-4.5
Jiu Xiang Chong/ Aspongopus	✓										●							3-6
Jiu Zi/ Allium	✓																	3-9
Ju He/ Citrus	✓																	3-9
Ju Hong/ Citrus	✓																	2-4.5
Ju Hua/ Chrysanthemum	✓																	4.5-15
Ju Ye San Qi/ Gynura	✓	○			○													6-9
Jue Ming Zi/ Cassia	✓																14	9-15
Ku Lian Gen Pi/ Melia	✓				○										✿			6-15

Legend for symbols used in the table:

- Powder/Pills taken internally: ○ may be ◎ commonly ● always
- External use: ○ possible ◎ mainly (internal caution) ● only
- Do not cook substance: ◎ / Refrigerate ●
- Add near end of cooking: ○ last 5 min ◎ 10 min ● 15 min
- Slice or Crush: ◎ small pieces ● powder
- May be used: ◎ fresh or dried ● fresh only
- May be available in prepared form — less toxic or stronger this way
- Toxic: ◎ slightly ● very toxic
- Contraindicated in pregnancy: ◎ caution ● never use
- Combining Cautions... See page 620

Name of herb or substance	Decoction	Powder/Pills taken internally	Used with wine or extracted	Whole substance often eaten separately	External use	Do not cook substance / Refrigerate	Add near end of cooking	Cook 30–60 minutes before adding other herbs	Dissolve/steep in strained previously cooked decoction	Wrap in separate porous bag (cheesecloth)	Slice or Crush	May be used	May be available in prepared form	Available in charred form	Toxic	Contraindicated in pregnancy	Combining Cautions	Standard Dosage Range in Grams
Ku Lian Mu Pi/ Melia	✓				○										◎			6-15
Ku Shen/ Sophora	✓	◎	✓		○												42	3-15
Kuan Dong Hua/ Tussilago	✓																49	3-9
Kuan Jin Teng/ Tinospora	✓				○											●		15-30
Kun Bu/ Laminaria	✓																	4.5-15
Lai Fu Zi/ Raphanus	✓																	6-12
Lao Guan Cao/ Geranium	✓				○													9-30
Lei Wan/ Omphalia		◎		✓							●				◎		68	6-9
Li Lu/ Veratrum		●			◎										●	●	15	0.3-0.9
Li Pi/ Pyrus	✓		✓									◎						9-15
Li Zhi He/ Litchi	✓											◎						6-15
Lian Fang/ Nelumbo	✓											◎		✓				4.5-9
Lian Geng/ Nelumbo	✓																	9-15
Lian Qiao/ Forsythia	✓																	6-16
Lian Xin/ Nelumbo	✓																	1.5-6
Lian Xu/ Nelumbo	✓																16	1.5-9

K, L

Name of herb or substance	Decoction	Powder/Pills taken internally: ○ may be ✿ commonly ● always	Used with wine or extracted	Whole substance often eaten separately	External use: ○ possible ✿ mainly (internal caution) ● only	✿ Do not cook substance ● Refrigerate	Add near end of cooking: ○ last 5 min ✿ 10 min ● 15 min	Cook 30 - 60 minutes before adding other herbs	Dissolve/steep in strained previously cooked decoction	Wrap in separate porous bag (cheesecloth)	Slice or Crush: ✿ small pieces ● powder	May be used: ✿ fresh or dried ● fresh only	May be available in prepared form - less toxic or stronger this way	Available in charred form	Toxic: ✿ slightly ● very toxic	Contraindicated in pregnancy: ✿ caution ● never use	Combining Cautions... See page 620	Standard Dosage Range in Grams
Lian Zi/ Nelumbo	✓										✿							6-15
Ling Yang Jiao/ Saiga	✓	✿					✓				✿							1.5-3
Ling Zhi/ Ganoderma	✓	✿	✓	✓							✿							3-15
Liu Huang/ Sulphur		●			✿	✿									✿	●	52	0.15-0.6
Liu Ji Nu/ Artemisia	✓				○													5-9
Long Chi/ Dens Draconis	✓							✓			✿							9-15
Long Dan Cao/ Gentiana	✓																	3-9
Long Gu/ Os Draconis	✓				○			✓			✿			✓				9-30
Long Yan Rou/ Euphoria	✓			✓														6-15
Lou Gu/ Gryllotalpa	✓	○	✓								●					✿		3-4.5
Lou Lu/ Rhaponticum	✓															●		3-12
Lu Dou/ Phaseolus	✓			✓	○													25-50
Lu Feng Fang/ Polistes	✓				✿											●	65	1.5-3
Lu Gan Shi/ Smithsonitum					●								✓			●		
Lu Gen/ Phragmites	✓											✿						15-30
Lu Hui/ Aloe		●			○	✿					●					●		0.3-1.5

Legend — Powder/Pills taken internally: ○ may be ✪ commonly ● always · External use: ○ possible ✪ mainly (internal caution) ● only · Do not cook substance: ✪ / ● Refrigerate · Add near end of cooking: ○ last 5 min ✪ 10 min ● 15 min · Slice or Crush: ✪ small pieces ● powder · May be used: ✪ fresh or dried ● fresh only · Toxic: ✪ slightly ● very toxic · Contraindicated in pregnancy: ✪ caution ● never use · Combining Cautions… See page 620

Name of herb or substance	Decoction	Powder/Pills taken internally	Used with wine or extracted	Whole substance often eaten separately	External use	Do not cook substance / Refrigerate	Add near end of cooking	Cook 30-60 minutes before adding other herbs	Dissolve/steep in strained previously cooked decoction	Wrap in separate porous bag (cheesecloth)	Slice or Crush	May be used	May be available in prepared form - less toxic or stronger this way	Available in charred form	Toxic	Contraindicated in pregnancy	Combining Cautions… See page 620	Standard Dosage Range in Grams
Lu Jiao/ Cervus	✓	✪		✓	○			✓			✪							4.5-9
Lu Jiao Jiao/ Cervus		✪	✓	✓	✪				✓		●							6-12
Lu Jiao Shuang/ Cervus	✓				○						●		✓					15-30
Lu Lu Tong/ Liquidambar	✓				○											●		3-9
Lu Rong/ Cervus	✓	✪	✓	✓							✪							1-4.5
Lu Xian Cao/ Pyrola	✓				○													15-30
Lu Ying/ Sambucus	✓				○													9-15
Luo Bu Ma/ Apocynum	✓																	6-9
Luo Han Guo/ Momordica	✓			✓														9-15
Luo Han Ye/ Momordica																		
Luo Shi Teng/ Trachelospermum	✓																47	6-15
Ma Bian Cao/ Verbena	✓				○						✪					●		9-30
Ma Bo/ Lasiosphaera	✓				○					✓								1.5-3
Ma Chi Xian/ Portulaca	✓				○						✪					●		15-60
Ma Dou Ling/ Aristolochia	✓																	3-9

L, M

Legend:
- Powder/Pills taken internally: ○ may be ✿ commonly ● always
- External use: ○ possible ✿ mainly (internal caution) ● only
- Do not cook substance ● Refrigerate
- Add near end of cooking: ○ last 5 min ✿ 10 min ● 15 min
- Slice or Crush: ✿ small pieces ● powder
- May be used: ✿ fresh or dried ● fresh only
- Toxic: ✿ slightly ● very toxic
- Contraindicated in pregnancy: ✿ caution ● never use
- Combining Cautions... See page 620

Name of herb or substance	Decoction	Powder/Pills taken internally	Used with wine or extracted	Whole substance often eaten separately	External use	Do not cook substance / Refrigerate	Add near end of cooking	Cook 30-60 min before adding other herbs	Dissolve/steep in strained previously cooked decoction	Wrap in separate porous bag (cheesecloth)	Slice or Crush	May be used	May be available in prepared form - less toxic or stronger this way	Available in charred form	Toxic	Contraindicated in pregnancy	Combining Cautions	Standard Dosage Range in Grams
Ma Huang/ Ephedra	✓																	3-9
Ma Huang Gen/ Ephedra	✓																	3-9
Ma Qian Zi/ Strychnos		○			✿						●				●	●		0.3-0.6
Mai Men Dong/ Ophiopogon	✓																61	6-12
Mai Ya/ Hordeum	✓	✿						✓										9-30
Man Jing Zi/ Vitex	✓		✓														36	6-9
Man Shan Hong/ Rhododendron	✓				○													25-50
Mang Xiao/ Mirabilitum	✓	○			○				✓							●		4.5-9
Mao Dong Qing/ Ilex	✓																	30-60
Mao Mei/ Rubus	✓				○							✿						15-60
Mao Zhao Cao/ Ranunculus	✓																	20-50
Mei Gui Hua/ Rosa	✓		✓															3-6
Meng Chong/ Tabanus	✓	○									●				✿	●		1.5-3
Meng Shi/ Lapis Micae seu Chloriti	✓	○					✓			✓	●		✓			●		1.5-3

Name of herb or substance	Decoction	Powder/Pills taken internally	Used with wine or extracted	Whole substance often eaten separately	External use	Do not cook substance / Refrigerate	Add near end of cooking	Cook 30-60 min before adding other herbs	Dissolve/steep in strained previously cooked decoction	Wrap in separate porous bag (cheesecloth)	Slice or Crush	May be used	May be available in prepared form - less toxic or stronger this way	Available in charred form	Toxic	Contraindicated in pregnancy	Combining Cautions... See page 620	Standard Dosage Range in Grams
Mi Meng Hua/ Buddleia	✓																	3-9
Mi Tuo Seng/ Lithargyrum		○			✿										●			0.3-1
Mian Hua Gen/ Gossypium	✓															●		50-100
Ming Dang Shen/ Changium	✓															●		6-9
Ming Fan/ Alumen		○			✿						●				✿		67	0.5-3
Mo Yao/ Commiphora	✓				○											●		3-12
Mu Bie Zi/ Momordica		○			✿										●	●		0.6-1.2
Mu Dan Pi/ Paeonia	✓															●	38	6-12
Mu Gua/ Chaenomeles	✓																	4.5-12
Mu Hu Die/ Oroxylum	✓				○													1.5-6
Mu Li/ Ostrea	✓							✓			✿		✓				17	15-30
Mu Tong/ Akebia	✓															●		3-9
Mu Xiang/ Saussurea	✓						○											1.5-9
Mu Zei/ Equisetum	✓				○												✿	3-9
Nan Gua Zi/ Cucurbita	✓	○									✿							30-60

M, N

Legend: Powder/Pills taken internally: ○ may be ⊘ commonly ● always — External use: ○ possible ⊘ mainly (internal caution) ● only — ⊘ Do not cook substance ● Refrigerate — Add near end of cooking: ○ last 5 min ⊘ 10 min ● 15 min — Slice or Crush: ⊘ small pieces ● powder — May be used: ⊘ fresh or dried ● fresh only — Toxic: ⊘ slightly ● very toxic — Contraindicated in pregnancy: ⊘ caution ● never use — Combining Cautions... See page 620

Name of herb or substance	Decoction	Powder/Pills taken internally	Used with wine or extracted	Whole substance often eaten separately	External use	⊘ Do not cook substance ● Refrigerate	Add near end of cooking	Cook 30 - 60 minutes before adding other herbs	Dissolve/steep in strained previously cooked decoction	Wrap in separate porous bag (cheesecloth)	Slice or Crush	May be used	May be available in prepared form - less toxic or stronger this way	Available in charred form	Toxic	Contraindicated in pregnancy	Combining Cautions... See page 620	Standard Dosage Range in Grams
Nan Sha Shen/ Adenophora	✓																4	9-15
Niu Bang Zi/ Arctium	✓																	4.5-9
Niu Dan/ Bos		●			○													
Niu Huang/ Bos		●		✓	○	⊘					●					●	20	0.15-1
Nu Zhen Zi/ Ligustrum	✓																	4.5-15
Nuo Dao Gen/ Oryza	✓																	25-50
Ou Jie/ Nelumbo	✓										⊘							9-15
Pang Da Hai/ Sterculia	✓				○													4.5-9
Pao Jiang/ Zingiber	✓															⊘		3-6
Pei Lan/ Eupatorium	✓																	5-9
Peng Sha/ Borax		○			⊘						●					●		1.5-3
Pi Pa Ye/ Eriobotrya	✓											⊘						4.5-9
Pi Shi/ Arsenolite					●										●	●		0.03-0.08
Pu Gong Ying/ Taraxacum	✓				○							⊘						9-30
Pu Huang/ Typha	✓		✓		○						✓	●			✓		⊘	4.5-9
Pu Hui/ Typha	✓													✓				

Name of herb or substance	Decoction	Powder/Pills taken internally: ○ may be ◉ commonly ● always	Used with wine or extracted	Whole substance often eaten separately	External use: ○ possible ◉ mainly (internal caution) ● only	◉ Do not cook substance ● Refrigerate	Add near end of cooking: ○ last 5 min ◉ 10 min ● 15 min	Cook 30-60 minutes before adding other herbs	Dissolve/steep in strained previously cooked decoction	Wrap in separate porous bag (cheesecloth)	Slice or Crush: ◉ small pieces ● powder	May be used: ◉ fresh or dried ● fresh only	May be available in prepared form - less toxic or stronger this way	Available in charred form	Toxic: ◉ slightly ● very toxic	Contraindicated in pregnancy: ◉ caution ● never use	Combining Cautions... See page 620	Standard Dosage Range in Grams
Qian Cao Gen/ Rubia	✓																	6-9
Qian Dan/ Minium		○			◉											●		0.3-0.6
Qian Hu/ Peucedanum	✓																4	4.5-9
Qian Li Guang/ Senecio	✓												◉					9-15
Qian Niu Zi/ Pharbitis	✓	○													◉	●		1.5-9
Qian Shi/ Euryale	✓										◉							9-15
Qiang Huo/ Notopterygium	✓																	6-15
Qiao Mai/ Fagopyrum	✓																	3-50
Qin Jiao/ Gentiana	✓																	4.5-9
Qin Pi/ Fraxinus	✓																	4.5-9
Qing Dai/ Indigo		◉			○					✓								1.5-2.5
Qing Fen/ Calomelas		○			◉							●			●	●		0.06-0.15
Qing Hao/ Artemisia	✓																18	4.5-9
Qing Mu Xiang/ Aristolochia	✓																	3-9
Qing Pi/ Citrus	✓						●											3-9
Qing Xiang Zi/ Celosia	✓																	9-15

Q, R

Legend (column symbols):
- Powder/Pills taken internally: ○ may be ✿ commonly ● always
- External use: ○ possible ✿ mainly (internal caution) ● only
- ✿ Do not cook substance ● Refrigerate
- Add near end of cooking: ○ last 5 min ✿ 10 min ● 15 min
- Slice or Crush: ✿ small pieces ● powder
- May be used: ✿ fresh or dried ● fresh only
- Toxic: ✿ slightly ● very toxic
- Contraindicated in pregnancy: ✿ caution ● never use
- Combining Cautions... See page 620

Name of herb or substance	Decoction	Powder/Pills taken internally	Used with wine or extracted	Whole substance often eaten separately	External use	Do not cook / Refrigerate	Add near end of cooking	Cook 30-60 minutes before adding other herbs	Dissolve/steep in strained previously cooked decoction	Wrap in separate porous bag (cheesecloth)	Slice or Crush	May be used fresh/dried	May be available in prepared form - less toxic or stronger this way	Available in charred form	Toxic	Contraindicated in pregnancy	Combining Cautions	Standard Dosage Range in Grams
Qu Mai/ Dianthus	✓															●	45	6-12
Quan Xie/ Buthus	✓	✿			○						●			●				0.6-0.9
Ren Shen/ Panax	✓	○		✓									✓				19	1.5-9
Ren Shen Lu/ Panax	✓																	3-9
Ren Shen Ye/ Panax	✓																	3-9
Rou Cong Rong/ Cistanche	✓																	9-21
Rou Dou Kou/ Myristica	✓										✿			✿				1.5-9
Rou Gui/ Cinnamomum	✓	✿	✓				○		✓		●					✿	31	1.5-4.5
Ru Xiang/ Boswellia	✓				○											●		3-9
San Bai Cao/ Saururus	✓				○													9-15
San Leng/ Sparganium	✓															●	53	4.5-9
San Qi/ Panax	✓	✿	✓		○											●		1-9
San Qi Hua/ Panax	✓																	6-15
Sang Bai Pi/ Morus	✓																	6-15
Sang Ji Sheng/ Loranthus	✓																	9-30

Legend:
- Powder/Pills taken internally: ○ may be, ❂ commonly, ● always
- External use: ○ possible, ❂ mainly (internal caution), ● only
- Do not cook substance ❂; Refrigerate ●
- Add near end of cooking: ○ last 5 min, ❂ 10 min, ● 15 min
- Slice or Crush: ❂ small pieces, ● powder
- May be used: ❂ fresh or dried, ● fresh only
- Toxic: ❂ slightly, ● very toxic
- Contraindicated in pregnancy: ❂ caution, ● never use
- Combining Cautions... See page 620

Name of herb or substance	Decoction	Powder/Pills taken internally	Used with wine or extracted	Whole substance often eaten separately	External use	Do not cook substance / Refrigerate	Add near end of cooking	Cook 30-60 minutes before adding other herbs	Dissolve/steep in strained previously cooked decoction	Wrap in separate porous bag (cheesecloth)	Slice or Crush	May be used	May be available in prepared form - less toxic or stronger this way	Available in charred form	Toxic	Contraindicated in pregnancy	Combining Cautions... See page 620	Standard Dosage Range in Grams
Sang Piao Xiao/ Paratenodera	✓	❂															34	5-9
Sang Shen/ Morus	✓																	9-15
Sang Ye/ Morus	✓			○														5-15
Sang Zhi/ Morus	✓																	10-30
Sha Ren/ Amomum	✓						○				❂							1.5-6
Sha Ren Ke/ Amomum	✓			○			○				❂							2.5-4.5
Sha Yuan Ji Li/ Astragalus	✓																	6-15
Shan Ci Gu/ Tulipa	✓			❂							❂					●		3-9
Shan Dou Gen/ Sophora	✓			○														3-9
Shan Li Hong/ Crataegus	✓																	3-9
Shan Yang Jiao/ Naemorhedis	✓	❂	✓				✓				❂							9-15
Shan Yao/ Dioscorea	✓																	9-30
Shan Zha/ Crataegus	✓																	9-15
Shan Zha Rou/ Crataegus	✓																	12-15
Shan Zha Tan/ Crataegus	✓													✓				12-15

S

Name of herb or substance	Decoction	Powder/Pills taken internally: ○ may be ⊙ commonly ● always	Used with wine or extracted	Whole substance often eaten separately	External use: ○ possible ⊙ mainly (internal caution) ● only	⊙ Do not cook substance ● Refrigerate	Add near end of cooking: ○ last 5 min ⊙ 10 min ● 15 min	Cook 30 - 60 minutes before adding other herbs	Dissolve/steep in strained previously cooked decoction	Wrap in separate porous bag (cheesecloth)	Slice or Crush: ⊙ small pieces ● powder	May be used: ⊙ fresh or dried ● fresh only	May be available in prepared form - less toxic or stronger this way	Available in charred form	Toxic: ⊙ slightly ● very toxic	Contraindicated in pregnancy: ⊙ caution ● never use	Combining Cautions... See page 620	Standard Dosage Range in Grams
Shan Zhu Yu/ Cornus	✓																64	3-12
Shang Lu/ Phytolacca	✓				○							⊙			●	●		4.5-9
She Chuang Zi/ Cnidium	✓	○			⊙												69	3-9
She Gan/ Belamcanda	✓															●		1.5-9
She Xiang/ Moschus		●	✓	○	⊙						●					●		0.06-0.15
She Tui/ Zaocys	✓	○														●		0.3-3
Shen Jin Cao/ Lycopodium	✓															●		9-15
Shen Qu/ Massa Fermentata	✓	○											✓			⊙		6-12
Sheng Di Huang/ Rehmannia	✓										⊙					⊙		9-30
Sheng Jiang/ Zingiber	✓				○							●						3-9
Sheng Jiang Pi/ Zingiber	✓											●						3-9
Sheng Ma/ Cimicifuga	✓																	1.5-9
Sheng Tie Luo/ Frusta Ferri	✓							✓			⊙							9-30
Shi Chang Pu/ Acorus	✓	○			○							⊙	✓				67	3-9
Shi Da Gong Lao/ Mahonia	✓																	6-9

Name of herb or substance	Decoction	Powder/Pills taken internally: ○ may be ✪ commonly ● always	Used with wine or extracted	Whole substance often eaten separately	External use: ○ possible ✪ mainly (internal caution) ● only	Do not cook substance ● Refrigerate	Add near end of cooking: ○ last 5 min ✪ 10 min ● 15 min	Cook 30 - 60 minutes before adding other herbs	Dissolve/steep in strained previously cooked decoction	Wrap in separate porous bag (cheesecloth)	Slice or Crush: ✪ small pieces ● powder	May be used: ✪ fresh or dried ● fresh only	May be available in prepared form - less toxic or stronger this way	Available in charred form	Toxic: ✪ slightly ● very toxic	Contraindicated in pregnancy: ✪ caution ● never use	Combining Cautions... See page 620	Standard Dosage Range in Grams
Shi Di/ Diospyros	✓																	6-12
Shi Gao/ Gypsum	✓				○			✓			✪							9-30
Shi Hu/ Dendrobium	✓																32	6-15
Shi Jue Ming/ Haliotis	✓	○			○			✓			✪						34	9-30
Shi Jun Zi/ Quisqualis	✓										✪	✪			✪			4.5-12
Shi Liu Gen Pi/ Punica	✓														✪			1.5-9
Shi Liu Pi/ Punica	✓														✪		21	3-9
Shi Shang Bai/ Selaginella	✓		✓															15-30
Shi Wei/ Pyrrosia	✓																	4.5-9
Shu Di Huang/ Rehmannia	✓																	9-30
Shu Qi/ Dichroa	✓														✪			3-6
Shu Yi Ren/ Coix	✓																	9-30
Shui Niu Jiao/ Bubalus	✓	✪		✓				✓								✪		6-120
Shui Yin/ Hydrargyrum					●										●	●	22	
Shui Zhi/ Hirudo		●										●			✪	●		1.5-3
Si Gua Luo/ Luffa	✓																	6-12

Name of herb or substance	Decoction	Powder/Pills taken internally	Used with wine or extracted	Whole substance often eaten separately	External use	Do not cook substance	Add near end of cooking	Cook 30-60 minutes before adding other herbs	Dissolve/steep in strained previously cooked decoction	Wrap in separate porous bag (cheesecloth)	Slice or Crush	May be used	May be available in prepared form - less toxic or stronger this way	Available in charred form	Toxic	Contraindicated in pregnancy	Combining Cautions... See page 620	Standard Dosage Range in Grams
Song Jie/ Pinus	✓										✪							9-15
Su He Xiang/ Liquidambar		●			○													0.3-1
Su Mu/ Caesalpinia	✓										✪					●		3-9
Suan Jiang/ Physalis	✓				○							✪				✪		9-15
Suan Zao Ren/ Ziziphus	✓	○									✪							1.5-18
Suo Yang/ Cynomorium	✓	○																5-15
Tai Zi Shen/ Pseudostellaria	✓																4	9-30
Tan Xiang/ Santalum	✓	○					●				✪							1.5-9
Tang Song Cao/ Thalictrum	✓																	3-9
Tao Ren/ Prunus	✓										✪					●		5-9
Tian Hua Fen/ Trichosanthes	✓				○											●		9-15
Tian Ma/ Gastrodia	✓	○																0.9-9
Tian Men Dong/ Asparagus	✓																	6-15
Tian Nan Xing/ Arisaema	✓	●			✪						●				●	●	23	0.3-1
Tian Zhu Huang/ Bambusa	✓	○														✪		0.6-9

Name of herb or substance	Decoction	Powder/Pills taken internally: ○ may be ❂ commonly ● always	Used with wine or extracted	Whole substance often eaten separately	External use: ○ possible ❂ mainly (internal caution) ● only	Do not cook substance	Refrigerate	Add near end of cooking: ○ last 5 min ❂ 10 min ● 15 min	Cook 30 - 60 minutes before adding other herbs	Dissolve/steep in strained previously cooked decoction	Wrap in separate porous bag (cheesecloth)	Slice or Crush: ❂ small pieces ● powder	May be used: ❂ fresh or dried ● fresh only	May be available in prepared form - less toxic or stronger this way	Available in charred form	Toxic: ❂ slightly ● very toxic	Contraindicated in pregnancy: ❂ caution ● never use	Combining Cautions... See page 620	Standard Dosage Range in Grams
Tie Xian/ Acalypha	✓				○							❂					●		9-15
Ting Li Zi/ Lepidium	✓										✓								4.5-9
Tong Cao/ Tetrapanax	✓																	❂	3-6
Tu Bie Chong/ Eupolyphaga	✓	○			○								●			❂	●		1-6
Tu Fu Ling/ Smilax	✓																		15-60
Tu Niu Xi/ Achyranthes	✓																●		15-30
Tu Si Zi/ Cuscuta	✓																	❂	9-15
Wa Leng Zi/ Arca	✓								✓			❂							9-15
Wan Nian Qing/ Rhodea	✓												❂			❂			3-9
Wang Bu Liu Xing/ Vaccaria	✓																●		4.5-9
Wei Jiang/ Zingiber	✓																	❂	6-12
Wei Ling Xian/ Clematis	✓		✓																6-12
Wu Bei Zi/ Rhus/ Melaphis	✓	❂			○														1-6
Wu Gong/ Scolopendra	✓	❂			○								●			●	●		0.6-3
Wu Jia Pi/ Acanthopanax	✓		✓																4.5-15

T, U, V, W

Name of herb or substance	Decoction	Powder/Pills taken internally: ○ may be ◐ commonly ● always	Used with wine or extracted	Whole substance often eaten separately	External use: ○ possible ◐ mainly (internal caution) ● only	Do not cook substance ● / Refrigerate	Add near end of cooking: ○ last 5 min ◐ 10 min ● 15 min	Cook 30 - 60 minutes before adding other herbs	Dissolve/steep in strained previously cooked decoction	Wrap in separate porous bag (cheesecloth)	Slice or Crush: ◐ small pieces ● powder	May be used: ◐ fresh or dried ● fresh only	May be available in prepared form - less toxic or stronger this way	Available in charred form	Toxic: ◐ slightly ● very toxic	Contraindicated in pregnancy: ◐ caution ● never use	Combining Cautions... See page 620	Standard Dosage Range in Grams
Wu Jiu Gen Pi/ Sapium	✓														◐	●		4.5-9
Wu Ling Zhi/ Trogopterus	✓									✓						◐	24	4.5-9
Wu Mei/ Prunus	✓				○													3-9
Wu Shao She/ Zaocys	✓	◐	✓															3-9
Wu Tou/ Aconitum	✓				○			✓					✓		●	●	25	3-9
Wu Wei Zi/ Schisandra	✓		✓															1.5-9
Wu Yao/ Lindera	✓																	4.5-9
Wu Zhi Mao Tao/ Ficus	✓																	
Wu Zhu Yu/ Evodia	✓														◐		55	3-9
Xi Gua/ Citrullus	✓					◐						●						1 cup juice
Xi Hong Hua/ Crocus	✓															●		0.9-1.5
Xi Jiao/ Rhinoceros		●		✓												◐	9	1-2
Xi Xian Cao/ Siegesbeckia	✓		✓															9-15
Xi Xin/ Asarum	✓				○												35	1-3
Xi Yang Shen/ Panax	✓			✓													4	2.5-9
Xia Ku Cao/ Prunella	✓																	6-15

Name of herb or substance	Decoction	Powder/Pills taken internally: ○ may be ☼ commonly ● always	Used with wine or extracted	Whole substance often eaten separately	External use: ○ possible ☼ mainly (internal caution) ● only	☼ Do not cook substance ● Refrigerate	Add near end of cooking: ○ last 5 min ☼ 10 min ● 15 min	Cook 30 - 60 minutes before adding other herbs	Dissolve/steep in strained previously cooked decoction	Wrap in separate porous bag (cheesecloth)	Slice or Crush: ☼ small pieces ● powder	May be used: ☼ fresh or dried ● fresh only	May be available in prepared form - less toxic or stronger this way	Available in charred form	Toxic: ☼ slightly ● very toxic	Contraindicated in pregnancy: ☼ caution ● never use	Combining Cautions... See page 620	Standard Dosage Range in Grams
Xian He Cao/ Agrimonia	✓				○						☼							9-15
Xian Mao/ Curculigo	✓		✓												☼			4.5-9
Xiang Fu/ Cyperus	✓																	4.5-12
Xiang Ru/ Elsholtzia	✓						○											3-9
Xiao Hui Xiang/ Foeniculum	✓				○													3-9
Xiao Ji/ Cephalanoplos	✓				○						☼							10-15
Xie Bai/ Allium	✓										☼							4.5-9
Xin Yi Hua/ Magnolia	✓	○			○					✓								3-9
(Ku) Xing Ren/ Prunus	✓										☼				☼		48	3-9
(Tian) Xing Ren/ Prunus	✓										☼				☼			3-9
Xiong Dan/ Ursus		●		✓	○							●					26	1-2.5
Xiong Huang/ Realgar		●			☼							●			●	●		0.15-0.6
Xu Duan/ Dipsacus	✓				○												58	6-21
Xu Sui Zi/ Euphorbia		●													☼	●		1.5-3
Xuan Fu Hua/ Inula	✓									✓								3-12
Xuan Ming Fen/ Mirabilitum					●	☼												

Legend for symbols used in column headers:
- Powder/Pills taken internally: ○ may be　◎ commonly　● always
- External use: ○ possible　◎ mainly (internal caution)　● only
- Do not cook substance: ◎　● Refrigerate
- Add near end of cooking: ○ last 5 min　◎ 10 min　● 15 min
- Slice or Crush: ◎ small pieces　● powder
- May be used: ◎ fresh or dried　● fresh only
- Toxic: ◎ slightly　● very toxic
- Contraindicated in pregnancy: ◎ caution　● never use

Name of herb or substance	Decoction	Powder/Pills taken internally	Used with wine or extracted	Whole substance often eaten separately	External use	Do not cook substance	Add near end of cooking	Cook 30-60 minutes before adding other herbs	Dissolve/steep in strained previously cooked decoction	Wrap in separate porous bag (cheesecloth)	Slice or Crush	May be used	May be available in prepared form - less toxic or stronger this way	Available in charred form	Toxic	Contraindicated in pregnancy	Combining Cautions... See page 620	Standard Dosage Range in Grams
Xuan Shen/ Scrophularia	✓																29	9-30
Xue Jie/ Dracaena		●			○											●		0.3-1.5
Xue Yu Tan/ HomoSapiens	✓	◎			○									✓				1.5-9
Xun Gu Feng/ Aristolochia	✓																	9-15
Ya Dan Zi/ Brucea		●			○										●	◎		10-30 pieces
Ya Zhi Cao/ Commelina	✓				○						◎							9-15
Yan Fu Mu/ Rhus	✓				○													9-15
Yan Hu Suo/ Corydalis	✓	○														●		4.5-12
Yang Qi Shi/ Actinolitum		●											✓				60	3-4.5
Ye Jiao Teng/ Polygonum	✓				○													9-30
Ye Ju Hua/ Chrysanthemum	✓				○													6-12
Ye Ming Sha/ Vespertilio	✓															◎	37	3-9
Yi Mu Cao/ Leonurus	✓															●		9-30
Yi Tang/ Saccharum Granorum					◎				✓									30-60
Yi Yi Ren/ Coix	✓										◎					◎		9-30

Name of herb or substance	Decoction	Powder/Pills taken internally: ○ may be ✿ commonly ● always	Used with wine or extracted	Whole substance often eaten separately	External use: ○ possible ✿ mainly (internal caution) ● only	✿ Do not cook substance ● Refrigerate	Add near end of cooking: ○ last 5 min ✿ 10 min ● 15 min	Cook 30 - 60 minutes before adding other herbs	Dissolve/steep in strained previously cooked decoction	Wrap in separate porous bag (cheesecloth)	Slice or Crush: ✿ small pieces ● powder	May be used: ✿ fresh or dried ● fresh only	May be available in prepared form - less toxic or stronger this way	Available in charred form	Toxic: ✿ slightly ● very toxic	Contraindicated in pregnancy: ✿ caution ● never use	Combining Cautions... See page 620	Standard Dosage Range in Grams
Yi Zhi Ren/ Alpinia	✓										✿							3-9
Yin Chai Hu/ Stellaria	✓																	3-9
Yin Chen Hao/ Artemisia	✓																	9-15
Yin Yang Huo/ Epimedium	✓		✓															6-15
Ying Su Ke/ Papaver	✓															●		1.5-6
Yu Jin/ Curcuma	✓															✿	51	4.5-9
Yu Li Ren/ Prunus	✓										✿					✿		3-9
Yu Mi Xu/ Zea	✓																	15-30
Yu Xing Cao/ Houttuynia	✓				○							✿						15-30
Yu Zhu/ Polygonatum	✓																	9-15
Yuan Hua/ Daphne	✓	✿			○										✿	●	8	1.5-3
Yuan Zhi/ Polygala	✓		✓		○													3-9
Yue Ji Hua/ Rosa	✓		✓													●		3-6
Zao Jiao/ Gleditsia		●			○						●				✿	●		0.6-1.5
Zao Jiao Ci/ Gleditsia	✓	○			○										✿	●		3-9
Zao Xiu/ Paris	✓				○										✿	●		3-9

Y, Z

Name of herb or substance	Decoction	Powder/Pills taken internally: (O may be ◉ commonly ● always)	Used with wine or extracted	Whole substance often eaten separately	External use: (O possible ◉ mainly (internal caution) ● only)	Do not cook substance ◉ / Refrigerate ●	Add near end of cooking: (O last 5 min ◉ 10 min ● 15 min)	Cook 30-60 minutes before adding other herbs	Dissolve/steep in strained previously cooked decoction	Wrap in separate porous bag (cheesecloth)	Slice or Crush: (◉ small pieces ● powder)	May be used: (◉ fresh or dried ● fresh only)	May be available in prepared form - less toxic or stronger this way	Available in charred form	Toxic: (◉ slightly ● very toxic)	Contraindicated in pregnancy: (◉ caution ● never use)	Combining Cautions... See page 620	Standard Dosage Range in Grams
Ze Lan/ Lycopus	✓				O											◉		4.5-9
Ze Qi/ Euphorbia	✓				O										◉			3-15
Ze Xie/ Alisma	✓																	6-15
Zhang Nao/ Cinnamomum		O	✓		◉										●	●		0.06-0.15
Zhe Bei Mu/ Fritillaria	✓																9	4.5-9
Zhen Zhu/ Pteria		●		✓	O		✓				●							0.6-1
Zhen Zhu Mu/ Pteria	✓	O					✓				◉							15-30
Zhi Gan Cao/ Glycyrrhiza	✓												✓					2-12
Zhi Ke/ Citrus	✓															◉		3-9
Zhi Mu/ Anemarrhena	✓																	6-15
Zhi Shi/ Citrus	✓															◉		3-9
Zhi Nan Xing/ Arisaema	✓														◉	●		4.5-9
Zhi Zi/ Gardenia	✓				O						◉							6-12
Zhu Ling/ Polyporus	✓																	6-15
Zhu Li/ Bambusa		◉		✓								◉						9-60
Zhu Ma Gen/ Boehmeria	✓				O													5-15
Zhu Ru/ Bambusa	✓																	4.5-9

Name of herb or substance	Decoction	Powder/Pills taken internally: (O may be · ✿ commonly · ● always)	Used with wine or extracted	Whole substance often eaten separately	External use: (O possible · ✿ mainly (internal caution) · ● only)	Do not cook substance / Refrigerate (✿ Do not cook substance · ● Refrigerate)	Add near end of cooking: (O last 5 min · O 10 min · ● 15 min)	Cook 30 - 60 minutes before adding other herbs	Dissolve/steep in strained previously cooked decoction	Wrap in separate porous bag (cheesecloth)	Slice or Crush: (✿ small pieces · ● powder)	May be used: (✿ fresh or dried · ● fresh only)	May be available in prepared form - less toxic or stronger this way	Available in charred form	Toxic: (✿ slightly · ● very toxic)	Contraindicated in pregnancy: (✿ caution · ● never use)	Combining Cautions... See page 620	Standard Dosage Range in Grams
Zhu Sha/ Cinnabaris		✿			O	✿			✓		●				●	●		0.3-1
Zhu Sha Gen/ Ardisia	✓				O													9-15
Zi Cao/ Lithospermum	✓				O													3-9
Zi He Che/ Homo Sapiens		✿		✓							●							2.5-4.5
Zi Hua Di Ding/ Viola	✓				O							✿						10-16
Zi Ran Tong/ Pyritum	✓	O			O			✓			✿							0.3-9
Zi Shi Ying/ Fluoritum	✓							✓			●							6-15
Zi Su Geng/ Perilla	✓																	4.5-9
Zi Su Ye/ Perilla	✓						●											6-9
Zi Su Zi/ Perilla	✓											●						4.5-9
Zi Wan/ Aster	✓																	1.5-9
Zi Zhu / Callicarpa	✓	O			O													1.5-30
Zong Lu Pi Tan/ Trachycarpus	✓	O												✓				1-15

N

Combining Cautions as Listed in Column 17

1. Do not use with *Fu Zi / Aconitum* or *Wu Tou / Aconitum*.

2. Do not use with *Qian Niu Zi / Pharbitis*.

3. Do not use with *Yu Jin / Curcuma*.

4. Do not use with *Li Lu / Veratrum*.

5. Do not use with *Long Dan Cao / Gentiana*.

6. Do not use with *Bai Ji / Bletilla, (Fa) Ban Xia / Pinellia, Bei Mu / Fritillaria, Gua Lou / Trichosanthes, Xi Jiao / Rhinoceros, Wu Gong / Scolopendra, Bai Wei / Cynanchum* or *Lu Dou / Phaseolus*.

7. Do not use with *Jing Da Ji / Euphorbia, Yuan Hua / Daphne, Gan Sui / Euphorbia, Hai Zao / Sargassum* or *Yuan Zhi / Polygala*.

8. Do not use with *Gan Cao / Glycyrrhiza*.

9. Do not use with *Wu Tou / Aconitum*.

10. Do not use with *Gan Jiang / Zingiber, Huai Niu Xi / Achyranthes* or *Wu Tou / Aconitum*.

11. Do not use with *Fu Zi / Aconitum* or *Bai Ji / Bletilla*.

12. Do not cook in steel or iron pot.

13. Do not use with *Gan Cao / Glycyrrhiza, Yuan Hua / Daphne*, or *Hai Zao / Sargassum*.

14. Do not use with *Huo Ma Ren / Cannabis* or *Li Lu / Veratrum*.

15. Do not use with *Xi Xin / Asarum, Bai Shao Yao / Paeonia, Dan Shen / Salvia, Dang Shen / Codonopsis, Ren Shen / Panax, Ku Shen / Sophora, Nan Sha Shen / Adenophora* or *Bei Sha Shen / Glehnia*.

16. Do not use with *Sheng Di Huang / Rehmannia, Cong Bai / Allium* or *Da Suan / Allium*.

17. Do not use with *Ma Huang / Ephedra, Wu Zhu Yu / Evodia*, or *Xi Xin / Asarum*.

18. Do not use with *Sheng Di Huang / Rehmannia* or *Dang Gui / Angelica*.

19. Do not use with *Wu Ling Zhi / Trogopterus* or *Li Lu / Veratrum*. Note: this herb is usually decocted separately.

20. Do not use with *Long Dan Cao / Gentiana, Huai Niu Xi / Achyranthes, Chang Shan / Dichroa, Long Gu / Os Draconis* or *Sheng Di Huang / Rehmannia*.

21. Do not use with fat or oil.

22. Do not use with *Pi Shi / Arsenolite*.

23. Do not use with *Fu Zi / Aconitum, Gan Jiang / Zingiber*, or *Sheng Jiang / Zingiber*.

24. Do not use with *Ren Shen / Panax*.

25. Do not use with *Gua Lou / Trichosanthes, Bai Lian / Ampelopsis, Bei Mu / Fritillaria, Bai Ji / Bletilla* or *(Fa) Ban Xia / Pinellia*.

26. Do not use with *Sheng Di Huang / Rehmannia* or *Han Fang Ji / Stephania*.

27.   Do not use with *Huang Jing Ye / Polygonatum.*

28.   Do not use with *Shi Hu / Dendrobium, Mang Xiao / Mirabilitum, Bie Jia / Amyda, Xiao Ji / Cephalanoplos* or *Li Lu / Veratrum.*

29.   Do not use with *Gan Jiang / Zingiber, Li Lu / Veratrum, Huang Qi / Astragalus, Da Zao / Ziziphus* or *Shan Zhu Yu / Cornus.*

30.   Do not use with *Wu Tou / Aconitum* or *Qin Jiao / Gentiana.*

31.   Do not use with *Chi Shi Zi / Halloysitum Rubrum.*

32.   Do not use with *Ba Dou / Croton* or *Lei Wan / Omphalia.*

33.   Do not use with *Li Lu / Veratrum, Gan Jiang / Zingiber* or *Bei Xie / Dioscorea.*

34.   Do not use with *Xuan Fu Hua / Inula.*

35.   Do not use with *Hua Shi / Talcum, Shan Zhu Yu / Cornus*, or *Huang Qi / Astragalus.*

36.   Do not use with *Shi Gao / Gypsum* or *Wu Tou / Aconitum.*

37.   Do not use with *Bai Wei / Cynanchum.*

38.   Do not use with *Tu Si Zi / Cuscuta, Bei Mu / Fritillaria*, or *Da Huang / Rheum.*

39.   Do not use with *Jing Da Ji / Euphorbia, Da Huang / Rheum, Huang Qi / Astragalus, Da Zao / Ziziphus, Shan Zhu Yu / Cornus*, or *Gan Jiang / Zingiber.*

40.   Do not use with *Li Lu / Veratrum* or *Mu Dan Pi / Paeonia.*

41.   Do not use with *Huai Niu Xi / Achyranthes, Bai Xian Pi / Dictamnus, Ju Hua / Chrysanthemum, Xuan Shen / Scrophularia, Jiang Can / Bombyx*, or *Kuan Dong Hua / Tussilago.*

42.   Do not use with *Li Lu / Veratrum, Bei Mu / Fritillaria* or *Tu Si Zi / Cuscuta.*

43.   Do not use with *Gan Cao / Glycyrrhiza* or *Yuan Zhi / Polygala.*

44.   Do not use with *Bie Jia / Amyda, Qin Jiao / Gentiana*, or *Di Yu / Sanguisorba.*

45.   Do not use with *Sang Piao Xiao / Paratenodera.*

46.   Do not use with *Hai Piao Xiao / Sepia.*

47.   Do not use with *Bei Mu / Fritillaria* or *Shi Chang Pu / Acorus.*

48.   Do not use with *Huang Qin / Scutellaria, Ge Gen / Pueraria* or *Huang Qi / Astragalus.*

49.   Do not use with *Ma Huang / Ephedra, Huang Qin / Scutellaria, Xuan Shen / Scrophularia, Bei Mu / Fritillaria, Huang Lian / Coptis, Huang Qi / Astragalus*, or *Xin Yi Hua / Magnolia.*

50.   Do not use with *Ze Xie / Alisma* or *Han Shui Shi / Calcitum.*

51.   Do not use with *Ding Xiang / Eugenia.*

52.   Do not use with *Po Xiao / Sal Glauberis.*

53.   Do not use with *Ya Xiao / Nitrum.*

54.   Do not use with *Bai Qian / Cynanchum.*

55.   Do not use with *Dan Shen / Salvia* or *Zi Shi Ying / Fluoritum.*

56.   Do not use with *Kuan Dong Hua / Tussilago, Gua Lou / Trichosanthes, Fang Feng / Ledebouriella* or *Fu Zi / Aconitum.*

57.   Do not use with *Da Huang / Rheum.*

58. Do not use with *Lei Wan / Omphalia.*

59. Do not use with *Bai Jiang Cao / Patrinia.*

60. Do not use with *Lei Wan / Omphalia, Ze Xie / Alisma, Tu Si Zi / Cuscuta,* or *Chan Tui / Cryptotympana.*

61. Do not use with *Bai Mu Er / Tremella, Ku Shen / Sophora,* or *Kuan Dong Hua / Tussilago.*

62. Do not use with *Ren Shen / Panax, Nan Sha Shen / Adenophora,* or *Bei Sha Shen / Glehnia.*

63. Do not use with *Ming Fan / Alumen.*

64. Do not use with *Fang Feng / Ledebouriella, Guang Fang Ji / Aristolochia,* or *Jie Geng / Platycodon.*

65. Do not use with *Dan Shen / Salvia, Mu Li / Ostrea, Shao Yao / Paeonia,* or *Gan Jiang / Zingiber.*

66. Do not use with *Rou Gui / Cinnamomum, Huang Qin / Scutellaria, Yuan Hua / Daphne,* or *Da Huang / Rheum.*

67. Do not use with *Ma Huang / Ephedra.*

68. Do not use with *Ge Gen / Pueraria* or *Bian Xu / Polygonum.*

69. Do not use with *Mu Dan Pi / Paeonia, Ba Dou / Croton,* or *Bei Mu / Fritillaria.*

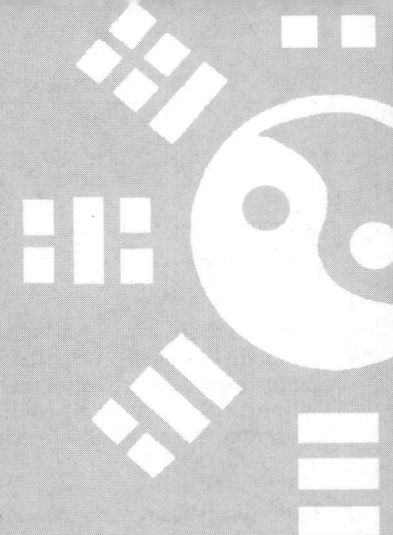

Part 4

Naming Convention
Cross Reference

This chapter allows instant cross-referencing by latinate botanical, latinate pharmaceutical, common, and Pinyin names of over 480 Chinese herbs.

Because there is not yet standardization of herbal nomenclature in Oriental medical schools, practitioners and students face confusion. Some programs may use only common and botanical names, while others teach Pinyin and pharmaceutical names. Practitioners are often at a loss when presented with an herb in a naming convention with which they are unfamiliar.

This chapter contains tables of the herbs listed alphabetically by the four most commonly used naming conventions (botanical, pharmaceutical, common, and Pinyin). The herbs in the first column of the table are alphabetized and then the tables are re-sorted four times, so that each naming convention appears in the first column once.

The Pinyin names of herbs are relatively standard. The botanical names are shortened to their genus form and do not necessarily indicate differences in species. For plant substances, the pharmaceutical nomenclature represents the genus, the part of the plant used, and usually the species, as well as adjectival information, such as location of discovery. As the most specific nomenclature, the pharmaceutical name may be considered the most useful, but it is not necessarily the most widely used. There are often two or three common names for an herb, representing geographical and folkloric diversity. The common names tend to be the least reliable, due to the variety of names any single herb may be called across the continent, or in other countries.

For non-plant substances in the botanical name column, there are some points to note. Animal substances are given their zoological name in the botanical column. Mineral substances are given their pharmaceutical name in the botanical column.

In the pharmaceutical name column, the reader will find that some herbs are marked with an asterisk (*). These pharmaceutical names are disputed or are from obscure sources. The authors have chosen to include and mark disputable pharmaceutical names rather than omit the herbs from the listings.

Herb Name Cross Reference Keyed to Pinyin Names

Pinyin	Botanical	Pharmaceutical	Common
Ai Ye	Artemisia	Folium Artemisiae Argyi	Mugwort Leaf
An Xi Xiang	Styrax	Benzoinum	Processed Resin of Styrax Benzoin
Ba Dou	Croton	Semen Croton Tiglii	Croton Seed
Ba Ji Tian	Morinda	Radix Morindae Officinalis	Morinda Root
Ba Jiao Hui Xiang	Illicium	Fructus Illicii*	Star Anise Fruit
Ba Qia	Smilax	Rhizoma Smilacis China*	Smilax Rhizome
Ba Xian Hua	Hydrangea	Flos Hydrangeae Macrophyllae*	Hydrangea Flower
Ba Yue Zha	Akebia	Fructus Akebiae	Akebia Fruit
Bai Bu	Stemona	Radix Stemonae	Stemona Root
Bai Dou Kou	Amomum	Fructus Amomi Kravanh	Round Cardamon Fruit; Cluster Fruit
Bai Fu Zi	Typhonium	Rhizoma Typhonii Gigantei	Typhonium Rhizome
Bai Guo	Ginkgo	Semen Ginkgo Bilobae	Ginkgo Nut
Bai He	Lilium	Bulbus Lilii	Lily Bulb
Bai Hua She	Agkistrodon	Agkistrodon seu Bungarus	Long-noded Pit Viper Snake
Bai Hua She She Cao	Oldenlandia	Herba Oldenlandiae Diffusae	Oldenlandia
Bai Ji	Bletilla	Rhizoma Bletillae Striatae	Bletilla Rhizome
Bai Ji Li	Tribulus	Fructus Tribuli Terrestris	Puncture Vine Fruit; Caltrop Fruit
Bai Jiang Cao	Patrinia or Thiaspi	Herba cum Radice Patriniae	Patrinia; Thiaspi
Bai Jie Zi	Brassica	Semen Sinapsis Albae	White Mustard Seed
Bai Lian	Ampelopsis	Radix Ampelopsis Japonicae*	Ampelopsis Root
Bai Mao Gen	Imperata	Rhizoma Imperatae Cylindricae	Woolly Grass Rhizome; White Grass Rhizome
Bai Mao Hua	Imperata	Flos Imperatae Cylindricae	Wooly Grass Flower; White Grass Flower
Bai Mao Xia Ku Cao	Ajuga	Herba Ajugae Decumbentis*	Ajuga
Bai Mu Er	Tremella	Fructificatio Tremellae Fuciformis	Tremella Fungus Fruiting Body
Bai Qian	Cynanchum	Rhizoma et Radix Cynanchi Baiqian	Cynanchum Rhizome and Root
Bai Shao	Paeonia	Radix Paeoniae Lactiflorae	White Peony Root
Bai Shen	Panax	Radix Ginseng	Rock Candy cured White Ginseng Root
Bai Tou Weng	Pulsatilla	Radix Pulsatillae Chinensis	Pulsatilla Root; Anemone Root

Pinyin

Pinyin	Botanical	Pharmaceutical	Common
Bai Wei	*Cynanchum*	*Radix Cynanchi Baiwei*	*Swallowort Root*
Bai Xian Pi	*Dictamnus*	*Cortex Dictamni Dasycarpi Radicis*	*Dittany Root Bark*
Bai Zhi	*Angelica*	*Radix Angelicae Dahuricae*	*Angelica Root*
Bai Zhu	*Atractylodes*	*Rhizoma Atractylodis Macrocephalae*	*White Atractylodes Rhizome*
Bai Zi Ren	*Biota*	*Semen Biotae Orientalis*	*Arbor-Vitae Seed*
Ban Bian Lian	*Lobelia*	*Herba Lobeliae Chinensis cum Radice*	*Chinese Lobelia*
Ban Lan Gen	*Isatis*	*Radix Isatidis seu Baphicacanthi*	*Isatis Root; Woad Root*
Ban Mao	*Mylabris*	*Mylabris*	*Cantharides; Chinese Blistering Beetle*
(Fa) Ban Xia	*Pinellia*	*Rhizoma Pinelliae Ternatae*	*Prepared Pinellia Rhizome*
(Sheng) Ban Xia	*Pinellia*	*Rhizoma Pinelliae Ternatae*	*Raw Pinellia Rhizome*
Ban Zhi Lian	*Scutellaria*	*Herba Scutellariae Barbatae*	*Barbat Scullcap*
Bao Gu	*Panthera*	*Os Leopardis*	*Leopard Bone*
Bao Ma Zi	*Syringa*	*Cortex Syringae**	*Manchurian Lilac Bark*
Bei Sha Shen	*Glehnia*	*Radix Glehniae Littoralis*	*Beech Silver-top Root; Northern Sand Root*
Bei Xie	*Dioscorea*	*Rhizoma Dioscoreae Hypoglaucae*	*Hypoglauca Yam Rhizome; Fish-poison Yam Rhizome*
Bi Ba	*Piper*	*Fructus Piperis Longi*	*Long Pepper Fruit*
Bi Cheng Qie	*Piper*	*Fructus Cubebae*	*Cubeba Fruit*
Bian Dou	*Dolichos*	*Semen Dolichoris Lablab*	*Hyacinth Bean*
Bian Dou Hua	*Dolichos*	*Flos Dolichoris Lablab*	*Hyacinth Bean Flower*
Bian Xu	*Polygonum*	*Herba Polygoni Avicularis*	*Avicularis; Knotweed*
Bie Jia	*Amyda*	*Carapax Amydae Sinensis*	*Chinese Soft-shell Turtle Shell*
Bing Lang	*Areca*	*Semen Arecae Catechu*	*Betel Nut*
Bing Pian	*Dryobalanops*	*Borneol*	*Processed Resin of Borneol Camphor*
Bo He	*Mentha*	*Herba Menthae Haplocalycis*	*Peppermint; Spearmint; Field Mint*
Bu Gu Zhi	*Psoralea*	*Fructus Psoraleae Corylifoliae*	*Scurfy Pea Fruit*
Can Sha	*Bombyx*	*Excrementum Bombycis Mori*	*Silkworm Feces*
Cang Er Zi	*Xanthium*	*Fructus Xanthii Sibirici*	*Xanthium Fruit; Cocklebur Fruit*
Cang Zhu	*Atractylodes*	*Rhizoma Atractylodis*	*Atractylodes Rhizome*
Cao Dou Kou	*Alpinia*	*Semen Alpiniae Katsumadai*	*Wild Cardamon Seed; Katsumada's Galangal Seed*
Cao Guo	*Amomum*	*Fructus Amomi Tsao-Ko*	*Chinese Cardamon Fruit*

Pinyin	Botanical	Pharmaceutical	Common
Cao Wu	Aconitum	Radix Aconiti Kusnezoffii	Wild Aconite
Ce Bai Ye	Biota	Cacumen Biotae Orientalis	Arborvitae Leafy Twig
Chai Hu	Bupleurum	Radix Bupleuri	Thorowax Root; Hare's Ear Root
Chan Su	Bufo	Secretio Bufonis	Dried Skin Secretion of Toad
Chan Tui	Cryptotympana	Periostracum Cicadae	Cicada Skin; Cicada Moulting
Chang Chun Teng	Hedera	Herba Hederae Nepalensis*	Ivy
Chang Shan	Dichroa	Radix Dichroae Febrifugae	Dichroa Root
Che Qian Cao	Plantago	Herba Plantaginis	Plantago; Plantain
Che Qian Zi	Plantago	Semen Plantaginis	Plantago Seed; Plantain Seed
Chen Pi	Citrus	Pericarpium Citri Reticulatae	Tangerine Peel
Chen Shi Huei	Calcaria	Calcaria*	Calcium Hydroxide
Chen Xiang	Aquilaria	Lignum Aquilariae	Aloeswood Secretion or Sap
Cheng Liu	Tamarix	Cacumen Tamaricis Chinensis*	Tamarisk
Chi Fu Ling	Poria	Sclerotium Poriae Cocos Rubrae	Red Hoelen; Red Tuckahoe
Chi Shao	Paeonia	Radix Paeoniae Rubra	Red Peony Root
Chi Shi Zhi	Halloysitum Rubrum	Halloysitum Rubrum	Halloysite; Red Kaolin
Chi Xiao Dou	Phaseolus	Semen Phaseoli Calcarati	Aduki Bean
Chong Wei Zi	Leonurus	Semen Leonuri Heterophylli	Motherwort Seed
Chou Wu Tong	Clerodendron	Folium Clerodendri Trichotomi	Glorybower Leaf
Chu Shi Zi	Broussonetia	Semen Broussonetiae Papyriferae*	Broussonetia Seed
Chuan Bei Mu	Fritillaria	Bulbus Fritillariae Cirrhosae	Tendrilled Fritillary Bulb
Chuan Jiao	Zanthoxylum	Pericarpum Zanthoxyli Bungeani	Sichuan Pepper Fruit
Chuan Jiao Mu	Zanthoxylum	Semen Zanthoxyli Bungeani	Sichuan Pepper Seed
Chuan Lian Zi	Melia	Fructus Meliae Toosendan	Sichuan Chinaberry Fruit; Sichuan Pagoda Tree Fruit; Neem Fruit
Chuan Niu Xi	Cyathula	Radix Cyathulae Officinalis	Cyathula Root
Chuan Shan Jia	Manis	Squama Manitis Pentadactylae	Anteater-Scales; Pangolin Scales
Chuan Shan Long	Dioscorea	Rhizoma Dioscoreae Nipponicae*	Japanese Dioscorea Rhizome
Chuan Wu	Aconitum	Radix Aconite Carmichaeli	Sichuan Aconite
Chuan Xin Lian	Andrographis	Herba Andrographitis Paniculatae	Kariyat; Green Chiretta
Chuan Xiong	Ligusticum	Radix Ligustici Wallichii	Sichuan Lovage Root
Chui Pen Cao	Sedum	Herba Sedii Sarmentosi*	Stonecrop

Pinyin

Pinyin	Botanical	Pharmaceutical	Common
Chun Pi	Ailanthus	Cortex Ailanthi Altissimae	Tree of Heaven Bark
Ci Shi	Magnetitum	Magnetitum	Magnetite; Magnetic Iron Ore; Loadstone
Cong Bai	Allium	Bulbus Allii Fistulosi	White Bulb of Green Onion or Scallion
Da Feng Zi	Hydnocarpus	Semen Hydnocarpi Anthelminticae	Chaulmoogra Seed
Da Fu Pi	Areca	Pericarpium Arecae Catechu	Betelnut Husk
Da Huang	Rheum	Radix et Rhizoma Rhei	Rhubarb Root and Rhizome
Da Ji	Cirsium	Herba seu Radix Cirsii Japonici	Japanese Thistle
Da Qing Ye	Isatis	Folium Daqingye	Isatis Leaf; Woad Leaf
Da Suan	Allium	Bulbus Allii Sativi	Garlic Bulb
Da Zao	Ziziphus	Fructus Ziziphi Jujubae	Jujube Fruit; Chinese Black Date
Dai Mao	Eretmochelys	Carapax Eretmochelydis Imbricatae*	Hawksbill Turtle Shell
Dai Zhe Shi	Haematitum	Haematitum	Hematite; Iron Ore
Dan Dou Chi	Glycine	Semen Sojae Praeparatum	Prepared (Fermented) Soybean
Dan Fan	Chalcanthitum	Chalcanthitum*	Copper Sulphate; Blue Vitriol
Dan Nan Xing	Arisaema	Pulvis Arisaemae cum Felle Bovis	Powdered Jack-in-the-Pulpit Rhizome mixed with Cow Bile
Dan Shen	Salvia	Radix Salviae Miltiorrhizae	Red Sage Root
Dan Zhu Ye	Lophatherum	Herba Lophatheri Gracilis	Bland Bamboo Leaf and Stem
Dang Gui	Angelica	Radix Angelicae Sinensis	Tangkuei Root
Dang Gui Tou	Angelica	Caput Radicis Angelicae Sinensis	Tangkuei Head
Dang Gui Wei	Angelica	Extremas Radicis Angelicae Sinensis	Tangkuei Tail
Dang Shen	Codonopsis	Radix Codonopsitis Pilosulae	Asiabell Root
Deng Xin Cao	Juncus	Medulla Junci Effusi	Rush Pith
Di Fu Zi	Kochia	Fructus Kochiae Scopariae	Broom Cyperus Seed
Di Gu Pi	Lycium	Cortex Lycii Radicis	Matrimony-vine Rootbark, Wolfberry Bark
Di Long	Pheretima	Lumbricus	Earthworm
Di Yu	Sanguisorba	Radix Sanguisorbae Officinalis	Burnet-bloodwort Root
Dian Di Mei	Androsace	Herba Androsacae Umbellatae*	Androsace
Ding Xiang	Eugenia	Flos Caryophylli	Clove Flower-bud
Dong Bei Guan Zhong	Dryopteris	Rhizoma Dryopteridis	Dryopteris Rhizome

Pinyin	Botanical	Pharmaceutical	Common
Dong Chong Xia Cao	Cordyceps	Cordyceps Sinensis	Chinese Caterpillar Fungus
Dong Gua Pi	Benincasa	Epicarpium Benincasae Hispidae	Wintermelon Fruit Peel; Wax Gourd Fruit Peel
Dong Gua Ren	Benincasa	Semen Benincasae Hispidae	Wintermelon Seed; Wax Gourd Seed
Dong Kui Zi	Malva or Abutilon	Semen Albutili seu Malvae	Musk Mallow Seed; Malva Seed
Dou Chi Jiang	Litsea	Radix et Ramus Litseae Cubebae	Aromatic Litsea Root and Stem
Dou Juan	Glycine	Semen Glycines Germinatum	Young Soybean Sprout
Du Huo	Angelica	Radix Angelicae Pubescentis	Pubescent Angelica Root
Du Zhong	Eucommia	Cortex Eucommiae Ulmoidis	Eucommia Bark
Duan Long Gu	Os Draconis	Os Draconis	Calcined Dragon Bone; Calcined Fossilized Bone
Duan Mu Li	Ostrea	Concha Ostreae	Calcined Oyster Shell
E Bu Shi Cao	Centipeda	Herba Centipedae Minimae*	Centipeda Herb
E Guan Shi	Stalactitum	Stalactitum	Stalactite Tubular Tip
E Jiao	Equus	Gelatinum Corii Asini	Donkey Hide Gelatin; Ass Skin Glue
E Wei	Ferula	Resinae Asafoetidae*	Asafoetida Gum-resin; Devil's Dung
E Zhu	Curcuma	Rhizoma Curcumae	Zedoary Tumeric Rhizome
Er Cha	Acacia or Uncaria	Pasta Acacia seu Uncaria	Dried Paste of Concentrated Decoction of Black or White Cutch
Fan Bai Cao	Potentilla	Herba Potentillae Discoloris*	Potentilla
Fan Xie Ye	Cassia	Folium Sennae	Senna Leaf
Fang Feng	Ledebouriella	Radix Ledebouriella Divaricatae	Siler Root; Ledebouriella Root
Fei Zi	Torreya	Semen Torreyae Grandis	Torrreya Seed
Feng Mi	Mel	Mel*	Honey
Feng Wei Cao	Pteris	Herba Pterii*	Pteris
Fo Shou	Citrus	Fructus Citri Sarcodactylis	Finger Citron Fruit
Fo Shou Hua	Citrus	Flos Citri Sarcodactylis	Finger Citron Flower
Fu Hai Shi	Pumice	Pumice	Pumice
Fu Ling	Poria	Sclerotium Poriae Cocos	Hoelen; China Root; Tuckahoe; Indian Bread
Fu Ling Pi	Poria	Cortex Poriae Cocos	Tuckahoe Skin
Fu Long Gan	Terra Flava Usta	Terra Flava Usta	Ignited Wood Stove Earth
Fu Pen Zi	Rubus	Fructus Rubi Chingii	Raspberry Fruit Bud
Fu Ping	Spirodela or Lemna	Herba Lemnae seu Spirodelae	Duckweed

Pinyin

Pinyin	Botanical	Pharmaceutical	Common
Fu Shen	Poria Cocos	Sclerotium Poriae Cocos Pararadicis	Tuckahoe Spirit
Fu Xiao Mai	Triticum	Semen Tritici Aestivi Levis	Wheat Chaff/Grain
(Hei)Fu Zi	Aconitum	Radix Lateralis Aconiti Carmichaeli Praeparata	Prepared Sichuan Aconite Root
Gan Cao	Glycyrhiza	Radix Glycyrrhizae Uralensis	Licorice Root
Gan Jiang	Zingiber	Rhizoma Zingiberis Officinalis	Dried Ginger Rhizome
Gan Jie Geng	Adenophora	Radix Adenophorae Trachelioidis	Sweet Jie Geng
Gan Qi	Rhus	Lacca Sinica Exsiccatae	Laquer
Gan Sui	Euphorbia	Radix Euphorbiae Kansui	Kansui Spurge Root
Gao Ben	Ligusticum	Rhizoma et Radix Ligustici	Straw Weed Rhizome and Root; Chinese Lovage Rhizome and Root
Gao Liang Jiang	Alpinia	Rhizoma Alpiniae Officinari	Lesser Galangal Rhizome
Ge Gen	Pueraria	Radix Puerariae	Kudzu Root
Ge Hua	Pueraria	Flos Puerariae	Kudzu Flower
Ge Jie	Gekko	Gekko	Gecko Lizard
Ge Shan Xiang	Cynanchum	Radix Cynanchi Auriculati	Cynanchum Root
Gou Gu	Canis	Os Canine	Dog Bone
Gou Ji	Cibotium	Rhizoma Cibotii Barometz	Chain Fern Rhizome
Gou Qi Zi	Lycium	Fructus Lycii	Matrimony Vine Fruit; Wolfberry Fruit
Gou Teng	Uncaria	Ramulus cum Uncis Uncariae	Gambir vine Stems and Hooks
Gu Jing Cao	Eriocaulon	Scapus et Inflorescentia Eriocaulonis Buergeriani	Pipewort Scapus
Gu Sui Bu	Drynaria	Rhizoma Drynariae	Drynaria Rhizome
Gu Ya	Oryza	Fructus Oryzae Sativae Germinatus	Rice Sprout
Gua Di	Cucumis	Pedicellus Cucumeris	Melon Pedicle
Gua Lou	Trichosanthes	Fructus Trichosanthis	Snakegourd Fruit
Gua Lou Pi	Trichosanthes	Pericarpium Trichosanthis	Snakegourd Peel
Gua Lou Ren	Trichosanthes	Semen Trichosanthis	Snakegourd Seed
Guan Gui	Cinnamomum	Cortex Tubiformis Cinnamomi Cassiae	Thin Cinnamon Bark from Young Trees
Guan Ye Liao	Polygonum	Herba Polygoni Perfoliati*	Polygonum
Guan Zhong	Dryopteris	Rhizoma Guanzhong	Shield-fern Rhizome
Guang Fang Ji	Aristolochia or Cocculus	Radix Aristolochiae Fangchi	Aristolochia Root
Guang Gou Shen	Canis	Testis et Penis Canis*	Male Dog Sexual Organs
Gui Ban	Chinemys	Plastrum Testudinis	Fresh Water Turtle Shell
Gui Zhi	Cinnamomum	Ramulus Cinnamomi Cassiae	Cinnamon Twig

Pinyin	Botanical	Pharmaceutical	Common
Hai Dai	Laminaria	Herba Laminaria Japonicae	Algae
Hai Feng Teng	Piper	Caulis Piperis Futokadsurae	Kadsura Stem
Hai Ge Ke	Cyclina	Concha Cyclinae Sinensis	Clam Shell
Hai Gou Shen	Phoca	Testes et Penis Otariae*	Male Seal Sexual Organs
Hai Jin Sha	Lygodium	Spora Lygodii Japonici	Japanese Climbing Fern Spore
Hai Long	Solenognathus	Hailong	Pipe-fish
Hai Ma	Hippocampus	Hippocampus	Sea Horse
Hai Piao Xiao	Sepia or Sepiella	Os Sepiae seu Sepiellae	Cuttle-fish Bone
Hai Shen	Strichopus	Strichopus Japonicus	Sea Cucumber, Sea Slug
Hai Tong Pi	Erythrina	Cortex Erythrinae	Coral-bean Bark
Hai Zao	Sargassum	Herba Sargassii	Sargassum Seaweed
Han Cai	Rorippa	Herba Rorippae*	Rorippa
Han Fang Ji	Stephania	Radix Stephaniae Tetrandrae	Stephania Root
Han Lian Cao	Eclipta	Herba Ecliptae Prostratae	Eclipta
Han Shui Shi	Calcitum	Calcitum	Calcite
He Huan Hua	Albizzia	Flos Albizziae Julibrissin*	Mimosa Tree Flower; Silktree Flower
He Huan Pi	Albizzia	Cortex Albizziae Julibrissin	Mimosa Tree Bark; Silktree Bark
He Shi	Carpesium or Daucus	Fructus Carpesii seu Daucusi	Carpesium Fruit
He Shou Wu	Polygonum	Radix Polygoni Multiflori	Fleeceflower Root; Fo-Ti Root
He Ye	Nelumbo	Folium Nelumbinis Nuciferae	Lotus Leaf
He Zi	Terminalia	Fructus Terminaliae Chebulae	Myrobalan Fruit
Hei Lu Shen	Equus	Testis et Penis Equii*	Male Horse Sexual Organs
Hei Zhi Ma	Sesamum	Semen Sesami Indici	Black Sesame Seed
Hong Hua	Carthamus	Flos Carthami Tinctorii	Safflower
Hong Teng	Sargentodoxa	Caulis Sargentodoxae Cuneatae	Sargentodoxa Stem
Hong Zao	Ziziphus	Fructus Ziziphi Jujubae	Jujube Fruit; Chinese Red Date
Hou Po	Magnolia	Cortex Magnoliae Officinalis	Magnolia Bark
Hou Po Hua	Magnolia	Flos Magnoliae Officinalis	Magnolia Flower
Hou Zao	Macaca	Calculus Macacae Mulattae	Macaque Gallstone
Hu Er Cao	Saxifrage	Herba Saxifragae Stoloniferae*	Saxifrage
Hu Gu	Panthera	Os Tigris	Tiger Bone
Hu Huang Lian	Picrorhiza	Rhizoma Picrorhizae	Picrorhiza Rhizome
Hu Jiao	Piper	Fructus Piperis Nigri	Black Pepper Fruit

Pinyin	Botanical	Pharmaceutical	Common
Hu Lu Ba	Trigonella	Semen Trigonellae Foeni-graeci	Fenugreek Seed
Hu Po	Succinum	Succinum	Amber; Fossilized Resin of Pine Tree
Hu Tao Ren	Juglans	Semen Juglandis Regiae	Walnut
Hu Tui Ye	Eleagnus	Folium Eleagni Pungens	Eleagnus Leaf
Hu Zhang	Polygonum	Radix et Rhizoma Polygoni Cuspidati	Giant Knotweed Rhizome
Hua Lu Shen	Cervus	Testis et Penis Cervi*	Male Deer Sexual Organs
Hua Rui Shi	Ophicalcitum	Ophicalcitum	Ophicalcite
Hua Sheng Yi	Arachis	Pericarpium Arachi*	Peanut Skin
Hua Shi	Talcum	Talcum	Talc; Soapstone
Huai Hua Mi	Sophora	Flos Sophorae Japonicae Immaturus	Pagoda Tree Flower Bud
Huai Jiao	Sophora	Fructus Sophorae Japonicae	Pagoda Tree Fruit
Huai Niu Xi	Achyranthes	Radix Achyranthis Bidentatae	Achyranthes Root
Huang Bai	Phellodendron	Cortex Phellodendri	Amur Cork-tree Bark
Huang Jin	Aurum	Aurum*	Gold
Huang Jing	Polygonatum	Rhizoma Polygonati	Siberian Solomon Seal Rhizome
Huang Lian	Coptis	Rhizoma Coptidis	Coptis; Golden Thread Rhizome
Huang Qi	Astragalus	Radix Astragali Membranaceus	Yellow Milk-vetch Root
Huang Qin	Scutellaria	Radix Scutellariae Baicalensis	Scute; Baical Skullcap Root
Huang Yao Zi	Dioscorea	Tuber Dioscoreae Bulbiferae	Dioscorea Tuber
Huo Ma Ren	Cannabis	Semen Cannabis Sativae	Hemp Seed; Marihuana Seed
Huo Xiang	Agastache or Pogostemon	Herba Agastaches seu Pogostemi	Patchouli, Agastache
Ji Cai	Capsella	Herba Capsellae*	Shepherd's Purse
Ji Guan Hua	Celosia	Flos Celosiae Cristatae	Cockscomb Flower
Ji Lin Shen	Panax	Radix Ginseng	Jilin Wild Ginseng
Ji Mu	Loropetalum	Cortex Loropetali*	Loropetalum Bark
Ji Nei Jin	Gallus	Endothelium Corneum Gigeriae Galli	Chicken Gizard Lining
Ji Ning	Salvia	Herba Salviae Plebeia*	Salvia
Ji Shi Teng	Paederia	Caulis Paederiae*	Paederia Stem
Ji Xue Teng	Millettia	Radix et Caulis Jixueteng	Millettia Root and Vine; Chicken Blood Vine
Jiang Can	Bombyx	Bombyx Batryticatus	Dead Stiff Body of Sick Silkworm Larvae

Pinyin	Botanical	Pharmaceutical	Common
Jiang Huang	Curcuma	Rhizoma Curcumae Longae	Tumeric Rhizome
Jiang Xiang	Dalbergia	Lignum Dalbergiae Odoriferae	Dalbergia Heartwood
(Chuan) Jiao Mu	Zanthoxylum	Semen Zanthoxyli Bungeani	Sichuan Pepper Seed
(Ku) Jie Geng	Platycodon	Radix Platycodi Grandiflori	Ballonflower Root; Bellflower Root; Bitter Jie Geng
Jin Fei Cao	Inula	Herba Inulae	Elecampane
Jin Guo Lan	Tinospora	Radix Tinosporae Capillipes*	Tinospora Root
Jin Qian Cao	Lysimachia	Herba Lysimachiae	Lysimachia
Jin Qiao Mai	Fagopyrum	Rhizoma Fagopyri Cynosi*	Wild Buckwheat Rhizome
Jin Sha Teng	Lygodium	Herba Lygodii Japonici	Japanese Climbing Fern
Jin Yin Hua	Lonicera	Flos Lonicerae Japonicae	Honeysuckle Flower
Jin Yin Teng	Lonicera	Ramus Lonicerae Japonicae	Honeysuckle Stem
Jin Ying Zi	Rosa	Fructus Rosae Laevigatae	Cherokee Rose Fruit / Rosehip
Jing Da Ji	Euphorbia or Knoxia	Radix Euphorbiae seu Knoxiae	Peking Spurge Root
Jing Jie	Schizonepeta	Herba Schizonepetae Tenuifoliae	Schizonepeta Stem or Bud
Jing Mi	Oryza	Semen Oryzae Sativae*	Rice Grain
Jing Tian San Qi	Sedum	Herba Sedi*	Sedum
Jiu Jie Chang Pu	Anemone	Rhizoma Anemoni Attaicae*	Altaica Rhizome
Jiu Xiang Chong	Aspongopus	Aspongopus*	Stink Bug
Jiu Zi	Allium	Semen Allii Tuberosi	Chinese Leek Seed
Ju He	Citrus	Semen Citri Reticulatae*	Tangerine Seed
Ju Hong	Citrus	Pars Rubra Epicarpii Citri Erythrocarpae	Red Tangerine Peel
(Bai) Ju Hua	Chrysanthemum	Flos Chrysanthemi Morifolii	White Chrysanthemum Flower
(Huang) Ju Hua	Chrysanthemum	Flos Chrysanthemi Morifolii	Yellow Chrysanthemum Flower
Ju Ye San Qi	Gynura	Folium Gynurae*	Gynura Leaf
Jue Ming Zi	Cassia	Semen Cassiae	Cassia Seed
Ku Fan	Alumen Praeparatum	Alumen Praeparatum	Prepared Alum
Ku Lian Gen Pi	Melia	Cortex Meliae Radicis	Sichuan Chinaberry Root Bark; Sichuan Pagoda Tree Root Bark; Neem Root Bark
Ku Lian Mu Pi	Melia	Cortex Meliae	Sichuan Chinaberry Tree Bark; Sichuan Pagoda Tree Bark; Neem Tree Bark
Ku Shen	Sophora	Radix Sophorae Flavenscentis	Bitter Ginseng Root
Kuan Dong Hua	Tussilago	Flos Tussilaginis Farfarae	Coltsfoot Flower

Pinyin

Pinyin	Botanical	Pharmaceutical	Common
Kuan Jin Teng	Tinospora	Ramus Tinosporae Sinensis	Tinospora Stem
Kun Bu	Laminaria or Ecklonia	Thallus Algae	Kelp Thallus; Kombu Thallus
Lai Fu Zi	Raphanus	Semen Raphani Satavi	Radish Seed
Lao Guan Cao	Erodium or Geranium	Herba Erodii seu Geranii*	Geranium; Heronbill; Cranebill
Lei Wan	Omphalia	Sclerotium Omphaliae Lapidescens	Omphalia Fungus Fruiting Body
Li Lu	Veratrum	Radix et Rhizoma Veratri	Veratrum Root
Li Pi	Pyrus	Pericarpium Pyri*	Pear Peel
Li Zhi He	Litchi	Semen Litchi Chinensis	Leechee Nut
Lian Fang	Nelumbo	Receptaculum Nelumbinis Nuciferae	Mature Lotus Receptacle
Lian Geng	Nelumbo	Ramulus Nelumbinis Nuciferae	Lotus Stem
Lian Qiao	Forsythia	Fructus Forsythiae Suspensae	Forsythia Fruit; Golden Bells
Lian Xin	Nelumbo	Plumula Nelumbinis Nuciferae	Lotus Plumule
Lian Xu	Nelumbo	Stamen Nelumbinis Nuciferae	Lotus Stamen
Lian Zi	Nelumbo	Semen Nelumbinis Nuciferae	Lotus Seed
Ling Yang Jiao	Saiga	Cornu Antelopis	Antelope Horn
Ling Zhi	Ganoderma	Fructificatio Ganodermae Lucidi*	Lucid Ganoderma; Reishi
Liu Huang	Sulphur	Sulphur	Sulphur
Liu Ji Nu	Artemisia	Herba Artemisiae Anomalae	Artemisia
Long Chi	Dens Draconis	Dens Draconis	Dragon Tooth; Fossilized Tooth
Long Dan Cao	Gentiana	Radix Gentianae Longdancao	Chinese Gentian Root
Long Gu	Os Draconis	Os Draconis	Dragon Bone; Fossilized Bone
Long Yan Rou	Euphoria	Arillus Euphoriae Longanae	Longan Fruit Flesh
Lou Lu	Rhaponticum or Echinops	Radix Rhapontici seu Echinops	Rhaponticum Root, Echinops Root
Lu Dou	Phaseolus	Semen Phaseoli Radiati	Mung Bean
Lu Feng Fang	Polistes	Nidus Vespae	Hornet Nest; Wasp Nest
Lu Gan Shi	Smithsonitum	Smithsonitum	Smithsonite; Calamine
Lu Gen	Phragmites	Rhizoma Phragmitis Communis	Reed Rhizome; Corrizo Rhizome
Lu Hui	Aloe	Herba Aloes	Aloe Vera Leaf
Lu Jiao	Cervus	Cornu Cervi	Antler; Deerhorn; Ossified Horn of the Mature Male Deer

Pinyin	Botanical	Pharmaceutical	Common
Lu Jiao Jiao	Cervus	Colla Cornu Cervi	Mature Antler Glue; Mature Antler Gelatin
Lu Jiao Shuang	Cervus	Cornu Cervi Degelatinatium	Antler Powder from the dregs of cooking Antler Glue
Lu Lu Tong	Liquidambar	Fructus Liquidambaris Taiwanianae	Sweetgum Fruit
Lu Rong	Cervus	Cornu Cervi Parvum	Young Deer Antler Velvet
Lu Xian Cao	Pyrola	Herba Pyrolae*	Pyrola
Lu Ying	Sambucus	Cortex Sambuci*	Japanese Elder Bark
Luo Bu Ma	Apocynum	Herba seu Folium Apocyni Veneti*	Red Dogbane Whole Herb or Leaf
Luo Han Guo	Momordica	Fructus Momordicae Grosvenori	Momordica Fruit
Luo Huo Guo Ye	Momordica	Folium Momordicae Grosvenori	Momordica Leaf
Luo Shi Teng	Trachelospermum	Caulis Trachelospermi Jasminoidis	Star Jasmine Stem
Ma Bian Cao	Verbena	Herba Verbenae*	Vervain
Ma Bo	Lasiosphaera	Fructificatio Lasiosphaerae seu Calvatiae	Puffball Fruiting Body
Ma Chi Xian	Portulaca	Herba Portulacae Oleraceae	Purslane
Ma Dou Ling	Aristolochia	Fructus Aristolochiae	Birthwort Fruit
Ma Huang	Ephedra	Herba Ephedrae	Ephedra Stem
Ma Huang Gen	Ephedra	Radix Ephedrae	Ephedra Root
Ma Qian Zi	Strychnos	Semen Strychni	Nux-vomica Seed
Mai Men Dong	Ophiopogon	Tuber Ophiopogonis Japonici	Creeping Lily-turf Tuber
Mai Ya	Hordeum	Fructus Hordei Vulgaris Germinatus	Barley Sprout, Malted Barley
Man Jing Zi	Vitex	Fructus Viticis	Vitex Fruit
Man Shan Hong	Rhododendron	Folium Rhododendri*	Rhododendron Leaf
Mang Xiao	Mirabilitum	Mirabilitum	Mirabilite; Glauber's Salt
Mao Dong Qing	Ilex	Radix Ilicis Pubescentis*	Pubescent Holly Root
Mao Mei	Rubus	Herba Rubi Parvifolii*	Thimbleberry
Mao Zhao Cao	Ranunculus	Radix Ranunculi Ternati*	Buttercup Root
Mei Gui Hua	Rosa	Flos Rosae Rugosae	Young Chinese Rose Flower
Meng Chong	Tabanus	Tabani Bivittati*	Gadfly
Meng Shi	Lapis Micae seu Chloriti	Lapis Micae seu Chloriti	Chlorite Schist; Lapis
Mi Meng Hua	Buddleia	Flos Buddleiae Officinalis Immaturus	Buddleia Flower
Mi Tuo Seng	Lithargyrum	Lithargyrum	Litharge; Galena
Mian Hua Gen	Gossypium	Radix Gossypii Hirsuti*	Cotton Root
Ming Dang Shen	Changium	Radix Changii*	Changium Root

Pinyin	Botanical	Pharmaceutical	Common
Ming Fan	Alumen	Alumen	Alum; Potassium Aluminum Sulfate
Mo Yao	Commiphora	Resinae Myrrhae	Myrrh Gum-resin
Mu Bie Zi	Momordica	Semen Momordicae Cochinchinensis	Momordica Seed
Mu Dan Pi	Paeonia	Cortex Moutan Radicis	Tree Peony Rootbark
Mu Gua	Chaenomeles	Frutus Chaenomelis	Chinese Quince Fruit
Mu Hu Die	Oroxylum	Semen Oroxyli Indici	Oroxylum Seed
Mu Li	Ostrea	Concha Ostreae	Oyster Shell
Mu Tong	Akebia	Caulis Mutong	Akebia Stem
Mu Xiang	Saussurea	Radix Saussureae Lappae	Costus Root, Aucklandia
Mu Zei	Equisetum	Herba Equiseti Hiemalis	Horsetail, Scouring Rush; Shavegrass
Nan Gua Zi	Cucurbita	Semen Cucurbitae Moschatae	Pumpkin Seed and Husk
Nan Sha Shen	Adenophora	Radix Adenophorae	Ladybell Root, Southern Sand Root
Nan Wu Wei Zi	Schisandra	Fructus Schisandrae Sphenantherae	Southern Schisandra Fruit
Niu Bang Zi	Arctium	Fructus Arctii Lappae	Burdock Seed
Niu Dan	Bos	Vesica Fellea Bovus	Cow Gallbladder
Niu Huang	Bos or Bubalis	Calculus Bovis seu Calculus Bubali	Ox or Water Buffalo Gallstone
Nu Zhen Zi	Ligustrum	Fructus Ligustri Lucidi	Privet Fruit; Waxtree Fruit
Nuo Dao Gen Xu	Oryza	Radix et Rhizoma Oryzae Glutinosae	Sweet Rice Root and Rhizome
Ou Jie	Nelumbo	Nodus Nelumbinis Nuciferae Rhizomatis	Lotus Rhizome Node
Pang Da Hai	Sterculia	Semen Sterculiae Scaphigerae	Sterculia Seed
Pao Jiang	Zingiber	Rhizoma Zingiberis*	Quick-fried Ginger Rhizome
Pei Lan	Eupatorium	Herba Eupatorii Fortunei	Boneset; Thoroughwort; Feverwort
Peng Sha	Borax	Borax	Borax; Sodium Tetraborate
Pi Pa Ye	Eriobotrya	Folium Eriobotryae Japonicae	Loquat Leaf
Pi Shi	Arsenolite	Arsenicum	White Arsenic
Pu Gong Ying	Taraxacum	Herba Taraxaci Mongolici cum Radice	Dandelion
(Sheng) Pu Huang	Typha	Pollen Typhae	Raw Cattail Pollen
Pu Huang Tan	Typha	Pollen Typhae Carbonisatus	Charred Cattail Pollen
Pu Hui	Typha	Folium Typhae	Cattail Leaves
Qian Cao Gen	Rubia	Radix Rubiae Cordifoliae	Madder Root
Qian Dan	Minium	Minium	Red Lead Oxide

Pinyin	Botanical	Pharmaceutical	Common
Qian Hu	Peucedanum	Radix Peucedani	Hogfennel Root
Qian Li Guang	Senecio	Herba Senecionis Scandentis*	Groundsel
Qian Nian Jian	Homalomena	Rhizoma Homalomenae Occultae	Homalomena Rhizome
Qian Niu Zi	Pharbitis	Semen Pharbitidis	Morning Glory Seed
Qian Shi	Euryale	Semen Euryales Ferocis	Euryale Seed
Qiang Huo	Notopterygium	Rhizoma et Radix Notopterygii	Notopterygium Rhizome and Root
Qin Jiao	Gentiana	Radix Gentianae Qinjiao	Large-Leaf Gentian Root
Qin Pi	Fraxinus	Cortex Fraxini	Korean Ash Bark
Qing Dai	Indigo	Indigo Pulverata Levis	Indigo
Qing Fen	Calomelas	Calomelas	Calomel; Mercurous Chloride
Qing Hao	Artemisia	Herba Artemisiae Annuae	Sweet Wormwood; Southernwood
Qing Mu Xiang	Aristolochia	Radix Aristolochiae	Birthwort Root
Qing Pi	Citrus	Pericarpium Citri Reticulatae Viride	Immature (Green) Tangerine Peel
Qing Xiang Zi	Celosia	Semen Celosiae Argenteae	Celosia Seed
Qu Mai	Dianthus	Herba Dianthi	Pink Flower Herb
Quan Xie	Buthus	Buthus Martensi	Scorpion
Ren Gong Niu Huang	Bos	Calculus Artificialis	Artificially Induced Cow Gallstons
(Hong) Ren Shen	Panax	Radix Ginseng	Ginseng Root steamed until red
Ren Shen Lu	Panax	Cervix Ginseng	Ginseng Root Neck
Ren Shen Ye	Panax	Folium Ginseng	Ginseng Leaf
Rou Cong Rong	Cistanche	Herba Cistanches Deserticolae	Broomrape Fleshy Stem
Rou Dou Kou	Myristica	Semen Myristicae Fragrantis	Nutmeg Seed
Rou Gui	Cinnamomum	Cortex Cinnamomi Cassiae	Cinnamon Bark
Ru Xiang	Boswellia	Gummi Olibanum	Frankincense Gum-resin
San Bai Cao	Saururus	Herba Saururi Chinensis*	Saururus
San Leng	Sparganium	Rhizoma Sparganii Stoloniferi	Bur-reed Rhizome
San Qi	Panax	Radix Pseudoginseng	Pseudoginseng Root; Notoginseng Root
San Qi Hua	Panax	Flos Pseudoginseng	Pseudoginseng Flower; Notoginseng Flower
Sang Bai Pi	Morus	Cortex Mori Albae Radicis	Mulberry Rootbark
Sang Ji Sheng	Loranthus or Viscum	Ramulus Sangjishang	Mulberry Mistletoe Stem
Sang Piao Xiao	Paratenodera	Ootheca Mantidis	Praying Mantis Egg Case
Sang Shen	Morus	Fructus Mori Albae	Mulberry Fruit Bud

Pinyin	Botanical	Pharmaceutical	Common
Sang Ye	Morus	Folium Mori Albae	Mulberry Leaf
Sang Zhi	Morus	Ramulus Mori Albae	Mulberry Twig
Sha Ren	Amomum	Fructus seu Semen Amomi	Grains-of-Paradise Fruit or Seeds
Sha Ren Hua	Amomum	Flos Amomi	Grains-of-Paradise Flower
Sha Ren Ke	Amomum	Pericarpium Amomi	Grains-of-Paradise Shell
Sha Yuan Ji Li	Astragalus	Semen Astragali Complanati	Flattened Milk-vetch Seed
Shan Ci Gu	Tulipa	Pseudobulbus Shancigu	Chinese Tulip Bulb
Shan Dou Gen	Sophora	Radix Sophorae Tonkinensis	Pigeon Pea Root
Shan Yang Jiao	Naemorhedis	Cornu Naemorhedis	Goat Horn
Shan Yao	Dioscorea	Radix Dioscoreae Oppositae	Chinese Wild Yam Root
Shan Zha	Crataegus	Fructus Crataegi	Hawthorn Unripe Fruit or Berry
Shan Zha Rou	Crataegus	Fructus Crataegi	Hawthorn Ripe Fruit or Berry
Shan Zha Tan	Crataegus	Fructus Crataegi Carbonisatus	Charred Hawthorn Fruit or Berry
Shan Zhu Yu	Cornus	Fructus Corni Officinalis	Dogwood Fruit; Asiatic Cornelian Cherry Fruit
Shang Lu	Phytolacca	Radix Phytolaccae	Poke Root
She Chuang Zi	Cnidium	Fructus Cnidii Monnieri	Cnidium Seed
She Gan	Belamcanda	Rhizoma Belamcandae Chinensis	Belamcanda Rhizome; Blackberry Lily Rhizome
She Tui	Zaocys	Exuviae Serpentis	Snake Skin Slough
She Xiang	Moschus	Secretio Moschus	Musk; Musk Deer Navel Gland Secretion
Shen Jin Cao	Lycopodium	Herba Lycopodii Clavati*	Clubmoss
Shen Qu	Massa Fermentata	Massa Fermentata	Medicated Leaven
Shen Xu	Panax	Radix Ginseng	Rock Candy cured White Ginseng Root Tail
Sheng Di Huang	Rehmannia	Radix Rehmanniae Glutinosae	Fresh Chinese Foxglove Root
Sheng Jiang	Zingiber	Rhizoma Zingiberis Officinalis Recens	Fresh Ginger Rhizome
Sheng Jiang Pi	Zingiber	Cortex Zingiberis Officinalis Recens	Fresh Ginger Skin
Sheng Ma	Cimicifuga	Rhizoma Cimicifugae	Black Cohosh Rhizome; Bugbane Rhizome
Sheng Shai Shen	Panax	Radix Ginseng	Fresh Dried Ginseng Root
Sheng Tie Luo	Frusta Ferri	Frusta Ferri	Iron Filing
Shi Bing	Diospyros	Fructus Diospyri Kaki*	Dried Persimmon Fruit
Shi Chang Pu	Acorus	Rhizoma Acori Graminei	Sweetflag Rhizome
Shi Da Gong Lao	Mahonia	Folium Mahoniae*	Mahonia Leaf
Shi Di	Diospyros	Calyx Diospyri Kaki	Persimmon Calyx

Pinyin	Botanical	Pharmaceutical	Common
Shi Gao	Gypsum	Gypsum Fibrosum	Gypsum; Calcium Sulphate
Shi Hu	Dendrobium	Herba Dendrobii	Dendrobium Stem
Shi Jue Ming	Haliotis	Concha Haliotidis	Abalone Shell
Shi Jun Zi	Quisqualis	Fructus Quisqualis Indicae	Rangoon Creeper Fruit
Shi Liu Gen Pi	Punica	Cortex Punicae Granati Radicis	Pomegranate Root Bark
Shi Liu Pi	Punica	Pericarpium Punicae Granati	Pomegranate Husk or Rind
Shi Shang Bai	Selaginella	Herba Selaginellae Doederleinii	Selaginella
Shi Wei	Pyrrosia	Folium Pyrrosiae	Pyrrosia Leaf
Shu Di Huang	Rehmannia	Radix Rehmanniae Glutinosae Conquitae	Wine-cooked Chinese Foxglove Root
Shu Qi	Dichroa	Folium Dichroae Febrifugae	Dichroa Leaf
Shu Yi Ren	Coix	Semen Coicis Lachryma-jobi	Dry-Fried Coix Seed
Shui Niu Jiao	Bubalus	Cornu Bubali	Waterbuffalo Horn
Shui Yin	Hydrargyrum	Hydrargyrum	Mercury
Shui Zhi	Hirudo	Hirudo seu Whitmania	Leech
Si Gua Lou	Luffa	Fasciculus Vascularis Luffae	Dried Skeleton of Luffa Sponge
Si Gua Pi	Luffa	Pericarpium Luffae Acutangulae	Luffa Skin
Si Ji Qing	Ilex	Folium Ilicis Chinensis*	Holly Leaf
Song Jie	Pinus	Lignum Pini Nodi	Knotty Pine Wood
Su He Xiang	Liquidambar	Styrax Liquidis	Rose Maloes Resin
Su Mu	Caesalpinia	Lignum Sappan	Sappan Heartwood
Suan Jiang	Physalis	Calyx seu Fructus Physalis*	Wintercherry Calyx or Fruit
Suan Zao Ren	Ziziphus	Semen Ziziphi Spinosae	Sour Jujube Seed; Zizyphus
Suo Yang	Cynomorium	Herba Cynomorii Songarici	Cynomorium Fleshy Stem
Tai Zi Shen	Pseudostellaria	Radix Pseudostellariae Heterophyllae	Prince Ginseng Root
Tan Xiang	Santalum	Lignum Santali Albi	Sandalwood Heartwood
Tang Song Cao	Thalictrum	Herba Thalictri Foliolosi*	Thalictrum
Tao Ren	Prunus	Semen Persicae	Peach Seed (Kernel)
Tian Hua Fen	Trichosanthes	Radix Trichosanthis Kirilowii	Snakegourd Root
Tian Ma	Gastrodia	Rhizoma Gastrodiae Elatae	Gastrodia Rhizome
Tian Men Dong	Asparagus	Tuber Asparagi Cochinchinensis	Chinese Asparagus Tuber
Tian Ming Jing	Carpesium	Herba Carpesii	Carpesium
(Sheng) Tian Nan Xing	Arisaema	Rhizoma Arisaematis	Raw Jack-in-the-Pulpit Rhizome
Tian Zhu Huang	Bambusa	Concretio Silicea Bambusae Textillis	Siliceous Secretions of Bamboo

Pinyin

Pinyin	Botanical	Pharmaceutical	Common
Tie Xian	Acalypha	Herba Acalypae Australis*	Acalypha
Ting Li Zi	Lepidium or Descurainia	Semen Lepidii seu Descurainiae	Tansy Mustard Seed
Tong Cao	Tetrapanax	Medulla Tetrapanacis Papyriferi	Rice Paper Pith
Tu Bie Chong	Eupolyphaga	Eupolyphaga seu Opisthoplatia	Wingless Cockroach
Tu Fu Ling	Smilax	Rhizoma Smilacis Glabrae	Glabrous Greenbrier Rhizome
Tu Niu Xi	Achyranthes	Radix Achyranthis Aspera	Achyranthes Root
Tu Si Zi	Cuscuta	Semen Cuscutae Chinensis	Dodder Seed
Wa Leng Zi	Arca	Concha Arcae	Cockle Shell; Ark Shell
Wan Nian Qing	Rhodea	Herba Rhodeae Japonicae*	Rhodea
Wang Bu Liu Xing	Vaccaria	Semen Vaccariae Segetalis	Cow Soapwort Seed
Wei Ling Xian	Clematis	Radix Clematidis	Clematis Root
Wu Bei Zi	Rhus/Melaphis	Galla Rhois Chinensis	Gallnut of Chinese Sumac
Wu Gong	Scolopendra	Scolopendra Subspinipes	Centipede
Wu Jia Pi	Acanthopanax	Cortex Acanthopanacis Gracilistyli Radicis	Acanthopanax Rootbark.
Wu Jiu Gen Pi	Sapium	Cortex Sappii Sebiferi Radicis*	Tallow Tree Root Bark
Wu Ling Zhi	Trogopterus or Pteromys	Excrementum Trogopteri seu Pteromi	Flying Squirrel Feces
Wu Mei	Prunus	Fructus Pruni Mume	Ume Plum Fruit; Black Plum Fruit
Wu Shao She	Zaocys	Zaocys Dhumnades	Black-striped Snake
Wu Tou	Aconitum	Radix Aconiti	Aconite Root
Wu Wei Zi	Schisandra	Fructus Schisandrae Chinensis	Northern Schisandra Fruit
Wu Yao	Lindera	Radix Linderae Strychnifoliae	Spicebush Root
Wu Yi	Ulmus	Praepartio Fructus Ulmi Macrocarpi	Stinking Elm Fruit Paste
Wu Zhu Yu	Evodia	Fructus Evodiae Rutaecarpae	Evodia Fruit
Xi Gua	Citrullus	Fructus Citrulli Vulgaris	Watermelon Fruit and Peel or Rind
Xi Hong Hua	Crocus	Stigma Crocus Sativae	Stigma of the True Saffron Flower
Xi Jiao	Rhinoceros	Cornu Rhinoceri	Rhinoceros Horn
Xi Xian Cao	Siegesbeckia	Herba Siegesbeckiae	St. Paul's Wort

Pinyin	Botanical	Pharmaceutical	Common
Xi Xin	Asarum	Herba cum Radice Asari	Asarum; Chinese Wild Ginger
Xi Yang Shen	Panax	Radix Panacis Quinquefolii	American Ginseng Root
Xia Ku Cao	Prunella	Spica Prunellae Vulgaris	Selfheal Spike; Heal all Spike
Xian He Cao	Agrimonia	Herba Agrimoniae Pilosae	Agrimony
Xian Mao	Curculigo	Rhizoma Curculiginis Orchioidis	Golden Eye-grass Rhizome
Xiang Fu	Cyperus	Rhizoma Cyperi Rotundi	Cyperus Rhizome; Nut-grass Rhizome; Sedge Rhizome
Xiang Ru	Elsholtzia	Herba Elsholtziae seu Moslae	Aromatic Madder
Xiao Hui Xiang	Foeniculum	Fructus Foeniculi Vulgaris	Fennel Fruit
Xiao Ji	Cephalanoplos	Herba Cephalanoplos	Small Thistle; Field Thistle
Xiao Shi	Niter	Niter*	Silver
Xie Bai	Allium	Bulbus Allii	Chinese Chive Bulb
Xin Yi Hua	Magnolia	Flos Magnoliae	Magnolia Flower
(Bei) Xing Ren	Prunus	Semen Pruni Armeniacae	(Northern) Apricot Seed
(Nan) Xing Ren	Prunus	Semen Pruni Armeniacae	(Southern) Apricot Seed
Xiong Dan	Ursus	Vesica Fellea Ursi	Bear Gallbladder
Xiong Huang	Realgar	Realgar	Realgar; Arsenic Disulfide
Xu Duan	Dipsacus	Radix Dipsaci Asperi	Teasel Root
Xu Sui Zi	Euphorbia	Semen Euphorbiae Lathyridis*	Caper Spurge Seed; Moleplant Seed
Xuan Fu Hua	Inula	Flos Inulae	Elecampane Flower
Xuan Ming Fen	Mirabilitum	Mirabilitum Purum	Pure Mirabilite; Pure Sodium Sulphate; Pure Glauber's Salt
Xuan Shen	Scrophularia	Radix Scrophulariae Ningpoensis	Figwort Root
Xue Jie	Dracaena	Sanguis Draconis	Dragon's Blood Resin
Xue Yu Tan	Homo Sapiens	Crinis Carbonisatus Hominis	Charred Human Hair
Ya Dan Zi	Brucea	Fructus Bruceae Javanicae	Brucea Fruit
Ya Zhi Cao	Commelina	Herba Commelinae*	Commelina
Yan Fu Mu	Rhus	Cortex Rhois Chinensis*	Chinese Sumac Bark
Yan Hu Suo	Corydalis	Rhizoma Corydalis Yanhusuo	Corydalis Rhizome
Yang Qi Shi	Actinolitum	Actinolitum	Actinolite
Ye Jiao Teng	Polygonum	Caulis Polygoni Multiflori	Fleeceflower Stem; Fo-Ti Stem
Ye Ju Hua	Chrysanthemum	Flos Chrysanthemi Indici	Wild Chrysanthemum Flower
Ye Ming Sha	Vespertilio	Excrementum Vespertilionis Murini	Bat Dung or Feces

Pinyin	Botanical	Pharmaceutical	Common
Ye Shan Shen	Panax	Radix Ginseng	Wild Ginseng
Yi Mu Cao	Leonurus	Herba Leonuri Heterophylli	Motherwort
Yi Tang	Saccharum Granorum	Saccharum Granorum	Barley Malt Sugar/Syrup
Yi Yi Ren	Coix	Semen Coicis Lachryma-jobi	Coix Seed; Job's Tears Seed
Yi Zhi Ren	Alpinia	Fructus Alpiniae Oxyphyllae	Black Cardamon Fruit
Yin Chai Hu	Stellaria	Radix Stellariae Dichotomae	Stellaria Root
Yin Chen Hao	Artemisia	Herba Artemisiae Yinchenhao	Oriental Wormwood
Yin Guo Ye	Ginkgo	Folium Ginkgo Bilobae	Ginkgo Leaf
Yin Yang Huo	Epimedium	Herba Epimedii	Epimedium
Ying Su Ke	Papaver	Pericarpium Papaveris Somniferi	Opium Poppy Husk
Yu Jin	Curcuma	Tuber Curcumae	Tumeric Tuber
Yu Li Ren	Prunus	Semen Pruni	Bush Cherry Seed
Yu Liang Shi	Limonite	Limonite	Limonite
Yu Mi Xu	Zea	Stylus Zeae Mays	Cornsilk
Yu Xing Cao	Houttuynia	Herba cum Radice Houttuyniae Cordatae	Houttuynia; Fish Smell Plant
Yu Zhu	Polygonatum	Rhizoma Polygonati Odorati	Fragrant Solomon's Seal Rhizome; Polygonatum
Yuan Hua	Daphne	Flos Daphnes Genkwa	Daphne Flower
Yuan Zhi	Polygala	Radix Polygalae Tenuifoliae	Chinese Senega Root; Seneca Snakeroot
Yue Ji Hua	Rosa	Flos et Fructus Rosae Chinensis	Partially-blossoming Chinese Tea Rose Flower
Zao Jiao	Gleditsia	Fructus Gleditsiae Sinensis	Honeylocust Fruit; Soap Bean Fruit
Zao Jiao Ci	Gleditsia	Spina Gleditsiae Sinensis	Honeylocust Spine; Soap Bean Spine
Zao Xiu	Paris	Rhizoma Paridis Polyphyllae*	Paris Rhizome
Ze Lan	Lycopus	Herba Lycopi Lucidi	Bugleweed
Ze Qi	Euphorbia	Herba Euphorbiae Helioscopiae	Pill-bearing Spurge
Ze Xie	Alisma	Rhizoma Alismatis Orientalitis	Water Plantain Rhizome
Zhang Nao	Cinnamomum	Camphora	Crystalized Volatile Oil of the Camphor Tree
Zhe Bei Mu	Fritillaria	Bulbus Fritillariae Thunbergii	Thunberg Fritillary Bulb
Zhen Zhu	Pteria	Margarita	Pearl
Zhen Zhu Mu	Pteria	Concha Margaritiferae	Mother-of-Pearl Shell
Zhi Gan Cao	Glycyrrhiza	Radix Glycyrrhizae Praeparata*	Honey-fried Licorice Root

Pinyin	Botanical	Pharmaceutical	Common
Zhi Ke	Citrus or Poncirus	Fructus Citri Aurantii	Bitter Orange Fruit
Zhi Mu	Anemarrhena	Radix Anemarrhenae Asphodeloidis	Anemarrhena Root
Zhi Nan Xing	Arisaema	Rhizoma Arisaematis Praeparatae	Prepared Jack-in-the-Pulpit Rhizome
Zhi Shi	Citrus or Poncirus	Fructus Immaturus Citri Aurantii	Immature Bitter Orange Fruit
Zhi Zi	Gardenia	Fructus Gardeniae Jasminoidis	Gardenia Fruit
Zhu Li	Bambusa	Succus Bambusae	Dried Bamboo Sap
Zhu Ling	Polyporus	Sclerotium Polypori Umbellati	Polyporus Sclerotium
Zhu Ma Gen	Boehmeria	Radix Boehmeriae Niveae*	Ramie Root
Zhu Ru	Bambusa	Caulis Bambusae in Taeniis	Bamboo Shavings
Zhu Sha	Cinnabaris	Cinnabaris	Cinnabar; Red Mercury Sulfide
Zhu Sha Gen	Ardisia	Radix Ardisiae Crenatae*	Ardisia Root
Zi Bei Tian Kuei	Begonia	Herba Begoniae Fimbristipulatae	Begonia
Zi Cao	Lithospermum	Radix Lithospermi seu Arnebiae	Groomwell Root
Zi He Che	Homo Sapiens	Placenta Hominis	Human Placenta
Zi Hua Di Ding	Viola	Herba cum Radice Violae Yedoensitis	Viola
Zi Ran Tong	Pyritum	Pyritum	Pyrite
Zi Shi Ying	Fluoritum	Fluoritum	Fluorite
Zi Su Geng	Perilla	Ramulus Perillae*	Perilla Stem
Zi Su Ye	Perilla	Folium Perillae Frutescentis	Perilla Leaf
Zi Su Zi	Perilla	Semen Perillae Frutescentis	Perilla Seed
Zi Wan	Aster	Radix Asteris Tatarici	Purple Aster Root
Zi Zhu	Callicarpa	Folium Callicarpae	Callicarpa Leaf
Zong Lu Pi Tan	Trachycarpus	Fibra Stipulae Trachycarpi Carbonisatus	Charred Windmill Palm Petiole

Pinyin

Herb Name Cross Reference
Keyed to Botanical Names

Botanical	Pinyin	Pharmaceutical	Common
Abrus	Ji Gu Cao	Herba Abri*	Chicken Bone Vine
Acacia or Uncaria	Er Cha	Pasta Acacia seu Uncaria	Dried Paste of Concentrated Decoction of Black or White Cutch
Acalypha	Tie Xian	Herba Acalypae Australis*	Acalypha
Acanthopanax	Wu Jia Pi	Cortex Acanthopanacis Gracilistyli Radicis	Acanthopanax Rootbark.
Achyranthes	Huai Niu Xi	Radix Achyranthis Bidentatae	Achyranthes Root
Achyranthes	Tu Niu Xi	Radix Achyranthis Aspera	Achyranthes Root
Aconitum	Cao Wu	Radix Aconiti Kusnezoffii	Wild Aconite
Aconitum	Chuan Wu	Radix Aconite Carmichaeli	Sichuan Aconite
Aconitum	(Hei)Fu Zi	Radix Lateralis Aconiti Carmichaeli Praeparata	Prepared Sichuan Aconite Root
Aconitum	Wu Tou	Radix Aconiti	Aconite Root
Acorus	Shi Chang Pu	Rhizoma Acori Graminei	Sweetflag Rhizome
Actinolitum	Yang Qi Shi	Actinolitum	Actinolite
Adenophora	Gan Jie Geng	Radix Adenophorae Trachelioidis	Sweet Jie Geng
Adenophora	Nan Sha Shen	Radix Adenophorae	Ladybell Root; Southern Sand Root
Agastache or Pogostemon	Huo Xiang	Herba Agastaches seu Pogostemi	Patchouli; Agastache
Agkistrodon	Bai Hua She	Agkistrodon seu Bungarus	Long-noded Pit Viper Snake
Agrimonia	Xian He Cao	Herba Agrimoniae Pilosae	Agrimony
Ailanthus	Chun Pi	Cortex Ailanthi Altissimae	Tree of Heaven Bark
Ajuga	Bai Mao Xia Ku Cao	Herba Ajugae Decumbentis*	Ajuga
Akebia	Ba Yue Zha	Fructus Akebiae	Akebia Fruit
Akebia	Mu Tong	Caulis Mutong	Akebia Stem
Albizzia	He Huan Hua	Flos Albizziae Julibrissin*	Mimosa Tree Flower; Silktree Flower
Albizzia	He Huan Pi	Cortex Albizziae Julibrissin	Mimosa Tree Bark; Silktree Bark
Alisma	Ze Xie	Rhizoma Alismatis Orientalitis	Water Plantain Rhizome

Botanical	Pinyin	Pharmaceutical	Common
Allium	Cong Bai	Bulbus Allii Fistulosi	White Bulb of Green Onion or Scallion
Allium	Da Suan	Bulbus Allii Sativi	Garlic Bulb
Allium	Jiu Zi	Semen Allii Tuberosi	Chinese Leek Seed
Allium	Xie Bai	Bulbus Allii	Chinese Chive Bulb
Aloe	Lu Hui	Herba Aloes	Aloe Vera Leaf
Alpinia	Cao Dou Kou	Semen Alpiniae Katsumadai	Wild Cardamon Seed; Katsumada's Galangal Seed
Alpinia	Gao Liang Jiang	Rhizoma Alpiniae Officinari	Lesser Galangal Rhizome
Alpinia	Yi Zhi Ren	Fructus Alpiniae Oxyphyllae	Black Cardamon Fruit
Alumen	Ming Fan	Alumen	Alum; Potassium Aluminum Sulfate
Alumen Praeparatum	Ku Fan	Alumen Praeparatum	Prepared Alum
Amomum	Bai Dou Kou	Fructus Amomi Kravanh	Round Cardamon Fruit; Cluster Fruit
Amomum	Cao Guo	Fructus Amomi Tsao-Ko	Chinese Cardamon Fruit
Amomum	Sha Ren	Fructus seu Semen Amomi	Grains-of-Paradise Fruit or Seeds
Amomum	Sha Ren Hua	Flos Amomi	Grains-of-Paradise Flower
Amomum	Sha Ren Ke	Pericarpium Amomi	Grains-of-Paradise Shell
Ampelopsis	Bai Lian	Radix Ampelopsis Japonicae*	Ampelopsis Root
Amyda	Bie Jia	Carapax Amydae Sinensis	Chinese Soft-shell Turtle Shell
Andrographis	Chuan Xin Lian	Herba Andrographitis Paniculatae	Kariyat; Green Chiretta
Androsace	Dian Di Mei	Herba Androsacae Umbellatae*	Androsace
Anemarrhena	Zhi Mu	Radix Anemarrhenae Asphodeloidis	Anemarrhena Root
Anemone	Jiu Jie Chang Pu	Rhizoma Anemoni Attaicae*	Altaica Rhizome
Angelica	Bai Zhi	Radix Angelicae Dahuricae	Angelica Root
Angelica	Dang Gui	Radix Angelicae Sinensis	Tangkuei Root
Angelica	Dang Gui Tou	Caput Radicis Angelicae Sinensis	Tangkuei Head
Angelica	Dang Gui Wei	Extremas Radicis Angelicae Sinensis	Tangkuei Tail
Angelica	Du Huo	Radix Angelicae Pubescentis	Pubescent Angelica Root
Apocynum	Luo Bu Ma	Herba seu Folium Apocyni Veneti*	Red Dogbane Whole Herb or Leaf
Aquilaria	Chen Xiang	Lignum Aquilariae	Aloeswood Secretion or Sap
Arachis	Hua Sheng Yi	Pericarpium Arachi*	Peanut Skin
Arca	Wa Leng Zi	Concha Arcae	Cockle Shell; Ark Shell

Botanical	Pinyin	Pharmaceutical	Common
Arctium	Niu Bang Zi	Fructus Arctii Lappae	Burdock Seed
Ardisia	Zhu Sha Gen	Radix Ardisiae Crenatae*	Ardisia Root
Areca	Bing Lang	Semen Arecae Catechu	Betel Nut
Areca	Da Fu Pi	Pericarpium Arecae Catechu	Betelnut Husk
Arisaema	Dan Nan Xing	Pulvis Arisaemae cum Felle Bovis	Powdered Jack-in-the-Pulpit Rhizome mixed with Cow Bile
Arisaema	(Sheng) Tian Nan Xing	Rhizoma Arisaematis	Raw Jack-in-the-Pulpit Rhizome
Arisaema	Zhi Nan Xing	Rhizoma Arisaematis Praeparatae	Prepared Jack-in-the-Pulpit Rhizome
Aristolochia	Ma Dou Ling	Fructus Aristolochiae	Birthwort Fruit
Aristolochia	Qing Mu Xiang	Radix Aristolochiae	Birthwort Root
Aristolochia or Cocculus	Guang Fang Ji	Radix Aristolochiae Fangchi	Aristolochia Root
Arsenolite	Pi Shi	Arsenicum	White Arsenic
Artemisia	Ai Ye	Folium Artemisiae Argyi	Mugwort Leaf
Artemisia	Liu Ji Nu	Herba Artemisiae Anomalae	Artemisia
Artemisia	Qing Hao	Herba Artemisiae Annuae	Sweet Wormwood; Southernwood
Artemisia	Yin Chen Hao	Herba Artemisiae Yinchenhao	Oriental Wormwood
Asarum	Xi Xin	Herba cum Radice Asari	Asarum; Chinese Wild Ginger
Asparagus	Tian Men Dong	Tuber Asparagi Cochinchinensis	Chinese Asparagus Tuber
Aspongopus	Jiu Xiang Chong	Aspongopus*	Stink Bug
Aster	Zi Wan	Radix Asteris Tatarici	Purple Aster Root
Astragalus	Huang Qi	Radix Astragali Membranaceus	Yellow Milk-vetch Root
Astragalus	Sha Yuan Ji Li	Semen Astragali Complanati	Flattened Milk-vetch Seed
Atractylodes	Bai Zhu	Rhizoma Atractylodis Macrocephalae	White Atractylodes Rhizome
Atractylodes	Cang Zhu	Rhizoma Atractylodis	Atractylodes Rhizome
Aurum	Huang Jin	Aurum*	Gold
Bambusa	Tian Zhu Huang	Concretio Silicea Bambusae Textillis	Siliceous Secretions of Bamboo
Bambusa	Zhu Li	Succus Bambusae	Dried Bamboo Sap
Bambusa	Zhu Ru	Caulis Bambusae in Taeniis	Bamboo Shavings
Begonia	Zi Bei Tian Kuei	Herba Begoniae Fimbristipulatae	Begonia
Belamcanda	She Gan	Rhizoma Belamcandae Chinensis	Belamcanda Rhizome; Blackberry Lily Rhizome
Benincasa	Dong Gua Pi	Epicarpium Benincasae Hispidae	Wintermelon Fruit Peel; Wax Gourd Fruit Peel

Botanical

Botanical	Pinyin	Pharmaceutical	Common
Benincasa	Dong Gua Ren	Semen Benincasae Hispidae	Wintermelon Seed; Wax Gourd Seed
Biota	Bai Zi Ren	Semen Biotae Orientalis	Arbor-Vitae Seed
Biota	Ce Bai Ye	Cacumen Biotae Orientalis	Arborvitae Leafy Twig
Bletilla	Bai Ji	Rhizoma Bletillae Striatae	Bletilla Rhizome
Boehmeria	Zhu Ma Gen	Radix Boehmeriae Niveae*	Ramie Root
Bombyx	Can Sha	Excrementum Bombycis Mori	Silkworm Feces
Bombyx	Jiang Can	Bombyx Batryticatus	Dead Stiff Body of Sick Silkworm Larvae
Borax	Peng Sha	Borax	Borax; Sodium Tetraborate
Bos	Niu Dan	Vesica Fellea Bovus	Cow Gallbladder
Bos	Ren Gong Niu Huang	Calculus Artificialis	Artificially Induced Cow Gallstons
Bos or Bubalis	Niu Huang	Calculus Bovis seu Calculus Bubali	Ox or Water Buffalo Gallstone
Boswellia	Ru Xiang	Gummi Olibanum	Frankincense Gum-resin
Brassica	Bai Jie Zi	Semen Sinapsis Albae	White Mustard Seed
Broussonetia	Chu Shi Zi	Semen Broussonetiae Papyriferae*	Broussonetia Seed
Brucea	Ya Dan Zi	Fructus Bruceae Javanicae	Brucea Fruit
Bubalus	Shui Niu Jiao	Cornu Bubali	Waterbuffalo Horn
Buddleia	Mi Meng Hua	Flos Buddleiae Officinalis Immaturus	Buddleia Flower
Bufo	Chan Su	Secretio Bufonis	Dried Skin Secretion of Toad
Bupleurum	Chai Hu	Radix Bupleuri	Thorowax Root; Hare's Ear Root
Buthus	Quan Xie	Buthus Martensi	Scorpion
Caesalpinia	Su Mu	Lignum Sappan	Sappan Heartwood
Calcaria	Chen Shi Huei	Calcaria*	Calcium Hydroxide
Calcitum	Han Shui Shi	Calcitum	Calcite
Callicarpa	Zi Zhu	Folium Callicarpae	Callicarpa Leaf
Calomelas	Qing Fen	Calomelas	Calomel; Mercurous Chloride
Canis	Gou Gu	Os Canine	Dog Bone
Canis	Guang Gou Shen	Testis et Penis Canis*	Male Dog Sexual Organs
Cannabis	Huo Ma Ren	Semen Cannabis Sativae	Hemp Seed; Marihuana Seed
Capsella	Ji Cai	Herba Capsellae*	Shepherd's Purse
Carpesium	Tian Ming Jing	Herba Carpesii	Carpesium
Carpesium or Daucus	He Shi	Fructus Carpesii seu Daucusi	Carpesium Fruit
Carthamus	Hong Hua	Flos Carthami Tinctorii	Safflower

Botanical	Pinyin	Pharmaceutical	Common
Cassia	Fan Xie Ye	*Folium Sennae*	Senna Leaf
Cassia	Jue Ming Zi	*Semen Cassiae*	Cassia Seed
Celosia	Ji Guan Hua	*Flos Celosiae Cristatae*	Cockscomb Flower
Celosia	Qing Xiang Zi	*Semen Celosiae Argenteae*	Celosia Seed
Centipeda	E Bu Shi Cao	*Herba Centipedae Minimae**	Centipeda Herb
Cephalanoplos	Xiao Ji	*Herba Cephalanoplos*	Small Thistle; Field Thistle
Cervus	Hua Lu Shen	*Testis et Penis Cervi**	Male Deer Sexual Organs
Cervus	Lu Jiao	*Cornu Cervi*	Antler; Deerhorn; Ossified Horn of the Mature Male Deer
Cervus	Lu Jiao Jiao	*Colla Cornu Cervi*	Mature Antler Glue; Mature Antler Gelatin
Cervus	Lu Jiao Shuang	*Cornu Cervi Degelatinatium*	Antler Powder from the dregs of cooking Antler Glue
Cervus	Lu Rong	*Cornu Cervi Parvum*	Young Deer Antler Velvet
Chaenomeles	Mu Gua	*Frutus Chaenomelis*	Chinese Quince Fruit
Chalcanthitum	Dan Fan	*Chalcanthitum**	Copper Sulphate; Blue Vitriol
Changium	Ming Dang Shen	*Radix Changii**	Changium Root
Chinemys	Gui Ban	*Plastrum Testudinis*	Fresh Water Turtle Shell
Chrysanthemum	(Bai) Ju Hua	*Flos Chrysanthemi Morifolii*	White Chrysanthemum Flower
Chrysanthemum	(Huang) Ju Hua	*Flos Chrysanthemi Morifolii*	Yellow Chrysanthemum Flower
Chrysanthemum	Ye Ju Hua	*Flos Chrysanthemi Indici*	Wild Chrysanthemum Flower
Cibotium	Gou Ji	*Rhizoma Cibotii Barometz*	Chain Fern Rhizome
Cimicifuga	Sheng Ma	*Rhizoma Cimicifugae*	Black Cohosh Rhizome; Bugbane Rhizome
Cinnabaris	Zhu Sha	*Cinnabaris*	Cinnabar; Red Mercury Sulfide
Cinnamomum	Guan Gui	*Cortex Tubiformis Cinnamomi Cassiae*	Thin Cinnamon Bark from Young Trees
Cinnamomum	Gui Zhi	*Ramulus Cinnamomi Cassiae*	Cinnamon Twig
Cinnamomum	Rou Gui	*Cortex Cinnamomi Cassiae*	Cinnamon Bark
Cinnamomum	Zhang Nao	*Camphora*	Crystalized Volatile Oil of the Camphor Tree
Cirsium	Da Ji	*Herba seu Radix Cirsii Japonici*	Japanese Thistle
Cistanche	Rou Cong Rong	*Herba Cistanches Deserticolae*	Broomrape Fleshy Stem
Citrullus	Xi Gua	*Fructus Citrulli Vulgaris*	Watermelon Fruit and Peel or Rind
Citrus	Chen Pi	*Pericarpium Citri Reticulatae*	Tangerine Peel
Citrus	Fo Shou	*Fructus Citri Sarcodactylis*	Finger Citron Fruit

Botanical

Botanical	Pinyin	Pharmaceutical	Common
Citrus	Fo Shou Hua	Flos Citri Sarcodactylis	Finger Citron Flower
Citrus	Ju He	Semen Citri Reticulatae*	Tangerine Seed
Citrus	Ju Hong	Pars Rubra Epicarpii Citri Erythrocarpae	Red Tangerine Peel
Citrus	Qing Pi	Pericarpium Citri Reticulatae Viride	Immature (Green) Tangerine Peel
Citrus or Poncirus	Zhi Ke	Fructus Citri Aurantii	Bitter Orange Fruit
Citrus or Poncirus	Zhi Shi	Fructus Immaturus Citri Aurantii	Immature Bitter Orange Fruit
Clematis	Wei Ling Xian	Radix Clematidis	Clematis Root
Clerodendron	Chou Wu Tong	Folium Clerodendri Trichotomi	Glorybower Leaf
Cnidium	She Chuang Zi	Fructus Cnidii Monnieri	Cnidium Seed
Codonopsis	Dang Shen	Radix Codonopsitis Pilosulae	Asiabell Root
Coix	Shu Yi Ren	Semen Coicis Lachryma-jobi	Dry-Fried Coix Seed
Coix	Yi Yi Ren	Semen Coicis Lachryma-jobi	Coix Seed; Job's Tears Seed
Commelina	Ya Zhi Cao	Herba Commelinae*	Commelina
Commiphora	Mo Yao	Resinae Myrrhae	Myrrh Gum-resin
Coptis	Huang Lian	Rhizoma Coptidis	Coptis; Golden Thread Rhizome
Cordyceps	Dong Chong Xia Cao	Cordyceps Sinensis	Chinese Caterpillar Fungus
Cornus	Shan Zhu Yu	Fructus Corni Officinalis	Dogwood Fruit; Asiatic Cornelian Cherry Fruit
Corydalis	Yan Hu Suo	Rhizoma Corydalis Yanhusuo	Corydalis Rhizome
Crataegus	Shan Zha	Fructus Crataegi	Hawthorn Unripe Fruit or Berry
Crataegus	Shan Zha Rou	Fructus Crataegi	Hawthorn Ripe Fruit or Berry
Crataegus	Shan Zha Tan	Fructus Crataegi Carbonisatus	Charred Hawthorn Fruit or Berry
Crocus	Xi Hong Hua	Stigma Crocus Sativae	Stigma of the True Saffron Flower
Croton	Ba Dou	Semen Croton Tiglii	Croton Seed
Cryptotympana	Chan Tui	Periostracum Cicadae	Cicada Skin; Cicada Moulting
Cucumis	Gua Di	Pedicellus Cucumeris	Melon Pedicle
Cucurbita	Nan Gua Zi	Semen Cucurbitae Moschatae	Pumpkin Seed and Husk
Curculigo	Xian Mao	Rhizoma Curculiginis Orchioidis	Golden Eye-grass Rhizome
Curcuma	E Zhu	Rhizoma Curcumae	Zedoary Tumeric Rhizome
Curcuma	Jiang Huang	Rhizoma Curcumae Longae	Tumeric Rhizome
Curcuma	Yu Jin	Tuber Curcumae	Tumeric Tuber

Botanical	Pinyin	Pharmaceutical	Common
Cuscuta	Tu Si Zi	Semen Cuscutae Chinensis	Dodder Seed
Cyathula	Chuan Niu Xi	Radix Cyathulae Officinalis	Cyathula Root
Cyclina	Hai Ge Ke	Concha Cyclinae Sinensis	Clam Shell
Cynanchum	Bai Qian	Rhizoma et Radix Cynanchi Baiqian	Cynanchum Rhizome and Root
Cynanchum	Bai Wei	Radix Cynanchi Baiwei	Swallowort Root
Cynanchum	Ge Shan Xiang	Radix Cynanchi Auriculati	Cynanchum Root
Cynomorium	Suo Yang	Herba Cynomorii Songarici	Cynomorium Fleshy Stem
Cyperus	Xiang Fu	Rhizoma Cyperi Rotundi	Cyperus Rhizome; Nutgrass Rhizome; Sedge Rhizome
Dalbergia	Jiang Xiang	Lignum Dalbergiae Odoriferae	Dalbergia Heartwood
Daphne	Yuan Hua	Flos Daphnes Genkwa	Daphne Flower
Dendrobium	Shi Hu	Herba Dendrobii	Dendrobium Stem
Dens Draconis	Long Chi	Dens Draconis	Dragon Tooth; Fossilized Tooth
Dianthus	Qu Mai	Herba Dianthi	Pink Flower Herb
Dichroa	Chang Shan	Radix Dichroae Febrifugae	Dichroa Root
Dichroa	Shu Qi	Folium Dichroae Febrifugae	Dichroa Leaf
Dictamnus	Bai Xian Pi	Cortex Dictamni Dasycarpi Radicis	Dittany Root Bark
Dioscorea	Bei Xie	Rhizoma Dioscoreae Hypoglaucae	Hypoglauca Yam Rhizome; Fish-poison Yam Rhizome
Dioscorea	Chuan Shan Long	Rhizoma Dioscoreae Nipponicae*	Japanese Dioscorea Rhizome
Dioscorea	Huang Yao Zi	Tuber Dioscoreae Bulbiferae	Dioscorea Tuber
Dioscorea	Shan Yao	Radix Dioscoreae Oppositae	Chinese Wild Yam Root
Diospyros	Shi Bing	Fructus Diospyri Kaki*	Dried Persimmon Fruit
Diospyros	Shi Di	Calyx Diospyri Kaki	Persimmon Calyx
Dipsacus	Xu Duan	Radix Dipsaci Asperi	Teasel Root
Dolichos	Bian Dou	Semen Dolichoris Lablab	Hyacinth Bean
Dolichos	Bian Dou Hua	Flos Dolichoris Lablab	Hyacinth Bean Flower
Dracaena	Xue Jie	Sanguis Draconis	Dragon's Blood Resin
Drynaria	Gu Sui Bu	Rhizoma Drynariae	Drynaria Rhizome
Dryobalanops	Bing Pian	Borneol	Processed Resin of Borneol Camphor
Dryopteris	Dong Bei Guan Zhong	Rhizoma Dryopteridis	Dryopteris Rhizome
Dryopteris	Guan Zhong	Rhizoma Guanzhong	Shield-fern Rhizome
Eclipta	Han Lian Cao	Herba Ecliptae Prostratae	Eclipta
Eleagnus	Hu Tui Ye	Folium Eleagni Pungens	Eleagnus Leaf
Elsholtzia	Xiang Ru	Herba Elsholtziae seu Moslae	Aromatic Madder

Botanical	Pinyin	Pharmaceutical	Common
Ephedra	Ma Huang	Herba Ephedrae	Ephedra Stem
Ephedra	Ma Huang Gen	Radix Ephedrae	Ephedra Root
Epimedium	Yin Yang Huo	Herba Epimedii	Epimedium
Equisetum	Mu Zei	Herba Equiseti Hiemalis	Horsetail; Scouring Rush; Shavegrass
Equus	E Jiao	Gelatinum Corii Asini	Donkey Hide Gelatin; Ass Skin Glue
Equus	Hei Lu Shen	Testis et Penis Equii*	Male Horse Sexual Organs
Eretmochelys	Dai Mao	Carapax Eretmochelydis Imbricatae*	Hawksbill Turtle Shell
Eriobotrya	Pi Pa Ye	Folium Eriobotryae Japonicae	Loquat Leaf
Eriocaulon	Gu Jing Cao	Scapus et Inflorescentia Eriocaulonis Buergeriani	Pipewort Scapus
Erodium or Geranium	Lao Guan Cao	Herba Erodii seu Geranii*	Geranium; Heronbill; Cranebill
Erythrina	Hai Tong Pi	Cortex Erythrinae	Coral-bean Bark
Eucommia	Du Zhong	Cortex Eucommiae Ulmoidis	Eucommia Bark
Eugenia	Ding Xiang	Flos Caryophylli	Clove Flower-bud
Eupatorium	Pei Lan	Herba Eupatorii Fortunei	Boneset; Thoroughwort; Feverwort
Euphorbia	Gan Sui	Radix Euphorbiae Kansui	Kansui Spurge Root
Euphorbia	Xu Sui Zi	Semen Euphorbiae Lathyridis*	Caper Spurge Seed; Moleplant Seed
Euphorbia	Ze Qi	Herba Euphorbiae Helioscopiae	Pill-bearing Spurge
Euphorbia or Knoxia	Jing Da Ji	Radix Euphorbiae seu Knoxiae	Peking Spurge Root
Euphoria	Long Yan Rou	Arillus Euphoriae Longanae	Longan Fruit Flesh
Eupolyphaga	Tu Bie Chong	Eupolyphaga seu Opisthoplatia	Wingless Cockroach
Euryale	Qian Shi	Semen Euryales Ferocis	Euryale Seed
Evodia	Wu Zhu Yu	Fructus Evodiae Rutaecarpae	Evodia Fruit
Fagopyrum	Jin Qiao Mai	Rhizoma Fagopyri Cynosi*	Wild Buckwheat Rhizome
Ferula	E Wei	Resinae Asafoetidae*	Asafoetida Gum-resin; Devil's Dung
Fluoritum	Zi Shi Ying	Fluoritum	Fluorite
Foeniculum	Xiao Hui Xiang	Fructus Foeniculi Vulgaris	Fennel Fruit
Forsythia	Lian Qiao	Fructus Forsythiae Suspensae	Forsythia Fruit; Golden Bells
Fraxinus	Qin Pi	Cortex Fraxini	Korean Ash Bark
Fritillaria	Chuan Bei Mu	Bulbus Fritillariae Cirrhosae	Tendrilled Fritillary Bulb
Fritillaria	Zhe Bei Mu	Bulbus Fritillariae Thunbergii	Thunberg Fritillary Bulb

Botanical	Pinyin	Pharmaceutical	Common
Frusta Ferri	Sheng Tie Luo	Frusta Ferri	Iron Filing
Gallus	Ji Nei Jin	Endothelium Corneum Gigeriae Galli	Chicken Gizard Lining
Ganoderma	Ling Zhi	Fructificatio Ganodermae Lucidi*	Lucid Ganoderma; Reishi
Gardenia	Zhi Zi	Fructus Gardeniae Jasminoidis	Gardenia Fruit
Gastrodia	Tian Ma	Rhizoma Gastrodiae Elatae	Gastrodia Rhizome
Gekko	Ge Jie	Gekko	Gecko Lizard
Gentiana	Long Dan Cao	Radix Gentianae Longdancao	Chinese Gentian Root
Gentiana	Qin Jiao	Radix Gentianae Qinjiao	Large-Leaf Gentian Root
Ginkgo	Bai Guo	Semen Ginkgo Bilobae	Ginkgo Nut
Ginkgo	Yin Guo Ye	Folium Ginkgo Bilobae	Ginkgo Leaf
Gleditsia	Zao Jiao	Fructus Gleditsiae Sinensis	Honeylocust Fruit; Soap Bean Fruit
Gleditsia	Zao Jiao Ci	Spina Gleditsiae Sinensis	Honeylocust Spine; Soap Bean Spine
Glehnia	Bei Sha Shen	Radix Glehniae Littoralis	Beech Silver-top Root; Northern Sand Root
Glycine	Dan Dou Chi	Semen Sojae Praeparatum	Prepared (Fermented) Soybean
Glycine	Dou Juan	Semen Glycines Germinatum	Young Soybean Sprout
Glycyrrhiza	Gan Cao	Radix Glycyrrhizae Uralensis	Licorice Root
Glycyrrhiza	Zhi Gan Cao	Radix Glycyrrhizae Praeparata*	Honey-fried Licorice Root
Gossypium	Mian Hua Gen	Radix Gossypii Hirsuti*	Cotton Root
Gynura	Ju Ye San Qi	Folium Gynurae*	Gynura Leaf
Gypsum	Shi Gao	Gypsum Fibrosum	Gypsum; Calcium Sulphate
Haematitum	Dai Zhe Shi	Haematitum	Hematite; Iron Ore
Haliotis	Shi Jue Ming	Concha Haliotidis	Abalone Shell
Halloysitum Rubrum	Chi Shi Zhi	Halloysitum Rubrum	Halloysite; Red Kaolin
Hedera	Chang Chun Teng	Herba Hederae Nepalensis*	Ivy
Hippocampus	Hai Ma	Hippocampus	Sea Horse
Hirudo	Shui Zhi	Hirudo seu Whitmania	Leech
Homalomena	Qian Nian Jian	Rhizoma Homalomenae Occultae	Homalomena Rhizome
Homo Sapiens	Xue Yu Tan	Crinis Carbonisatus Hominis	Charred Human Hair
Homo Sapiens	Zi He Che	Placenta Hominis	Human Placenta
Hordeum	Mai Ya	Fructus Hordei Vulgaris Germinatus	Barley Sprout; Malted Barley
Houttuynia	Yu Xing Cao	Herba cum Radice Houttuyniae Cordatae	Houttuynia; Fish Smell Plant

Botanical

Botanical	Pinyin	Pharmaceutical	Common
Hydnocarpus	Da Feng Zi	Semen Hydnocarpi Anthelminticae	Chaulmoogra Seed
Hydrangea	Ba Xian Hua	Flos Hydrangeae Macrophyllae*	Hydrangea Flower
Hydrargyrum	Shui Yin	Hydrargyrum	Mercury
Ilex	Mao Dong Qing	Radix Ilicis Pubescentis*	Pubescent Holly Root
Ilex	Si Ji Qing	Folium Ilicis Chinensis*	Holly Leaf
Illicium	Ba Jiao Hui Xiang	Fructus Illicii*	Star Anise Fruit
Imperata	Bai Mao Gen	Rhizoma Imperatae Cylindricae	Woolly Grass Rhizome; White Grass Rhizome
Imperata	Bai Mao Hua	Flos Imperatae Cylindricae	Wooly Grass Flower; White Grass Flower
Indigo	Qing Dai	Indigo Pulverata Levis	Indigo
Inula	Jin Fei Cao	Herba Inulae	Elecampane
Inula	Xuan Fu Hua	Flos Inulae	Elecampane Flower
Isatis	Ban Lan Gen	Radix Isatidis seu Baphicacanthi	Isatis Root; Woad Root
Isatis	Da Qing Ye	Folium Daqingye	Isatis Leaf; Woad Leaf
Juglans	Hu Tao Ren	Semen Juglandis Regiae	Walnut
Juncus	Deng Xin Cao	Medulla Junci Effusi	Rush Pith
Kochia	Di Fu Zi	Fructus Kochiae Scopariae	Broom Cyperus Seed
Laminaria	Hai Dai	Herba Laminaria Japonicae	Algae
Laminaria or Ecklonia	Kun Bu	Thallus Algae	Kelp Thallus; Kombu Thallus
Lapis Micae seu Chloriti	Meng Shi	Lapis Micae seu Chloriti	Chlorite Schist; Lapis
Lasiosphaera	Ma Bo	Fructificatio Lasiosphaerae seu Calvatiae	Puffball Fruiting Body
Ledebouriella	Fang Feng	Radix Ledebouriella Divaricatae	Siler Root; Ledebouriella Root
Leonurus	Chong Wei Zi	Semen Leonuri Heterophylli	Motherwort Seed
Leonurus	Yi Mu Cao	Herba Leonuri Heterophylli	Motherwort
Lepidium or Descurainia	Ting Li Zi	Semen Lepidii seu Descurainiae	Tansy Mustard Seed
Ligusticum	Chuan Xiong	Radix Ligustici Wallichii	Sichuan Lovage Root
Ligusticum	Gao Ben	Rhizoma et Radix Ligustici	Straw Weed Rhizome and Root; Chinese Lovage Rhizome and Root
Ligustrum	Nu Zhen Zi	Fructus Ligustri Lucidi	Privet Fruit; Waxtree Fruit
Lilium	Bai He	Bulbus Lilii	Lily Bulb
Limonite	Yu Liang Shi	Limonite	Limonite
Lindera	Wu Yao	Radix Linderae Strychnifoliae	Spicebush Root
Liquidambar	Lu Lu Tong	Fructus Liquidambaris Taiwanianae	Sweetgum Fruit
Liquidambar	Su He Xiang	Styrax Liquidis	Rose Maloes Resin

Botanical	Pinyin	Pharmaceutical	Common
Litchi	Li Zhi He	Semen Litchi Chinensis	Leechee Nut
Lithargyrum	Mi Tuo Seng	Lithargyrum	Litharge; Galena
Lithospermum	Zi Cao	Radix Lithospermi seu Arnebiae	Groomwell Root
Litsea	Dou Chi Jiang	Radix et Ramus Litseae Cubebae	Aromatic Litsea Root and Stem
Lobelia	Ban Bian Lian	Herba Lobeliae Chinensis cum Radice	Chinese Lobelia
Lonicera	Jin Yin Hua	Flos Lonicerae Japonicae	Honeysuckle Flower
Lonicera	Jin Yin Teng	Ramus Lonicerae Japonicae	Honeysuckle Stem
Lophatherum	Dan Zhu Ye	Herba Lophatheri Gracilis	Bland Bamboo Leaf and Stem
Loranthus or Viscum	Sang Ji Sheng	Ramulus Sangjishang	Mulberry Mistletoe Stem
Loropetalum	Ji Mu	Cortex Loropetali*	Loropetalum Bark
Luffa	Si Gua Lou	Fasciculus Vascularis Luffae	Dried Skeleton of Luffa Sponge
Luffa	Si Gua Pi	Pericarpium Luffae Acutangulae	Luffa Skin
Lycium	Di Gu Pi	Cortex Lycii Radicis	Matrimony-vine Rootbark; Wolfberry Bark
Lycium	Gou Qi Zi	Fructus Lycii	Matrimony Vine Fruit; Wolfberry Fruit
Lycopodium	Shen Jin Cao	Herba Lycopodii Clavati*	Clubmoss
Lycopus	Ze Lan	Herba Lycopi Lucidi	Bugleweed
Lygodium	Hai Jin Sha	Spora Lygodii Japonici	Japanese Climbing Fern Spore
Lygodium	Jin Sha Teng	Herba Lygodii Japonici	Japanese Climbing Fern
Lysimachia	Jin Qian Cao	Herba Lysimachiae	Lysimachia
Macaca	Hou Zao	Calculus Macacae Mulattae	Macaque Gallstone
Magnetitum	Ci Shi	Magnetitum	Magnetite; Magnetic Iron Ore; Loadstone
Magnolia	Hou Po	Cortex Magnoliae Officinalis	Magnolia Bark
Magnolia	Hou Po Hua	Flos Magnoliae Officinalis	Magnolia Flower
Magnolia	Xin Yi Hua	Flos Magnoliae	Magnolia Flower
Mahonia	Shi Da Gong Lao	Folium Mahoniae*	Mahonia Leaf
Malva or Abutilon	Dong Kui Zi	Semen Albutili seu Malvae	Musk Mallow Seed; Malva Seed
Manis	Chuan Shan Jia	Squama Manitis Pentadactylae	Anteater-Scales; Pangolin Scales
Massa Fermentata	Shen Qu	Massa Fermentata	Medicated Leaven
Mel	Feng Mi	Mel*	Honey
Melia	Chuan Lian Zi	Fructus Meliae Toosendan	Sichuan Chinaberry Fruit; Sichuan Pagoda Tree Fruit; Neem Fruit

Botanical

Botanical	Pinyin	Pharmaceutical	Common
Melia	Ku Lian Gen Pi	Cortex Meliae Radicis	Sichuan Chinaberry Root Bark; Sichuan Pagoda Tree Root Bark; Neem Root Bark
Melia	Ku Lian Mu Pi	Cortex Meliae	Sichuan Chinaberry Tree Bark; Sichuan Pagoda Tree Bark; Neem Tree Bark
Mentha	Bo He	Herba Menthae Haplocalycis	Peppermint; Spearmint; Field Mint
Millettia	Ji Xue Teng	Radix et Caulis Jixueteng	Millettia Root and Vine; Chicken Blood Vine
Minium	Qian Dan	Minium	Red Lead Oxide
Mirabilitum	Mang Xiao	Mirabilitum	Mirabilite; Glauber's Salt
Mirabilitum	Xuan Ming Fen	Mirabilitum Purum	Pure Mirabilite; Pure Sodium Sulphate; Pure Glauber's Salt
Momordica	Luo Han Guo	Fructus Momordicae Grosvenori	Momordica Fruit
Momordica	Luo Huo Guo Ye	Folium Momordicae Grosvenori	Momordica Leaf
Momordica	Mu Bie Zi	Semen Momordicae Cochinchinensis	Momordica Seed
Morinda	Ba Ji Tian	Radix Morindae Officinalis	Morinda Root
Morus	Sang Bai Pi	Cortex Mori Albae Radicis	Mulberry Rootbark
Morus	Sang Shen	Fructus Mori Albae	Mulberry Fruit Bud
Morus	Sang Ye	Folium Mori Albae	Mulberry Leaf
Morus	Sang Zhi	Ramulus Mori Albae	Mulberry Twig
Moschus	She Xiang	Secretio Moschus	Musk; Musk Deer Navel Gland Secretion
Mylabris	Ban Mao	Mylabris	Cantharides; Chinese Blistering Beetle
Myristica	Rou Dou Kou	Semen Myristicae Fragrantis	Nutmeg Seed
Naemorhedis	Shan Yang Jiao	Cornu Naemorhedis	Goat Horn
Nelumbo	He Ye	Folium Nelumbinis Nuciferae	Lotus Leaf
Nelumbo	Lian Fang	Receptaculum Nelumbinis Nuciferae	Mature Lotus Receptacle
Nelumbo	Lian Geng	Ramulus Nelumbinis Nuciferae	Lotus Stem
Nelumbo	Lian Xin	Plumula Nelumbinis Nuciferae	Lotus Plumule
Nelumbo	Lian Xu	Stamen Nelumbinis Nuciferae	Lotus Stamen
Nelumbo	Lian Zi	Semen Nelumbinis Nuciferae	Lotus Seed
Nelumbo	Ou Jie	Nodus Nelumbinis Nuciferae Rhizomatis	Lotus Rhizome Node
Niter	Xiao Shi	Niter*	Silver

Botanical	Pinyin	Pharmaceutical	Common
Notopterygium	Qiang Huo	Rhizoma et Radix Notopterygii	Notopterygium Rhizome and Root
Oldenlandia	Bai Hua She She Cao	Herba Oldenlandiae Diffusae	Oldenlandia
Omphalia	Lei Wan	Sclerotium Omphaliae Lapidescens	Omphalia Fungus Fruiting Body
Ophicalcitum	Hua Rui Shi	Ophicalcitum	Ophicalcite
Ophiopogon	Mai Men Dong	Tuber Ophiopogonis Japonici	Creeping Lily-turf Tuber
Oroxylum	Mu Hu Die	Semen Oroxyli Indici	Oroxylum Seed
Oryza	Gu Ya	Fructus Oryzae Sativae Germinatus	Rice Sprout
Oryza	Jing Mi	Semen Oryzae Sativae*	Rice Grain
Oryza	Nuo Dao Gen Xu	Radix et Rhizoma Oryzae Glutinosae	Sweet Rice Root and Rhizome
Os Draconis	Duan Long Gu	Os Draconis	Calcined Dragon Bone; Calcined Fossilized Bone
Os Draconis	Long Gu	Os Draconis	Dragon Bone; Fossilized Bone
Ostrea	Duan Mu Li	Concha Ostreae	Calcined Oyster Shell
Ostrea	Mu Li	Concha Ostreae	Oyster Shell
Paederia	Ji Shi Teng	Caulis Paederiae*	Paederia Stem
Paeonia	Bai Shao	Radix Paeoniae Lactiflorae	White Peony Root
Paeonia	Chi Shao	Radix Paeoniae Rubra	Red Peony Root
Paeonia	Mu Dan Pi	Cortex Moutan Radicis	Tree Peony Rootbark
Panax	Bai Shen	Radix Ginseng	Rock Candy cured White Ginseng Root
Panax	Ji Lin Shen	Radix Ginseng	Jilin Wild Ginseng
Panax	(Hong) Ren Shen	Radix Ginseng	Ginseng Root steamed until red
Panax	Ren Shen Lu	Cervix Ginseng	Ginseng Root Neck
Panax	Ren Shen Ye	Folium Ginseng	Ginseng Leaf
Panax	San Qi	Radix Pseudoginseng	Pseudoginseng Root; Notoginseng Root
Panax	San Qi Hua	Flos Pseudoginseng	Pseudoginseng Flower; Notoginseng Flower
Panax	Shen Xu	Radix Ginseng	Rock Candy cured White Ginseng Root Tail
Panax	Sheng Shai Shen	Radix Ginseng	Fresh Dried Ginseng Root
Panax	Xi Yang Shen	Radix Panacis Quinquefolii	American Ginseng Root
Panax	Ye Shan Shen	Radix Ginseng	Wild Ginseng
Panthera	Bao Gu	Os Leopardis	Leopard Bone
Panthera	Hu Gu	Os Tigris	Tiger Bone
Papaver	Ying Su Ke	Pericarpium Papaveris Somniferi	Opium Poppy Husk

Botanical	Pinyin	Pharmaceutical	Common
Paratenodera	Sang Piao Xiao	Ootheca Mantidis	Praying Mantis Egg Case
Paris	Zao Xiu	Rhizoma Paridis Polyphyllae*	Paris Rhizome
Patrinia or Thiaspi	Bai Jiang Cao	Herba cum Radice Patriniae	Patrinia; Thiaspi
Perilla	Zi Su Geng	Ramulus Perillae*	Perilla Stem
Perilla	Zi Su Ye	Folium Perillae Frutescentis	Perilla Leaf
Perilla	Zi Su Zi	Semen Perillae Frutescentis	Perilla Seed
Peucedanum	Qian Hu	Radix Peucedani	Hogfennel Root
Pharbitis	Qian Niu Zi	Semen Pharbitidis	Morning Glory Seed
Phaseolus	Chi Xiao Dou	Semen Phaseoli Calcarati	Aduki Bean
Phaseolus	Lu Dou	Semen Phaseoli Radiati	Mung Bean
Phellodendron	Huang Bai	Cortex Phellodendri	Amur Cork-tree Bark
Pheretima	Di Long	Lumbricus	Earthworm
Phoca	Hai Gou Shen	Testes et Penis Otariae*	Male Seal Sexual Organs
Phragmites	Lu Gen	Rhizoma Phragmitis Communis	Reed Rhizome; Corrizo Rhizome
Physalis	Suan Jiang	Calyx seu Fructus Physalis*	Wintercherry Calyx or Fruit
Phytolacca	Shang Lu	Radix Phytolaccae	Poke Root
Picrorhiza	Hu Huang Lian	Rhizoma Picrorhizae	Picrorhiza Rhizome
Pinellia	(Fa) Ban Xia	Rhizoma Pinelliae Ternatae	Prepared Pinellia Rhizome
Pinellia	(Sheng) Ban Xia	Rhizoma Pinelliae Ternatae	Raw Pinellia Rhizome
Pinus	Song Jie	Lignum Pini Nodi	Knotty Pine Wood
Piper	Bi Ba	Fructus Piperis Longi	Long Pepper Fruit
Piper	Bi Cheng Qie	Fructus Cubebae	Cubeba Fruit
Piper	Hai Feng Teng	Caulis Piperis Futokadsurae	Kadsura Stem
Piper	Hu Jiao	Fructus Piperis Nigri	Black Pepper Fruit
Plantago	Che Qian Cao	Herba Plantaginis	Plantago; Plantain
Plantago	Che Qian Zi	Semen Plantaginis	Plantago Seed; Plantain Seed
Platycodon	(Ku) Jie Geng	Radix Platycodi Grandiflori	Ballonflower Root; Bellflower Root; Bitter Jie Geng
Polistes	Lu Feng Fang	Nidus Vespae	Hornet Nest; Wasp Nest
Polygala	Yuan Zhi	Radix Polygalae Tenuifoliae	Chinese Senega Root; Seneca Snakeroot
Polygonatum	Huang Jing	Rhizoma Polygonati	Siberian Solomon Seal Rhizome
Polygonatum	Yu Zhu	Rhizoma Polygonati Odorati	Fragrant Solomon's Seal Rhizome; Polygonatum
Polygonum	Bian Xu	Herba Polygoni Avicularis	Avicularis; Knotweed
Polygonum	Guan Ye Liao	Herba Polygoni Perfoliati*	Polygonum

Botanical	Pinyin	Pharmaceutical	Common
Polygonum	Hu Zhang	Radix et Rhizoma Polygoni Cuspidati	Giant Knotweed Rhizome
Polygonum	Ye Jiao Teng	Caulis Polygoni Multiflori	Fleeceflower Stem; Fo-Ti Stem
Polygonum	He Shou Wu	Radix Polygoni Multiflori	Fleeceflower Root; Fo-Ti Root
Polyporus	Zhu Ling	Sclerotium Polypori Umbellati	Polyporus Sclerotium
Poria	Chi Fu Ling	Sclerotium Poriae Cocos Rubrae	Red Hoelen; Red Tuckahoe
Poria	Fu Ling	Sclerotium Poriae Cocos	Hoelen; China Root; Tuckahoe; Indian Bread
Poria	Fu Ling Pi	Cortex Poriae Cocos	Tuckahoe Skin
Poria Cocos	Fu Shen	Sclerotium Poriae Cocos Pararadicis	Tuckahoe Spirit
Portulaca	Ma Chi Xian	Herba Portulacae Oleraceae	Purslane
Potentilla	Fan Bai Cao	Herba Potentillae Discoloris*	Potentilla
Prunella	Xia Ku Cao	Spica Prunellae Vulgaris	Selfheal Spike; Heal all Spike
Prunus	Tao Ren	Semen Persicae	Peach Seed (Kernel)
Prunus	Wu Mei	Fructus Pruni Mume	Ume Plum Fruit; Black Plum Fruit
Prunus	(Bei) Xing Ren	Semen Pruni Armeniacae	(Northern) Apricot Seed
Prunus	(Nan) Xing Ren	Semen Pruni Armeniacae	(Southern) Apricot Seed
Prunus	Yu Li Ren	Semen Pruni	Bush Cherry Seed
Pseudostellaria	Tai Zi Shen	Radix Pseudostellariae Heterophyllae	Prince Ginseng Root
Psoralea	Bu Gu Zhi	Fructus Psoraleae Corylifoliae	Scurfy Pea Fruit
Pteria	Zhen Zhu	Margarita	Pearl
Pteria	Zhen Zhu Mu	Concha Margaritiferae	Mother-of-Pearl Shell
Pteris	Feng Wei Cao	Herba Pterii*	Pteris
Pueraria	Ge Gen	Radix Puerariae	Kudzu Root
Pueraria	Ge Hua	Flos Puerariae	Kudzu Flower
Pulsatilla	Bai Tou Weng	Radix Pulsatillae Chinensis	Pulsatilla Root; Anemone Root
Pumice	Fu Hai Shi	Pumice	Pumice
Punica	Shi Liu Gen Pi	Cortex Punicae Granati Radicis	Pomegranate Root Bark
Punica	Shi Liu Pi	Pericarpium Punicae Granati	Pomegranate Husk or Rind
Pyritum	Zi Ran Tong	Pyritum	Pyrite
Pyrola	Lu Xian Cao	Herba Pyrolae*	Pyrola
Pyrrosia	Shi Wei	Folium Pyrrosiae	Pyrrosia Leaf
Pyrus	Li Pi	Pericarpium Pyri*	Pear Peel

Botanical	Pinyin	Pharmaceutical	Common
Quisqualis	Shi Jun Zi	Fructus Quisqualis Indicae	Rangoon Creeper Fruit
Ranunculus	Mao Zhao Cao	Radix Ranunculi Ternati*	Buttercup Root
Raphanus	Lai Fu Zi	Semen Raphani Satavi	Radish Seed
Realgar	Xiong Huang	Realgar	Realgar; Arsenic Disulfide
Rehmannia	Sheng Di Huang	Radix Rehmanniae Glutinosae	Fresh Chinese Foxglove Root
Rehmannia	Shu Di Huang	Radix Rehmanniae Glutinosae Conquitae	Wine-cooked Chinese Foxglove Root
Rhaponticum or Echinops	Lou Lu	Radix Rhapontici seu Echinops	Rhaponticum Root; Echinops Root
Rheum	Da Huang	Radix et Rhizoma Rhei	Rhubarb Root and Rhizome
Rhinoceros	Xi Jiao	Cornu Rhinoceri	Rhinoceros Horn
Rhodea	Wan Nian Qing	Herba Rhodeae Japonicae*	Rhodea
Rhododendron	Man Shan Hong	Folium Rhododendri*	Rhododendron Leaf
Rhus	Gan Qi	Lacca Sinica Exsiccatae	Laquer
Rhus	Yan Fu Mu	Cortex Rhois Chinensis*	Chinese Sumac Bark
Rhus/Melaphis	Wu Bei Zi	Galla Rhois Chinensis	Gallnut of Chinese Sumac
Rorippa	Han Cai	Herba Rorippae*	Rorippa
Rosa	Jin Ying Zi	Fructus Rosae Laevigatae	Cherokee Rose Fruit / Rosehip
Rosa	Mei Gui Hua	Flos Rosae Rugosae	Young Chinese Rose Flower
Rosa	Yue Ji Hua	Flos et Fructus Rosae Chinensis	Partially-blossoming Chinese Tea Rose Flower
Rubia	Qian Cao Gen	Radix Rubiae Cordifoliae	Madder Root
Rubus	Fu Pen Zi	Fructus Rubi Chingii	Raspberry Fruit Bud
Rubus	Mao Mei	Herba Rubi Parvifolii*	Thimbleberry
Saccharum Granorum	Yi Tang	Saccharum Granorum	Barley Malt Sugar/Syrup
Saiga	Ling Yang Jiao	Cornu Antelopis	Antelope Horn
Salvia	Dan Shen	Radix Salviae Miltiorrhizae	Red Sage Root
Salvia	Ji Ning	Herba Salviae Plebeia*	Salvia
Sambucus	Lu Ying	Cortex Sambuci*	Japanese Elder Bark
Sanguisorba	Di Yu	Radix Sanguisorbae Officinalis	Burnet-bloodwort Root
Santalum	Tan Xiang	Lignum Santali Albi	Sandalwood Heartwood
Sapium	Wu Jiu Gen Pi	Cortex Sappii Sebiferi Radicis*	Tallow Tree Root Bark
Sargassum	Hai Zao	Herba Sargassii	Sargassum Seaweed
Sargentodoxa	Hong Teng	Caulis Sargentodoxae Cuneatae	Sargentodoxa Stem
Saururus	San Bai Cao	Herba Saururi Chinensis*	Saururus
Saussurea	Mu Xiang	Radix Saussureae Lappae	Costus Root; Aucklandia

Botanical	Pinyin	Pharmaceutical	Common
Saxifrage	Hu Er Cao	Herba Saxifragae Stoloniferae*	Saxifrage
Schisandra	Nan Wu Wei Zi	Fructus Schisandrae Sphenantherae	Southern Schisandra Fruit
Schisandra	Wu Wei Zi	Fructus Schisandrae Chinensis	Northern Schisandra Fruit
Schizonepeta	Jing Jie	Herba Schizonepetae Tenuifoliae	Schizonepeta Stem or Bud
Scolopendra	Wu Gong	Scolopendra Subspinipes	Centipede
Scrophularia	Xuan Shen	Radix Scrophulariae Ningpoensis	Figwort Root
Scutellaria	Ban Zhi Lian	Herba Scutellariae Barbatae	Barbat Scullcap
Scutellaria	Huang Qin	Radix Scutellariae Baicalensis	Scute; Baical Skullcap Root
Sedum	Chui Pen Cao	Herba Sedii Sarmentosi*	Stonecrop
Sedum	Jing Tian San Qi	Herba Sedi*	Sedum
Selaginella	Shi Shang Bai	Herba Selaginellae Doederleinii	Selaginella
Senecio	Qian Li Guang	Herba Senecionis Scandentis*	Groundsel
Sepia or Sepiella	Hai Piao Xiao	Os Sepiae seu Sepiellae	Cuttle-fish Bone
Sesamum	Hei Zhi Ma	Semen Sesami Indici	Black Sesame Seed
Siegesbeckia	Xi Xian Cao	Herba Siegesbeckiae	St. Paul's Wort
Smilax	Ba Qia	Rhizoma Smilacis China*	Smilax Rhizome
Smilax	Tu Fu Ling	Rhizoma Smilacis Glabrae	Glabrous Greenbrier Rhizome
Smithsonitum	Lu Gan Shi	Smithsonitum	Smithsonite; Calamine
Solenognathus	Hai Long	Hailong	Pipe-fish
Sophora	Huai Hua Mi	Flos Sophorae Japonicae Immaturus	Pagoda Tree Flower Bud
Sophora	Huai Jiao	Fructus Sophorae Japonicae	Pagoda Tree Fruit
Sophora	Ku Shen	Radix Sophorae Flavenscentis	Bitter Ginseng Root
Sophora	Shan Dou Gen	Radix Sophorae Tonkinensis	Pigeon Pea Root
Sparganium	San Leng	Rhizoma Sparganii Stoloniferi	Bur-reed Rhizome
Spirodela or Lemna	Fu Ping	Herba Lemnae seu Spirodelae	Duckweed
Stalactitum	E Guan Shi	Stalactitum	Stalactite Tubular Tip
Stellaria	Yin Chai Hu	Radix Stellariae Dichotomae	Stellaria Root
Stemona	Bai Bu	Radix Stemonae	Stemona Root
Stephania	Han Fang Ji	Radix Stephaniae Tetrandrae	Stephania Root
Sterculia	Pang Da Hai	Semen Sterculiae Scaphigerae	Sterculia Seed

Botanical

Botanical	Pinyin	Pharmaceutical	Common
Strichopus	Hai Shen	Strichopus Japonicus	Sea Cucumber; Sea Slug
Strychnos	Ma Qian Zi	Semen Strychni	Nux-vomica Seed
Styrax	An Xi Xiang	Benzoinum	Processed Resin of Styrax Benzoin
Succinum	Hu Po	Succinum	Amber; Fossilized Resin of Pine Tree
Sulphur	Liu Huang	Sulphur	Sulphur
Syringa	Bao Ma Zi	Cortex Syringae*	Manchurian Lilac Bark
Tabanus	Meng Chong	Tabani Bivittati*	Gadfly
Talcum	Hua Shi	Talcum	Talc; Soapstone
Tamarix	Cheng Liu	Cacumen Tamaricis Chinensis*	Tamarisk
Taraxacum	Pu Gong Ying	Herba Taraxaci Mongolici cum Radice	Dandelion
Terminalia	He Zi	Fructus Terminaliae Chebulae	Myrobalan Fruit
Terra Flava Usta	Fu Long Gan	Terra Flava Usta	Ignited Wood Stove Earth
Tetrapanax	Tong Cao	Medulla Tetrapanacis Papyriferi	Rice Paper Pith
Thalictrum	Tang Song Cao	Herba Thalictri Foliolosi*	Thalictrum
Tinospora	Jin Guo Lan	Radix Tinosporae Capillipes*	Tinospora Root
Tinospora	Kuan Jin Teng	Ramus Tinosporae Sinensis	Tinospora Stem
Torreya	Fei Zi	Semen Torreyae Grandis	Torreya Seed
Trachelospermum	Luo Shi Teng	Caulis Trachelospermi Jasminoidis	Star Jasmine Stem
Trachycarpus	Zong Lu Pi Tan	Fibra Stipulae Trachycarpi Carbonisatus	Charred Windmill Palm Petiole
Tremella	Bai Mu Er	Fructificatio Tremellae Fuciformis	Tremella Fungus Fruiting Body
Tribulus	Bai Ji Li	Fructus Tribuli Terrestris	Puncture Vine Fruit; Caltrop Fruit
Trichosanthes	Gua Lou	Fructus Trichosanthis	Snakegourd Fruit
Trichosanthes	Gua Lou Pi	Pericarpium Trichosanthis	Snakegourd Peel
Trichosanthes	Gua Lou Ren	Semen Trichosanthis	Snakegourd Seed
Trichosanthes	Tian Hua Fen	Radix Trichosanthis Kirilowii	Snakegourd Root
Trigonella	Hu Lu Ba	Semen Trigonellae Foeni-graeci	Fenugreek Seed
Triticum	Fu Xiao Mai	Semen Tritici Aestivi Levis	Wheat Chaff/Grain
Trogopterus or Pteromys	Wu Ling Zhi	Excrementum Trogopteri seu Pteromi	Flying Squirrel Feces
Tulipa	Shan Ci Gu	Pseudobulbus Shancigu	Chinese Tulip Bulb
Tussilago	Kuan Dong Hua	Flos Tussilaginis Farfarae	Coltsfoot Flower
Typha	(Sheng) Pu Huang	Pollen Typhae	Raw Cattail Pollen
Typha	Pu Huang Tan	Pollen Typhae Carbonisatus	Charred Cattail Pollen

Botanical	Pinyin	Pharmaceutical	Common
Typha	Pu Hui	Folium Typhae	Cattail Leaves
Typhonium	Bai Fu Zi	Rhizoma Typhonii Gigantei	Typhonium Rhizome
Ulmus	Wu Yi	Praepartio Fructus Ulmi Macrocarpi	Stinking Elm Fruit Paste
Uncaria	Gou Teng	Ramulus cum Uncis Uncariae	Gambir vine Stems and Hooks
Ursus	Xiong Dan	Vesica Fellea Ursi	Bear Gallbladder
Vaccaria	Wang Bu Liu Xing	Semen Vaccariae Segetalis	Cow Soapwort Seed
Veratrum	Li Lu	Radix et Rhizoma Veratri	Veratrum Root
Verbena	Ma Bian Cao	Herba Verbenae*	Vervain
Vespertilio	Ye Ming Sha	Excrementum Vespertilionis Murini	Bat Dung or Feces
Viola	Zi Hua Di Ding	Herba cum Radice Violae Yedoensitis	Viola
Vitex	Man Jing Zi	Fructus Viticis	Vitex Fruit
Xanthium	Cang Er Zi	Fructus Xanthii Sibirici	Xanthium Fruit; Cocklebur Fruit
Zanthoxylum	Chuan Jiao	Pericarpum Zanthoxyli Bungeani	Sichuan Pepper Fruit
Zanthoxylum	Chuan Jiao Mu	Semen Zanthoxyli Bungeani	Sichuan Pepper Seed
Zanthoxylum	(Chuan) Jiao Mu	Semen Zanthoxyli Bungeani	Sichuan Pepper Seed
Zaocys	She Tui	Exuviae Serpentis	Snake Skin Slough
Zaocys	Wu Shao She	Zaocys Dhumnades	Black-striped Snake
Zea	Yu Mi Xu	Stylus Zeae Mays	Cornsilk
Zingiber	Gan Jiang	Rhizoma Zingiberis Officinalis	Dried Ginger Rhizome
Zingiber	Pao Jiang	Rhizoma Zingiberis*	Quick-fried Ginger Rhizome
Zingiber	Sheng Jiang	Rhizoma Zingiberis Officinalis Recens	Fresh Ginger Rhizome
Zingiber	Sheng Jiang Pi	Cortex Zingiberis Officinalis Recens	Fresh Ginger Skin
Ziziphus	Da Zao	Fructus Ziziphi Jujubae	Jujube Fruit; Chinese Black Date
Ziziphus	Hong Zao	Fructus Ziziphi Jujubae	Jujube Fruit; Chinese Red Date
Ziziphus	Suan Zao Ren	Semen Ziziphi Spinosae	Sour Jujube Seed; Zizyphus

Botanical

Herb Name Cross Reference Keyed to Pharmaceutical Names

Pharmaceutical	Pinyin	Botanical	Common
Actinolitum	Yang Qi Shi	Actinolitum	Actinolite
Agkistrodon seu Bungarus	Bai Hua She	Agkistrodon	Long-noded Pit Viper Snake
Alumen	Ming Fan	Alumen	Alum; Potassium Aluminum Sulfate
Alumen Praeparatum	Ku Fan	Alumen Praeparatum	Prepared Alum
Arillus Euphoriae Longanae	Long Yan Rou	Euphoria	Longan Fruit Flesh
Arsenicum	Pi Shi	Arsenolite	White Arsenic
Aspongopus*	Jiu Xiang Chong	Aspongopus	Stink Bug
Aurum*	Huang Jin	Aurum	Gold
Benzoinum	An Xi Xiang	Styrax	Processed Resin of Styrax Benzoin
Bombyx Batryticatus	Jiang Can	Bombyx	Dead Stiff Body of Sick Silkworm Larvae
Borax	Peng Sha	Borax	Borax; Sodium Tetraborate
Borneol	Bing Pian	Dryobalanops	Processed Resin of Borneol Camphor
Bulbus Allii	Xie Bai	Allium	Chinese Chive Bulb
Bulbus Allii Fistulosi	Cong Bai	Allium	White Bulb of Green Onion or Scallion
Bulbus Allii Sativi	Da Suan	Allium	Garlic Bulb
Bulbus Fritillariae Cirrhosae	Chuan Bei Mu	Fritillaria	Tendrilled Fritillary Bulb
Bulbus Fritillariae Thunbergii	Zhe Bei Mu	Fritillaria	Thunberg Fritillary Bulb
Bulbus Lilii	Bai He	Lilium	Lily Bulb
Buthus Martensi	Quan Xie	Buthus	Scorpion
Cacumen Biotae Orientalis	Ce Bai Ye	Biota	Arborvitae Leafy Twig
Cacumen Tamaricis Chinensis*	Cheng Liu	Tamarix	Tamarisk
Calcaria*	Chen Shi Huei	Calcaria	Calcium Hydroxide
Calcitum	Han Shui Shi	Calcitum	Calcite
Calculus Artificialis	Ren Gong Niu Huang	Bos	Artificially Induced Cow Gallstons
Calculus Bovis seu Calculus Bubali	Niu Huang	Bos or Bubalis	Ox or Water Buffalo Gallstone
Calculus Macacae Mulattae	Hou Zao	Macaca	Macaque Gallstone
Calomelas	Qing Fen	Calomelas	Calomel; Mercurous Chloride
Calyx Diospyri Kaki	Shi Di	Diospyros	Persimmon Calyx
Calyx seu Fructus Physalis*	Suan Jiang	Physalis	Wintercherry Calyx or Fruit

Pharmaceutical

Pharmaceutical	Pinyin	Botanical	Common
Camphora	Zhang Nao	Cinnamomum	Crystalized Volatile Oil of the Camphor Tree
Caput Radicis Angelicae Sinensis	Dang Gui Tou	Angelica	Tangkuei Head
Carapax Amydae Sinensis	Bie Jia	Amyda	Chinese Soft-shell Turtle Shell
Carapax Eretmochelydis Imbricatae*	Dai Mao	Eretmochelys	Hawksbill Turtle Shell
Caulis Bambusae in Taeniis	Zhu Ru	Bambusa	Bamboo Shavings
Caulis Mutong	Mu Tong	Akebia	Akebia Stem
Caulis Paederiae*	Ji Shi Teng	Paederia	Paederia Stem
Caulis Piperis Futokadsurae	Hai Feng Teng	Piper	Kadsura Stem
Caulis Polygoni Multiflori	Ye Jiao Teng	Polygonum	Fleeceflower Stem; Fo-Ti Stem
Caulis Sargentodoxae Cuneatae	Hong Teng	Sargentodoxa	Sargentodoxa Stem
Caulis Trachelospermi Jasminoidis	Luo Shi Teng	Trachelospermum	Star Jasmine Stem
Cervix Ginseng	Ren Shen Lu	Panax	Ginseng Root Neck
Chalcanthitum*	Dan Fan	Chalcanthitum	Copper Sulphate; Blue Vitriol
Cinnabaris	Zhu Sha	Cinnabaris	Cinnabar; Red Mercury Sulfide
Colla Cornu Cervi	Lu Jiao Jiao	Cervus	Mature Antler Glue; Mature Antler Gelatin
Concha Arcae	Wa Leng Zi	Arca	Cockle Shell; Ark Shell
Concha Cyclinae Sinensis	Hai Ge Ke	Cyclina	Clam Shell
Concha Haliotidis	Shi Jue Ming	Haliotis	Abalone Shell
Concha Margaritiferae	Zhen Zhu Mu	Pteria	Mother-of-Pearl Shell
Concha Ostreae	Mu Li	Ostrea	Oyster Shell
Concha Ostreae	Duan Mu Li	Ostrea	Calcined Oyster Shell
Concretio Silicea Bambusae Textillis	Tian Zhu Huang	Bambusa	Siliceous Secretions of Bamboo
Cordyceps Sinensis	Dong Chong Xia Cao	Cordyceps	Chinese Caterpillar Fungus
Cornu Antelopis	Ling Yang Jiao	Saiga	Antelope Horn
Cornu Bubali	Shui Niu Jiao	Bubalus	Waterbuffalo Horn
Cornu Cervi	Lu Jiao	Cervus	Antler; Deerhorn; Ossified Horn of the Mature Male Deer
Cornu Cervi Degelatinatium	Lu Jiao Shuang	Cervus	Antler Powder from the dregs of cooking Antler Glue
Cornu Cervi Parvum	Lu Rong	Cervus	Young Deer Antler Velvet
Cornu Naemorhedis	Shan Yang Jiao	Naemorhedis	Goat Horn
Cornu Rhinoceri	Xi Jiao	Rhinoceros	Rhinoceros Horn

Pharmaceutical	Pinyin	Botanical	Common
Cortex Acanthopanacis Gracilistyli Radicis	Wu Jia Pi	Acanthopanax	Acanthopanax Rootbark.
Cortex Ailanthi Altissimae	Chun Pi	Ailanthus	Tree of Heaven Bark
Cortex Albizziae Julibrissin	He Huan Pi	Albizzia	Mimosa Tree Bark; Silktree Bark
Cortex Cinnamomi Cassiae	Rou Gui	Cinnamomum	Cinnamon Bark
Cortex Dictamni Dasycarpi Radicis	Bai Xian Pi	Dictamnus	Dittany Root Bark
Cortex Erythrinae	Hai Tong Pi	Erythrina	Coral-bean Bark
Cortex Eucommiae Ulmoidis	Du Zhong	Eucommia	Eucommia Bark
Cortex Fraxini	Qin Pi	Fraxinus	Korean Ash Bark
Cortex Loropetali*	Ji Mu	Loropetalum	Loropetalum Bark
Cortex Lycii Radicis	Di Gu Pi	Lycium	Matrimony-vine Rootbark; Wolfberry Bark
Cortex Magnoliae Officinalis	Hou Po	Magnolia	Magnolia Bark
Cortex Meliae	Ku Lian Mu Pi	Melia	Sichuan Chinaberry Tree Bark; Sichuan Pagoda Tree Bark; Neem Tree Bark
Cortex Meliae Radicis	Ku Lian Gen Pi	Melia	Sichuan Chinaberry Root Bark; Sichuan Pagoda Tree Root Bark; Neem Root Bark
Cortex Mori Albae Radicis	Sang Bai Pi	Morus	Mulberry Rootbark
Cortex Moutan Radicis	Mu Dan Pi	Paeonia	Tree Peony Rootbark
Cortex Phellodendri	Huang Bai	Phellodendron	Amur Cork-tree Bark
Cortex Poriae Cocos	Fu Ling Pi	Poria	Tuckahoe Skin
Cortex Punicae Granati Radicis	Shi Liu Gen Pi	Punica	Pomegranate Root Bark
Cortex Rhois Chinensis*	Yan Fu Mu	Rhus	Chinese Sumac Bark
Cortex Sambuci*	Lu Ying	Sambucus	Japanese Elder Bark
Cortex Sappii Sebiferi Radicis*	Wu Jiu Gen Pi	Sapium	Tallow Tree Root Bark
Cortex Syringae*	Bao Ma Zi	Syringa	Manchurian Lilac Bark
Cortex Tubiformis Cinnamomi Cassiae	Guan Gui	Cinnamomum	Thin Cinnamon Bark from Young Trees
Cortex Zingiberis Officinalis Recens	Sheng Jiang Pi	Zingiber	Fresh Ginger Skin
Crinis Carbonisatus Hominis	Xue Yu Tan	Homo Sapiens	Charred Human Hair
Dens Draconis	Long Chi	Dens Draconis	Dragon Tooth; Fossilized Tooth
Endothelium Corneum Gigeriae Galli	Ji Nei Jin	Gallus	Chicken Gizard Lining

Pharmaceutical

Pharmaceutical	Pinyin	Botanical	Common
Epicarpium Benincasae Hispidae	Dong Gua Pi	Benincasa	Wintermelon Fruit Peel; Wax Gourd Fruit Peel
Eupolyphaga seu Opisthoplatia	Tu Bie Chong	Eupolyphaga	Wingless Cockroach
Excrementum Bombycis Mori	Can Sha	Bombyx	Silkworm Feces
Excrementum Trogopteri seu Pteromi	Wu Ling Zhi	Trogopterus or Pteromys	Flying Squirrel Feces
Excrementum Vespertilionis Murini	Ye Ming Sha	Vespertilio	Bat Dung or Feces
Extremas Radicis Angelicae Sinensis	Dang Gui Wei	Angelica	Tangkuei Tail
Exuviae Serpentis	She Tui	Zaocys	Snake Skin Slough
Fasciculus Vascularis Luffae	Si Gua Lou	Luffa	Dried Skeleton of Luffa Sponge
Fibra Stipulae Trachycarpi Carbonisatus	Zong Lu Pi Tan	Trachycarpus	Charred Windmill Palm Petiole
Flos Albizziae Julibrissin*	He Huan Hua	Albizzia	Mimosa Tree Flower; Silktree Flower
Flos Amomi	Sha Ren Hua	Amomum	Grains-of-Paradise Flower
Flos Buddleiae Officinalis Immaturus	Mi Meng Hua	Buddleia	Buddleia Flower
Flos Carthami Tinctorii	Hong Hua	Carthamus	Safflower
Flos Caryophylli	Ding Xiang	Eugenia	Clove Flower-bud
Flos Celosiae Cristatae	Ji Guan Hua	Celosia	Cockscomb Flower
Flos Chrysanthemi Indici	Ye Ju Hua	Chrysanthemum	Wild Chrysanthemum Flower
Flos Chrysanthemi Morifolii	(Bai) Ju Hua	Chrysanthemum	White Chrysanthemum Flower
Flos Chrysanthemi Morifolii	(Huang) Ju Hua	Chrysanthemum	Yellow Chrysanthemum Flower
Flos Citri Sarcodactylis	Fo Shou Hua	Citrus	Finger Citron Flower
Flos Daphnes Genkwa	Yuan Hua	Daphne	Daphne Flower
Flos Dolichoris Lablab	Bian Dou Hua	Dolichos	Hyacinth Bean Flower
Flos et Fructus Rosae Chinensis	Yue Ji Hua	Rosa	Partially-blossoming Chinese Tea Rose Flower
Flos Hydrangeae Macrophyllae*	Ba Xian Hua	Hydrangea	Hydrangea Flower
Flos Imperatae Cylindricae	Bai Mao Hua	Imperata	Wooly Grass Flower; White Grass Flower
Flos Inulae	Xuan Fu Hua	Inula	Elecampane Flower
Flos Lonicerae Japonicae	Jin Yin Hua	Lonicera	Honeysuckle Flower
Flos Magnoliae	Xin Yi Hua	Magnolia	Magnolia Flower
Flos Magnoliae Officinalis	Hou Po Hua	Magnolia	Magnolia Flower
Flos Pseudoginseng	San Qi Hua	Panax	Pseudoginseng Flower; Notoginseng Flower
Flos Puerariae	Ge Hua	Pueraria	Kudzu Flower

Pharmaceutical	Pinyin	Botanical	Common
Flos Rosae Rugosae	Mei Gui Hua	Rosa	Young Chinese Rose Flower
Flos Sophorae Japonicae Immaturus	Huai Hua Mi	Sophora	Pagoda Tree Flower Bud
Flos Tussilaginis Farfarae	Kuan Dong Hua	Tussilago	Coltsfoot Flower
Fluoritum	Zi Shi Ying	Fluoritum	Fluorite
Folium Artemisiae Argyi	Ai Ye	Artemisia	Mugwort Leaf
Folium Callicarpae	Zi Zhu	Callicarpa	Callicarpa Leaf
Folium Clerodendri Trichotomi	Chou Wu Tong	Clerodendron	Glorybower Leaf
Folium Daqingye	Da Qing Ye	Isatis	Isatis Leaf; Woad Leaf
Folium Dichroae Febrifugae	Shu Qi	Dichroa	Dichroa Leaf
Folium Eleagni Pungens	Hu Tui Ye	Eleagnus	Eleagnus Leaf
Folium Eriobotryae Japonicae	Pi Pa Ye	Eriobotrya	Loquat Leaf
Folium Ginkgo Bilobae	Yin Guo Ye	Ginkgo	Ginkgo Leaf
Folium Ginseng	Ren Shen Ye	Panax	Ginseng Leaf
Folium Gynurae*	Ju Ye San Qi	Gynura	Gynura Leaf
Folium Ilicis Chinensis*	Si Ji Qing	Ilex	Holly Leaf
Folium Mahoniae*	Shi Da Gong Lao	Mahonia	Mahonia Leaf
Folium Momordicae Grosvenori	Luo Huo Guo Ye	Momordica	Momordica Leaf
Folium Mori Albae	Sang Ye	Morus	Mulberry Leaf
Folium Nelumbinis Nuciferae	He Ye	Nelumbo	Lotus Leaf
Folium Perillae Frutescentis	Zi Su Ye	Perilla	Perilla Leaf
Folium Pyrrosiae	Shi Wei	Pyrrosia	Pyrrosia Leaf
Folium Rhododendri*	Man Shan Hong	Rhododendron	Rhododendron Leaf
Folium Sennae	Fan Xie Ye	Cassia	Senna Leaf
Folium Typhae	Pu Hui	Typha	Cattail Leaves
Fructificatio Ganodermae Lucidi*	Ling Zhi	Ganoderma	Lucid Ganoderma; Reishi
Fructificatio Lasiosphaerae seu Calvatiae	Ma Bo	Lasiosphaera	Puffball Fruiting Body
Fructificatio Tremellae Fuciformis	Bai Mu Er	Tremella	Tremella Fungus Fruiting Body
Fructus Akebiae	Ba Yue Zha	Akebia	Akebia Fruit
Fructus Alpiniae Oxyphyllae	Yi Zhi Ren	Alpinia	Black Cardamon Fruit
Fructus Amomi Kravanh	Bai Dou Kou	Amomum	Round Cardamon Fruit; Cluster Fruit
Fructus Amomi Tsao-Ko	Cao Guo	Amomum	Chinese Cardamon Fruit
Fructus Arctii Lappae	Niu Bang Zi	Arctium	Burdock Seed
Fructus Aristolochiae	Ma Dou Ling	Aristolochia	Birthwort Fruit
Fructus Bruceae Javanicae	Ya Dan Zi	Brucea	Brucea Fruit

Pharmaceutical

Pharmaceutical	Pinyin	Botanical	Common
Fructus Carpesii seu Daucusi	He Shi	Carpesium or Daucus	Carpesium Fruit
Fructus Citri Aurantii	Zhi Ke	Citrus or Poncirus	Bitter Orange Fruit
Fructus Citri Sarcodactylis	Fo Shou	Citrus	Finger Citron Fruit
Fructus Citrulli Vulgaris	Xi Gua	Citrullus	Watermelon Fruit and Peel or Rind
Fructus Cnidii Monnieri	She Chuang Zi	Cnidium	Cnidium Seed
Fructus Corni Officinalis	Shan Zhu Yu	Cornus	Dogwood Fruit; Asiatic Cornelian Cherry Fruit
Fructus Crataegi	Shan Zha	Crataegus	Hawthorn Unripe Fruit or Berry
Fructus Crataegi	Shan Zha Rou	Crataegus	Hawthorn Ripe Fruit or Berry
Fructus Crataegi Carbonisatus	Shan Zha Tan	Crataegus	Charred Hawthorn Fruit or Berry
Fructus Cubebae	Bi Cheng Qie	Piper	Cubeba Fruit
Fructus Diospyri Kaki*	Shi Bing	Diospyros	Dried Persimmon Fruit
Fructus Evodiae Rutaecarpae	Wu Zhu Yu	Evodia	Evodia Fruit
Fructus Foeniculi Vulgaris	Xiao Hui Xiang	Foeniculum	Fennel Fruit
Fructus Forsythiae Suspensae	Lian Qiao	Forsythia	Forsythia Fruit; Golden Bells
Fructus Gardeniae Jasminoidis	Zhi Zi	Gardenia	Gardenia Fruit
Fructus Gleditsiae Sinensis	Zao Jiao	Gleditsia	Honeylocust Fruit; Soap Bean Fruit
Fructus Hordei Vulgaris Germinatus	Mai Ya	Hordeum	Barley Sprout; Malted Barley
Fructus Illicii*	Ba Jiao Hui Xiang	Illicium	Star Anise Fruit
Fructus Immaturus Citri Aurantii	Zhi Shi	Citrus or Poncirus	Immature Bitter Orange Fruit
Fructus Kochiae Scopariae	Di Fu Zi	Kochia	Broom Cyperus Seed
Fructus Ligustri Lucidi	Nu Zhen Zi	Ligustrum	Privet Fruit; Waxtree Fruit
Fructus Liquidambaris Taiwanianae	Lu Lu Tong	Liquidambar	Sweetgum Fruit
Fructus Lycii	Gou Qi Zi	Lycium	Matrimony Vine Fruit; Wolfberry Fruit
Fructus Meliae Toosendan	Chuan Lian Zi	Melia	Sichuan Chinaberry Fruit; Sichuan Pagoda Tree Fruit; Neem Fruit
Fructus Momordicae Grosvenori	Luo Han Guo	Momordica	Momordica Fruit
Fructus Mori Albae	Sang Shen	Morus	Mulberry Fruit Bud
Fructus Oryzae Sativae Germinatus	Gu Ya	Oryza	Rice Sprout
Fructus Piperis Longi	Bi Ba	Piper	Long Pepper Fruit
Fructus Piperis Nigri	Hu Jiao	Piper	Black Pepper Fruit

Pharmaceutical	Pinyin	Botanical	Common
Fructus Pruni Mume	Wu Mei	Prunus	Ume Plum Fruit; Black Plum Fruit
Fructus Psoraleae Corylifoliae	Bu Gu Zhi	Psoralea	Scurfy Pea Fruit
Fructus Quisqualis Indicae	Shi Jun Zi	Quisqualis	Rangoon Creeper Fruit
Fructus Rosae Laevigatae	Jin Ying Zi	Rosa	Cherokee Rose Fruit / Rosehip
Fructus Rubi Chingii	Fu Pen Zi	Rubus	Raspberry Fruit Bud
Fructus Schisandrae Chinensis	Wu Wei Zi	Schisandra	Northern Schisandra Fruit
Fructus Schisandrae Sphenantherae	Nan Wu Wei Zi	Schisandra	Southern Schisandra Fruit
Fructus seu Semen Amomi	Sha Ren	Amomum	Grains-of-Paradise Fruit or Seeds
Fructus Sophorae Japonicae	Huai Jiao	Sophora	Pagoda Tree Fruit
Fructus Terminaliae Chebulae	He Zi	Terminalia	Myrobalan Fruit
Fructus Tribuli Terrestris	Bai Ji Li	Tribulus	Puncture Vine Fruit; Caltrop Fruit
Fructus Trichosanthis	Gua Lou	Trichosanthes	Snakegourd Fruit
Fructus Viticis	Man Jing Zi	Vitex	Vitex Fruit
Fructus Xanthii Sibirici	Cang Er Zi	Xanthium	Xanthium Fruit; Cocklebur Fruit
Fructus Ziziphi Jujubae	Da Zao	Ziziphus	Jujube Fruit; Chinese Black Date
Fructus Ziziphi Jujubae	Hong Zao	Ziziphus	Jujube Fruit; Chinese Red Date
Frusta Ferri	Sheng Tie Luo	Frusta Ferri	Iron Filing
Frutus Chaenomelis	Mu Gua	Chaenomeles	Chinese Quince Fruit
Galla Rhois Chinensis	Wu Bei Zi	Rhus/Melaphis	Gallnut of Chinese Sumac
Gekko	Ge Jie	Gekko	Gecko Lizard
Gelatinum Corii Asini	E Jiao	Equus	Donkey Hide Gelatin; Ass Skin Glue
Gummi Olibanum	Ru Xiang	Boswellia	Frankincense Gum-resin
Gypsum Fibrosum	Shi Gao	Gypsum	Gypsum; Calcium Sulphate
Haematitum	Dai Zhe Shi	Haematitum	Hematite; Iron Ore
Hailong	Hai Long	Solenognathus	Pipe-fish
Halloysitum Rubrum	Chi Shi Zhi	Halloysitum Rubrum	Halloysite; Red Kaolin
Herba Acalypae Australis*	Tie Xian	Acalypha	Acalypha
Herba Agastaches seu Pogostemi	Huo Xiang	Agastache or Pogostemon	Patchouli; Agastache
Herba Agrimoniae Pilosae	Xian He Cao	Agrimonia	Agrimony
Herba Ajugae Decumbentis*	Bai Mao Xia Ku Cao	Ajuga	Ajuga
Herba Aloes	Lu Hui	Aloe	Aloe Vera Leaf

Pharmaceutical	Pinyin	Botanical	Common
Herba Andrographitis Paniculatae	Chuan Xin Lian	Andrographis	Kariyat; Green Chiretta
Herba Androsacae Umbellatae*	Dian Di Mei	Androsace	Androsace
Herba Artemisiae Annuae	Qing Hao	Artemisia	Sweet Wormwood; Southernwood
Herba Artemisiae Anomalae	Liu Ji Nu	Artemisia	Artemisia
Herba Artemisiae Yinchenhao	Yin Chen Hao	Artemisia	Oriental Wormwood
Herba Begoniae Fimbristipulatae	Zi Bei Tian Kuei	Begonia	Begonia
Herba Capsellae*	Ji Cai	Capsella	Shepherd's Purse
Herba Carpesii	Tian Ming Jing	Carpesium	Carpesium
Herba Centipedae Minimae*	E Bu Shi Cao	Centipeda	Centipeda Herb
Herba Cephalanoplos	Xiao Ji	Cephalanoplos	Small Thistle; Field Thistle
Herba Cistanches Deserticolae	Rou Cong Rong	Cistanche	Broomrape Fleshy Stem
Herba Commelinae*	Ya Zhi Cao	Commelina	Commelina
Herba cum Radice Asari	Xi Xin	Asarum	Asarum; Chinese Wild Ginger
Herba cum Radice Houttuyniae Cordatae	Yu Xing Cao	Houttuynia	Houttuynia; Fish Smell Plant
Herba cum Radice Patriniae	Bai Jiang Cao	Patrinia or Thiaspi	Patrinia; Thiaspi
Herba cum Radice Violae Yedoensitis	Zi Hua Di Ding	Viola	Viola
Herba Cynomorii Songarici	Suo Yang	Cynomorium	Cynomorium Fleshy Stem
Herba Dendrobii	Shi Hu	Dendrobium	Dendrobium Stem
Herba Dianthi	Qu Mai	Dianthus	Pink Flower Herb
Herba Ecliptae Prostratae	Han Lian Cao	Eclipta	Eclipta
Herba Elsholtziae seu Moslae	Xiang Ru	Elsholtzia	Aromatic Madder
Herba Ephedrae	Ma Huang	Ephedra	Ephedra Stem
Herba Epimedii	Yin Yang Huo	Epimedium	Epimedium
Herba Equiseti Hiemalis	Mu Zei	Equisetum	Horsetail; Scouring Rush; Shavegrass
Herba Erodii seu Geranii*	Lao Guan Cao	Erodium or Geranium	Geranium; Heronbill; Cranebill
Herba Eupatorii Fortunei	Pei Lan	Eupatorium	Boneset; Thoroughwort; Feverwort
Herba Euphorbiae Helioscopiae	Ze Qi	Euphorbia	Pill-bearing Spurge
Herba Hederae Nepalensis*	Chang Chun Teng	Hedera	Ivy
Herba Inulae	Jin Fei Cao	Inula	Elecampane
Herba Laminaria Japonicae	Hai Dai	Laminaria	Algae

Pharmaceutical	Pinyin	Botanical	Common
Herba Lemnae seu Spirodelae	Fu Ping	Spirodela or Lemna	Duckweed
Herba Leonuri Heterophylli	Yi Mu Cao	Leonurus	Motherwort
Herba Lobeliae Chinensis cum Radice	Ban Bian Lian	Lobelia	Chinese Lobelia
Herba Lophatheri Gracilis	Dan Zhu Ye	Lophatherum	Bland Bamboo Leaf and Stem
Herba Lycopi Lucidi	Ze Lan	Lycopus	Bugleweed
Herba Lycopodii Clavati*	Shen Jin Cao	Lycopodium	Clubmoss
Herba Lygodii Japonici	Jin Sha Teng	Lygodium	Japanese Climbing Fern
Herba Lysimachiae	Jin Qian Cao	Lysimachia	Lysimachia
Herba Menthae Haplocalycis	Bo He	Mentha	Peppermint; Spearmint; Field Mint
Herba Oldenlandiae Diffusae	Bai Hua She She Cao	Oldenlandia	Oldenlandia
Herba Plantaginis	Che Qian Cao	Plantago	Plantago; Plantain
Herba Polygoni Avicularis	Bian Xu	Polygonum	Avicularis; Knotweed
Herba Polygoni Perfoliati*	Guan Ye Liao	Polygonum	Polygonum
Herba Portulacae Oleraceae	Ma Chi Xian	Portulaca	Purslane
Herba Potentillae Discoloris*	Fan Bai Cao	Potentilla	Potentilla
Herba Pterii*	Feng Wei Cao	Pteris	Pteris
Herba Pyrolae*	Lu Xian Cao	Pyrola	Pyrola
Herba Rhodeae Japonicae*	Wan Nian Qing	Rhodea	Rhodea
Herba Rorippae*	Han Cai	Rorippa	Rorippa
Herba Rubi Parvifolii*	Mao Mei	Rubus	Thimbleberry
Herba Salviae Plebeia*	Ji Ning	Salvia	Salvia
Herba Sargassii	Hai Zao	Sargassum	Sargassum Seaweed
Herba Saururi Chinensis*	San Bai Cao	Saururus	Saururus
Herba Saxifragae Stoloniferae*	Hu Er Cao	Saxifrage	Saxifrage
Herba Schizonepetae Tenuifoliae	Jing Jie	Schizonepeta	Schizonepeta Stem or Bud
Herba Scutellariae Barbatae	Ban Zhi Lian	Scutellaria	Barbat Scullcap
Herba Sedi*	Jing Tian San Qi	Sedum	Sedum
Herba Sedii Sarmentosi*	Chui Pen Cao	Sedum	Stonecrop
Herba Selaginellae Doederleinii	Shi Shang Bai	Selaginella	Selaginella
Herba Senecionis Scandentis*	Qian Li Guang	Senecio	Groundsel
Herba seu Folium Apocyni Veneti*	Luo Bu Ma	Apocynum	Red Dogbane Whole Herb or Leaf
Herba seu Radix Cirsii Japonici	Da Ji	Cirsium	Japanese Thistle
Herba Siegesbeckiae	Xi Xian Cao	Siegesbeckia	St. Paul's Wort

Pharmaceutical

Pharmaceutical	Pinyin	Botanical	Common
Herba Taraxaci Mongolici cum Radice	Pu Gong Ying	Taraxacum	Dandelion
Herba Thalictri Foliolosi*	Tang Song Cao	Thalictrum	Thalictrum
Herba Verbenae*	Ma Bian Cao	Verbena	Vervain
Hippocampus	Hai Ma	Hippocampus	Sea Horse
Hirudo seu Whitmania	Shui Zhi	Hirudo	Leech
Hydrargyrum	Shui Yin	Hydrargyrum	Mercury
Indigo Pulverata Levis	Qing Dai	Indigo	Indigo
Lacca Sinica Exsiccatae	Gan Qi	Rhus	Laquer
Lapis Micae seu Chloriti	Meng Shi	Lapis Micae seu Chloriti	Chlorite Schist; Lapis
Lignum Aquilariae	Chen Xiang	Aquilaria	Aloeswood Secretion or Sap
Lignum Dalbergiae Odoriferae	Jiang Xiang	Dalbergia	Dalbergia Heartwood
Lignum Pini Nodi	Song Jie	Pinus	Knotty Pine Wood
Lignum Santali Albi	Tan Xiang	Santalum	Sandalwood Heartwood
Lignum Sappan	Su Mu	Caesalpinia	Sappan Heartwood
Limonite	Yu Liang Shi	Limonite	Limonite
Lithargyrum	Mi Tuo Seng	Lithargyrum	Litharge; Galena
Lumbricus	Di Long	Pheretima	Earthworm
Magnetitum	Ci Shi	Magnetitum	Magnetite; Magnetic Iron Ore; Loadstone
Margarita	Zhen Zhu	Pteria	Pearl
Massa Fermentata	Shen Qu	Massa Fermentata	Medicated Leaven
Medulla Junci Effusi	Deng Xin Cao	Juncus	Rush Pith
Medulla Tetrapanacis Papyriferi	Tong Cao	Tetrapanax	Rice Paper Pith
Mel*	Feng Mi	Mel	Honey
Minium	Qian Dan	Minium	Red Lead Oxide
Mirabilitum	Mang Xiao	Mirabilitum	Mirabilite; Glauber's Salt
Mirabilitum Purum	Xuan Ming Fen	Mirabilitum	Pure Mirabilite; Pure Sodium Sulphate; Pure Glauber's Salt
Mylabris	Ban Mao	Mylabris	Cantharides; Chinese Blistering Beetle
Nidus Vespae	Lu Feng Fang	Polistes	Hornet Nest; Wasp Nest
Niter*	Xiao Shi	Niter	Silver
Nodus Nelumbinis Nuciferae Rhizomatis	Ou Jie	Nelumbo	Lotus Rhizome Node
Ootheca Mantidis	Sang Piao Xiao	Paratenodera	Praying Mantis Egg Case
Ophicalcitum	Hua Rui Shi	Ophicalcitum	Ophicalcite
Os Canine	Gou Gu	Canis	Dog Bone
Os Draconis	Duan Long Gu	Os Draconis	Calcined Dragon Bone; Calcined Fossilized Bone

Pharmaceutical	Pinyin	Botanical	Common
Os Draconis	Long Gu	Os Draconis	Dragon Bone; Fossilized Bone
Os Leopardis	Bao Gu	Panthera	Leopard Bone
Os Sepiae seu Sepiellae	Hai Piao Xiao	Sepia or Sepiella	Cuttle-fish Bone
Os Tigris	Hu Gu	Panthera	Tiger Bone
Pars Rubra Epicarpii Citri Erythrocarpae	Ju Hong	Citrus	Red Tangerine Peel
Pasta Acacia seu Uncaria	Er Cha	Acacia or Uncaria	Dried Paste of Concentrated Decoction of Black or White Cutch
Pedicellus Cucumeris	Gua Di	Cucumis	Melon Pedicle
Pericarpium Amomi	Sha Ren Ke	Amomum	Grains-of-Paradise Shell
Pericarpium Arachi*	Hua Sheng Yi	Arachis	Peanut Skin
Pericarpium Arecae Catechu	Da Fu Pi	Areca	Betelnut Husk
Pericarpium Citri Reticulatae	Chen Pi	Citrus	Tangerine Peel
Pericarpium Citri Reticulatae Viride	Qing Pi	Citrus	Immature (Green) Tangerine Peel
Pericarpium Luffae Acutangulae	Si Gua Pi	Luffa	Luffa Skin
Pericarpium Papaveris Somniferi	Ying Su Ke	Papaver	Opium Poppy Husk
Pericarpium Punicae Granati	Shi Liu Pi	Punica	Pomegranate Husk or Rind
Pericarpium Pyri*	Li Pi	Pyrus	Pear Peel
Pericarpium Trichosanthis	Gua Lou Pi	Trichosanthes	Snakegourd Peel
Pericarpum Zanthoxyli Bungeani	Chuan Jiao	Zanthoxylum	Sichuan Pepper Fruit
Periostracum Cicadae	Chan Tui	Cryptotympana	Cicada Skin; Cicada Moulting
Placenta Hominis	Zi He Che	Homo Sapiens	Human Placenta
Plastrum Testudinis	Gui Ban	Chinemys	Fresh Water Turtle Shell
Plumula Nelumbinis Nuciferae	Lian Xin	Nelumbo	Lotus Plumule
Pollen Typhae	(Sheng) Pu Huang	Typha	Raw Cattail Pollen
Pollen Typhae Carbonisatus	Pu Huang Tan	Typha	Charred Cattail Pollen
Praepartio Fructus Ulmi Macrocarpi	Wu Yi	Ulmus	Stinking Elm Fruit Paste
Pseudobulbus Shancigu	Shan Ci Gu	Tulipa	Chinese Tulip Bulb
Pulvis Arisaemae cum Felle Bovis	Dan Nan Xing	Arisaema	Powdered Jack-in-the-Pulpit Rhizome mixed with Cow Bile
Pumice	Fu Hai Shi	Pumice	Pumice
Pyritum	Zi Ran Tong	Pyritum	Pyrite
Radix Achyranthis Aspera	Tu Niu Xi	Achyranthes	Achyranthes Root
Radix Achyranthis Bidentatae	Huai Niu Xi	Achyranthes	Achyranthes Root

Pharmaceutical

Pharmaceutical	Pinyin	Botanical	Common
Radix Aconite Carmichaeli	Chuan Wu	Aconitum	Sichuan Aconite
Radix Aconiti	Wu Tou	Aconitum	Aconite Root
Radix Aconiti Kusnezoffii	Cao Wu	Aconitum	Wild Aconite
Radix Adenophorae	Nan Sha Shen	Adenophora	Ladybell Root; Southern Sand Root
Radix Adenophorae Trachelioidis	Gan Jie Geng	Adenophora	Sweet Jie Geng
Radix Ampelopsis Japonicae*	Bai Lian	Ampelopsis	Ampelopsis Root
Radix Anemarrhenae Asphodeloidis	Zhi Mu	Anemarrhena	Anemarrhena Root
Radix Angelicae Dahuricae	Bai Zhi	Angelica	Angelica Root
Radix Angelicae Pubescentis	Du Huo	Angelica	Pubescent Angelica Root
Radix Angelicae Sinensis	Dang Gui	Angelica	Tangkuei Root
Radix Ardisiae Crenatae*	Zhu Sha Gen	Ardisia	Ardisia Root
Radix Aristolochiae	Qing Mu Xiang	Aristolochia	Birthwort Root
Radix Aristolochiae Fangchi	Guang Fang Ji	Aristolochia or Cocculus	Aristolochia Root
Radix Asteris Tatarici	Zi Wan	Aster	Purple Aster Root
Radix Astragali Membranaceus	Huang Qi	Astragalus	Yellow Milk-vetch Root
Radix Boehmeriae Niveae*	Zhu Ma Gen	Boehmeria	Ramie Root
Radix Bupleuri	Chai Hu	Bupleurum	Thorowax Root; Hare's Ear Root
Radix Changii*	Ming Dang Shen	Changium	Changium Root
Radix Clematidis	Wei Ling Xian	Clematis	Clematis Root
Radix Codonopsitis Pilosulae	Dang Shen	Codonopsis	Asiabell Root
Radix Cyathulae Officinalis	Chuan Niu Xi	Cyathula	Cyathula Root
Radix Cynanchi Auriculati	Ge Shan Xiang	Cynanchum	Cynanchum Root
Radix Cynanchi Baiwei	Bai Wei	Cynanchum	Swallowort Root
Radix Dichroae Febrifugae	Chang Shan	Dichroa	Dichroa Root
Radix Dioscoreae Oppositae	Shan Yao	Dioscorea	Chinese Wild Yam Root
Radix Dipsaci Asperi	Xu Duan	Dipsacus	Teasel Root
Radix Ephedrae	Ma Huang Gen	Ephedra	Ephedra Root
Radix et Caulis Jixueteng	Ji Xue Teng	Millettia	Millettia Root and Vine; Chicken Blood Vine
Radix et Ramus Litseae Cubebae	Dou Chi Jiang	Litsea	Aromatic Litsea Root and Stem
Radix et Rhizoma Oryzae Glutinosae	Nuo Dao Gen Xu	Oryza	Sweet Rice Root and Rhizome
Radix et Rhizoma Polygoni Cuspidati	Hu Zhang	Polygonum	Giant Knotweed Rhizome
Radix et Rhizoma Rhei	Da Huang	Rheum	Rhubarb Root and Rhizome

Pharmaceutical	Pinyin	Botanical	Common
Radix et Rhizoma Veratri	Li Lu	Veratrum	Veratrum Root
Radix Euphorbiae Kansui	Gan Sui	Euphorbia	Kansui Spurge Root
Radix Euphorbiae seu Knoxiae	Jing Da Ji	Euphorbia or Knoxia	Peking Spurge Root
Radix Gentianae Longdancao	Long Dan Cao	Gentiana	Chinese Gentian Root
Radix Gentianae Qinjiao	Qin Jiao	Gentiana	Large-Leaf Gentian Root
Radix Ginseng	Bai Shen	Panax	Rock Candy cured White Ginseng Root
Radix Ginseng	Ji Lin Shen	Panax	Jilin Wild Ginseng
Radix Ginseng	(Hong) Ren Shen	Panax	Ginseng Root steamed until red
Radix Ginseng	Shen Xu	Panax	Rock Candy cured White Ginseng Root Tail
Radix Ginseng	Sheng Shai Shen	Panax	Fresh Dried Ginseng Root
Radix Ginseng	Ye Shan Shen	Panax	Wild Ginseng
Radix Glehniae Littoralis	Bei Sha Shen	Glehnia	Beech Silver-top Root; Northern Sand Root
Radix Glycyrrhizae Praeparata*	Zhi Gan Cao	Glycyrrhiza	Honey-fried Licorice Root
Radix Glycyrrhizae Uralensis	Gan Cao	Glycyrhiza	Licorice Root
Radix Gossypii Hirsuti*	Mian Hua Gen	Gossypium	Cotton Root
Radix Ilicis Pubescentis*	Mao Dong Qing	Ilex	Pubescent Holly Root
Radix Isatidis seu Baphicacanthi	Ban Lan Gen	Isatis	Isatis Root; Woad Root
Radix Lateralis Aconiti Carmichaeli Praeparata	(Hei)Fu Zi	Aconitum	Prepared Sichuan Aconite Root
Radix Ledebouriella Divaricatae	Fang Feng	Ledebouriella	Siler Root; Ledebouriella Root
Radix Ligustici Wallichii	Chuan Xiong	Ligusticum	Sichuan Lovage Root
Radix Linderae Strychnifoliae	Wu Yao	Lindera	Spicebush Root
Radix Lithospermi seu Arnebiae	Zi Cao	Lithospermum	Groomwell Root
Radix Morindae Officinalis	Ba Ji Tian	Morinda	Morinda Root
Radix Paeoniae Lactiflorae	Bai Shao	Paeonia	White Peony Root
Radix Paeoniae Rubra	Chi Shao	Paeonia	Red Peony Root
Radix Panacis Quinquefolii	Xi Yang Shen	Panax	American Ginseng Root
Radix Peucedani	Qian Hu	Peucedanum	Hogfennel Root
Radix Phytolaccae	Shang Lu	Phytolacca	Poke Root
Radix Platycodi Grandiflori	(Ku) Jie Geng	Platycodon	Ballonflower Root; Bellflower Root; Bitter Jie Geng
Radix Polygalae Tenuifoliae	Yuan Zhi	Polygala	Chinese Senega Root; Seneca Snakeroot

Pharmaceutical	Pinyin	Botanical	Common
Radix Polygoni Multiflori	He Shou Wu	Polygonum	Fleeceflower Root; Fo-Ti Root
Radix Pseudoginseng	San Qi	Panax	Pseudoginseng Root; Notoginseng Root
Radix Pseudostellariae Heterophyllae	Tai Zi Shen	Pseudostellaria	Prince Ginseng Root
Radix Puerariae	Ge Gen	Pueraria	Kudzu Root
Radix Pulsatillae Chinensis	Bai Tou Weng	Pulsatilla	Pulsatilla Root; Anemone Root
Radix Ranunculi Ternati*	Mao Zhao Cao	Ranunculus	Buttercup Root
Radix Rehmanniae Glutinosae	Sheng Di Huang	Rehmannia	Fresh Chinese Foxglove Root
Radix Rehmanniae Glutinosae Conquitae	Shu Di Huang	Rehmannia	Wine-cooked Chinese Foxglove Root
Radix Rhapontici seu Echinops	Lou Lu	Rhaponticum or Echinops	Rhaponticum Root; Echinops Root
Radix Rubiae Cordifoliae	Qian Cao Gen	Rubia	Madder Root
Radix Salviae Miltiorrhizae	Dan Shen	Salvia	Red Sage Root
Radix Sanguisorbae Officinalis	Di Yu	Sanguisorba	Burnet-bloodwort Root
Radix Saussureae Lappae	Mu Xiang	Saussurea	Costus Root; Aucklandia
Radix Scrophulariae Ningpoensis	Xuan Shen	Scrophularia	Figwort Root
Radix Scutellariae Baicalensis	Huang Qin	Scutellaria	Scute; Baical Skullcap Root
Radix Sophorae Flavenscentis	Ku Shen	Sophora	Bitter Ginseng Root
Radix Sophorae Tonkinensis	Shan Dou Gen	Sophora	Pigeon Pea Root
Radix Stellariae Dichotomae	Yin Chai Hu	Stellaria	Stellaria Root
Radix Stemonae	Bai Bu	Stemona	Stemona Root
Radix Stephaniae Tetrandrae	Han Fang Ji	Stephania	Stephania Root
Radix Tinosporae Capillipes*	Jin Guo Lan	Tinospora	Tinospora Root
Radix Trichosanthis Kirilowii	Tian Hua Fen	Trichosanthes	Snakegourd Root
Ramulus Cinnamomi Cassiae	Gui Zhi	Cinnamomum	Cinnamon Twig
Ramulus cum Uncis Uncariae	Gou Teng	Uncaria	Gambir vine Stems and Hooks
Ramulus Mori Albae	Sang Zhi	Morus	Mulberry Twig
Ramulus Nelumbinis Nuciferae	Lian Geng	Nelumbo	Lotus Stem
Ramulus Perillae*	Zi Su Geng	Perilla	Perilla Stem
Ramulus Sangjishang	Sang Ji Sheng	Loranthus or Viscum	Mulberry Mistletoe Stem
Ramus Lonicerae Japonicae	Jin Yin Teng	Lonicera	Honeysuckle Stem
Ramus Tinosporae Sinensis	Kuan Jin Teng	Tinospora	Tinospora Stem

Pharmaceutical	Pinyin	Botanical	Common
Realgar	Xiong Huang	Realgar	Realgar; Arsenic Disulfide
Receptaculum Nelumbinis Nuciferae	Lian Fang	Nelumbo	Mature Lotus Receptacle
Resinae Asafoetidae*	E Wei	Ferula	Asafoetida Gum-resin; Devil's Dung
Resinae Myrrhae	Mo Yao	Commiphora	Myrrh Gum-resin
Rhizoma Acori Graminei	Shi Chang Pu	Acorus	Sweetflag Rhizome
Rhizoma Alismatis Orientalitis	Ze Xie	Alisma	Water Plantain Rhizome
Rhizoma Alpiniae Officinari	Gao Liang Jiang	Alpinia	Lesser Galangal Rhizome
Rhizoma Anemoni Attaicae*	Jiu Jie Chang Pu	Anemone	Altaica Rhizome
Rhizoma Arisaematis	(Sheng) Tian Nan Xing	Arisaema	Raw Jack-in-the-Pulpit Rhizome
Rhizoma Arisaematis Praeparatae	Zhi Nan Xing	Arisaema	Prepared Jack-in-the-Pulpit Rhizome
Rhizoma Atractylodis	Cang Zhu	Atractylodes	Atractylodes Rhizome
Rhizoma Atractylodis Macrocephalae	Bai Zhu	Atractylodes	White Atractylodes Rhizome
Rhizoma Belamcandae Chinensis	She Gan	Belamcanda	Belamcanda Rhizome; Blackberry Lily Rhizome
Rhizoma Bletillae Striatae	Bai Ji	Bletilla	Bletilla Rhizome
Rhizoma Cibotii Barometz	Gou Ji	Cibotium	Chain Fern Rhizome
Rhizoma Cimicifugae	Sheng Ma	Cimicifuga	Black Cohosh Rhizome; Bugbane Rhizome
Rhizoma Coptidis	Huang Lian	Coptis	Coptis; Golden Thread Rhizome
Rhizoma Corydalis Yanhusuo	Yan Hu Suo	Corydalis	Corydalis Rhizome
Rhizoma Curculiginis Orchioidis	Xian Mao	Curculigo	Golden Eye-grass Rhizome
Rhizoma Curcumae	E Zhu	Curcuma	Zedoary Tumeric Rhizome
Rhizoma Curcumae Longae	Jiang Huang	Curcuma	Tumeric Rhizome
Rhizoma Cyperi Rotundi	Xiang Fu	Cyperus	Cyperus Rhizome; Nut-grass Rhizome; Sedge Rhizome
Rhizoma Dioscoreae Hypoglaucae	Bei Xie	Dioscorea	Hypoglauca Yam Rhizome; Fish-poison Yam Rhizome
Rhizoma Dioscoreae Nipponicae*	Chuan Shan Long	Dioscorea	Japanese Dioscorea Rhizome
Rhizoma Drynariae	Gu Sui Bu	Drynaria	Drynaria Rhizome
Rhizoma Dryopteridis	Dong Bei Guan Zhong	Dryopteris	Dryopteris Rhizome
Rhizoma et Radix Ligustici	Gao Ben	Ligusticum	Straw Weed Rhizome and Root; Chinese Lovage Rhizome and Root
Rhizoma et Radix Notopterygii	Qiang Huo	Notopterygium	Notopterygium Rhizome and Root

Pharmaceutical	Pinyin	Botanical	Common
Rhizoma Fagopyri Cynosi*	Jin Qiao Mai	Fagopyrum	Wild Buckwheat Rhizome
Rhizoma Gastrodiae Elatae	Tian Ma	Gastrodia	Gastrodia Rhizome
Rhizoma Guanzhong	Guan Zhong	Dryopteris	Shield-fern Rhizome
Rhizoma Homalomenae Occultae	Qian Nian Jian	Homalomena	Homalomena Rhizome
Rhizoma Imperatae Cylindricae	Bai Mao Gen	Imperata	Woolly Grass Rhizome; White Grass Rhizome
Rhizoma Paridis Polyphyllae*	Zao Xiu	Paris	Paris Rhizome
Rhizoma Phragmitis Communis	Lu Gen	Phragmites	Reed Rhizome; Corrizo Rhizome
Rhizoma Picrorhizae	Hu Huang Lian	Picrorhiza	Picrorhiza Rhizome
Rhizoma Pinelliae Ternatae	(Fa) Ban Xia	Pinellia	Prepared Pinellia Rhizome
Rhizoma Pinelliae Ternatae	(Sheng) Ban Xia	Pinellia	Raw Pinellia Rhizome
Rhizoma Polygonati	Huang Jing	Polygonatum	Siberian Solomon Seal Rhizome
Rhizoma Polygonati Odorati	Yu Zhu	Polygonatum	Fragrant Solomon's Seal Rhizome; Polygonatum
Rhizoma et Radix Cynanchi Baiqian	Bai Qian	Cynanchum	Cynanchum Rhizome and Root
Rhizoma Smilacis China*	Ba Qia	Smilax	Smilax Rhizome
Rhizoma Smilacis Glabrae	Tu Fu Ling	Smilax	Glabrous Greenbrier Rhizome
Rhizoma Sparganii Stoloniferi	San Leng	Sparganium	Bur-reed Rhizome
Rhizoma Typhonii Gigantei	Bai Fu Zi	Typhonium	Typhonium Rhizome
Rhizoma Zingiberis Officinalis	Gan Jiang	Zingiber	Dried Ginger Rhizome
Rhizoma Zingiberis Officinalis Recens	Sheng Jiang	Zingiber	Fresh Ginger Rhizome
Rhizoma Zingiberis*	Pao Jiang	Zingiber	Quick-fried Ginger Rhizome
Saccharum Granorum	Yi Tang	Saccharum Granorum	Barley Malt Sugar/Syrup
Sanguis Draconis	Xue Jie	Dracaena	Dragon's Blood Resin
Scapus et Inflorescentia Eriocaulonis Buergeriani	Gu Jing Cao	Eriocaulon	Pipewort Scapus
Sclerotium Omphaliae Lapidescens	Lei Wan	Omphalia	Omphalia Fungus Fruiting Body
Sclerotium Polypori Umbellati	Zhu Ling	Polyporus	Polyporus Sclerotium
Sclerotium Poriae Cocos	Fu Ling	Poria	Hoelen; China Root; Tuckahoe; Indian Bread
Sclerotium Poriae Cocos Pararadicis	Fu Shen	Poria Cocos	Tuckahoe Spirit
Sclerotium Poriae Cocos Rubrae	Chi Fu Ling	Poria	Red Hoelen; Red Tuckahoe
Scolopendra Subspinipes	Wu Gong	Scolopendra	Centipede

Pharmaceutical	Pinyin	Botanical	Common
Secretio Bufonis	Chan Su	Bufo	Dried Skin Secretion of Toad
Secretio Moschus	She Xiang	Moschus	Musk; Musk Deer Navel Gland Secretion
Semen Albutili seu Malvae	Dong Kui Zi	Malva or Abutilon	Musk Mallow Seed; Malva Seed
Semen Allii Tuberosi	Jiu Zi	Allium	Chinese Leek Seed
Semen Alpiniae Katsumadai	Cao Dou Kou	Alpinia	Wild Cardamon Seed; Katsumada's Galangal Seed
Semen Arecae Catechu	Bing Lang	Areca	Betel Nut
Semen Astragali Complanati	Sha Yuan Ji Li	Astragalus	Flattened Milk-vetch Seed
Semen Benincasae Hispidae	Dong Gua Ren	Benincasa	Wintermelon Seed; Wax Gourd Seed
Semen Biotae Orientalis	Bai Zi Ren	Biota	Arbor-Vitae Seed
Semen Broussonetiae Papyriferae*	Chu Shi Zi	Broussonetia	Broussonetia Seed
Semen Cannabis Sativae	Huo Ma Ren	Cannabis	Hemp Seed; Marihuana Seed
Semen Cassiae	Jue Ming Zi	Cassia	Cassia Seed
Semen Celosiae Argenteae	Qing Xiang Zi	Celosia	Celosia Seed
Semen Citri Reticulatae*	Ju He	Citrus	Tangerine Seed
Semen Coicis Lachryma-jobi	Shu Yi Ren	Coix	Dry-Fried Coix Seed
Semen Coicis Lachryma-jobi	Yi Yi Ren	Coix	Coix Seed; Job's Tears Seed
Semen Croton Tiglii	Ba Dou	Croton	Croton Seed
Semen Cucurbitae Moschatae	Nan Gua Zi	Cucurbita	Pumpkin Seed and Husk
Semen Cuscutae Chinensis	Tu Si Zi	Cuscuta	Dodder Seed
Semen Dolichoris Lablab	Bian Dou	Dolichos	Hyacinth Bean
Semen Euphorbiae Lathyridis*	Xu Sui Zi	Euphorbia	Caper Spurge Seed; Moleplant Seed
Semen Euryales Ferocis	Qian Shi	Euryale	Euryale Seed
Semen Ginkgo Bilobae	Bai Guo	Ginkgo	Ginkgo Nut
Semen Glycines Germinatum	Dou Juan	Glycine	Young Soybean Sprout
Semen Hydnocarpi Anthelminticae	Da Feng Zi	Hydnocarpus	Chaulmoogra Seed
Semen Juglandis Regiae	Hu Tao Ren	Juglans	Walnut
Semen Leonuri Heterophylli	Chong Wei Zi	Leonurus	Motherwort Seed
Semen Lepidii seu Descurainiae	Ting Li Zi	Lepidium or Descurainia	Tansy Mustard Seed
Semen Litchi Chinensis	Li Zhi He	Litchi	Leechee Nut
Semen Momordicae Cochinchinensis	Mu Bie Zi	Momordica	Momordica Seed
Semen Myristicae Fragrantis	Rou Dou Kou	Myristica	Nutmeg Seed

Pharmaceutical	Pinyin	Botanical	Common
Semen Nelumbinis Nuciferae	Lian Zi	Nelumbo	Lotus Seed
Semen Oroxyli Indici	Mu Hu Die	Oroxylum	Oroxylum Seed
Semen Oryzae Sativae*	Jing Mi	Oryza	Rice Grain
Semen Perillae Frutescentis	Zi Su Zi	Perilla	Perilla Seed
Semen Persicae	Tao Ren	Prunus	Peach Seed (Kernel)
Semen Pharbitidis	Qian Niu Zi	Pharbitis	Morning Glory Seed
Semen Phaseoli Calcarati	Chi Xiao Dou	Phaseolus	Aduki Bean
Semen Phaseoli Radiati	Lu Dou	Phaseolus	Mung Bean
Semen Plantaginis	Che Qian Zi	Plantago	Plantago Seed; Plantain Seed
Semen Pruni	Yu Li Ren	Prunus	Bush Cherry Seed
Semen Pruni Armeniacae	(Bei) Xing Ren	Prunus	(Northern) Apricot Seed
Semen Pruni Armeniacae	(Nan) Xing Ren	Prunus	(Southern) Apricot Seed
Semen Raphani Satavi	Lai Fu Zi	Raphanus	Radish Seed
Semen Sesami Indici	Hei Zhi Ma	Sesamum	Black Sesame Seed
Semen Sinapsis Albae	Bai Jie Zi	Brassica	White Mustard Seed
Semen Sojae Praeparatum	Dan Dou Chi	Glycine	Prepared (Fermented) Soybean
Semen Sterculiae Scaphigerae	Pang Da Hai	Sterculia	Sterculia Seed
Semen Strychni	Ma Qian Zi	Strychnos	Nux-vomica Seed
Semen Torreyae Grandis	Fei Zi	Torreya	Torrreya Seed
Semen Trichosanthis	Gua Lou Ren	Trichosanthes	Snakegourd Seed
Semen Trigonellae Foeni-graeci	Hu Lu Ba	Trigonella	Fenugreek Seed
Semen Tritici Aestivi Levis	Fu Xiao Mai	Triticum	Wheat Chaff/Grain
Semen Vaccariae Segetalis	Wang Bu Liu Xing	Vaccaria	Cow Soapwort Seed
Semen Zanthoxyli Bungeani	Chuan Jiao Mu	Zanthoxylum	Sichuan Pepper Seed
Semen Zanthoxyli Bungeani	(Chuan) Jiao Mu	Zanthoxylum	Sichuan Pepper Seed
Semen Ziziphi Spinosae	Suan Zao Ren	Ziziphus	Sour Jujube Seed; Zizyphus
Smithsonitum	Lu Gan Shi	Smithsonitum	Smithsonite; Calamine
Spica Prunellae Vulgaris	Xia Ku Cao	Prunella	Selfheal Spike; Heal all Spike
Spina Gleditsiae Sinensis	Zao Jiao Ci	Gleditsia	Honeylocust Spine; Soap Bean Spine
Spora Lygodii Japonici	Hai Jin Sha	Lygodium	Japanese Climbing Fern Spore
Squama Manitis Pentadactylae	Chuan Shan Jia	Manis	Anteater-Scales; Pangolin Scales
Stalactitum	E Guan Shi	Stalactitum	Stalactite Tubular Tip
Stamen Nelumbinis Nuciferae	Lian Xu	Nelumbo	Lotus Stamen

Pharmaceutical	Pinyin	Botanical	Common
Stigma Crocus Sativae	Xi Hong Hua	Crocus	Stigma of the True Saffron Flower
Strichopus Japonicus	Hai Shen	Strichopus	Sea Cucumber; Sea Slug
Stylus Zeae Mays	Yu Mi Xu	Zea	Cornsilk
Styrax Liquidis	Su He Xiang	Liquidambar	Rose Maloes Resin
Succinum	Hu Po	Succinum	Amber; Fossilized Resin of Pine Tree
Succus Bambusae	Zhu Li	Bambusa	Dried Bamboo Sap
Sulphur	Liu Huang	Sulphur	Sulphur
Tabani Bivittati*	Meng Chong	Tabanus	Gadfly
Talcum	Hua Shi	Talcum	Talc; Soapstone
Terra Flava Usta	Fu Long Gan	Terra Flava Usta	Ignited Wood Stove Earth
Testes et Penis Otariae*	Hai Gou Shen	Phoca	Male Seal Sexual Organs
Testis et Penis Canis*	Guang Gou Shen	Canis	Male Dog Sexual Organs
Testis et Penis Cervi*	Hua Lu Shen	Cervus	Male Deer Sexual Organs
Testis et Penis Equii*	Hei Lu Shen	Equus	Male Horse Sexual Organs
Thallus Algae	Kun Bu	Laminaria or Ecklonia	Kelp Thallus; Kombu Thallus
Tuber Asparagi Cochinchinensis	Tian Men Dong	Asparagus	Chinese Asparagus Tuber
Tuber Curcumae	Yu Jin	Curcuma	Tumeric Tuber
Tuber Dioscoreae Bulbiferae	Huang Yao Zi	Dioscorea	Dioscorea Tuber
Tuber Ophiopogonis Japonici	Mai Men Dong	Ophiopogon	Creeping Lily-turf Tuber
Vesica Fellea Bovus	Niu Dan	Bos	Cow Gallbladder
Vesica Fellea Ursi	Xiong Dan	Ursus	Bear Gallbladder
Zaocys Dhumnades	Wu Shao She	Zaocys	Black-striped Snake

Pharmaceutical

Herb Name Cross Reference Keyed to Common Names

Common	Pinyin	Botanical	Pharmaceutical
(Northern) Apricot Seed	(Bei) Xing Ren	Prunus	Semen Pruni Armeniacae
(Southern) Apricot Seed	(Nan) Xing Ren	Prunus	Semen Pruni Armeniacae
Abalone Shell	Shi Jue Ming	Haliotis	Concha Haliotidis
Acalypha	Tie Xian	Acalypha	Herba Acalypae Australis*
Acanthopanax Rootbark.	Wu Jia Pi	Acanthopanax	Cortex Acanthopanacis Gracilistyli Radicis
Achyranthes Root	Huai Niu Xi	Achyranthes	Radix Achyranthis Bidentatae
Achyranthes Root	Tu Niu Xi	Achyranthes	Radix Achyranthis Aspera
Aconite Root	Wu Tou	Aconitum	Radix Aconiti
Actinolite	Yang Qi Shi	Actinolitum	Actinolitum
Aduki Bean	Chi Xiao Dou	Phaseolus	Semen Phaseoli Calcarati
Agrimony	Xian He Cao	Agrimonia	Herba Agrimoniae Pilosae
Ajuga	Bai Mao Xia Ku Cao	Ajuga	Herba Ajugae Decumbentis*
Akebia Fruit	Ba Yue Zha	Akebia	Fructus Akebiae
Akebia Stem	Mu Tong	Akebia	Caulis Mutong
Algae	Hai Dai	Laminaria	Herba Laminaria Japonicae
Aloe Vera Leaf	Lu Hui	Aloe	Herba Aloes
Aloeswood Secretion or Sap	Chen Xiang	Aquilaria	Lignum Aquilariae
Altaica Rhizome	Jiu Jie Chang Pu	Anemone	Rhizoma Anemoni Attaicae*
Alum; Potassium Aluminum Sulfate	Ming Fan	Alumen	Alumen
Amber; Fossilized Resin of Pine Tree	Hu Po	Succinum	Succinum
American Ginseng Root	Xi Yang Shen	Panax	Radix Panacis Quinquefolii
Ampelopsis Root	Bai Lian	Ampelopsis	Radix Ampelopsis Japonicae*
Amur Cork-tree Bark	Huang Bai	Phellodendron	Cortex Phellodendri
Androsace	Dian Di Mei	Androsace	Herba Androsacae Umbellatae*
Anemarrhena Root	Zhi Mu	Anemarrhena	Radix Anemarrhenae Asphodeloidis
Angelica Root	Bai Zhi	Angelica	Radix Angelicae Dahuricae
Anteater-Scales; Pangolin Scales	Chuan Shan Jia	Manis	Squama Manitis Pentadactylae

Common

Common	Pinyin	Botanical	Pharmaceutical
Antelope Horn	Ling Yang Jiao	Saiga	Cornu Antelopis
Antler Powder from the dregs of cooking Antler Glue	Lu Jiao Shuang	Cervus	Cornu Cervi Degelatinatium
Antler; Deerhorn; Ossified Horn of the Mature Male Deer	Lu Jiao	Cervus	Cornu Cervi
Arbor-Vitae Seed	Bai Zi Ren	Biota	Semen Biotae Orientalis
Arborvitae Leafy Twig	Ce Bai Ye	Biota	Cacumen Biotae Orientalis
Ardisia Root	Zhu Sha Gen	Ardisia	Radix Ardisiae Crenatae*
Aristolochia Root	Guang Fang Ji	Aristolochia or Cocculus	Radix Aristolochiae Fangchi
Aromatic Litsea Root and Stem	Dou Chi Jiang	Litsea	Radix et Ramus Litseae Cubebae
Aromatic Madder	Xiang Ru	Elsholtzia	Herba Elsholtziae seu Moslae
Artemisia	Liu Ji Nu	Artemisia	Herba Artemisiae Anomalae
Artificially Induced Cow Gallstons	Ren Gong Niu Huang	Bos	Calculus Artificialis
Asafoetida Gum-resin; Devil's Dung	E Wei	Ferula	Resinae Asafoetidae*
Asarum; Chinese Wild Ginger	Xi Xin	Asarum	Herba cum Radice Asari
Asiabell Root	Dang Shen	Codonopsis	Radix Codonopsitis Pilosulae
Atractylodes Rhizome	Cang Zhu	Atractylodes	Rhizoma Atractylodis
Avicularis; Knotweed	Bian Xu	Polygonum	Herba Polygoni Avicularis
Ballonflower Root; Bellflower Root; Bitter Jie Geng	(Ku) Jie Geng	Platycodon	Radix Platycodi Grandiflori
Bamboo Shavings	Zhu Ru	Bambusa	Caulis Bambusae in Taeniis
Barbat Scullcap	Ban Zhi Lian	Scutellaria	Herba Scutellariae Barbatae
Barley Malt Sugar/Syrup	Yi Tang	Saccharum Granorum	Saccharum Granorum
Barley Sprout; Malted Barley	Mai Ya	Hordeum	Fructus Hordei Vulgaris Germinatus
Bat Dung or Feces	Ye Ming Sha	Vespertilio	Excrementum Vespertilionis Murini
Bear Gallbladder	Xiong Dan	Ursus	Vesica Fellea Ursi
Beech Silver-top Root; Northern Sand Root	Bei Sha Shen	Glehnia	Radix Glehniae Littoralis
Begonia	Zi Bei Tian Kuei	Begonia	Herba Begoniae Fimbristipulatae
Belamcanda Rhizome; Blackberry Lily Rhizome	She Gan	Belamcanda	Rhizoma Belamcandae Chinensis
Betel Nut	Bing Lang	Areca	Semen Arecae Catechu
Betelnut Husk	Da Fu Pi	Areca	Pericarpium Arecae Catechu
Birthwort Fruit	Ma Dou Ling	Aristolochia	Fructus Aristolochiae
Birthwort Root	Qing Mu Xiang	Aristolochia	Radix Aristolochiae

Common	Pinyin	Botanical	Pharmaceutical
Bitter Ginseng Root	Ku Shen	Sophora	Radix Sophorae Flavenscentis
Bitter Orange Fruit	Zhi Ke	Citrus or Poncirus	Fructus Citri Aurantii
Black Cardamon Fruit	Yi Zhi Ren	Alpinia	Fructus Alpiniae Oxyphyllae
Black Cohosh Rhizome; Bugbane Rhizome	Sheng Ma	Cimicifuga	Rhizoma Cimicifugae
Black Pepper Fruit	Hu Jiao	Piper	Fructus Piperis Nigri
Black Sesame Seed	Hei Zhi Ma	Sesamum	Semen Sesami Indici
Black-striped Snake	Wu Shao She	Zaocys	Zaocys Dhumnades
Bland Bamboo Leaf and Stem	Dan Zhu Ye	Lophatherum	Herba Lophatheri Gracilis
Bletilla Rhizome	Bai Ji	Bletilla	Rhizoma Bletillae Striatae
Boneset; Thoroughwort; Feverwort	Pei Lan	Eupatorium	Herba Eupatorii Fortunei
Borax; Sodium Tetraborate	Peng Sha	Borax	Borax
Broom Cyperus Seed	Di Fu Zi	Kochia	Fructus Kochiae Scopariae
Broomrape Fleshy Stem	Rou Cong Rong	Cistanche	Herba Cistanches Deserticolae
Broussonetia Seed	Chu Shi Zi	Broussonetia	Semen Broussonetiae Papyriferae*
Brucea Fruit	Ya Dan Zi	Brucea	Fructus Bruceae Javanicae
Buddleia Flower	Mi Meng Hua	Buddleia	Flos Buddleiae Officinalis Immaturus
Bugleweed	Ze Lan	Lycopus	Herba Lycopi Lucidi
Bur-reed Rhizome	San Leng	Sparganium	Rhizoma Sparganii Stoloniferi
Burdock Seed	Niu Bang Zi	Arctium	Fructus Arctii Lappae
Burnet-bloodwort Root	Di Yu	Sanguisorba	Radix Sanguisorbae Officinalis
Bush Cherry Seed	Yu Li Ren	Prunus	Semen Pruni
Buttercup Root	Mao Zhao Cao	Ranunculus	Radix Ranunculi Ternati*
Calcined Dragon Bone; Calcined Fossilized Bone	Duan Long Gu	Os Draconis	Os Draconis
Calcined Oyster Shell	Duan Mu Li	Ostrea	Concha Ostreae
Calcite	Han Shui Shi	Calcitum	Calcitum
Calcium Hydroxide	Chen Shi Huei	Calcaria	Calcaria*
Callicarpa Leaf	Zi Zhu	Callicarpa	Folium Callicarpae
Calomel; Mercurous Chloride	Qing Fen	Calomelas	Calomelas
Cantharides; Chinese Blistering Beetle	Ban Mao	Mylabris	Mylabris
Caper Spurge Seed; Moleplant Seed	Xu Sui Zi	Euphorbia	Semen Euphorbiae Lathyridis*
Carpesium	Tian Ming Jing	Carpesium	Herba Carpesii

Common

Common	Pinyin	Botanical	Pharmaceutical
Carpesium Fruit	He Shi	Carpesium or Daucus	Fructus Carpesii seu Daucusi
Cassia Seed	Jue Ming Zi	Cassia	Semen Cassiae
Cattail Leaves	Pu Hui	Typha	Folium Typhae
Celosia Seed	Qing Xiang Zi	Celosia	Semen Celosiae Argenteae
Centipeda Herb	E Bu Shi Cao	Centipeda	Herba Centipedae Minimae*
Centipede	Wu Gong	Scolopendra	Scolopendra Subspinipes
Chain Fern Rhizome	Gou Ji	Cibotium	Rhizoma Cibotii Barometz
Changium Root	Ming Dang Shen	Changium	Radix Changii*
Charred Cattail Pollen	Pu Huang Tan	Typha	Pollen Typhae Carbonisatus
Charred Hawthorn Fruit or Berry	Shan Zha Tan	Crataegus	Fructus Crataegi Carbonisatus
Charred Human Hair	Xue Yu Tan	Homo Sapiens	Crinis Carbonisatus Hominis
Charred Windmill Palm Petiole	Zong Lu Pi Tan	Trachycarpus	Fibra Stipulae Trachycarpi Carbonisatus
Chaulmoogra Seed	Da Feng Zi	Hydnocarpus	Semen Hydnocarpi Anthelminticae
Cherokee Rose Fruit / Rosehip	Jin Ying Zi	Rosa	Fructus Rosae Laevigatae
Chicken Gizard Lining	Ji Nei Jin	Gallus	Endothelium Corneum Gigeriae Galli
Chinese Asparagus Tuber	Tian Men Dong	Asparagus	Tuber Asparagi Cochinchinensis
Chinese Cardamon Fruit	Cao Guo	Amomum	Fructus Amomi Tsao-Ko
Chinese Caterpillar Fungus	Dong Chong Xia Cao	Cordyceps	Cordyceps Sinensis
Chinese Chive Bulb	Xie Bai	Allium	Bulbus Allii
Chinese Gentian Root	Long Dan Cao	Gentiana	Radix Gentianae Longdancao
Chinese Leek Seed	Jiu Zi	Allium	Semen Allii Tuberosi
Chinese Lobelia	Ban Bian Lian	Lobelia	Herba Lobeliae Chinensis cum Radice
Chinese Quince Fruit	Mu Gua	Chaenomeles	Frutus Chaenomelis
Chinese Senega Root; Seneca Snakeroot	Yuan Zhi	Polygala	Radix Polygalae Tenuifoliae
Chinese Soft-shell Turtle Shell	Bie Jia	Amyda	Carapax Amydae Sinensis
Chinese Sumac Bark	Yan Fu Mu	Rhus	Cortex Rhois Chinensis*
Chinese Tulip Bulb	Shan Ci Gu	Tulipa	Pseudobulbus Shancigu
Chinese Wild Yam Root	Shan Yao	Dioscorea	Radix Dioscoreae Oppositae
Chlorite Schist; Lapis	Meng Shi	Lapis Micae seu Chloriti	Lapis Micae seu Chloriti
Chlorite Schist; Phlogopitum; Lapis	Meng Shi	Lapis Micae seu Chloriti	Lapis Chloriti seu Micae
Cicada Skin; Cicada Moulting	Chan Tui	Cryptotympana	Periostracum Cicadae

Common	Pinyin	Botanical	Pharmaceutical
Cinnabar; Red Mercury Sulfide	Zhu Sha	Cinnabaris	Cinnabaris
Cinnamon Bark	Rou Gui	Cinnamomum	Cortex Cinnamomi Cassiae
Cinnamon Twig	Gui Zhi	Cinnamomum	Ramulus Cinnamomi Cassiae
Clam Shell	Hai Ge Ke	Cyclina	Concha Cyclinae Sinensis
Clematis Root	Wei Ling Xian	Clematis	Radix Clematidis
Clove Flower-bud	Ding Xiang	Eugenia	Flos Caryophylli
Clubmoss	Shen Jin Cao	Lycopodium	Herba Lycopodii Clavati*
Cnidium Seed	She Chuang Zi	Cnidium	Fructus Cnidii Monnieri
Cockle Shell; Ark Shell	Wa Leng Zi	Arca	Concha Arcae
Cockscomb Flower	Ji Guan Hua	Celosia	Flos Celosiae Cristatae
Coix Seed; Job's Tears Seed	Yi Yi Ren	Coix	Semen Coicis Lachryma-jobi
Coltsfoot Flower	Kuan Dong Hua	Tussilago	Flos Tussilaginis Farfarae
Commelina	Ya Zhi Cao	Commelina	Herba Commelinae*
Copper Sulphate; Blue Vitriol	Dan Fan	Chalcanthitum	Chalcanthitum*
Coptis; Golden Thread Rhizome	Huang Lian	Coptis	Rhizoma Coptidis
Coral-bean Bark	Hai Tong Pi	Erythrina	Cortex Erythrinae
Cornsilk	Yu Mi Xu	Zea	Stylus Zeae Mays
Corydalis Rhizome	Yan Hu Suo	Corydalis	Rhizoma Corydalis Yanhusuo
Costus Root; Aucklandia	Mu Xiang	Saussurea	Radix Saussureae Lappae
Cotton Root	Mian Hua Gen	Gossypium	Radix Gossypii Hirsuti*
Cow Gallbladder	Niu Dan	Bos	Vesica Fellea Bovus
Cow Soapwort Seed	Wang Bu Liu Xing	Vaccaria	Semen Vaccariae Segetalis
Creeping Lily-turf Tuber	Mai Men Dong	Ophiopogon	Tuber Ophiopogonis Japonici
Croton Seed	Ba Dou	Croton	Semen Croton Tiglii
Crystalized Volatile Oil of the Camphor Tree	Zhang Nao	Cinnamomum	Camphora
Cubeba Fruit	Bi Cheng Qie	Piper	Fructus Cubebae
Cuttle-fish Bone	Hai Piao Xiao	Sepia or Sepiella	Os Sepiae seu Sepiellae
Cyathula Root	Chuan Niu Xi	Cyathula	Radix Cyathulae Officinalis
Cynanchum Rhizome and Root	Bai Qian	Cynanchum	Rhizoma et Radix Cynanchi Baiqian
Cynanchum Root	Ge Shan Xiang	Cynanchum	Radix Cynanchi Auriculati
Cynomorium Fleshy Stem	Suo Yang	Cynomorium	Herba Cynomorii Songarici
Cyperus Rhizome; Nut-grass Rhizome; Sedge Rhizome	Xiang Fu	Cyperus	Rhizoma Cyperi Rotundi

Common

Common	Pinyin	Botanical	Pharmaceutical
Dalbergia Heartwood	Jiang Xiang	Dalbergia	Lignum Dalbergiae Odoriferae
Dandelion	Pu Gong Ying	Taraxacum	Herba Taraxaci Mongolici cum Radice
Daphne Flower	Yuan Hua	Daphne	Flos Daphnes Genkwa
Dead Stiff Body of Sick Silkworm Larvae	Jiang Can	Bombyx	Bombyx Batryticatus
Dendrobium Stem	Shi Hu	Dendrobium	Herba Dendrobii
Dichroa Leaf	Shu Qi	Dichroa	Folium Dichroae Febrifugae
Dichroa Root	Chang Shan	Dichroa	Radix Dichroae Febrifugae
Dioscorea Tuber	Huang Yao Zi	Dioscorea	Tuber Dioscoreae Bulbiferae
Dittany Root Bark	Bai Xian Pi	Dictamnus	Cortex Dictamni Dasycarpi Radicis
Dodder Seed	Tu Si Zi	Cuscuta	Semen Cuscutae Chinensis
Dog Bone	Gou Gu	Canis	Os Canine
Dogwood Fruit; Asiatic Cornelian Cherry Fruit	Shan Zhu Yu	Cornus	Fructus Corni Officinalis
Donkey Hide Gelatin; Ass Skin Glue	E Jiao	Equus	Gelatinum Corii Asini
Dragon Bone; Fossilized Bone	Long Gu	Os Draconis	Os Draconis
Dragon Tooth; Fossilized Tooth	Long Chi	Dens Draconis	Dens Draconis
Dragon's Blood Resin	Xue Jie	Dracaena	Sanguis Draconis
Dried Bamboo Sap	Zhu Li	Bambusa	Succus Bambusae
Dried Ginger Rhizome	Gan Jiang	Zingiber	Rhizoma Zingiberis Officinalis
Dried Paste of Concentrated Decoction of Black or White Cutch	Er Cha	Acacia or Uncaria	Pasta Acacia seu Uncaria
Dried Persimmon Fruit	Shi Bing	Diospyros	Fructus Diospyri Kaki*
Dried Skeleton of Luffa Sponge	Si Gua Lou	Luffa	Fasciculus Vascularis Luffae
Dried Skin Secretion of Toad	Chan Su	Bufo	Secretio Bufonis
Dry-Fried Coix Seed	Shu Yi Ren	Coix	Semen Coicis Lachryma-jobi
Drynaria Rhizome	Gu Sui Bu	Drynaria	Rhizoma Drynariae
Dryopteris Rhizome	Dong Bei Guan Zhong	Dryopteris	Rhizoma Dryopteridis
Duckweed	Fu Ping	Spirodela or Lemna	Herba Lemnae seu Spirodelae
Earthworm	Di Long	Pheretima	Lumbricus
Eclipta	Han Lian Cao	Eclipta	Herba Ecliptae Prostratae
Eleagnus Leaf	Hu Tui Ye	Eleagnus	Folium Eleagni Pungens
Elecampane	Jin Fei Cao	Inula	Herba Inulae
Elecampane Flower	Xuan Fu Hua	Inula	Flos Inulae

Common	Pinyin	Botanical	Pharmaceutical
Ephedra Root	Ma Huang Gen	Ephedra	Radix Ephedrae
Ephedra Stem	Ma Huang	Ephedra	Herba Ephedrae
Epimedium	Yin Yang Huo	Epimedium	Herba Epimedii
Eucommia Bark	Du Zhong	Eucommia	Cortex Eucommiae Ulmoidis
Euryale Seed	Qian Shi	Euryale	Semen Euryales Ferocis
Evodia Fruit	Wu Zhu Yu	Evodia	Fructus Evodiae Rutaecarpae
Fennel Fruit	Xiao Hui Xiang	Foeniculum	Fructus Foeniculi Vulgaris
Fenugreek Seed	Hu Lu Ba	Trigonella	Semen Trigonellae Foeni-graeci
Figwort Root	Xuan Shen	Scrophularia	Radix Scrophulariae Ningpoensis
Finger Citron Flower	Fo Shou Hua	Citrus	Flos Citri Sarcodactylis
Finger Citron Fruit	Fo Shou	Citrus	Fructus Citri Sarcodactylis
Flattened Milk-vetch Seed	Sha Yuan Ji Li	Astragalus	Semen Astragali Complanati
Fleeceflower Root; Fo-Ti Root	He Shou Wu	Polygonum	Radix Polygoni Multiflori
Fleeceflower Stem; Fo-Ti Stem	Ye Jiao Teng	Polygonum	Caulis Polygoni Multiflori
Fluorite	Zi Shi Ying	Fluoritum	Fluoritum
Flying Squirrel Feces	Wu Ling Zhi	Trogopterus or Pteromys	Excrementum Trogopteri seu Pteromi
Forsythia Fruit; Golden Bells	Lian Qiao	Forsythia	Fructus Forsythiae Suspensae
Fragrant Solomon's Seal Rhizome; Polygonatum	Yu Zhu	Polygonatum	Rhizoma Polygonati Odorati
Frankincense Gum-resin	Ru Xiang	Boswellia	Gummi Olibanum
Fresh Chinese Foxglove Root	Sheng Di Huang	Rehmannia	Radix Rehmanniae Glutinosae
Fresh Dried Ginseng Root	Sheng Shai Shen	Panax	Radix Ginseng
Fresh Ginger Rhizome	Sheng Jiang	Zingiber	Rhizoma Zingiberis Officinalis Recens
Fresh Ginger Skin	Sheng Jiang Pi	Zingiber	Cortex Zingiberis Officinalis Recens
Fresh Water Turtle Shell	Gui Ban	Chinemys	Plastrum Testudinis
Gadfly	Meng Chong	Tabanus	Tabani Bivittati*
Gallnut of Chinese Sumac	Wu Bei Zi	Rhus/Melaphis	Galla Rhois Chinensis
Gambir vine Stems and Hooks	Gou Teng	Uncaria	Ramulus cum Uncis Uncariae
Gardenia Fruit	Zhi Zi	Gardenia	Fructus Gardeniae Jasminoidis
Garlic Bulb	Da Suan	Allium	Bulbus Allii Sativi
Gastrodia Rhizome	Tian Ma	Gastrodia	Rhizoma Gastrodiae Elatae
Gecko Lizard	Ge Jie	Gekko	Gekko

Common	Pinyin	Botanical	Pharmaceutical
Geranium; Heronbill; Cranebill	Lao Guan Cao	Erodium or Geranium	Herba Erodii seu Geranii*
Giant Knotweed Rhizome	Hu Zhang	Polygonum	Radix et Rhizoma Polygoni Cuspidati
Ginkgo Leaf	Yin Guo Ye	Ginkgo	Folium Ginkgo Bilobae
Ginkgo Nut	Bai Guo	Ginkgo	Semen Ginkgo Bilobae
Ginseng Leaf	Ren Shen Ye	Panax	Folium Ginseng
Ginseng Root Neck	Ren Shen Lu	Panax	Cervix Ginseng
Ginseng Root steamed until red	(Hong) Ren Shen	Panax	Radix Ginseng
Glabrous Greenbrier Rhizome	Tu Fu Ling	Smilax	Rhizoma Smilacis Glabrae
Glorybower Leaf	Chou Wu Tong	Clerodendron	Folium Clerodendri Trichotomi
Goat Horn	Shan Yang Jiao	Naemorhedis	Cornu Naemorhedis
Gold	Huang Jin	Aurum	Aurum*
Golden Eye-grass Rhizome	Xian Mao	Curculigo	Rhizoma Curculiginis Orchioidis
Grains-of-Paradise Flower	Sha Ren Hua	Amomum	Flos Amomi
Grains-of-Paradise Fruit or Seeds	Sha Ren	Amomum	Fructus seu Semen Amomi
Grains-of-Paradise Shell	Sha Ren Ke	Amomum	Pericarpium Amomi
Groomwell Root	Zi Cao	Lithospermum	Radix Lithospermi seu Arnebiae
Groundsel	Qian Li Guang	Senecio	Herba Senecionis Scandentis*
Gynura Leaf	Ju Ye San Qi	Gynura	Folium Gynurae*
Gypsum; Calcium Sulphate	Shi Gao	Gypsum	Gypsum Fibrosum
Halloysite; Red Kaolin	Chi Shi Zhi	Halloysitum Rubrum	Halloysitum Rubrum
Hawksbill Turtle Shell	Dai Mao	Eretmochelys	Carapax Eretmochelydis Imbricatae*
Hawthorn Ripe Fruit or Berry	Shan Zha Rou	Crataegus	Fructus Crataegi
Hawthorn Unripe Fruit or Berry	Shan Zha	Crataegus	Fructus Crataegi
Hematite; Iron Ore	Dai Zhe Shi	Haematitum	Haematitum
Hemp Seed; Marihuana Seed	Huo Ma Ren	Cannabis	Semen Cannabis Sativae
Hoelen; China Root; Tuckahoe; Indian Bread	Fu Ling	Poria	Sclerotium Poriae Cocos
Hogfennel Root	Qian Hu	Peucedanum	Radix Peucedani
Holly Leaf	Si Ji Qing	Ilex	Folium Ilicis Chinensis*
Homalomena Rhizome	Qian Nian Jian	Homalomena	Rhizoma Homalomenae Occultae
Honey	Feng Mi	Mel	Mel*

Common	Pinyin	Botanical	Pharmaceutical
Honey-fried Licorice Root	Zhi Gan Cao	Glycyrrhiza	Radix Glycyrrhizae Praeparata*
Honeylocust Fruit; Soap Bean Fruit	Zao Jiao	Gleditsia	Fructus Gleditsiae Sinensis
Honeylocust Spine; Soap Bean Spine	Zao Jiao Ci	Gleditsia	Spina Gleditsiae Sinensis
Honeysuckle Flower	Jin Yin Hua	Lonicera	Flos Lonicerae Japonicae
Honeysuckle Stem	Jin Yin Teng	Lonicera	Ramus Lonicerae Japonicae
Hornet Nest; Wasp Nest	Lu Feng Fang	Polistes	Nidus Vespae
Horsetail; Scouring Rush; Shavegrass	Mu Zei	Equisetum	Herba Equiseti Hiemalis
Houttuynia; Fish Smell Plant	Yu Xing Cao	Houttuynia	Herba cum Radice Houttuyniae Cordatae
Human Placenta	Zi He Che	Homo Sapiens	Placenta Hominis
Hyacinth Bean	Bian Dou	Dolichos	Semen Dolichoris Lablab
Hyacinth Bean Flower	Bian Dou Hua	Dolichos	Flos Dolichoris Lablab
Hydrangea Flower	Ba Xian Hua	Hydrangea	Flos Hydrangeae Macrophyllae*
Hypoglauca Yam Rhizome; Fish-poison Yam Rhizome	Bei Xie	Dioscorea	Rhizoma Dioscoreae Hypoglaucae
Ignited Wood Stove Earth	Fu Long Gan	Terra Flava Usta	Terra Flava Usta
Immature (Green) Tangerine Peel	Qing Pi	Citrus	Pericarpium Citri Reticulatae Viride
Immature Bitter Orange Fruit	Zhi Shi	Citrus or Poncirus	Fructus Immaturus Citri Aurantii
Indigo	Qing Dai	Indigo	Indigo Pulverata Levis
Iron Filing	Sheng Tie Luo	Frusta Ferri	Frusta Ferri
Isatis Leaf; Woad Leaf	Da Qing Ye	Isatis	Folium Daqingye
Isatis Root; Woad Root	Ban Lan Gen	Isatis	Radix Isatidis seu Baphicacanthi
Ivy	Chang Chun Teng	Hedera	Herba Hederae Nepalensis*
Japanese Climbing Fern	Jin Sha Teng	Lygodium	Herba Lygodii Japonici
Japanese Climbing Fern Spore	Hai Jin Sha	Lygodium	Spora Lygodii Japonici
Japanese Dioscorea Rhizome	Chuan Shan Long	Dioscorea	Rhizoma Dioscoreae Nipponicae*
Japanese Elder Bark	Lu Ying	Sambucus	Cortex Sambuci*
Japanese Thistle	Da Ji	Cirsium	Herba seu Radix Cirsii Japonici
Jilin Wild Ginseng	Ji Lin Shen	Panax	Radix Ginseng
Jujube Fruit; Chinese Black Date	Da Zao	Ziziphus	Fructus Ziziphi Jujubae
Jujube Fruit; Chinese Red Date	Hong Zao	Ziziphus	Fructus Ziziphi Jujubae
Kadsura Stem	Hai Feng Teng	Piper	Caulis Piperis Futokadsurae

Common	Pinyin	Botanical	Pharmaceutical
Kansui Spurge Root	Gan Sui	Euphorbia	Radix Euphorbiae Kansui
Kariyat; Green Chiretta	Chuan Xin Lian	Andrographis	Herba Andrographitis Paniculatae
Kelp Thallus; Kombu Thallus	Kun Bu	Laminaria or Ecklonia	Thallus Algae
Knotty Pine Wood	Song Jie	Pinus	Lignum Pini Nodi
Korean Ash Bark	Qin Pi	Fraxinus	Cortex Fraxini
Kudzu Flower	Ge Hua	Pueraria	Flos Puerariae
Kudzu Root	Ge Gen	Pueraria	Radix Puerariae
Ladybell Root; Southern Sand Root	Nan Sha Shen	Adenophora	Radix Adenophorae
Laquer	Gan Qi	Rhus	Lacca Sinica Exsiccatae
Large-Leaf Gentian Root	Qin Jiao	Gentiana	Radix Gentianae Qinjiao
Leech	Shui Zhi	Hirudo	Hirudo seu Whitmania
Leechee Nut	Li Zhi He	Litchi	Semen Litchi Chinensis
Leopard Bone	Bao Gu	Panthera	Os Leopardis
Lesser Galangal Rhizome	Gao Liang Jiang	Alpinia	Rhizoma Alpiniae Officinari
Licorice Root	Gan Cao	Glycyrhiza	Radix Glycyrrhizae Uralensis
Lily Bulb	Bai He	Lilium	Bulbus Lilii
Limonite	Yu Liang Shi	Limonite	Limonite
Litharge; Galena	Mi Tuo Seng	Lithargyrum	Lithargyrum
Long Pepper Fruit	Bi Ba	Piper	Fructus Piperis Longi
Long-noded Pit Viper Snake	Bai Hua She	Agkistrodon	Agkistrodon seu Bungarus
Longan Fruit Flesh	Long Yan Rou	Euphoria	Arillus Euphoriae Longanae
Loquat Leaf	Pi Pa Ye	Eriobotrya	Folium Eriobotryae Japonicae
Loropetalum Bark	Ji Mu	Loropetalum	Cortex Loropetali*
Lotus Leaf	He Ye	Nelumbo	Folium Nelumbinis Nuciferae
Lotus Plumule	Lian Xin	Nelumbo	Plumula Nelumbinis Nuciferae
Lotus Rhizome Node	Ou Jie	Nelumbo	Nodus Nelumbinis Nuciferae Rhizomatis
Lotus Seed	Lian Zi	Nelumbo	Semen Nelumbinis Nuciferae
Lotus Stamen	Lian Xu	Nelumbo	Stamen Nelumbinis Nuciferae
Lotus Stem	Lian Geng	Nelumbo	Ramulus Nelumbinis Nuciferae
Lucid Ganoderma; Reishi	Ling Zhi	Ganoderma	Fructificatio Ganodermae Lucidi*
Luffa Skin	Si Gua Pi	Luffa	Pericarpium Luffa Acutangulae
Lysimachia	Jin Qian Cao	Lysimachia	Herba Lysimachiae
Macaque Gallstone	Hou Zao	Macaca	Calculus Macacae Mulattae
Madder Root	Qian Cao Gen	Rubia	Radix Rubiae Cordifoliae

Common	Pinyin	Botanical	Pharmaceutical
Magnetite; Magnetic Iron Ore; Loadstone	Ci Shi	Magnetitum	Magnetitum
Magnolia Bark	Hou Po	Magnolia	Cortex Magnoliae Officinalis
Magnolia Flower	Hou Po Hua	Magnolia	Flos Magnoliae Officinalis
Magnolia Flower	Xin Yi Hua	Magnolia	Flos Magnoliae
Mahonia Leaf	Shi Da Gong Lao	Mahonia	Folium Mahoniae*
Male Deer Sexual Organs	Hua Lu Shen	Cervus	Testis et Penis Cervi*
Male Dog Sexual Organs	Guang Gou Shen	Canis	Testis et Penis Canis*
Male Horse Sexual Organs	Hei Lu Shen	Equus	Testis et Penis Equii*
Male Seal Sexual Organs	Hai Gou Shen	Phoca	Testes et Penis Otariae*
Manchurian Lilac Bark	Bao Ma Zi	Syringa	Cortex Syringae*
Matrimony Vine Fruit; Wolfberry Fruit	Gou Qi Zi	Lycium	Fructus Lycii
Matrimony-vine Rootbark; Wolfberry Bark	Di Gu Pi	Lycium	Cortex Lycii Radicis
Mature Antler Glue; Mature Antler Gelatin	Lu Jiao Jiao	Cervus	Colla Cornu Cervi
Mature Lotus Receptacle	Lian Fang	Nelumbo	Receptaculum Nelumbinis Nuciferae
Medicated Leaven	Shen Qu	Massa Fermentata	Massa Fermentata
Melon Pedicle	Gua Di	Cucumis	Pedicellus Cucumeris
Mercury	Shui Yin	Hydrargyrum	Hydrargyrum
Millettia Root and Vine; Chicken Blood Vine	Ji Xue Teng	Millettia	Radix et Caulis Jixueteng
Mimosa Tree Bark; Silktree Bark	He Huan Pi	Albizzia	Cortex Albizziae Julibrissin
Mimosa Tree Flower; Silktree Flower	He Huan Hua	Albizzia	Flos Albizziae Julibrissin*
Mirabilite; Glauber's Salt	Mang Xiao	Mirabilitum	Mirabilitum
Momordica Fruit	Luo Han Guo	Momordica	Fructus Momordicae Grosvenori
Momordica Leaf	Luo Huo Guo Ye	Momordica	Folium Momordicae Grosvenori
Momordica Seed	Mu Bie Zi	Momordica	Semen Momordicae Cochinchinensis
Morinda Root	Ba Ji Tian	Morinda	Radix Morindae Officinalis
Morning Glory Seed	Qian Niu Zi	Pharbitis	Semen Pharbitidis
Mother-of-Pearl Shell	Zhen Zhu Mu	Pteria	Concha Margaritiferae
Motherwort	Yi Mu Cao	Leonurus	Herba Leonuri Heterophylli
Motherwort Seed	Chong Wei Zi	Leonurus	Semen Leonuri Heterophylli
Mugwort Leaf	Ai Ye	Artemisia	Folium Artemisiae Argyi
Mulberry Fruit Bud	Sang Shen	Morus	Fructus Mori Albae
Mulberry Leaf	Sang Ye	Morus	Folium Mori Albae

Common

Common	Pinyin	Botanical	Pharmaceutical
Mulberry Mistletoe Stem	Sang Ji Sheng	Loranthus or Viscum	Ramulus Sangjishang
Mulberry Rootbark	Sang Bai Pi	Morus	Cortex Mori Albae Radicis
Mulberry Twig	Sang Zhi	Morus	Ramulus Mori Albae
Mung Bean	Lu Dou	Phaseolus	Semen Phaseoli Radiati
Musk Mallow Seed; Malva Seed	Dong Kui Zi	Malva or Abutilon	Semen Albutili seu Malvae
Musk; Musk Deer Navel Gland Secretion	She Xiang	Moschus	Secretio Moschus
Myrobalan Fruit	He Zi	Terminalia	Fructus Terminaliae Chebulae
Myrrh Gum-resin	Mo Yao	Commiphora	Resinae Myrrhae
Northern Schisandra Fruit	Wu Wei Zi	Schisandra	Fructus Schisandrae Chinensis
Notopterygium Rhizome and Root	Qiang Huo	Notopterygium	Rhizoma et Radix Notopterygii
Nutmeg Seed	Rou Dou Kou	Myristica	Semen Myristicae Fragrantis
Nux-vomica Seed	Ma Qian Zi	Strychnos	Semen Strychni
Oldenlandia	Bai Hua She She Cao	Oldenlandia	Herba Oldenlandiae Diffusae
Omphalia Fungus Fruiting Body	Lei Wan	Omphalia	Sclerotium Omphaliae Lapidescens
Ophicalcite	Hua Rui Shi	Ophicalcitum	Ophicalcitum
Opium Poppy Husk	Ying Su Ke	Papaver	Pericarpium Papaveris Somniferi
Oriental Wormwood	Yin Chen Hao	Artemisia	Herba Artemisiae Yinchenhao
Oroxylum Seed	Mu Hu Die	Oroxylum	Semen Oroxyli Indici
Ox or Water Buffalo Gallstone	Niu Huang	Bos or Bubalis	Calculus Bovis seu Calculus Bubali
Oyster Shell	Mu Li	Ostrea	Concha Ostreae
Paederia Stem	Ji Shi Teng	Paederia	Caulis Paederiae*
Pagoda Tree Flower Bud	Huai Hua Mi	Sophora	Flos Sophorae Japonicae Immaturus
Pagoda Tree Fruit	Huai Jiao	Sophora	Fructus Sophorae Japonicae
Paris Rhizome	Zao Xiu	Paris	Rhizoma Paridis Polyphyllae*
Partially-blossoming Chinese Tea Rose Flower	Yue Ji Hua	Rosa	Flos et Fructus Rosae Chinensis
Patchouli; Agastache	Huo Xiang	Agastache or Pogostemon	Herba Agastaches seu Pogostemi
Patrinia; Thiaspi	Bai Jiang Cao	Patrinia or Thiaspi	Herba cum Radice Patriniae
Peach Seed (Kernel)	Tao Ren	Prunus	Semen Persicae
Peanut Skin	Hua Sheng Yi	Arachis	Pericarpium Arachi*
Pear Peel	Li Pi	Pyrus	Pericarpium Pyri*
Pearl	Zhen Zhu	Pteria	Margarita

Common	Pinyin	Botanical	Pharmaceutical
Peking Spurge Root	Jing Da Ji	Euphorbia or Knoxia	Radix Euphorbiae seu Knoxiae
Peppermint; Spearmint; Field Mint	Bo He	Mentha	Herba Menthae Haplocalycis
Perilla Leaf	Zi Su Ye	Perilla	Folium Perillae Frutescentis
Perilla Seed	Zi Su Zi	Perilla	Semen Perillae Frutescentis
Perilla Stem	Zi Su Geng	Perilla	Ramulus Perillae*
Persimmon Calyx	Shi Di	Diospyros	Calyx Diospyri Kaki
Picrorhiza Rhizome	Hu Huang Lian	Picrorhiza	Rhizoma Picrorhizae
Pigeon Pea Root	Shan Dou Gen	Sophora	Radix Sophorae Tonkinensis
Pill-bearing Spurge	Ze Qi	Euphorbia	Herba Euphorbiae Helioscopiae
Pink Flower Herb	Qu Mai	Dianthus	Herba Dianthi
Pipe-fish	Hai Long	Solenognathus	Hailong
Pipewort Scapus	Gu Jing Cao	Eriocaulon	Scapus et Inflorescentia Eriocaulonis Buergeriani
Plantago Seed; Plantain Seed	Che Qian Zi	Plantago	Semen Plantaginis
Plantago; Plantain	Che Qian Cao	Plantago	Herba Plantaginis
Poke Root	Shang Lu	Phytolacca	Radix Phytolaccae
Polygonum	Guan Ye Liao	Polygonum	Herba Polygoni Perfoliati*
Polyporus Sclerotium	Zhu Ling	Polyporus	Sclerotium Polypori Umbellati
Pomegranate Husk or Rind	Shi Liu Pi	Punica	Pericarpium Punicae Granati
Pomegranate Root Bark	Shi Liu Gen Pi	Punica	Cortex Punicae Granati Radicis
Potentilla	Fan Bai Cao	Potentilla	Herba Potentillae Discoloris*
Powdered Jack-in-the-Pulpit Rhizome mixed with Cow Bile	Dan Nan Xing	Arisaema	Pulvis Arisaemae cum Felle Bovis
Praying Mantis Egg Case	Sang Piao Xiao	Paratenodera	Ootheca Mantidis
Prepared Alum	Ku Fan	Alumen Praeparatum	Alumen Praeparatum
Prepared (Fermented) Soybean	Dan Dou Chi	Glycine	Semen Sojae Praeparatum
Prepared Jack-in-the-Pulpit Rhizome	Zhi Nan Xing	Arisaema	Rhizoma Arisaematis Praeparatae
Prepared Pinellia Rhizome	(Fa) Ban Xia	Pinellia	Rhizoma Pinelliae Ternatae
Prepared Sichuan Aconite Root	(Hei)Fu Zi	Aconitum	Radix Lateralis Aconiti Carmichaeli Praeparata
Prince Ginseng Root	Tai Zi Shen	Pseudostellaria	Radix Pseudostellariae Heterophyllae
Privet Fruit; Waxtree Fruit	Nu Zhen Zi	Ligustrum	Fructus Ligustri Lucidi
Processed Resin of Borneol Camphor	Bing Pian	Dryobalanops	Borneol

Common	Pinyin	Botanical	Pharmaceutical
Processed Resin of Styrax Benzoin	An Xi Xiang	Styrax	Benzoinum
Pseudoginseng Flower; Notoginseng Flower	San Qi Hua	Panax	Flos Pseudoginseng
Pseudoginseng Root; Notoginseng Root	San Qi	Panax	Radix Pseudoginseng
Pteris	Feng Wei Cao	Pteris	Herba Pterii*
Pubescent Angelica Root	Du Huo	Angelica	Radix Angelicae Pubescentis
Pubescent Holly Root	Mao Dong Qing	Ilex	Radix Ilicis Pubescentis*
Puffball Fruiting Body	Ma Bo	Lasiosphaera	Fructificatio Lasiosphaerae seu Calvatiae
Pulsatilla Root; Anemone Root	Bai Tou Weng	Pulsatilla	Radix Pulsatillae Chinensis
Pumice	Fu Hai Shi	Pumice	Pumice
Pumpkin Seed and Husk	Nan Gua Zi	Cucurbita	Semen Cucurbitae Moschatae
Puncture Vine Fruit; Caltrop Fruit	Bai Ji Li	Tribulus	Fructus Tribuli Terrestris
Pure Mirabilite; Pure Sodium Sulphate; Pure Glauber's Salt	Xuan Ming Fen	Mirabilitum	Mirabilitum Purum
Purple Aster Root	Zi Wan	Aster	Radix Asteris Tatarici
Purslane	Ma Chi Xian	Portulaca	Herba Portulacae Oleraceae
Pyrite	Zi Ran Tong	Pyritum	Pyritum
Pyrola	Lu Xian Cao	Pyrola	Herba Pyrolae*
Pyrrosia Leaf	Shi Wei	Pyrrosia	Folium Pyrrosiae
Quick-fried Ginger Rhizome	Pao Jiang	Zingiber	Rhizoma Zingiberis*
Radish Seed	Lai Fu Zi	Raphanus	Semen Raphani Satavi
Ramie Root	Zhu Ma Gen	Boehmeria	Radix Boehmeriae Niveae*
Rangoon Creeper Fruit	Shi Jun Zi	Quisqualis	Fructus Quisqualis Indicae
Raspberry Fruit Bud	Fu Pen Zi	Rubus	Fructus Rubi Chingii
Raw Cattail Pollen	(Sheng) Pu Huang	Typha	Pollen Typhae
Raw Jack-in-the-Pulpit Rhizome	(Sheng) Tian Nan Xing	Arisaema	Rhizoma Arisaematis
Raw Pinellia Rhizome	(Sheng) Ban Xia	Pinellia	Rhizoma Pinelliae Ternatae
Realgar; Arsenic Disulfide	Xiong Huang	Realgar	Realgar
Red Dogbane Whole Herb or Leaf	Luo Bu Ma	Apocynum	Herba seu Folium Apocyni Veneti*
Red Hoelen; Red Tuckahoe	Chi Fu Ling	Poria	Sclerotium Poriae Cocos Rubrae
Red Lead Oxide	Qian Dan	Minium	Minium
Red Peony Root	Chi Shao	Paeonia	Radix Paeoniae Rubra
Red Sage Root	Dan Shen	Salvia	Radix Salviae Miltiorrhizae

Common	Pinyin	Botanical	Pharmaceutical
Red Tangerine Peel	Ju Hong	Citrus	Pars Rubra Epicarpii Citri Erythrocarpae
Reed Rhizome; Corrizo Rhizome	Lu Gen	Phragmites	Rhizoma Phragmitis Communis
Rhaponticum Root; Echinops Root	Lou Lu	Rhaponticum or Echinops	Radix Rhapontici seu Echinops
Rhinoceros Horn	Xi Jiao	Rhinoceros	Cornu Rhinoceri
Rhodea	Wan Nian Qing	Rhodea	Herba Rhodeae Japonicae*
Rhododendron Leaf	Man Shan Hong	Rhododendron	Folium Rhododendri*
Rhubarb Root and Rhizome	Da Huang	Rheum	Radix et Rhizoma Rhei
Rice Grain	Jing Mi	Oryza	Semen Oryzae Sativae*
Rice Paper Pith	Tong Cao	Tetrapanax	Medulla Tetrapanacis Papyriferi
Rice Sprout	Gu Ya	Oryza	Fructus Oryzae Sativae Germinatus
Rock Candy cured White Ginseng Root	Bai Shen	Panax	Radix Ginseng
Rock Candy cured White Ginseng Root Tail	Shen Xu	Panax	Radix Ginseng
Rorippa	Han Cai	Rorippa	Herba Rorippae*
Rose Maloes Resin	Su He Xiang	Liquidambar	Styrax Liquidis
Round Cardamon Fruit; Cluster Fruit	Bai Dou Kou	Amomum	Fructus Amomi Kravanh
Rush Pith	Deng Xin Cao	Juncus	Medulla Junci Effusi
Safflower	Hong Hua	Carthamus	Flos Carthami Tinctorii
Salvia	Ji Ning	Salvia	Herba Salviae Plebeia*
Sandalwood Heartwood	Tan Xiang	Santalum	Lignum Santali Albi
Sappan Heartwood	Su Mu	Caesalpinia	Lignum Sappan
Sargassum Seaweed	Hai Zao	Sargassum	Herba Sargassii
Sargentodoxa Stem	Hong Teng	Sargentodoxa	Caulis Sargentodoxae Cuneatae
Saururus	San Bai Cao	Saururus	Herba Saururi Chinensis*
Saxifrage	Hu Er Cao	Saxifrage	Herba Saxifragae Stoloniferae*
Schizonepeta Stem or Bud	Jing Jie	Schizonepeta	Herba Schizonepetae Tenuifoliae
Scorpion	Quan Xie	Buthus	Buthus Martensi
Scurfy Pea Fruit	Bu Gu Zhi	Psoralea	Fructus Psoraleae Corylifoliae
Scute; Baical Skullcap Root	Huang Qin	Scutellaria	Radix Scutellariae Baicalensis
Sea Cucumber; Sea Slug	Hai Shen	Strichopus	Strichopus Japonicus
Sea Horse	Hai Ma	Hippocampus	Hippocampus
Sedum	Jing Tian San Qi	Sedum	Herba Sedi*

Common

Common	Pinyin	Botanical	Pharmaceutical
Selaginella	Shi Shang Bai	Selaginella	Herba Selaginellae Doederleinii
Selfheal Spike; Heal all Spike	Xia Ku Cao	Prunella	Spica Prunellae Vulgaris
Senna Leaf	Fan Xie Ye	Cassia	Folium Sennae
Shepherd's Purse	Ji Cai	Capsella	Herba Capsellae*
Shield-fern Rhizome	Guan Zhong	Dryopteris	Rhizoma Guanzhong
Siberian Solomon Seal Rhizome	Huang Jing	Polygonatum	Rhizoma Polygonati
Sichuan Aconite	Chuan Wu	Aconitum	Radix Aconite Carmichaeli
Sichuan Chinaberry Fruit; Sichuan Pagoda Tree Fruit; Neem Fruit	Chuan Lian Zi	Melia	Fructus Meliae Toosendan
Sichuan Chinaberry Root Bark; Sichuan Pagoda Tree Root Bark; Neem Root Bark	Ku Lian Gen Pi	Melia	Cortex Meliae Radicis
Sichuan Chinaberry Tree Bark; Sichuan Pagoda Tree Bark; Neem Tree Bark	Ku Lian Mu Pi	Melia	Cortex Meliae
Sichuan Lovage Root	Chuan Xiong	Ligusticum	Radix Ligustici Wallichii
Sichuan Pepper Fruit	Chuan Jiao	Zanthoxylum	Pericarpum Zanthoxyli Bungeani
Sichuan Pepper Seed	Chuan Jiao Mu	Zanthoxylum	Semen Zanthoxyli Bungeani
Sichuan Pepper Seed	(Chuan) Jiao Mu	Zanthoxylum	Semen Zanthoxyli Bungeani
Siler Root; Ledebouriella Root	Fang Feng	Ledebouriella	Radix Ledebouriella Divaricatae
Siliceous Secretions of Bamboo	Tian Zhu Huang	Bambusa	Concretio Silicea Bambusae Textillis
Silkworm Feces	Can Sha	Bombyx	Excrementum Bombycis Mori
Silver	Xiao Shi	Niter	Niter*
Small Thistle; Field Thistle	Xiao Ji	Cephalanoplos	Herba Cephalanoplos
Smilax Rhizome	Ba Qia	Smilax	Rhizoma Smilacis China*
Smithsonite; Calamine	Lu Gan Shi	Smithsonitum	Smithsonitum
Snake Skin Slough	She Tui	Zaocys	Exuviae Serpentis
Snakegourd Fruit	Gua Lou	Trichosanthes	Fructus Trichosanthis
Snakegourd Peel	Gua Lou Pi	Trichosanthes	Pericarpium Trichosanthis
Snakegourd Root	Tian Hua Fen	Trichosanthes	Radix Trichosanthis Kirilowii
Snakegourd Seed	Gua Lou Ren	Trichosanthes	Semen Trichosanthis
Sour Jujube Seed; Ziziphus	Suan Zao Ren	Ziziphus	Semen Ziziphi Spinosae
Southern Schisandra Fruit	Nan Wu Wei Zi	Schisandra	Fructus Schisandrae Sphenantherae
Spicebush Root	Wu Yao	Lindera	Radix Linderae Strychnifoliae
St. Paul's Wort	Xi Xian Cao	Siegesbeckia	Herba Siegesbeckiae

Common	Pinyin	Botanical	Pharmaceutical
Stalactite Tubular Tip	E Guan Shi	Stalactitum	Stalactitum
Star Anise Fruit	Ba Jiao Hui Xiang	Illicium	Fructus Illicii*
Star Jasmine Stem	Luo Shi Teng	Trachelospermum	Caulis Trachelospermi Jasminoidis
Stellaria Root	Yin Chai Hu	Stellaria	Radix Stellariae Dichotomae
Stemona Root	Bai Bu	Stemona	Radix Stemonae
Stephania Root	Han Fang Ji	Stephania	Radix Stephaniae Tetrandrae
Sterculia Seed	Pang Da Hai	Sterculia	Semen Sterculiae Scaphigerae
Stigma of the True Saffron Flower	Xi Hong Hua	Crocus	Stigma Crocus Sativae
Stink Bug	Jiu Xiang Chong	Aspongopus	Aspongopus*
Stinking Elm Fruit Paste	Wu Yi	Ulmus	Praepartio Fructus Ulmi Macrocarpi
Stonecrop	Chui Pen Cao	Sedum	Herba Sedii Sarmentosi*
Straw Weed Rhizome and Root; Chinese Lovage Rhizome and Root	Gao Ben	Ligusticum	Rhizoma et Radix Ligustici
Sulphur	Liu Huang	Sulphur	Sulphur
Swallowort Root	Bai Wei	Cynanchum	Radix Cynanchi Baiwei
Sweet Jie Geng	Gan Jie Geng	Adenophora	Radix Adenophorae Trachelioidis
Sweet Rice Root and Rhizome	Nuo Dao Gen Xu	Oryza	Radix et Rhizoma Oryzae Glutinosae
Sweet Wormwood; Southernwood	Qing Hao	Artemisia	Herba Artemisiae Annuae
Sweetflag Rhizome	Shi Chang Pu	Acorus	Rhizoma Acori Graminei
Sweetgum Fruit	Lu Lu Tong	Liquidambar	Fructus Liquidambaris Taiwanianae
Talc; Soapstone	Hua Shi	Talcum	Talcum
Tallow Tree Root Bark	Wu Jiu Gen Pi	Sapium	Cortex Sappii Sebiferi Radicis*
Tamarisk	Cheng Liu	Tamarix	Cacumen Tamaricis Chinensis*
Tangerine Peel	Chen Pi	Citrus	Pericarpium Citri Reticulatae
Tangerine Seed	Ju He	Citrus	Semen Citri Reticulatae*
Tangkuei Head	Dang Gui Tou	Angelica	Caput Radicis Angelicae Sinensis
Tangkuei Root	Dang Gui	Angelica	Radix Angelicae Sinensis
Tangkuei Tail	Dang Gui Wei	Angelica	Extremas Radicis Angelicae Sinensis
Tansy Mustard Seed	Ting Li Zi	Lepidium or Descurainia	Semen Lepidii seu Descurainiae
Teasel Root	Xu Duan	Dipsacus	Radix Dipsaci Asperi
Tendrilled Fritillary Bulb	Chuan Bei Mu	Fritillaria	Bulbus Fritillariae Cirrhosae

Common

Common	Pinyin	Botanical	Pharmaceutical
Thalictrum	Tang Song Cao	Thalictrum	Herba Thalictri Foliolosi*
Thimbleberry	Mao Mei	Rubus	Herba Rubi Parvifolii*
Thin Cinnamon Bark from Young Trees	Guan Gui	Cinnamomum	Cortex Tubiformis Cinnamomi Cassiae
Thorowax Root; Hare's Ear Root	Chai Hu	Bupleurum	Radix Bupleuri
Thunberg Fritillary Bulb	Zhe Bei Mu	Fritillaria	Bulbus Fritillariae Thunbergii
Tiger Bone	Hu Gu	Panthera	Os Tigris
Tinospora Root	Jin Guo Lan	Tinospora	Radix Tinosporae Capillipes*
Tinospora Stem	Kuan Jin Teng	Tinospora	Ramus Tinosporae Sinensis
Torrreya Seed	Fei Zi	Torreya	Semen Torreyae Grandis
Tree of Heaven Bark	Chun Pi	Ailanthus	Cortex Ailanthi Altissimae
Tree Peony Rootbark	Mu Dan Pi	Paeonia	Cortex Moutan Radicis
Tremella Fungus Fruiting Body	Bai Mu Er	Tremella	Fructificatio Tremellae Fuciformis
Tuckahoe Skin	Fu Ling Pi	Poria	Cortex Poriae Cocos
Tuckahoe Spirit	Fu Shen	Poria Cocos	Sclerotium Poriae Cocos Pararadicis
Tumeric Rhizome	Jiang Huang	Curcuma	Rhizoma Curcumae Longae
Tumeric Tuber	Yu Jin	Curcuma	Tuber Curcumae
Typhonium Rhizome	Bai Fu Zi	Typhonium	Rhizoma Typhonii Gigantei
Ume Plum Fruit; Black Plum Fruit	Wu Mei	Prunus	Fructus Pruni Mume
Veratrum Root	Li Lu	Veratrum	Radix et Rhizoma Veratri
Vervain	Ma Bian Cao	Verbena	Herba Verbenae*
Viola	Zi Hua Di Ding	Viola	Herba cum Radice Violae Yedoensitis
Vitex Fruit	Man Jing Zi	Vitex	Fructus Viticis
Walnut	Hu Tao Ren	Juglans	Semen Juglandis Regiae
Water Plantain Rhizome	Ze Xie	Alisma	Rhizoma Alismatis Orientalitis
Waterbuffalo Horn	Shui Niu Jiao	Bubalus	Cornu Bubali
Watermelon Fruit and Peel or Rind	Xi Gua	Citrullus	Fructus Citrulli Vulgaris
Wheat Chaff/Grain	Fu Xiao Mai	Triticum	Semen Tritici Aestivi Levis
White Arsenic	Pi Shi	Arsenolite	Arsenicum
White Atractylodes Rhizome	Bai Zhu	Atractylodes	Rhizoma Atractylodis Macrocephalae
White Bulb of Green Onion or Scallion	Cong Bai	Allium	Bulbus Allii Fistulosi
White Chrysanthemum Flower	(Bai) Ju Hua	Chrysanthemum	Flos Chrysanthemi Morifolii
White Mustard Seed	Bai Jie Zi	Brassica	Semen Sinapsis Albae

Common	Pinyin	Botanical	Pharmaceutical
White Peony Root	Bai Shao	Paeonia	Radix Paeoniae Lactiflorae
Wild Aconite	Cao Wu	Aconitum	Radix Aconiti Kusnezoffii
Wild Buckwheat Rhizome	Jin Qiao Mai	Fagopyrum	Rhizoma Fagopyri Cynosi*
Wild Cardamon Seed; Katsumada's Galangal Seed	Cao Dou Kou	Alpinia	Semen Alpiniae Katsumadai
Wild Chrysanthemum Flower	Ye Ju Hua	Chrysanthemum	Flos Chrysanthemi Indici
Wild Ginseng	Ye Shan Shen	Panax	Radix Ginseng
Wine-cooked Chinese Foxglove Root	Shu Di Huang	Rehmannia	Radix Rehmanniae Glutinosae Conquitae
Wingless Cockroach	Tu Bie Chong	Eupolyphaga	Eupolyphaga seu Opisthoplatia
Wintercherry Calyx or Fruit	Suan Jiang	Physalis	Calyx seu Fructus Physalis*
Wintermelon Fruit Peel; Wax Gourd Fruit Peel	Dong Gua Pi	Benincasa	Epicarpium Benincasae Hispidae
Wintermelon Seed; Wax Gourd Seed	Dong Gua Ren	Benincasa	Semen Benincasae Hispidae
Woolly Grass Rhizome; White Grass Rhizome	Bai Mao Gen	Imperata	Rhizoma Imperatae Cylindricae
Wooly Grass Flower; White Grass Flower	Bai Mao Hua	Imperata	Flos Imperatae Cylindricae
Xanthium Fruit; Cocklebur Fruit	Cang Er Zi	Xanthium	Fructus Xanthii Sibirici
Yellow Chrysanthemum Flower	(Huang) Ju Hua	Chrysanthemum	Flos Chrysanthemi Morifolii
Yellow Milk-vetch Root	Huang Qi	Astragalus	Radix Astragali Membranaceus
Young Chinese Rose Flower	Mei Gui Hua	Rosa	Flos Rosae Rugosae
Young Deer Antler Velvet	Lu Rong	Cervus	Cornu Cervi Parvum
Young Soybean Sprout	Dou Juan	Glycine	Semen Glycines Germinatum
Zedoary Tumeric Rhizome	E Zhu	Curcuma	Rhizoma Curcumae

Common

Appendices

Appendix A

Supplies Needed for a Start-Up Pharmacy

Setting up a Chinese herbal pharmacy need not be a complicated matter. There are few supplies needed other than a well-selected inventory of herbs.

Appendix B suggests 175 primary herbs used in the most common formulas. When developing an inventory, it is helpful to decide on a budget and compare prices between suppliers. Suppliers are listed in Appendix C. Most suppliers have catalogs, some may be in Chinese.

In Chinese pharmacies, wooden drawers are most commonly used to store herbs. However, we recommend one gallon glass jars as the storage method of choice. Glass jars prevent possible insect infestations from spreading between herbs. (Glass jar suppliers can be found in most major cities.) Containers should be labeled for each herb in the inventory. We suggest obtaining labeled samples or color pictures for all herbs in the pharmacy.

It is crucial that herb shipments be inspected carefully upon arrival from the supplier. This step ensures that the correct herbs have been sent, and that there are no possible insect infestations present in the shipment. The wrong herb can sometimes be sent, and it is important to be sure of what you are receiving. Herbs generally have a shelf life of about one year. Some last longer but potency may diminish with age. Inspect your stock frequently to check for insects or molds.

There are few other supplies needed to start up an herbal practice. A triple-beam scale is commonly used for weighing herbs. A mortar and pestle, preferably made of brass or marble for crushing heavier substances, is essential. A blender is used for grinding up softer herbs that need to be crushed or powdered. Finally, zip-lock bags or small paper bags work well to package herbal formulas for patients.

Appendix B

175 Herbs For A Start-up Pharmacy

This is a suggested list of herbs for practitioners who want to start a Chinese herbal pharmacy.

Ai Ye/ Artemisia	Chi Shao/ Paeonia
Ba Ji Tian/ Morinda	Chi Xiao Dou/ Phaseolus
Bai Dou Kou/ Amomum	Chuan Lian Zi/ Melia
Bai Jie Zi/ Brassica	Chuan Niu Xi/ Cyathula
Bai Mao Gen/ Imperata	Chuan Xiong/ Ligusticum
Bai Shao / Paeonia	Da Fu Pi/ Areca
Bai Tou Weng/ Pulsatilla	Da Huang/ Rheum
Bai Zhi/ Angelica	Da Qing Ye/ Isatis
Bai Zhu/ Atractylodes	Da Zao/ Ziziphus
Bai Zi Ren/ Biota	Dan Dou Chi/ Glycine
Ban Lan Gen/ Isatis	Dan Shen/ Salvia
Bei Sha Shen/ Glehnia	Dan Zhu Ye/ Lophatherum
Bei Xie/ Dioscorea	Dang Gui/ Angelica
Bi Ba/ Piper	Dang Shen/ Codonopsis
Bian Dou/ Dolichos	Di Fu Zi/ Kochia
Bing Lang/ Areca	Di Gu Pi/ Lycium
Bo He/ Mentha	Di Yu/ Sanguisorba
Cang Er Zi/ Xanthium	Dong Gua Ren/ Benincasa
Ce Bai Ye/ Biota	Du Huo/ Angelica
Chai Hu/ Bupleurum	Du Zhong/ Eucommia
Che Qian Zi/ Plantago	E Jiao/ Equus
Chen Pi/ Citrus	E Zhu/ Curcuma

(Fa) Ban Xia/ Pinellia

Fan Xie Ye/ Cassia

Fang Feng/ Ledebouriella

Fo Shou/ Citrus

Fu Ling/ Poria

Fu Pen Zi/ Rubus

Gan Cao/ Glycyrrhiza

Gan Jiang/ Zingiber

Gao Ben/ Ligusticum

Gao Liang Jiang/ Alpinia

Ge Gen/ Pueraria

Gou Qi Zi/ Lycium

Gou Teng/ Uncaria

Gua Lou Pi/ Trichosanthes

Gua Lou Ren/ Trichosanthes

Gui Zhi/ Cinnamomum

Hai Zao/ Sargassum

Han Fang Ji/ Stephania

He Shou Wu/ Polygonum

Hong Hua/ Carthamus

Hou Po/ Magnolia

Hu Huang Lian/ Picrorhiza

Hua Shi/ Talcum

Huai Niu Xi/ Achyranthes

Huang Bai/ Phellodendron

Huang Jing/ Polygonatum

Huang Lian/ Coptis

Huang Qi/ Astragalus

Huang Qin/ Scutellaria

Huo Ma Ren/ Cannabis

Huo Xiang/ Agastache

Ji Nei Jin/ Gallus

Ji Xue Teng/ Millettia

Jiang Huang/ Curcuma

Jie G eng/ Platycodon

Jin Qian Cao/ Lysimachia

Jin Yin Hua/ Lonicera

Jing Jie/ Schizonepeta

Ju Hua/ Chrysanthemum

Jue Ming Zi/ Cassia

Ku Shen/ Sophora

Kuan Dong Hua/ Tussilago

Kun Bu/ Laminaria

Lai Fu Zi/ Raphanus

Lian Qiao/ Forsythia

Lian Zi/ Nelumbo

Ling Zhi/ Ganoderma

Long Dan Cao/ Gentiana

Long Gu/ Os Draconis

Long Yan Rou/ Euphoria

Lu Gen/ Phragmites

Ma Huang/ Ephedra

Mai Men Dong/ Ophiopogon

Mai Ya/ Hordeum

Man Jing Zi/ Vitex

Mang Xiao/ Mirabilitum

Mu Dan Pi/ Paeonia

Mu Gua/ Chaenomeles

Mu Li/ Ostrea

Mu Tong/ Akebia

Mu Xiang/ Saussurea

Nan Sha Shen/ Adenophora

Niu Bang Zi/ Arctium

Pi Pa Ye/ Eriobotrya

Pu Gong Ying/ Taraxacum

Qian Cao Gen/ Rubia

Qian Hu/ Peucedanum

Qian Shi/ Euryale

Qiang Huo/ Notopterygium

Qin Jiao/ Gentiana

Qing Hao/ Artemisia

Qing Pi/ Citrus

Qu Mai/ Dianthus

Rou Cong Rong/ Cistanche

Rou Gui/ Cinnamonum

Sang Bai Pi/ Morus

Sang Ji Sheng/ Loranthus

Sang Ye/ Morus

Sha Ren/ Amomum

Shan Yao/ Dioscorea

Shan Zha/ Crataegus

Shan Zhu Yu/ Cornus

Shen Qu/ Massa Fermentata

Sheng Di Huang/ Rehmannia

Sheng Ma/ Cimicifuga

Shi Chang Pu/ Acorus

Shi Gao/ Gypsum

Shi Hu/ Dendrobium

Shi Wei/ Pyrrosia

Shu Di Huang/ Rehmannia

Suan Zao Ren/ Ziziphus

Tai Zi Shen/ Pseudostellaria

Tao Ren/ Prunus

Tian Hua Fen/ Trichosanthes

Tian Ma/ Gastrodia

Tian Nan Xing/ Arisaema

Tu Si Zi/ Cuscuta

Wei Ling Xian/ Clematis

Wu Jia Pi/ Acanthopanax

Wu Ling Zi/ Trogopterus

Wu Wei Zi/ Schisandra

Wu Yao/ Lindera

Wu Zhu Yu/ Evodia

Xi Xin/ Asarum

Xia Ku Cao/ Prunella

Xiang Fu/ Cyperus

Xiao Hui Xiang/ Foeniculum

Xin Yi Hua/ Magnolia

Xing Ren/ Prunus

Xu Duan/ Dipsacus

Xuan Shen/ Scrophularia

Yan Hu Suo/ Corydalis

Yi Mu Cao/ Leonurus

Yi Yi Ren/ Coix

Yi Zhi Ren/ Alpinia

Yin Chen Hao/ Artemisia

Yu Jin/ Curcuma

Yu Li Ren/ Prunus

Yu Zhu/ Polygonatum

Yuan Zhi/ Polygala

Ze Xie/ Alisma

Zhe Bei Mu/ Fritillaria

Zhi Ke/ Citrus

Zhi Mu/ Anemarrhena

Zhi Shi/ Citrus

Zhi Zi/ Gardenia

Zhu Ling/ Polyporus

Zhu Ru/ Bambusa

Zi Su Ye/ Perilla

Zi Su Zi/ Perilla

Zi Wan/ Aster

Appendix C

Suppliers of Chinese Herbs

Brion Herbs Corporation
9250 Jeronimo Road
Irvine, CA 92718
Tel: 800-333-Herb, 714-587-1238
Fax: 714-587-1260

Freeze-dried powdered & capsulated herbs only.

Mayhing Import & Export
7307 Edgewater Dr., Unit C
Oakland, CA 94621
Tel: 510-568-8052/8053
Fax: 510-568-8054

Mayway Corporation
1338 Cypress St.
Oakland, CA 94607
Tel: 510-208-3113
Fax: 510-208-3069/3070

Kwok Shing Import & Export
1818 Harrison St.
San Francisco, CA 94103
Tel: 800-326-1668, 415-861-1668

North South China Herbs, Inc.
1556 Stockton St.
San Francisco, CA 94133
Tel: 415-421-4907

Nu Herbs
3820 Penniman Ave.
Oakland, CA 94619
Tel: 800-233-4307, 510-534-HERB
Fax: 510-534-4384

Tashi Enterprise
4175 Lake Side Dr., Suite 120
Richmond, CA 94806
Tel: 800-562-4777, 510-262-6600

Powdered herbs only.

Traditional Chinese Medicine, Inc.
6837 Ramona Ave.
Alta Loma, CA 91701
Tel: 714-941-9989
Fax: 714-941-0030

Qualiherbs
13340 E. Firestone Blvd., Suite N
Santa Fe Springs, CA 90670
Tel: 1-800-533-5907, 213-802-0035
Fax: 213-802-0625

Source of capsulated or powdered extract herbs and formulas.

Appendix D

Instructions for Cooking Loose Herbs

Use a pot made of glass, pottery or porcelain; stainless steel is acceptable. Aluminium or iron pots will interfere with the effects of the herbs. Do not add honey, sugar, other sweeteners or anything else to the tea because these will change the property of the herbs. After taking the herbs if you find the taste unpleasant, you may put a drop of lemon juice on your tongue or eat a few raisins to get rid of the after-taste. As much as possible do not let the steam escape from the pot while the herbs are being cooked. Keep the lid on, but prevent overboiling.

Empty one bag of herbs into the pot and add _____ cups of water. Soak the herbs for 30 minutes. Bring herbs to a boil on a high flame, then lower to a medium/low flame and simmer for _____ minutes. Strain the liquid into a large container, preferably not aluminium or iron.

For the second boiling add _____ cups to the already wet herbs. Again bring to a boil and simmer for _____ minutes. Strain the liquid tea and combine with tea from the first boiling.

The tea should be stored in the refrigerator and will last for a week to ten days.

Drink _____ cup(s) _____ times a day before/after meals.

Each cup may be warmed or drunk cold. Do not use a microwave to warm up your tea.

Special Instructions: Follow Only if Checked!

_____ Cook _____ slices of fresh ginger with each bag.

_____ Add herb(s) from small bag _____ minutes before first cooking is finished.

_____ Cook herb(s) in small bag for _____ minutes before adding the remaining herbs.

NOTE: Chinese herbs are very strong, so sometimes their effects are felt immediately. However, in chronic cases, you may need to take herbs for several months. The prescription should be re-evaluated about every 2 weeks.

Should you experience any unpleasant side effects, please don't hesitate to call.

Bibliography

Chinese Herbal Medicine — Formulas and' Strategies
Bensky, Dan, and Barolet, Randall
Eastland Press, Seattle, WA, 1990

Chinese Herbal Medicine — Materia Medica
Bensky, Dan, and Gamble, Andrew
Eastland Press, Seattle, WA, 1986

Fire in the Valley — The TCM Diagnosis & Treatment of Vaginal Diseases
Flaws, Bob
Blue Poppy Press, Boulder, CO, 1991

Commonly Used Chinese Herb Formulas with Illustrations
Hsu, Hong-Yen
Oriental Healing Arts Institute, Long Beach, CA, 1980

Herbal Formulas — Practical Traditional Chinese Medicine and Pharmacology
Junying et al., Geng
New World Press, Beijing, China, 1991

Medicinal Herbs — Practical Traditional Chinese Medicine and Pharmacology
Junying, Geng; Wenquan, Huang; Tianchi, Ren; Xiufeng, Ma
New World Press, Beijing, China, 1991

Chinese Herbology Vols. 1, 2, and 3
Kim, Bong Dal
Emperor's College of Traditional Oriental Medicine, Santa Monica, CA, 1984, 1985

The Foundations of Chinese Medicine
Maciocia, Giovanni
Churchill Livingston, New York, NY, 1989

Outline Guide to Chinese Herbal Patent Medicines in Pill Form
Naeser, Margaret
Boston Chinese Medicine, Boston, MA, 1990

Chinese Herbology Made Easy
Ni, Maoshing
Union of Tao and Man, Los Angeles, CA

Herb Index
Rutiz, Jan; Karsten, Yuki; Kim, Bong Dal
Emperor's College of Traditional Oriental Medicine, Santa Monica, CA, 1985

Planetary Herbology
Tierra, Michael
Lotus Press, Santa Fe, NM, 1988

The Way of Herbs
Tierra, Michael
Pocket Books, New York, NY, 1990

Handbook of Chinese Herbs and Formulas, Vols. 1 and 2
Yeung, Him-che
Institute of Chinese Medicine, Los Angeles, CA, 1983

Class Notes:
Zeng, Nancy
International Institute of Chinese Medicine, Santa Fe, NM, 1989 – 1991

Treatise on Febrile Diseases Caused by Cold
Zhongjing, Zhang
New World Press, Beijing, China, 1986

Chinese Prepared Medicines
Zhu, Chun-Han
Paradigm Publications, Brookline, MA, 1989

A Comprehensive Guide to Chinese Herbal Medicine
Chen, Ze-Lin, M.D., Chen, Mei-fang, M.D.
Oriental Healing Arts Institute, Long Beach, CA, 1992

The Chinese Herbal Medicine
Chief Editor, Chengdu Institute of Traditional Chinese Medicine
Published by Shanghai Science and Technology Press
450 Ruijin Road, Shanghai, P.R. of China

Encyclopaedia of Chinese Herbal Medicine, 2nd edition
Jiangsu Institute of New Medicine
Published by Shanghai Science and Technology Press
450 Ruijin Road, Shanghai, P.R. of China, 1986

Chinese Herbal Medicine, 2nd edition
Chief Editor, Gansu Institute of New Medicine and Pharmacology
Published by The People's Medical Press, 10 Tiantan Xili, Beijing, P.R. of China, 1982

Traditional Chinese Internal Medicine, 8th edition
Chief Editor, Zhang Boyu
Published by Shanghai Science and Technology Press, 450 Ruijin Road, Shanghai, P.R. of China, 1985

Pinyin Index

* Indicates the most frequently used herbs that are cited throughout the book.
Note: Herbs that are cited on more than 10 pages but are less common than those marked with an * are broken out into disharmony subentries.

Six Divisions: 395, 397
Four Stages: 418, 420
OB/Gyn: 430
Internal & Misc. 493–497, 500,
501, 510, 513, 520, 522
Bu Dai Wan, 190
Bu Fei E Jiao Tang, 47
Bu Fei Tang, 41
Bu Gan Tang, 227, 238
Bu Gu Zhi
Lung Disharmonies: 58
Spleen Disharmonies: 124, 135
Stomach Disharmonies: 151
Liver Disharmonies: 232, 241
Kidney Disharmonies: 290,
295, 300, 302, 303, 308, 319
Bu Huan Jing Zheng Qi San, 5, 351
Bu Yang Huan Wu Tang, 207, 509
Bu Zhong Yi Qi Tang, 97, 111,
139, 142, 429

C

Can Sha, 168, 255, 282, 367, 489
Cang Er Zi, 27
Cang Er Zi San, 27
Cang Fu Dao Tan Tang, 352, 429
Cang Zhu
Lung Disharmonies: 5, 7, 12,
16, 60
Spleen Disharmonies: 105
Stomach Disharmonies: 155,
159, 165, 166
Liver Disharmonies: 206, 213,
217, 240, 249, 250, 252, 253
Jin Ye Disharmonies: 351, 352,
360, 361–363, 365, 366, 370,
377
Six Divisions: 388
Four Stages: 415
OB/Gyn: 429, 446, 453, 454,
457, 460, 461, 462, 469
Internal & Misc.: 474, 477, 482,
484, 486, 487, 490, 505, 522

Cao Dou Kou, 129, 152, 248, 355
Cao Guo, 104, 134, 155, 194, 291,
375, 384, 389–391
Cao Wu, 489, 523
Ce Bai Ye, 141, 187, 231, 261, 320,
341, 425
Ce Bai Ye Tan, 424, 441
Chai Ge Jie Ji Tang, 6, 27, 402
Chai Hu *
Chai Hu Bai Hu Tang, 383, 403, 417
Chai Hu Da Yuan Yin, 384
Chai Hu Gui Zhi Gan Jiang Tang,
368, 384
Chai Hu Gui Zhi Tang, 28, 37, 385
Chai Hu Jia Long Gu Mu Li Tang,
20, 385, 403
Chai Hu Jia Mang Xiao Tang, 386
Chai Hu Qing Gan Tang, 256
Chai Hu Qing Zao Tang, 386
Chai Hu Si Wu Tang, 387
Chai Hu Su Gan San, 198, 208
Chai Hu Xian Xiong Tang, 387
Chai Hu Zhi Jie Tang, 388
Chai Ping Tang, 388
Chai Shao Liu Jun Zi Tang, 219
Chai Zhi Ban Xia Tang, 369, 388
Chan Su, 494
Chan Tui, 243, 243, 520–522
Chang Ning Tang, 111, 466
Chang Shan, 194, 390
Che Qian Zi
Spleen Disharmonies: 105, 107
Liver Disharmonies: 236, 251,
252, 254, 259
Kidney Disharmonies: 293,
301, 327
Bladder Disharmonies: 329–332
Jin Ye Disharmonies: 359, 371
OB/Gyn: 451, 455, 456, 459,
460, 462, 463, 471
Internal & Misc.: 498
Chen Pi *

Chen Xiang
Lung Disharmonies: 58

N

English Index

C

Caesalpinia, 569
Calcaria, 582
Calcitum, 504, 516, 545
Callicarpa, 566
Calm Spirit and Stop Fear Decoction, 67, 283
Calm the Middle Powder, 123
Calm the Palace Pill with Cattle Gallstone, 88, 492, 509
Calm the Stomach and Poria Decoction, 362, 377, 461
Calm the Stomach Powder, 155, 360
Calomelas, 381, 581
Canis, 561, 573
Canopy Powder, 10
Capillaris and Hoelen Five Formula, 254, 281, 365
Capillaris Combination, 253, 281
Capillaris, Atractylodes and Aconite Combination, 137, 366, 379, 410
Capital Qi Pill, 49, 286, 313
Capsella, 567
Cardamon and Fennel Formula, 123
Cardamon Combination, 505
Carpesium, 191–192, 550, 580
Carthamus and Peach Seed Decoction, 210
Caryophyllum, 564
Cassia, 234, 264, 323, 545, 551
Cattle Gallstone Pill to Ascend and Clear, 495
Cattle Gallstone Pill to Clear the Heart, 512
Celosia, 234, 264, 323, 545, 567
Centipeda, 543
Cephalanoplos, 187, 261, 334, 567
Cephalanoplos Combination, 334
Cephalanoplos Decoction, 334
Chalcanthitum, 582
Change Yellow (Discharge) Decoction, 107, 451, 462

Changium, 571
Chianghuo and Turmeric Combination, 483
Chianghuo and Vitex Combination, 484
Chianghuo Combination, 12, 484
Chih-shih and Rhubarb Formula, 167, 347, 367
Chin-Chiu and T.S. Formula, 38, 51
Cibotium, 561, 573
Cimicifuga and Kudzu Decoction, 34
Cimicifuga and Pueraria Combination, 34
Cinnabaris Formula, 78, 85, 90
Cinnabaris Pill to Calm the Spirit, 78, 85, 90
Cinnamon and Anemarrhena Combination, 480
Cinnamon and Dragon Bone Combination, 75, 299
Cinnamon and Ginseng Combination, 23, 99, 408
Cinnamon and Hoelen Formula, 209, 354, 436, 517
Cinnamon and Ma-Huang Combination, 9
Cinnamon and Peony Combination, 22, 98, 407
Cinnamon and Poria Sweet Dew Decoction, 504
Cinnamon and Prepared Aconite Decoction to Regulate the Middle, 128, 298
Cinnamon and Pueraria Combination, 9, 22
Cinnamon Bark, Aconite, and Four-Substance Decoction, 114, 240, 435
Cinnamon Combination, 23
Cinnamon Twig and Ginseng Decoction, 23, 99, 408
Cinnamon Twig and Licorice Decoction, 68, 72
Cinnamon Twig and Poria Pill, 209, 354, 436, 517

Punica, 574, 580, 580
Purple Snow Special Pill, 516
Pyritum, 490, 569
Pyrola, 561
Pyrrosia, 331, 332, 554
Pyrrosia Leaf Powder, 332
Pyrus, 33, 39

Q

Quiet the Blood Decoction, 231
Quisqualis, 190–192, 580

R

Raise the Sinking Decoction, 45, 140
Rambling Powder, 206, 225
Ranunculus, 556
Raphanus, 60, 154, 158, 162, 396–397, 563
Reach the Membrane Source Decoction, 389
Realgar, 88, 186, 259, 275, 492, 494–495, 509, 515, 581
Rectify the Qi Powder Worth More Than Gold, 5, 351
Reduce Infantile Stagnation Pill, 165
Reduce Inflammation and Relieve Toxicity Pill, 500
Reduce Scrofula Pill, 364, 519
Reed Decoction, 65, 498
Regulate the Middle and Calm Roundworms Decoction, 192
Regulate the Middle and Transform Phlegm Pill, 131
Regulate the Middle Pill, 132, 174, 409
Regulate the Stomach and Order the Qi Decoction, 398
Regulating the Liver Decoction, 235, 325, 447
Rehmannia and Akebia Formula, 89, 331

Rehmannia and Gypsum Combination, 181, 188
Rehmannia and Schizandra Formula, 49, 286, 313
Rehmannia and Trichosanthes Formula, 55
Rehmannia Decoction, 510
Rehmannia Eight Formula, 289, 302
Rehmannia Six Formula, 230, 318
Relax the Channels and Invigorate the Blood Decoction, 213, 487
Remove Painful Obstruction Decoction from Selected Formulas, 483
Remove Painful Obstruction from Medical Revelations, 483
Renewal Powder, 26
Resistance Decoction, 339, 404, 431
Resistance Pill, 339, 405
Restore and Revive the Yang Decoction, 92, 131, 300, 408, 412–413
Restore the Left [Kidney] Decoction, 308, 328, 452, 473
Restore the Left [Kidney] Pill, 237, 327
Restore the Right Decoction, 305
Restore the Right Pill, 305, 451, 472
Restore the Spleen Decoction, 83, 98, 115, 143
Restrain the Liver Powder, 225
Return of the Spring Special Pill, 511
Revised Major Order the Qi Decoction, 396
Revive Health by Invigorating the Blood Decoction, 491
Rhaponticum, 548
Rhinoceros and Antelope Horn Formula, 516
Rhinoceros and Rehmannia Combination, 426
Rhinoceros and Scrophularia Combination, 322, 422
Rhinoceros and Succinum Formula, 275, 515

Disharmonies and Syndromes Index

More
InWord Press Titles

Oriental Medicine

The Chinese Herbalist's Handbook
ISBN 1-56690-312-2
Book $39.95

The Oriental Medicine Resource Guide
ISBN 1-56690-311-4
Book $29.95

Stress Management

How To Stay Stressed
ISBN 1-56690-325-4
Book $9.95

InWord Press Distribution

Individual and Corporate Sales

InWord Press books are available worldwide to individuals and corporate accounts from your local bookseller, or from SoftStore: call 1-800-223-6397 or 505-474-5120; fax 505-474-5020; write to Soft-Store, 2530 Camino Entrada, Santa Fe, NM 87505-4835, or e-mail ORDERS@HMP.COM. SoftStore, Inc., is a division of High Mountain Press.

Wholesale, Including Overseas Distribution

High Mountain Press distributes InWord Press books internationally. For terms call 1-800-466-9673 or 505-474-5130; fax to 505-474-5030; e-mail ORDERS@HMP.COM; or write to High Mountain Press, 2530 Camino Entrada, Santa Fe, NM 87505-4835, USA. Outside North America, call 505-474-5130.

Domestic Trade

InWord Press books are distributed to the U.S. domestic trade by Van Nostrand Reinhold. Call 1-800-842-3636, Fax 606/525-7778, or write Van Nostrand Reinhold at 115 Fifth Avenue, New York, NY 10003.

Europe, Middle East, and Africa

InWord Press books are distributed in Europe, the Middle East, and Africa by International Thomson Publishing. Call 071-497-1422, fax 071-497-1426, or write International Thomson Publishing at Berkshire House, 168-173 High Holborn, London WC1V 7AA, United Kingdom.

Asia, Pacific, Hawaii, Puerto Rico, and South America

InWord Press books are distributed in Asia, the Pacific, Puerto Rico, and South America by International Thomson Publishing. In Asia, call 2-272-6497, fax 2-272-6498, or write International Thomson Publishing at 38 Kim Tian Road #01-05, Kim Tian Plaza, Singapore 0316. In the U.S., call 617/423-4210, fax 617/423-4325, or write to International Thomson Publishing at 20 Park Plaza, 14th Floor, Boston, MA 02116.

InWord Press, 2530 Camino Entrada, Santa Fe, NM 87505-4835 USA